D0746080

DAT

MAR 0

Evidence-Based Nursing Guide to

Disease
Management

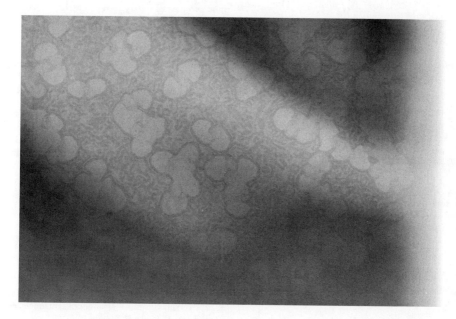

Wolters Kluwer | Lippincott Williams & Wilkins
Health

Philadelphia · Baltimore · New York · London
Buenos Aires · Hong Kong · Sydney · Tokyo

STAFF

EXECUTIVE PUBLISHER
Judith A. Schilling McCann, RN, MSN

EDITORIAL DIRECTOR
H. Nancy Holmes

CLINICAL DIRECTOR
Joan M. Robinson, RN, MSN

ART DIRECTOR
Mary Ludwicki

EDITORIAL PROJECT MANAGERS
Deborah Grandinetti, Sean Webb

CLINICAL PROJECT MANAGER
Jennifer Meyering, RN, BSN, MS, CCRN

EDITORS
Patricia Nale, Joysa Winter

CLINICAL EDITORS
Diane Hines, RN, BSN;
Anita Lockhart, RN, MS

COPY EDITORS
Kimberly Bilotta (supervisor), Scotti Cohn,
Amy Furman, Linda Hager, Dorothy P. Terry,
Pamela Wingrod

DESIGNERS
Deb Moloshok, Matie Ann Patterson

DIGITAL COMPOSITION SERVICES
Diane Paluba (manager), Joyce Rossi Biletz,
Donald G. Knauss, Donna S. Morris

ASSOCIATE MANUFACTURING MANAGER
Beth. J. Welsh

EDITORIAL ASSISTANTS
Karen J. Kirk, Jeri O'Shea, Linda K. Ruhf

DESIGN ASSISTANT
Kate Zulak

INDEXER
Deborah Tourtlotte

Library of Congress
Cataloging-in-Publication Data

The evidence-based nursing guide to disease management.
  p. ; cm.
Includes bibliographical references and index.
  1. Evidence-based nursing—Handbooks, manuals, etc. 2. Nursing diagnosis—Handbooks, manuals, etc.
I. Lippincott Williams & Wilkins.
  [DNLM: 1. Nursing Care—methods. 2. Evidence-Based Medicine. WY 100 E937 2009]
  RT51.E82 2009
  610.73—dc22
  ISBN-13: 978-0-7817-8826-7 (alk. paper)
  ISBN-10: 0-7817-8826-9 (alk. paper)
                                    2008022037

CONTENTS

CONTRIBUTORS
AND CONSULTANTS

DEBORAH HUTCHINSON ALLEN,
RN, MSN, FNP, APRN, BC, CCRN,
AOCNP
Family Nurse Practitioner
Duke Brain Tumor Center
Durham, N.C.

KATRINA D. ALLEN, RN, MSN,
CCRN
Nursing Instructor
Faulkner State Community
College
Bay Minette, Ala.

JO AZZARELLO, RN, PhD
Associate Professor
University of Oklahoma College
of Nursing
Oklahoma City

LINDA S. BAAS, RN, PhD, ACNP
Professor and Director of the
Acute Care Graduate Program
University of Cincinnati College
of Nursing

MICHAEL A. CARTER, APRN-BC,
DNSc, FAAN
University Distinguished
Professor
The University of Tennessee
Health Science Center
Memphis

MARSHA L. CONROY, RN, MSN,
APN
Nurse Educator
Cuyahoga Community College
Cleveland

ANNE WALENDY DAVIS, RN, PhD
Professor of Nursing
East Central University
Ada, Okla.

SUSAN DENMAN, RN, APRN-BC,
PhD, FNP-C
Assistant Professor
Duke School of Nursing
Durham, N.C.

STEPHEN GILLIAM, APRN-BC, PhD,
FNP
Assistant Professor
Medical College of Georgia
School of Nursing
Athens

MARGARET MARY HANSEN, RN,
MSN, EdD
Associate Professor
University of San Francisco

NANCY HUTTON HAYNES, RN,
PhD, CCRN
Assistant Professor
Saint Luke's College
Kansas City, Mo.

SHERYL A. INNERARITY, RN, PhD, FNP, CNS
Associate Professor for Clinical Nursing
The University of Texas at Austin

PATRICIA J. McBRIDE, RN, MSN, CIC
Infection Control Manager
Bryn Mawr (Pa.) Hospital

DARRELL OWENS, ARNP, PhD
Clinical Assistant Professor & Director of
    Palliative Care
Harborview Medical Center
Seattle

WILLIAM J. PAWLYSHYN, APRN, BC, BSN, MS,
    MN, MDiv, ANP-C
Nurse Practitioner
Mid and Upper Cape Community Health
    Center
Hyannis, Mass.

MONICA NARVAEZ RAMIREZ, RN, MSN
Nursing Instructor
University of the Incarnate Word School of
    Nursing & Health Professions
San Antonio, Tex.

DANA REEVES, RN, MSN
Assistant Professor
University of Arkansas
Fort Smith

DONNA SCEMONS, RN, MSN, CNS, CWOCN,
    FNP-C
Family Nurse Practitioner
Healthcare Systems, Inc.
Castaic, Calif.

JENNIFER K. SOFIE, APRN, MSN
Adjunct Assistant Professor & Nurse
    Practitioner
Montana State University
Bozeman

JANET SOMLYAY, CNS, MSN, CNE, CPNP-
    AC/PC
Faculty
Fay Whitney School of Nursing
University of Wyoming
Laramie

ANGELA STARKWEATHER, ACNP, PhD, CCRN,
    CNRN
Assistant Professor
Washington State University
Spokane

ALLISON J. TERRY, RN, MSN, PhD
Director, Center for Nursing
Alabama Board of Nursing
Montgomery

GAIL A. VIERGUTZ, ANP-C, MS
Nurse Practitioner—ER & Urgent Care
Ministry Corp/St. Michael's Hospital
Stevens Point, Wis.

CHERYL WESTLAKE, RN, APRN-BC, PhD
Professor
Azusa (Calif.) Pacific University
Associate Professor
California State University
Fullerton

SUSAN L. WOODS, RN, PhD, FAAN, FAHA
Professor & Associate Dean
University of Washington
Seattle

PATRICIA ZRELAK, CNRN, PhD, CNAA-BC
Administrative Nurse Research
University of California, Davis
Assistant Professor
Samuel Merritt College
Sacramento

FOREWORD

It is always a happy moment for me to discover another example of the growing general acceptance of evidence-based nursing practice. The *Evidence-Based Nursing Guide to Disease Management* provides comprehensive information on more than 150 diseases commonly encountered by nursing students and practicing nurses.

Readers with differing goals will find this book both practical and useful. The format lends itself to either a rapid scan for essentials only or a more leisurely examination if one wants to gain a more in-depth understanding.

Many of the entries include special evidence-based practice sidebars, which focus on a clinical question relevant to the disease covered in that entry. In an entry on cystic fibrosis, for instance, the evidence-based practice sidebar reports on a study that explored whether cystic fibrosis-related diabetes is common.

In addition to these evidence-based practice sidebars, the book contains three other recurring sidebars of interest to practicing nurses. One, identified by an *In the news* logo, summarizes current news reports on nursing-related topics. The second, identified by the *Health & safety* logo, covers issues such as infection control, injury, and risk reduction. The third, identified by an *Emerging infection* logo, provides relevant information on new infectious diseases.

Two appendices are also included, and give the reader additional resources for bolstering an evidence-based approach to practice. In summary, the *Evidence-Based Nursing Guide to Disease Management* has much to offer nurses with differing levels of experience. This book will be a valuable additional tool as nurses attempt to increase the evidence base of nursing practice.

Noreen R. Brady, PHD, CNS, LPCC
Assistant Professor in the School of Nursing
Director of the Sarah Cole Hirsh Institute
* for Best Nursing Practices Based on Evidence*
Frances Payne Bolton School of Nursing
Case Western Reserve University

Cardiovascular disorders

ABDOMINAL ANEURYSM

Abdominal aneurysm, an abnormal dilation in the arterial wall, generally occurs in the aorta between the renal arteries and iliac branches. Rupture—in which the aneurysm breaks open, resulting in profuse bleeding—is a common complication in larger aneurysms. Dissection is the term used when the artery's lining (intima) tears, and blood leaks into the walls.

Causes and incidence

Abdominal aortic aneurysms can result from arteriosclerosis, hypertension, congenital weakening, cystic medial necrosis, abdominal trauma, syphilis, and other infections. In children, this disorder can result from blunt abdominal injury or from Marfan syndrome. Abdominal aortic aneurysms develop slowly. At the onset, degenerative changes give rise to a focal weakness in the muscular layer of the aorta (the tunica media), allowing the inner layer (the tunica intima) and outer layer (tunica adventitia) to stretch outward. Blood pressure within the aorta causes progressive weakening of the vessel walls and enlarges the aneurysm.

Most abdominal aneurysms are fusiform, in which the arterial wall balloons on all sides. The resulting sac then fills with necrotic debris and thrombi.

This disorder is three times more common in males than in females and is most prevalent in whites between the ages of 50 and 80.[1] Research has also shown that there's a strong familial component to abdominal aneurysms. Smokers have a greater risk of developing abdominal aneurysms than nonsmokers.[2] Fewer than 50% of people with a ruptured, or dissected, abdominal aortic aneurysm survive.

There are three classification systems used to classify aortic aneurysms and dissections: the DeBakey, the Stanford, and one proposed by the European Society of Cardiology Task Force on Aortic Dissection. The DeBakey system classifies abdominal aneurysms into three types. The Stanford classification system recognizes abdominal aneurysms as type A or type B. Type A occurs in the ascending and descending aorta, and type B occurs only in the descending aorta. The European Society of Cardiology Task Force on Aortic Dissection classifies aortic dissection according to the type of aortic deformity and its cause. Class 1 refers to the classical dissection, which has a flap of the intima, or inner lining, between the true and false lumen. Class 2 includes disruption of the medial layer; intramural hematomas are formed. Class 3 refers to a discrete area of dissection without hematoma formation and anatomic disruption. Class 4 involves atherosclerotic plaque that has ruptured and causes aortic ulceration and hematoma. Class 5 includes aortic dissections that result from iatrogenic causes or trauma.[3]

Signs and symptoms

Although an abdominal aneurysm usually doesn't produce symptoms, it's likely to be evident (unless the patient is obese) as a pulsating mass in the periumbilical area, accompanied by a systolic bruit over the aorta. Pain is the most common symptom of abdominal aneurysm.[4] A large aneurysm may produce symptoms that mimic renal calculi, lumbar disk disease, and duodenal compression. Abdominal aneurysms rarely cause diminished peripheral pulses or claudication, unless embolization occurs.

The patient may complain of gnawing, generalized, steady abdominal pain or lower back pain that's unaffected by movement. He may feel gastric or abdominal fullness caused by pressure on the GI structures.

Sudden onset of severe abdominal pain or lumbar pain that radiates to the flank and groin from pressure on lumbar nerves may signify enlargement and imminent rupture. If the aneurysm ruptures into the peritoneal cavity, severe and persistent abdominal and back pain mimicking renal or ureteral colic occurs. If the aneurysm ruptures into the duodenum, GI bleeding occurs with massive hematemesis and melena.

The patient may have a history of syncopal episodes that occur when an aneurysm ruptures, causing hypovolemia and a subsequent drop in blood pressure. Once a clot forms and the bleeding stops, he may again be asymptomatic or have abdominal pain because of bleeding into the peritoneum.

Examination of the patient with an intact abdominal aneurysm usually reveals no significant finding. However, if the patient isn't obese, you may notice a pulsating mass in the periumbilical area. If the aneurysm has ruptured, you may notice signs of hypovolemic shock, such as skin mottling, decreased level of consciousness, diaphoresis, and oliguria. The abdomen may appear distended. Ecchymosis or a hematoma may be present in the abdominal, flank, or groin area.

Paraplegia may occur if an aneurysm rupture reduces blood flow to the spine. Auscultation of the abdomen may reveal a systolic bruit over the aorta caused by turbulent blood flow in the widened arterial segment. Hypotension occurs with aneurysm rupture.

Palpation of the abdomen may disclose some tenderness over the affected area. A pulsatile mass may be felt; however, avoid deep palpation to locate the mass because this may cause the aneurysm to rupture.

Although rare, embolization may occur and cause diminished peripheral pulses or claudication.[5]

Complications

▶ Rupture
▶ Obstruction of blood flow to other organs
▶ Embolization to a peripheral artery
▶ Diminished blood supply to vital organs resulting in organ failure (with rupture)

Diagnosis

Because abdominal aneurysms seldom produce symptoms, they're commonly detected accidentally as the result of an X-ray or a routine physical examination. X-rays aren't conclusive for determining the presence of an aortic aneurysm, but more than 90% of patients with an aortic aneurysm presented with an abnormal chest X-ray.[6]

Other tests that are recommended for diagnosis of abdominal aneurysms include transthoracic and transesophageal echocardiography, computed tomography (CT), magnetic resonance imaging, and aortography.[3] Echocardiography helps determine the size, shape, and location of the aneurysm. A CT scan is used to visualize the aneurysm's effect on nearby organs, particularly the position of the renal arteries in relation to the aneurysm. Aortography shows the condition of vessels proximal and distal to the aneurysm and the extent of the aneurysm.

Treatment

Usually, abdominal aneurysm requires resection of the aneurysm and replacement of the damaged aortic section with a Dacron graft. (See *Abdominal aneurysms: Before and after surgery,* page 4. Also see *Endovascular grafting for repair of an abdominal aortic aneurysm,* page 5.)

If the aneurysm is small and the patient is asymptomatic, surgery may be delayed and the aneurysm may be monitored and allowed to expand to a certain size because of possible surgical complications; however, small aneurysms may also rupture. Because of this risk, surgical repair or replacement is recommended for symptomatic patients or for patients with aneurysms greater than 2″ (5 cm) in diameter.[7]

Stenting is also a treatment option. It can be performed without an abdominal incision by introducing the catheters through arteries in the groin. However, not all patients with abdominal aortic aneurysms are candidates for this treatment.

For a patient with acute dissection, emergency treatment before surgery includes resuscitation with fluid and blood replacement, I.V. propranolol to reduce myocardial contractility, I.V. nitroprusside to reduce and maintain blood pressure to 100 to 120 mm Hg systolic, and an analgesic to relieve pain.[3]

Regular physical examination and ultrasound checks are necessary to detect enlargement, which may forewarn of rupture. Large aneurysms or those that produce symptoms pose a significant risk of rupture and necessitate immediate repair. In patients with poor distal runoff, external grafting may be done. Current recommendations are that all men between ages 65 and 74 who have a history of smoking should have an abdominal ultrasound to determine the presence or absence of an abdominal aneurysm.[8]

Risk factor modification is fundamental in the medical management of abdominal aneurysm, including control of hypocholesterolemia and hypertension. Angiotensin-converting enzyme inhibitors show promise in reducing the risk of aneurysm rupture.[9]

Special considerations

Abdominal aneurysm requires meticulous preoperative and postoperative care, psychological support, and comprehensive patient teaching. If rupture isn't imminent when the aneurysm is diagnosed, consider elective surgery, which allows time for additional preoperative tests to evaluate the patient's clinical status. Also:

▶ Monitor vital signs, and type and cross-match blood.

▶ Use only gentle abdominal palpation.

▶ As ordered, obtain renal function tests (blood urea nitrogen, creatinine, and electrolyte levels), blood samples (complete blood count with differential), electrocardiogram and cardiac evaluation, baseline pulmonary function tests, and arterial blood gas (ABG) analysis.

▶ Since rupture can be fatal, be alert for signs of rupture. Watch closely for signs of acute blood loss (decreasing blood pressure; increasing pulse and respiratory rate; cool, clammy skin; restlessness; and decreased sensorium).

▶ If rupture does occur, get the patient to surgery immediately. That's your first priority. A pneumatic antishock garment may be used while transporting him to surgery. Surgery allows direct compression of the aorta to control hemorrhage. Large amounts of blood may be needed during the resuscitative period to replace blood loss. In such a patient, renal failure caused by ischemia is a major postoperative complication, possibly requiring hemodialysis.

▶ Before elective surgery, weigh the patient, insert an indwelling urinary catheter and an

Abdominal aneurysms: Before and after surgery

During surgery, a prosthetic graft replaces or encloses the weakened area.

BEFORE SURGERY

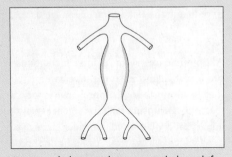

Aneurysm below renal arteries and above bifurcation

BEFORE SURGERY

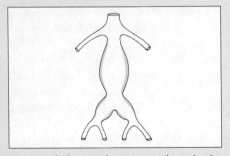

Aneurysm below renal arteries involving the iliac branches

BEFORE SURGERY

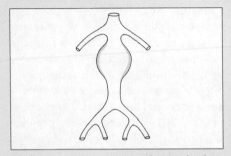

Small aneurysm in a patient with poor distal runoff (poor risk)

AFTER SURGERY

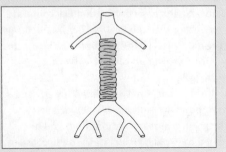

The prosthesis extends distal to the renal arteries to above the aortic bifurcation.

AFTER SURGERY

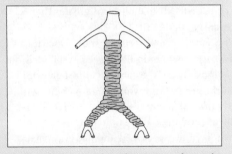

The prosthesis extends to the common femoral arteries.

AFTER SURGERY

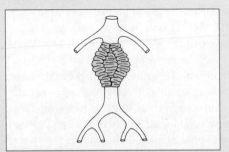

The external prosthesis encircles the aneurysm and is held in place with sutures.

I.V. line, and assist with insertion of an arterial line and pulmonary artery catheter to monitor fluid and hemodynamic balance. Give prophylactic antibiotics as ordered.

▶ Explain the surgical procedure and the expected postoperative care in the intensive care unit (ICU) for patients undergoing complex abdominal surgery (I.V. lines, endotracheal [ET] and nasogastric [NG] intubation, and mechanical ventilation).

▶ After surgery, in the ICU, closely monitor vital signs, intake and hourly output, neurologic status (level of consciousness, pupil size, and sensation in arms and legs), and ABG values. Assess the depth, rate, and character of respirations and breath sounds at least every hour.

▶ Watch for signs of bleeding (increased pulse and respiratory rates and hypotension) and back pain, which may indicate the graft is tearing. Check abdominal dressings for excessive bleeding or drainage. Be alert for temperature elevations and other signs of infection. After NG intubation for intestinal decompression, irrigate the tube frequently to ensure patency. Record the amount and type of drainage.

▶ Suction the ET tube often. If the patient can breathe unassisted and has good breath sounds and adequate ABG values, tidal volume, and vital capacity 24 hours after surgery, he will be extubated and may require supplemental oxygen.

▶ Weigh the patient daily to evaluate fluid balance.

▶ Help the patient walk as soon as he's able (generally the second day after surgery).

▶ Provide psychological support for the patient and his family. Help ease their fears about the ICU, the threat of impending rupture, and surgery by providing appropriate explanations and answering all questions.

Endovascular grafting for repair of an abdominal aortic aneurysm

Endovascular grafting is a minimally invasive procedure for the repair of an abdominal aortic aneurysm. This procedure reinforces the walls of the aorta to prevent rupture and prevent expansion of the aneurysm.

Endovascular grafting is performed with fluoroscopic guidance: Using a guide wire, a delivery catheter with an attached compressed graft is inserted through a small incision into the femoral or iliac artery. The delivery catheter is advanced into the aorta, where it's positioned across the aneurysm. A balloon on the catheter expands the graft and affixes it to the vessel wall.

The procedure generally takes 2 to 3 hours to perform. Patients are instructed to walk the first day after surgery and are generally discharged from the facility in 1 to 3 days.

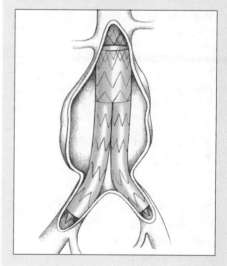

REFERENCES

1. The Merck Manuals Online Medical Library (2008 January). "Aneurysms" [Online]. Available at *www.merck.com/mmhe/sec03/ch035/ch035b.html.*
2. Blanchard, J.F., et al. "Risk Factors for Abdominal Aortic Aneurysm: Results of a Case-Control Study," *American Journal of Epidemiology* 151(6):575-83, March 2000.
3. Erbel, R., et al. "Diagnosis and Management of Aortic Dissection," *European Heart Journal* 22(18):1642-81, September 2001.
4. Khan, I.A., and Nair, C.K. "Clinical, Diagnostic, and Management Perspectives of Aortic Dissection," *Chest* 122(1):311-28, July 2002.
5. Bower, T.C., et al. "Unusual Manifestations of Abdominal Aortic Aneurysms," *Surgical Clinics of North America* 69(4):745-54, August 1989.
6. Klompas, M. "Does This Patient Have an Acute Thoracic Aortic Dissection?" *JAMA* 287(17):2262-72, May 2002.
7. Lederle, F.A., et al. "Systematic Review: Repair of Unruptured Abdominal Aortic Aneurysm," *Annals of Internal Medicine* 146(10):735-41, May 2007.
8. Birkmeyer, J.D., and Upchurch, G.R. "Evidence-Based Screening and Management of Abdominal Aortic Aneurysm," *Annals of Internal Medicine* 146(10):749-50, May 2007.
9. Hackam, H.G., et al. "Angiotensin-Converting Enzyme Inhibitors and Aortic Rupture: A Population-Based Case-Control Study," *Lancet* 368(9536):659-65, August 2006.

ARTERIAL OCCLUSIVE DISEASE

Arterial occlusive disease is the obstruction or narrowing of the lumen of the aorta and its major branches, causing an interruption of blood flow, usually to the legs and feet. This disorder may affect the carotid, vertebral, innominate, subclavian, and mesenteric arteries. (See *Types of arterial occlusive disease.*) Occlusions may be acute or chronic, and commonly cause severe ischemia, skin ulceration, and gangrene.

The prognosis depends on the occlusion's location, the development of collateral circulation to counteract reduced blood flow and, in acute disease, the time elapsed between occlusion and its removal.

Causes and incidence

Arterial occlusive disease is a common complication of atherosclerosis. The occlusive mechanism may be endogenous, due to emboli formation or thrombosis, or exogenous, due to trauma or fracture. Predisposing factors include smoking; aging; such conditions as hypertension, hyperlipidemia, and diabetes; and a family history of vascular disorders, myocardial infarction, or stroke.

Arterial occlusive disease has no racial predilection. Men older than 50 are at increased risk for intermittent claudication, a common sign of arterial occlusive disease.

Signs and symptoms

The signs and symptoms will vary based on the vessel that is occluded. Acute arterial occlusion occurs suddenly, in many cases without warning. However, peripheral occlusion can usually be recognized by the 5 P's:

▶ Pain, the most common symptom, occurs suddenly and is localized to the affected arm or leg.
▶ Pallor results from vasoconstriction distal to the occlusion.
▶ Pulselessness occurs distal to the occlusion.
▶ Paralysis and paresthesia occur in the affected arm or leg from disturbed nerve endings or skeletal muscle.

A sixth "P," known as poikilothermy, refers to temperature changes that occur distal to the occlusion, making the skin feel cool.

Complications

▶ Severe ischemia and necrosis
▶ Skin ulceration
▶ Gangrene, which can lead to limb amputation
▶ Impaired nail and hair growth
▶ Stroke or transient ischemic attack
▶ Peripheral or systemic embolism

Types of arterial occlusive disease

SITE OF OCCLUSION	SIGNS AND SYMPTOMS
Carotid arterial system	
• Internal carotids • External carotids	• Absent or decreased pulsation with an auscultatory bruit over the affected vessels • Neurologic dysfunction: transient ischemic attacks (TIAs) due to reduced cerebral circulation producing unilateral sensory or motor dysfunction (transient monocular blindness, and hemiparesis), possible aphasia or dysarthria, confusion, decreased mentation, and headache (These are recurrent features that usually last 5 to 10 minutes but may persist up to 24 hours and may herald a stroke.)
Vertebrobasilar system	
• Vertebral arteries • Basilar arteries	• Neurologic dysfunction: TIAs of the brain stem and cerebellum producing binocular vision disturbances, vertigo, dysarthria, and "drop attacks" (falling down without loss of consciousness); less common than carotid TIA
Innominate	
• Brachiocephalic artery	• Indications of ischemia (claudication) of the right arm • Neurologic dysfunction: signs and symptoms of vertebrobasilar occlusion • Possible bruit over the right side of the neck
Subclavian artery	
	• Clinical effects of vertebrobasilar occlusion and exercise-induced arm claudication • Subclavian steal syndrome (characterized by the backflow of blood from the brain through the vertebral artery on the same side as the occlusion, into the subclavian artery distal to the occlusion) • Possibly gangrene (usually limited to the digits)
Mesenteric artery	
• Superior (most commonly affected) • Celiac axis • Inferior	• Bowel ischemia, infarct necrosis, and gangrene • Diarrhea • Leukocytosis • Nausea and vomiting • Shock due to massive intraluminal fluid and plasma loss • Sudden, acute abdominal pain
Aortic bifurcation	
(saddle block occlusion, a medical emergency associated with cardiac embolization)	• Sensory and motor deficits (muscle weakness, numbness, paresthesias, and paralysis) in both legs • Signs of ischemia (sudden pain and cold, pale legs with decreased or absent peripheral pulses) in both legs

(continued)

Types of arterial occlusive disease *(continued)*

SITE OF OCCLUSION	SIGNS AND SYMPTOMS
Iliac artery (Leriche's syndrome)	● Absent or reduced femoral or distal pulses ● Impotence ● Intermittent claudication of the lower back, buttocks, and thighs, relieved by rest ● Possible bruit over femoral arteries
Femoral and popliteal artery (associated with aneurysm formation)	● Gangrene ● Intermittent claudication of the calves on exertion ● Ischemic pain in feet ● Leg pallor and coolness; blanching of the feet on elevation ● No palpable pulses in the ankles and feet ● Pretrophic pain (heralds necrosis and ulceration)

Diagnosis

Diagnosis of arterial occlusive disease is usually indicated by patient history and physical examination.

Pertinent supportive diagnostic tests include the following:

▶ Arteriography demonstrates the type (thrombus or embolus), location, and degree of obstruction and the collateral circulation. It's particularly useful in chronic disease or for evaluating candidates for reconstructive surgery.[1]

▶ Doppler ultrasonography and plethysmography are noninvasive tests that show decreased blood flow distal to the occlusion in acute disease.

▶ Ankle-brachial index (ABI) decreases with worsening arterial occlusive disease. An ABI less than 0.9 indicates some degree of arterial occlusive disease. However, new studies have shown that an ABI of 1.10 increases the patient's risk for carotid atherosclerosis.[2]

▶ Segmental limb pressures and pulse volume measurements help evaluate the location and extent of the occlusion.

▶ Ophthalmodynamometry helps determine the degree of obstruction in the internal carotid artery by comparing ophthalmic artery pressure to brachial artery pressure on the affected side. More than a 20% difference between pressures suggests insufficiency.

▶ EEG and computed tomography scan may be necessary to rule out brain lesions.

Treatment

Treatment depends on the obstruction's cause, location, and size. For mild chronic disease, supportive measures include hypertension control, walking for exercise, and eliminating smoking. For carotid artery occlusion, antiplatelet therapy may begin with ticlopidine or clopidogrel and aspirin. For intermittent claudication of chronic occlusive disease, pentoxifylline may improve blood flow through the capillaries, particularly for patients who are poor candidates for surgery.[3]

Acute arterial occlusive disease usually requires surgery to restore circulation to the affected area, for example:

▶ atherectomy—the excision of plaque using a drill or slicing mechanism

▶ balloon angioplasty—compression of the obstruction using balloon inflation

▶ bypass graft—the diversion of blood flow through an anastomosed autogenous or Dacron graft past the thrombosed segment

▶ combined therapy—the concomitant use of any of the above treatments

▶ embolectomy—the removal of thrombotic material from the artery, via a balloon-tipped catheter. Embolectomy is used mainly for mesenteric, femoral, or popliteal artery occlusion.

▶ laser angioplasty—the use of excision and hot tip lasers to vaporize the obstruction

▶ lumbar sympathectomy—an adjunct to surgery, depending on the sympathetic nervous system's condition

▶ patch grafting—the removal of the thrombosed arterial segment (which is then replaced with an autogenous vein or Dacron graft)

▶ stents—the insertion of a mesh of wires that stretch and mold to the arterial wall to prevent reocclusion. This adjunct treatment follows laser angioplasty or atherectomy.

▶ thromboendarterectomy—the opening of the occluded artery and direct removal of the obstructing thrombus and the medial layer of the arterial wall. This is usually performed after angiography and is commonly used with autogenous vein or Dacron bypass surgery (femoral-popliteal or aortofemoral).[4]

▶ thrombolytic therapy—the lysis of any clot around or in the plaque by urokinase, streptokinase, or alteplase.

Amputation becomes necessary with failure of arterial reconstructive surgery or with the development of gangrene, persistent infection, or intractable pain.

Other therapy includes heparin to prevent emboli (for embolic occlusion) and bowel resection after restoration of blood flow (for mesenteric artery occlusion).

Special considerations

▶ Provide comprehensive patient teaching, including proper foot care. Explain diagnostic tests and procedures. Advise the patient to stop smoking and to follow the prescribed medical regimen.

Preoperatively, during an acute episode:

▶ Assess the patient's circulatory status by checking for the most distal pulses and by inspecting his skin color and temperature.

▶ Provide pain relief as needed.

▶ Administer heparin by continuous I.V. drip as ordered. Use an infusion monitor or pump to ensure the proper flow rate.[3]

▶ Wrap the patient's affected foot in soft cotton batting, and reposition it frequently to prevent pressure on any one area. Strictly avoid elevating or applying heat to the affected leg.

▶ Watch for signs of fluid and electrolyte imbalance, and monitor intake and output for signs of renal failure (urine output less than 30 ml/hour).

▶ If the patient has carotid, innominate, vertebral, or subclavian artery occlusion, monitor him for signs of stroke, such as numbness in an arm or leg and intermittent blindness.

Postoperatively:

▶ Monitor the patient's vital signs. Continuously assess his circulatory function by inspecting skin color and temperature and by checking for distal pulses. In charting, compare earlier assessments and observations. Watch closely for signs of hemorrhage (tachycardia and hypotension), and check dressings for excessive bleeding.

▶ In carotid, innominate, vertebral, or subclavian artery occlusion, assess neurologic status frequently for changes in level of consciousness or muscle strength and pupil size.

▶ In mesenteric artery occlusion, connect the nasogastric tube to low intermittent suction. Monitor intake and output (low urine output may indicate damage to renal arteries during surgery). Check bowel sounds for return of peristalsis. Increasing abdominal distention and tenderness may indicate extension of bowel ischemia with resulting gan-

grene, necessitating further excision; or it may indicate peritonitis.

▶ In saddle block occlusion, check distal pulses for adequate circulation. Watch for signs of renal failure and mesenteric artery occlusion (severe abdominal pain) and for cardiac arrhythmias, which may precipitate embolus formation.

▶ In iliac artery occlusion, monitor urine output for signs of renal failure from decreased perfusion to the kidneys as a result of surgery. Provide meticulous catheter care.

▶ In both femoral and popliteal artery occlusions, assist with early ambulation, but discourage prolonged sitting.

▶ After amputation, check the patient's stump carefully for drainage, and record its color and amount and the time. Elevate the stump as ordered, and administer adequate analgesic medication. Because phantom limb pain is common, explain this phenomenon to the patient.

▶ When preparing the patient for discharge, instruct him to watch for signs of recurrence (pain, pallor, numbness, paralysis, and absence of pulse) that can result from graft occlusion or occlusion at another site. Warn him against wearing constrictive clothing.

REFERENCES

1. Schertler, T., et al. "Sixteen-Detector Row CT Angiography for Lower-Leg Arterial Occlusive Disease: Analysis of Section Width," *Radiology* 237(2):649-56, November 2005.
2. Allison, M.A., et al. "Association between the Ankle-Brachial Index and Carotid Intimal Medial Thickness in the Rancho Bernardo Study," *American Journal of Cardiology* 98(8):1105-109, October 2006.
3. Clagett, G.P., et al. "Antithrombotic Therapy in Peripheral Arterial Occlusive Disease: The Seventh ACCP Conference on Antithrombotic and Thrombolytic Therapy," *Chest* 126(3 Suppl):609S-26S, September 2004.
4. Schmittling, Z.C., et al. "Thrombolysis and Mechanical Thrombectomy for Arterial Disease," *Surgical Clinics of North America* 84(5):1237-66, v-vi, October 2004.

CORONARY ARTERY DISEASE

Coronary artery disease (CAD) occurs when the arteries that supply blood to the heart muscle harden and narrow. The diminished coronary blood flow results in a loss of oxygen and nutrients to the myocardial tissue, and can also lead to coronary syndrome (angina or myocardial infarction [MI]).

Causes and incidence

Atherosclerosis is the usual cause of CAD. In this form of arteriosclerosis, fatty, fibrous plaques, which may even include calcium deposits, narrow the lumen of the coronary arteries, reduce the volume of blood that can flow through them, and lead to myocardial ischemia. Plaque formation also predisposes individuals to thrombosis, which can provoke MI.

Atherosclerosis usually develops in high-flow, high-pressure arteries, such as those in the heart, brain, kidneys, and aorta, especially at bifurcation points. It has been linked to many risk factors: family history, male gender, age (risk increased in those ages 65 or older), hypertension, obesity, smoking, diabetes mellitus, stress, sedentary lifestyle, high serum cholesterol (particularly high low-density lipoprotein [LDL] cholesterol) or triglyceride levels, low high-density lipoprotein cholesterol levels, high blood homocysteine levels, menopause and, possibly, infections producing inflammatory responses in the artery walls.

Uncommon causes of reduced coronary artery blood flow include dissecting aneurysms, infectious vasculitis, syphilis, and congenital defects in the coronary vascular system. Coronary artery spasms may also impede blood flow. (See *Coronary artery spasm.*)

Coronary artery disease is the leading cause of death in the United States. About 13 millions Americans have CAD, and it's

Coronary artery spasm

In coronary artery spasm, a spontaneous, sustained contraction of one or more coronary arteries causes ischemia and dysfunction of the heart muscle. This disorder also causes Prinzmetal's angina and even myocardial infarction in patients with unoccluded coronary arteries. Its cause is unknown but possible contributing factors include:

• intimal hemorrhage into the medial layer of the blood vessel
• hyperventilation
• elevated catecholamine levels
• fatty buildup in lumen
• cocaine use.

SIGNS AND SYMPTOMS

The major symptom of coronary artery spasm is angina. But unlike classic angina, this pain often occurs spontaneously and may not be related to physical exertion or emotional stress; it's also more severe, usually lasts longer, and may be cyclic, frequently recurring every day at the same time. Such ischemic episodes may cause arrhythmias, altered heart rate, lower blood pressure and, occasionally, fainting due to diminished cardiac output. Spasm in the left coronary artery may result in mitral insufficiency, producing a loud systolic murmur and, possibly, pulmonary edema, with dyspnea, crackles, hemoptysis, or sudden death.

TREATMENT

After diagnosis by coronary angiography and electrocardiography, the patient may receive calcium channel blockers (verapamil, nifedipine, or diltiazem) to reduce coronary artery spasm and vascular resistance; and nitrates (nitroglycerin or isosorbide dinitrate) to relieve chest pain.

When caring for a patient with coronary artery spasm, explain all necessary procedures, and teach him how to take his medications safely. For calcium antagonist therapy, monitor blood pressure, pulse rate, and electrocardiogram patterns to detect arrhythmias. For nifedipine and verapamil therapy, monitor digoxin levels, and check for signs of digoxin toxicity. Because nifedipine may cause peripheral and periorbital edema, watch for fluid retention.

Because coronary artery spasm is commonly associated with atherosclerotic disease, advise the patient to stop smoking, avoid overeating, maintain a low-fat diet, use alcohol sparingly, and maintain a balance between exercise and rest.

---

more common in males, whites, and middle-age and elderly people. Researchers have identified more than 250 genes that may play a role in CAD. It commonly results from the combined effects of multiple genes, making it difficult to determine the impact of specific genes that can influence a person's risk for the disease. Some of the best understood genes linked to CAD include:

▶ LDL receptor—a protein that removes LDL from the bloodstream; a mutation in this gene is responsible for familial hypercholesterolemia[1]

▶ apolipoprotein E—mutations in this gene, commonly called *apo E*, also affect blood levels of LDL

▶ apolipoprotein B-100—a component of LDL; mutations of this gene cause LDL to stay in the blood longer than normal, leading to high LDL levels

▶ apolipoprotein A—a glycoprotein that combines with LDL to form a particle called *Lp(a)*; it appears as part of plaque on blood vessels

▶ MTHFR—an enzyme that clears homocysteine from the blood; mutations in MTHFR genes may cause higher homocysteine levels[2]

▶ cystathionine B-synthase—also known as CBS, another enzyme involved in homocysteine metabolism. CBS mutations cause a condition known as homocystinuria (homo-

cysteine levels are so high that homocysteine can be detected in the urine).

Signs and symptoms

The classic symptom of CAD is angina, the direct result of inadequate oxygen flow to the myocardium. Anginal pain is usually described as a burning, squeezing, or tight feeling in the substernal or precordial chest that may radiate to the left arm, neck, jaw, or shoulder blade. Typically, the patient clenches his fist over his chest or rubs his left arm when describing the pain, which may be accompanied by nausea, vomiting, shortness of breath, fainting, sweating, and cool extremities. Anginal episodes most commonly follow physical exertion but may also follow emotional excitement, exposure to cold, or a large meal.

Angina has four major forms: stable (pain is predictable in frequency and duration and can be relieved with nitrates and rest), unstable (pain increases in frequency and duration and is more easily induced), Prinzmetal's or variant (from unpredictable coronary artery spasm), and microvascular (in which impairment of vasodilator reserve causes angina-like chest pain in a patient with normal coronary arteries). Severe and prolonged anginal pain generally suggests MI, with potentially fatal arrhythmias and mechanical failure. Women are more likely to experience atypical pain, which may occur in the abdomen, back, or arm.[3]

Inspection may reveal evidence of atherosclerotic disease, such as xanthelasma and xanthoma. Ophthalmoscopic inspection may show increased light reflexes and arteriovenous nicking, suggesting hypertension, an important risk factor of coronary artery disease. Palpation can uncover thickened or absent peripheral arteries, signs of cardiac enlargement, and abnormal contraction of the cardiac impulse, such as left ventricular akinesia or dyskinesia. Auscultation may detect bruits, an S_3, an S_4, or a late systolic murmur (if mitral insufficiency is present).

Complications

- ▶ Angina
- ▶ Arrhythmias
- ▶ MI
- ▶ Ischemic cardiomyopathy

Diagnosis

The patient history—including the frequency and duration of angina and the presence of associated risk factors—is crucial in evaluating CAD. Additional diagnostic measures include the following:

▶ Electrocardiogram (ECG) during angina shows ischemia as demonstrated by T-wave inversion or ST-segment depression and possible arrhythmias, such as premature ventricular contractions. ECG results may be normal during pain-free periods. Arrhythmias may occur without infarction, secondary to ischemia. A Holter monitor may be used to obtain continuous graphic tracing of the ECG as the patient performs daily activities.

▶ A treadmill or exercise stress test may provoke chest pain and ECG signs of myocardial ischemia. Monitoring of electrical rhythm may demonstrate T-wave inversion or ST-segment depression in the ischemic areas.

▶ Coronary angiography reveals coronary artery stenosis or obstruction, possible collateral circulation, and the arteries' condition beyond the narrowing.

▶ Myocardial perfusion imaging with thallium-201, Cardiolite, or Myoview during treadmill exercise detects ischemic areas of the myocardium, visualized as "cold spots."

▶ Rest perfusion imaging with sestamibi can be used to rule out myocardial ischemia in the patient with a chest pain syndrome that isn't clearly cardiac in nature.

▶ Stress echocardiography may show wall motion abnormalities.

▶ Electron-beam computed tomography scanning identifies calcium within arterial plaque; the more calcium seen, the higher the likelihood of CAD.[4]

▶ Multiple-gated acquisition scanning demonstrates cardiac-wall motion and reflects injury to cardiac tissue.

Treatment

The goal of treatment in patients with angina is to either reduce myocardial oxygen demand or increase oxygen supply. Therapy consists primarily of nitrates such as nitroglycerin (given sublingually, orally, transdermally, or topically in ointment form) to dilate coronary arteries and improve blood supply to the heart. Glycoprotein IIb-IIIa inhibitors and antithrombin drugs may be used to reduce the risk of blood clots. Beta-adrenergic blockers may be used to decrease heart rate and lower the heart's oxygen use. Calcium channel blockers may be used to relax the coronary arteries and all systemic arteries, reducing the heart's workload. Angiotensin-converting enzyme inhibitors, diuretics, or other medications may be used to lower blood pressure.[5]

Percutaneous transluminal coronary angioplasty (PTCA) may be performed during cardiac catheterization to compress fatty deposits and relieve occlusion in patients with no calcification and partial occlusion. PTCA carries a certain risk but its morbidity is lower than that for surgery. (See *Relieving occlusions with angioplasty,* page 14.)

Laser angioplasty corrects occlusion by vaporizing fatty deposits. In addition, a stent may be placed in the artery to act as a scaffold to hold the artery open. Another procedure is rotational atherectomy, which removes arterial plaque with a high-speed burr. Obstructive lesions may necessitate coronary artery bypass graft (CABG) surgery and the use of vein grafts.

A surgical technique available as an alternative to traditional CABG surgery is minimally invasive coronary artery bypass surgery, also known as "keyhole" surgery. This procedure requires a shorter recovery period and has fewer postoperative complications. Instead of sawing open the patient's sternum

IN THE NEWS

New ways to treat CAD

Researchers are continuing to look for new ways to treat patients with coronary artery disease. One technique that's showing promise is gene therapy, where genes and growth factors are injected either through a catheter or directly into the heart. The hope is that the genes and growth factor will stimulate the growth of new blood vessels to restore blood flow. Gene-coated stents are also being researched, with the hope that they too will help stimulate the growth of new blood vessels.

and spreading the ribs apart, several small cuts are made in the torso through which small surgical instruments and fiber-optic cameras are inserted. This procedure was initially designed to correct blockages in just one or two easily-reached arteries; it may not be suitable for more complicated cases.

Coronary brachytherapy, which involves delivering beta or gamma radiation into the coronary arteries, may be used in patients who have undergone stent implantation in a coronary artery but then developed such problems as diffuse in-stent restenosis.[6] Brachytherapy is a promising technique, but its use is restricted to the treatment of stent-related problems because of complications and the unknown long-term effects of the radiation. However, in some facilities, brachytherapy is being studied as a first-line treatment of coronary disease. Research is continuing into new ways to treat coronary artery disease. (See *New ways to treat CAD.*)

Because CAD is so widespread, prevention is of incalculable importance. Dietary restrictions aimed at reducing intake of calories (in obesity), salt, saturated fats, and cholesterol serve to minimize the risk, especially when supplemented with regular exercise. Stress reduction and abstention from smoking are also beneficial. Other preventive ac-

Relieving occlusions with angioplasty

Percutaneous transluminal coronary angioplasty can open an occluded coronary without opening the chest—an important advantage over bypass surgery. First, coronary angiography must confirm the presence and location of the arterial occlusion. Then, the physician threads a guide catheter through the patient's femoral artery into the coronary artery under fluoroscopic guidance, as shown at right.

When angiography shows the guide catheter positioned at the occlusion site, the physician carefully inserts a smaller double-lumen balloon catheter through the guide catheter and directs the balloon through the occlusion (below, left). A marked pressure gradient will be obvious.

The physician alternately inflates and deflates the balloon until an angiogram verifies successful arterial dilation (below, right) and the pressure gradient has decreased.

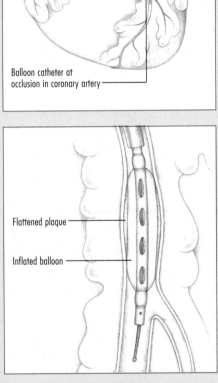

Guide catheter

Balloon catheter at occlusion in coronary artery

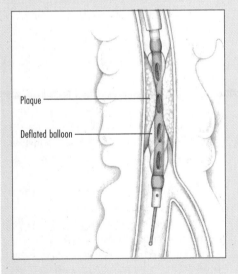

Plaque

Deflated balloon

Flattened plaque

Inflated balloon

tions include control of hypertension, control of elevated serum cholesterol or triglyceride levels (with antilipemics), and measures to minimize platelet aggregation and the danger of blood clots (with aspirin or other antiplatelet agents).

Special considerations

▶ During anginal episodes, monitor blood pressure and heart rate. Take an ECG during anginal episodes and before administering nitroglycerin or other nitrates. Record duration of pain, amount of medication required to relieve it, and accompanying symptoms.

▸ Keep nitroglycerin available for immediate use. Instruct the patient to call immediately whenever he feels chest, arm, or neck pain.

▸ Before cardiac catheterization, explain the procedure to the patient. Make sure he knows why it's necessary, understands the risks, and realizes that it may indicate a need for surgery.

▸ After catheterization, review the expected course of treatment with the patient and his family. Monitor the catheter site for bleeding. Also, check for distal pulses. To counter the dye's diuretic effect, make sure the patient drinks plenty of fluids. Assess potassium levels.

▸ If the patient is scheduled for surgery, explain the procedure to him and his family. Give them a tour of the intensive care unit and introduce them to the staff.

▸ After surgery, monitor blood pressure, intake and output, breath sounds, chest tube drainage, and ECG, watching for signs of ischemia and arrhythmias. Also, observe for and treat chest pain. Give vigorous chest physiotherapy, and guide the patient in removal of secretions through deep breathing, coughing, and expectoration of mucus.

▸ Before discharge, stress the need to follow the prescribed drug regimen (antihypertensives, nitrates, and antilipemics, for example), exercise program, and diet. Encourage regular, moderate exercise. Refer the patient to a self-help program to stop smoking.

REFERENCES

1. Yuan, G., et al. "Heterozygous Familial Hypercholesterolemia: An Underrecognized Cause of Early Cardiovascular Disease," *Canadian Medical Association Journal* 174(8):1124-29, April 2006.
2. Mager, A., et al. "Family History, Plasma Homocysteine, and Age at Onset of Symptoms of Myocardial Ischemia in Patients with Different Methylenetetrahydrofolate Reductase Genotypes," *American Journal of Cardiology* 95(12):1420-24, June 2005.
3. Douglas, P.S., and Ginsberg, G.S. "The Evaluation of Chest Pain in Women," *New England Journal of Medicine* 334(20):1311-15, May 1996.
4. Arad, Y., et al. "Coronary Calcification, Coronary Disease Risk Factors, C-Reactive Protein, and Atherosclerotic Cardiovascular Disease Events: The St. Francis Heart Study," *Journal of the American College of Cardiology* 46(1):158-65, July 2005.
5. American Heart Association. "2005 American Heart Association Guidelines for Cardiopulmonary Resuscitation and Emergency Cardiovascular Care: International Consensus on Science," *Circulation* 112(22Suppl):IV-1-IV-221, November 2005.
6. Torguson, R., et al. "Intravascular Brachytherapy versus Drug-Eluting Stents for the Treatment of Patients with Drug-Eluting Stent Restenosis," *American Journal of Cardiology* 98(10):1340-44, November 2006.

DILATED CARDIOMYOPATHY

Dilated cardiomyopathy results from extensively damaged myocardial muscle fibers. This disorder interferes with myocardial metabolism and grossly dilates all four chambers of the heart, giving the heart a globular appearance and shape. In this disorder, hypertrophy may be present. Dilated cardiomyopathy leads to intractable heart failure, arrhythmias, and emboli. Because this disease isn't usually diagnosed until it's in the advanced stages, the patient's prognosis is generally poor.

Causes and incidence

The cause of most cardiomyopathies is unknown. Occasionally, dilated cardiomyopathy results from myocardial destruction by toxic, infectious, or metabolic agents, such as certain viruses, endocrine and electrolyte disorders, and nutritional deficiencies. Other causes include muscle disorders (myasthenia gravis, progressive muscular dystrophy, and myotonic dystrophy), infiltrative disorders

(hemochromatosis and amyloidosis), and sarcoidosis.

Cardiomyopathy may also be a complication of alcoholism. In such cases, it may improve with abstinence from alcohol but recurs when the patient resumes drinking. How viruses induce cardiomyopathy is unclear, but researchers suspect a link between viral myocarditis and subsequent dilated cardiomyopathy, especially after infection with poliovirus, coxsackievirus B, influenza virus, or human immunodeficiency virus.

Metabolic cardiomyopathies are related to endocrine and electrolyte disorders and nutritional deficiencies. Thus, dilated cardiomyopathy may develop in patients with hyperthyroidism, pheochromocytoma, beriberi (thiamine deficiency), or kwashiorkor (protein deficiency). Cardiomyopathy may also result from rheumatic fever, especially among children with myocarditis. Newer studies suggest that dilated cardiomyopathy may be related to genetic mutations.[1]

Antepartal or postpartal cardiomyopathy may develop during the last trimester or within months after delivery. Its cause is unknown, but it occurs most frequently in multiparous women older than age 30, particularly those with malnutrition or preeclampsia. In these patients, cardiomegaly and heart failure may reverse with treatment, allowing a subsequent normal pregnancy.[2] If cardiomegaly persists despite treatment, the prognosis is poor.

Dilated cardiomyopathy most commonly affects middle-age men but can occur in any age-group. Because it usually isn't diagnosed until the advanced stages, the prognosis is generally poor. Most patients, especially those older than age 55, die within 2 years of symptom onset.

Signs and symptoms

In dilated cardiomyopathy, the heart ejects blood less efficiently than normal. Consequently, a large volume of blood remains in the left ventricle after systole, causing signs of heart failure—both left-sided (shortness of breath, orthopnea, dyspnea on exertion, paroxysmal nocturnal dyspnea, fatigue, and an irritating dry cough at night) and right-sided (edema, liver engorgement, and jugular vein distention). Dilated cardiomyopathy also produces peripheral cyanosis and sinus tachycardia or atrial fibrillation at rest in some patients secondary to low cardiac output. Auscultation reveals diffuse apical impulses, pansystolic murmur (mitral and tricuspid insufficiency secondary to cardiomegaly and weak papillary muscles), and S_3 and S_4 gallop rhythms. Worsening renal function will be present as decreased cardiac output produces decreased renal perfusion.

Complications

▶ Intractable heart failure
▶ Arrhythmias
▶ Emboli
▶ Ventricular arrhythmias that may lead to syncope and sudden death

Diagnosis

No single test confirms dilated cardiomyopathy. Diagnosis requires elimination of other possible causes of heart failure and arrhythmias.

▶ Electrocardiography and angiography rule out ischemic heart disease; an electrocardiogram may also show biventricular hypertrophy, sinus tachycardia, atrial enlargement, ST-segment and T-wave abnormalities and, in 20% of patients, atrial fibrillation and bundle-branch block. QRS complexes are decreased in amplitude.[3]

▶ Chest X-ray shows moderate to marked cardiomegaly—usually affecting all heart chambers—and may demonstrate pulmonary congestion, pleural or pericardial effusion, or pulmonary venous hypertension.

▶ Chest computed tomography scan or echocardiography identifies left ventricular thrombi, global hypokinesia, and degree of left ventricular dilation.

▶ Cardiac catheterization shows left ventricular dilation and dysfunction, elevated left ventricular and possible right ventricular filling pressures, and diminished cardiac output.

▶ Gallium scans may identify patients with dilated cardiomyopathy and myocarditis.[4]

▶ Cardiac magnetic resonance imaging is being used in some situations to determine the extent of cardiomyopathy and myocarditis.[5]

▶ Transvenous endomyocardial biopsy may be useful in some patients to determine the underlying disorder, such as amyloidosis or myocarditis.

Treatment

In patient with dilated cardiomyopathy, the goal of treatment is to correct the underlying causes and to improve the heart's pumping ability with a cardiac glycoside, a diuretic, oxygen, an anticoagulant, a vasodilator, and a low-sodium diet supplemented by vitamin therapy. An antiarrhythmic may be used to treat arrhythmias. In some cases, an implanted cardiac defibrillator may be placed to help control lethal arrhythmias. If the cardiomyopathy stems from alcoholism, alcohol consumption must be stopped. A woman of childbearing age should avoid pregnancy.

Therapy may also include prolonged bed rest and selective use of a corticosteroid, particularly when myocardial inflammation is present.

A vasodilator can help reduce preload and afterload, thereby decreasing congestion and increasing cardiac output. Acute heart failure necessitates vasodilation with I.V. nitroprusside, I.V. nesiritide, or I.V. nitroglycerin. Long-term treatment may include prazosin, hydralazine, isosorbide dinitrate, an angiotensin-converting enzyme inhibitor and, if the patient is on prolonged bed rest, an anticoagulant. Dopamine, dobutamine, and amrinone may be useful during the acute stage. Beta-adrenergic blockers help increase myo-cardial contractility in patients with a normal QRS.[6]

When these treatments fail, therapy may require heart transplantation for carefully selected patients.

Cardiomyoplasty may be used for those who aren't candidates for transplants and who are symptomatic at rest. During cardiomyoplasty, the latissimus dorsi muscle is wrapped around the ventricle, helping the ventricle to effectively pump blood. A cardiomyostimulator delivers bursts of electrical activity during systole to contract the muscle.

Special considerations

▶ Alternate periods of rest with required activities of daily living and treatments.

▶ Provide active or passive range-of-motion exercises to prevent muscle atrophy while the patient is on bed rest.

▶ Monitor for signs of progressive failure (increasing crackles and dyspnea and increased jugular vein distention) and compromised renal perfusion (oliguria, elevated blood urea nitrogen and creatinine levels, and electrolyte imbalances). Weigh the patient daily.

▶ Administer oxygen as needed.

▶ If the patient is receiving vasodilators, check blood pressure and heart rate. If he becomes hypotensive, stop the infusion and place him in a supine position, with legs elevated to increase venous return and to ensure cerebral blood flow.

▶ If the patient is receiving diuretics, monitor for signs of resolving congestion (decreased crackles and dyspnea) or too vigorous diuresis. Check serum potassium level for hypokalemia, especially if therapy includes digoxin.

▶ Therapeutic restrictions and an uncertain prognosis usually cause profound anxiety and depression, so offer support and let the patient express his feelings. Be flexible with visiting hours.

▶ Before discharge, teach the patient about his illness and its treatment. Emphasize the need to avoid alcohol and smoking, to restrict sodium intake, to watch for weight gain (a weight gain of 3 lb [1.4 kg] over 1 to 2 days indicates fluid accumulation), to take digoxin as prescribed and watch for its adverse effects (anorexia, nausea, vomiting, and yellow vision).

▶ Encourage family members to learn cardiopulmonary resuscitation.

REFERENCES

1. Taylor, M.R., et al. "Prevalence of Desmin Mutations in Dilated Cardiomyopathy," *Circulation* 115(10):1244-51, March 2007.
2. Murali, S., and Baldisseri, M.R. "Peripartum Cardiomyopathy," *Critical Care Medicine* 33(10 Suppl):S340-46, October 2005.
3. Rapezzi, C., et al. "Echocardiographic Clues to Diagnosis of Dystrophin Related Dilated Cardiomyopathy," *Heart* 93(1):10, January 2007.
4. Rigo, F., et al. "The Independent Prognostic Value of Contractile and Coronary Flow Reserve Determined by Dipyridamole Stress Echocardiography in Patients with Idiopathic Dilated Cardiomyopathy," *American Journal of Cardiology* 99(8):1154-58, April 2007.
5. Skouri, H.N., et al. "Noninvasive Imaging in Myocarditis," *Journal of the American College of Cardiology* 48(10):2085-93, November 2006.
6. Takemoto, Y., et al. "Beta-Blocker Therapy Induces Ventricular Resynchronization in Dilated Cardiomyopathy with Narrow QRS Complex," *Journal of the American College of Cardiology* 49(7):778-88, February 2007.

ENDOCARDITIS

Endocarditis (also known as *infective* or *bacterial endocarditis*) is an infection of the endocardium, heart valves, or cardiac prosthesis caused by bacterial or fungal invasion. This invasion produces vegetative growths on the heart valves, endocardial lining of a heart chamber, or endothelium of a blood vessel that may embolize to the spleen, kidneys, central nervous system, and lungs. In endocarditis, fibrin and platelets aggregate on the valve tissue and engulf circulating bacteria or fungi that flourish and produce friable verrucous vegetations. (See *Degenerative changes in endocarditis.*)

Such vegetations may cover the valve surfaces, causing ulceration and necrosis; they may also extend to the chordae tendineae, leading to their rupture and subsequent valvular insufficiency. Untreated endocarditis is usually fatal, but with proper treatment, 70% of patients recover. The prognosis is worst when endocarditis causes severe valvular damage, leading to insufficiency and heart failure, or when it involves a prosthetic valve.

Causes and incidence

Most cases of endocarditis occur in I.V. drug abusers, patients with prosthetic heart valves, and those with mitral valve prolapse (especially males with a systolic murmur). These conditions have surpassed rheumatic heart disease as the leading risk factor. Other predisposing conditions include coarctation of the aorta, tetralogy of Fallot, subaortic and valvular aortic stenosis, ventricular septal defects, pulmonary stenosis, Marfan syndrome, degenerative heart disease (especially calcific aortic stenosis) and, rarely, syphilitic aortic valve. However, some patients with endocarditis have no underlying heart disease.

Infecting organisms differ among these groups. In patients with native valve endocarditis who aren't I.V. drug abusers, causative organisms usually include—in order of frequency—streptococci (especially *Streptococcus viridans*), staphylococci, or enterococci. Although many other bacteria occasionally cause the disorder, fungal causes are rare in this group. The mitral valve is involved most commonly, followed by the aortic valve.

In patients who are I.V. drug abusers, *Staphylococcus aureus* is the most common infecting organism.[1] Less commonly, streptococci, enterococci, gram-negative bacilli, or fungi cause the disorder. The tricuspid valve is involved most commonly, followed by the aortic and then the mitral valve.

In patients with prosthetic valve endocarditis, early cases (those that develop within 60 days of valve insertion) are usually due to staphylococcal infection. However, gram-negative aerobic organisms, fungi, streptococci, enterococci, or diphtheroids may also cause the disorder. The course is usually fulminant and is associated with a high mortality. Late cases (occurring after 60 days) present similarly to native valve endocarditis.

In the United States, endocarditis affects 1.4 to 4.2 people out of every 100,000. Males are twice as likely as females to acquire this infection, and the mean age of onset is 50. Mortality is associated with increased age, infection of the aortic valve, heart failure and underlying heart disease, and central nervous system complications; mortality rates vary with the infecting organism.

Signs and symptoms

Early clinical features of endocarditis are usually nonspecific and include malaise, weakness, fatigue, weight loss, anorexia, arthralgia, night sweats, chills, valvular insufficiency and, in 90% of patients, an intermittent fever that may recur for weeks. A more acute onset is associated with organisms of high pathogenicity such as *S. aureus*. Endocarditis commonly causes a loud, regurgitant murmur typical of the underlying heart lesion. A suddenly changing murmur or the discovery of a new murmur in the presence of fever is a classic physical sign of endocarditis.

In about 30% of patients, embolization from vegetating lesions or diseased valvular tissue may produce typical features of splenic, renal, cerebral, or pulmonary infarc-

Degenerative changes in endocarditis

This illustration shows typical vegetations on the endocardium produced by fibrin and platelet deposits on infection sites.

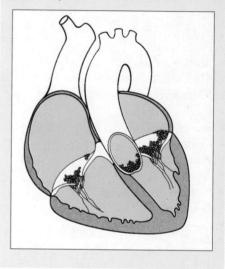

tion or of peripheral vascular occlusion. Here are typical features of each:
▶ splenic infarction—pain in the left upper quadrant, radiating to the left shoulder; abdominal rigidity
▶ renal infarction—hematuria, pyuria, flank pain, and decreased urine output
▶ cerebral infarction—hemiparesis, aphasia, or other neurologic deficits
▶ pulmonary infarction (most common in right-sided endocarditis, which commonly occurs among I.V. drug abusers and after cardiac surgery)—cough, pleuritic pain, pleural friction rub, dyspnea, and hemoptysis
▶ peripheral vascular occlusion—numbness and tingling in an arm, leg, finger, or toe, or signs of impending peripheral gangrene.

Other signs may include splenomegaly; petechiae of the skin (especially common on the upper anterior trunk) and the buccal,

pharyngeal, or conjunctival mucosa; and splinter hemorrhages under the nails. Rarely, endocarditis produces Osler's nodes (tender, raised, subcutaneous lesions on the fingers or toes), Roth's spots (hemorrhagic areas with white centers on the retina), and Janeway lesions (purplish macules on the palms or soles).

Complications

▶ Heart failure
▶ Aortic root abscesses
▶ Myocardial abscesses
▶ Pericarditis
▶ Cardiac arrhythmia
▶ Meningitis
▶ Cerebral emboli
▶ Brain abscesses
▶ Septic pulmonary infarcts
▶ Arthritis
▶ Glomerulonephritis
▶ Acute renal failure
▶ Death

Diagnosis

Three or more blood cultures in a 24- to 48-hour period (each from a separate venipuncture) identify the causative organism in up to 90% of patients. Blood cultures should be drawn from three different sites with at least 1 hour between each draw.

The remaining 10% may have negative blood cultures, possibly suggesting fungal infection or infections that are difficult to diagnose such as *Haemophilus parainfluenzae.*

Other abnormal but nonspecific laboratory test results include:
▶ normal or elevated white blood cell count
▶ abnormal histiocytes (macrophages)
▶ elevated erythrocyte sedimentation rate
▶ normocytic, normochromic anemia (in 70% to 90% of patients)
▶ proteinuria and microscopic hematuria (in about 50% of patients)
▶ positive serum rheumatoid factor (in about 50% of patients after endocarditis is present for 3 to 6 weeks).

Echocardiography (particularly trans-esophageal) may identify valvular damage; electrocardiography may show atrial fibrillation and other arrhythmias that accompany valvular disease.[2]

With the incidence of antibiotic-resistant organisms on the rise, some physicians are biopsying the infected valve to isolate the infectious organism in order to prescribe antibiotics that will treat the organism.[3]

Treatment

The goal of treatment is to eradicate the infecting organism with appropriate antimicrobial therapy, which should start promptly and continue over 4 to 6 weeks. Selection of an antibiotic is based on identification of the infecting organism and on sensitivity studies. While awaiting results, or if blood cultures are negative, empiric antimicrobial therapy is based on the likely infecting organism.[4]

Supportive treatment includes bed rest, aspirin for fever and aches, and sufficient fluid intake. Severe valvular damage, especially aortic or mitral insufficiency, may require corrective surgery if refractory heart failure develops, or in cases requiring that an infected prosthetic valve be replaced.

Special considerations

▶ Before giving antibiotics, obtain a patient history of allergies. Administer antibiotics on time to maintain consistent antibiotic blood levels.
▶ Observe for signs of infiltration or inflammation at the venipuncture site, possible complications of long-term I.V. drug administration. To reduce the risk of these complications, rotate venous access sites.
▶ Watch for signs of embolization (hematuria, pleuritic chest pain, left upper quadrant pain, or paresis), a common occurrence during the first 3 months of treatment. Tell the patient to watch for and report these signs, which may indicate impending peripheral vascular occlusion or splenic, renal, cerebral, or pulmonary infarction.

▶ Monitor the patient's renal status (blood urea nitrogen levels, creatinine clearance, and urine output) to check for signs of renal emboli or evidence of drug toxicity.

▶ Observe for signs of heart failure, such as dyspnea, tachypnea, tachycardia, crackles, jugular vein distention, edema, and weight gain.

▶ Provide reassurance by teaching the patient and his family about this disease and the need for prolonged treatment. Tell them to watch closely for fever, anorexia, and other signs of relapse about 2 weeks after treatment stops. Suggest quiet diversionary activities to prevent excessive physical exertion.

▶ Make sure high-risk patients understand the need for prophylactic antibiotics before, during, and after dental work, childbirth, and genitourinary, GI, or gynecologic procedures.

▶ Teach patients how to recognize symptoms of endocarditis, and tell them to notify the physician at once if such symptoms occur.

REFERENCES

1. Wang, A., et al. "Contemporary Clinical Profile and Outcome of Prosthetic Valve Endocarditis," *JAMA* 297(12):1354-61, March 2007.
2. Lester, S.J., and Wilansky, S. "Endocarditis and Associated Complications," *Critical Care Medicine* 35(8 Suppl):S384-91, August 2007.
3. Marin, M., et al. "Molecular Diagnosis of Infective Endocarditis by Real-Time Broad-Range Polymerase Chain Reaction (PCR) and Sequencing Directly from Heart Valve Tissue," *Medicine* 86(4):195-202, July 2007.
4. Wilson, W., et al. "Prevention of Infective Endocarditis: Guidelines from the American Heart Association: A Guideline from the American Heart Association Rheumatic Fever, Endocarditis, and Kawasaki Disease Committee, Council on Cardiovascular Disease in the Young, and the Council on Clinical Cardiology, Council on Cardiovascular Surgery and Anesthesia, and the Quality of Care and Outcomes Research Interdisciplinary Working Group," *Circulation* 116(15):1736-54, October 2007.

FEMORAL AND POPLITEAL ANEURYSMS

Femoral and popliteal aneurysms, sometimes called peripheral arterial aneurysms, are the end result of progressive atherosclerotic changes occurring in the walls (medial layer) of these major peripheral arteries. These aneurysm formations may be fusiform (spindle-shaped) or saccular (pouchlike); the fusiform type is three times more common. They may have singular or multiple segmental lesions, often affecting both legs, and may accompany other arterial aneurysms located in the abdominal aorta or iliac arteries. (See *Arteries of the leg*, page 22.)

Causes and incidence

This condition occurs most frequently in men older than age 50. The clinical course is usually progressive, eventually ending in thrombosis, embolization, and gangrene. Elective surgery before complications arise greatly improves the prognosis.

Femoral and popliteal aneurysms may be secondary to atherosclerosis or result from underlying hereditary or acquired causes.[1] Acquired causes may include trauma (blunt or penetrating), smoking, bacterial infection, or peripheral vascular reconstructive surgery (which causes "suture line" aneurysms, or false aneurysms, in which a blood clot forms a second lumen).

Signs and symptoms

Popliteal aneurysms may cause pain in the popliteal space when they're large enough to compress the medial popliteal nerve and edema and venous distention if the vein is compressed. Femoral and popliteal aneurysms can produce symptoms of severe ischemia in the leg or foot due to acute thrombosis with-

Arteries of the leg

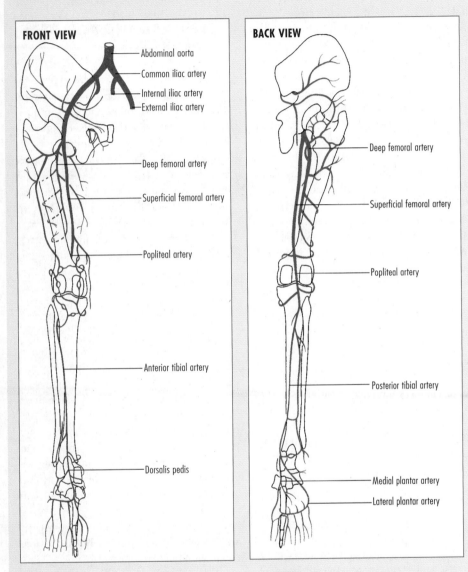

FRONT VIEW

- Abdominal aorta
- Common iliac artery
- Internal iliac artery
- External iliac artery
- Deep femoral artery
- Superficial femoral artery
- Popliteal artery
- Anterior tibial artery
- Dorsalis pedis

BACK VIEW

- Deep femoral artery
- Superficial femoral artery
- Popliteal artery
- Posterior tibial artery
- Medial plantar artery
- Lateral plantar artery

in the aneurysmal sac, embolization of mural thrombus fragments and, rarely, rupture. Symptoms of acute aneurysmal thrombosis include severe pain, loss of pulse and color, coldness in the affected leg or foot, and gangrene. Distal petechial hemorrhages may develop from aneurysmal emboli.

Complications

▶ Thrombosis
▶ Emboli
▶ Gangrene
▶ Amputation

Diagnosis

Diagnosis is usually confirmed by bilateral palpation that reveals a pulsating mass above or below the inguinal ligament in femoral aneurysm. When thrombosis has occurred, palpation detects a firm, nonpulsating mass. Arteriography or ultrasound may be indicated in doubtful situations. Arteriography may also detect associated aneurysms, especially those in the abdominal aorta and the iliac arteries. Ultrasound may be helpful in determining the size of the popliteal or femoral artery.

Treatment

Femoral and popliteal aneurysms require surgical bypass and reconstruction of the artery, usually with an autogenous saphenous vein graft replacement. Arterial occlusion that causes severe ischemia and gangrene may require leg amputation.

Special considerations

Before corrective surgery:
▶ Assess and record circulatory status, noting the location and quality of peripheral pulses in the affected arm or leg.
▶ Administer prophylactic antibiotics or anticoagulants, as ordered.
▶ Discuss expected postoperative procedures, and review the explanation of the surgery.

After arterial surgery:
▶ Monitor carefully for early signs of thrombosis or graft occlusion (loss of pulse, decreased skin temperature and sensation, and severe pain) and infection (fever).
▶ Palpate distal pulses at least every hour for the first 24 hours and then as frequently as ordered. Correlate these findings with preoperative circulatory assessment. Mark the sites on the patient's skin where pulses are palpable to facilitate repeated checks.
▶ Help the patient walk soon after surgery to prevent venostasis and possible thrombus formation.

To prepare the patient for discharge:

▶ Tell the patient to immediately report any recurrence of symptoms because the saphenous vein graft replacement can fail or another aneurysm may develop.
▶ Explain to the patient with popliteal artery resection that swelling may persist for some time. If antiembolism stockings are ordered, make sure they fit properly, and teach the patient how to apply them. Warn against wearing constrictive apparel.
▶ If the patient is receiving anticoagulants, suggest measures to prevent bleeding such as using an electric razor. Tell him to report any signs of bleeding immediately (bleeding gums, tarry stools, and easy bruising). Explain the importance of follow-up blood studies to monitor anticoagulant therapy. Warn him to avoid trauma, tobacco, and aspirin.[2]

REFERENCES

1. Hirsch, A., et al. "ACC/AHA 2005 Practice Guidelines for the Management of Patients with Peripheral Arterial Disease," *Circulation* 113(11):e463-54, March 2006.
2. Lee, T.L., and Bokovov, J. "Understanding Discharge Instructions after Vascular Surgery: An Observational Study," *Journal of Vascular Nursing* 23(1):25-29, March 2005.

HEART FAILURE

Heart failure is a syndrome characterized by myocardial dysfunction that leads to impaired pump performance (diminished cardiac output) or to frank heart failure and abnormal circulatory congestion. Congestion of systemic venous circulation may result in peripheral edema or hepatomegaly; congestion of pulmonary circulation may cause pulmonary edema, an acute life-threatening emergency. Pump failure usually occurs in a damaged left ventricle (left-sided heart failure) but may occur in the right ventricle (right-sided heart failure) either as a primary disorder or secondary to

What happens in heart failure

Heart failure occurs when cardiac output is inadequate to meet the body's needs. The pathophysiology of heart failure is shown in the flow chart below.

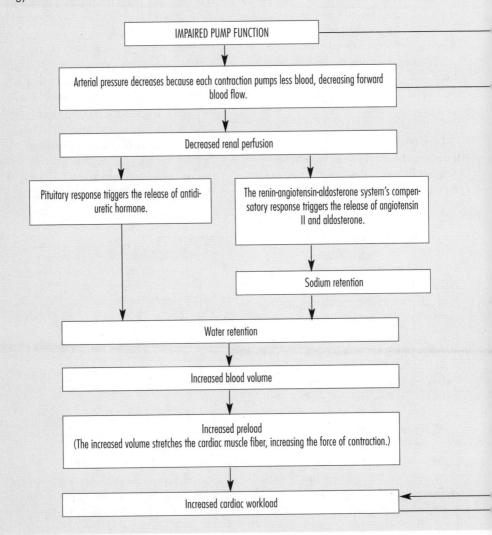

left-sided heart failure. Sometimes, left- and right-sided heart failure develop simultaneously. (See *What happens in heart failure*.) Although heart failure may be acute (as a direct result of myocardial infarction [MI]), it's generally a chronic disorder associated with sodium and water retention by the kidneys.

Advances in diagnostic and therapeutic techniques have greatly improved the outlook for patients with heart failure, but the prognosis still depends on the underlying cause and the patient's response to treatment. Survival after diagnosis is poorer in men;

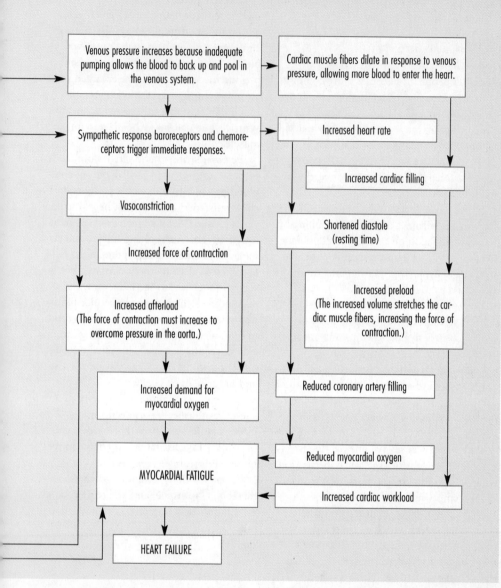

80% of men and 70% of women younger than age 65 will die within 8 years.[1]

The ACC/AHA 2005 Guideline for heart failure classifies heart failure in four stages:

Stage A: Includes patients who are at high risk for heart failure but don't have structural heart disease or symptoms.

Stage B: Includes patients who have structural heart disease but don't have signs or symptoms of heart failure.

Stage C: Includes patients who have structural heart disease with prior or current symptoms of heart failure.

Stage D: Includes patients who have refractory heart failure that requires special interventions such as heart transplant or permanent mechanical support.[2]

Causes and incidence

Heart failure affects approximately 1 of every 100 people. It becomes more common with advancing age.[3] The lifetime risk at age 40 for both men and women is 1 in 5.[1]

Heart failure may result from a primary abnormality of the heart muscle such as an infarction, inadequate myocardial perfusion due to coronary artery disease, or cardiomyopathy. Other causes include:

▶ diastolic dysfunction, decreased ejection fraction, impairment of ventricular filling by diminished relaxation or reduced compliance seen with hypertrophic cardiomyopathy, myocardial hypertrophy, and pericardial restriction

▶ mechanical disturbances as in mitral stenosis secondary to rheumatic heart disease or constrictive pericarditis and atrial fibrillation

▶ systolic hemodynamic disturbances, such as excessive cardiac workload due to volume overloading or pressure overload that limit the heart's pumping ability. These disturbances can result from mitral or aortic insufficiency, which causes volume overloading, and aortic stenosis or systemic hypertension, which result in increased resistance to ventricular emptying.

Reduced cardiac output triggers compensatory mechanisms, such as ventricular dilation, hypertrophy, increased sympathetic activity, and activation of the renin-angiotensin-aldosterone system. These mechanisms improve cardiac output at the expense of increased ventricular work. In cardiac dilation, an increase in end-diastolic ventricular volume (preload) causes increased stroke work and stroke volume during contraction, stretching cardiac muscle fibers beyond optimum limits and producing pulmonary congestion and pulmonary hypertension, which in turn may lead to right-sided heart failure.

In ventricular hypertrophy, an increase in muscle mass or diameter of the left ventricle allows the heart to pump against increased resistance (impedance) to the outflow of blood. An increase in ventricular diastolic pressure necessary to fill the enlarged ventricle may compromise diastolic coronary blood flow, limiting the oxygen supply to the ventricle and causing ischemia and impaired muscle contractility.

Increased sympathetic activity occurs as a response to decreased cardiac output and blood pressure by enhancing peripheral vascular resistance, contractility, heart rate, and venous return. Signs of increased sympathetic activity, such as cool extremities and clamminess, may indicate impending heart failure. Increased sympathetic activity also restricts blood flow to the kidneys, which respond by reducing the glomerular filtration rate and increasing tubular reabsorption of salt and water, in turn expanding the circulating blood volume. This renal mechanism, if unchecked, can aggravate congestion and produce overt edema.

Chronic heart failure may worsen as a result of respiratory tract infections, pulmonary embolism, stress, increased sodium or water intake, or failure to adhere to the prescribed treatment regimen.

Patients with hypertension, diabetes, metabolic syndrome, and atherosclerotic disease and those who smoke, drink alcohol, or take illicit drugs are at a higher risk for heart failure.[2]

Signs and symptoms

Left-sided heart failure primarily produces pulmonary signs and symptoms; right-sided heart failure, primarily systemic signs and symptoms. However, heart failure commonly affects both sides of the heart.

Clinical signs of left-sided heart failure include dyspnea, orthopnea, crackles, possibly wheezing, hypoxia, respiratory acidosis,

Classifying heart failure

Heart failure is classified according to its pathophysiology. It may be right- or left-sided, systolic or diastolic, and acute or chronic.

RIGHT-SIDED OR LEFT-SIDED
Right-sided heart failure is the result of ineffective right ventricular contraction. It may be caused by an acute right ventricular infarction or pulmonary embolus. However, the most common cause is profound backward flow due to left-sided heart failure.

Left-sided heart failure is the result of ineffective left ventricular contraction. It may lead to pulmonary congestion or pulmonary edema and decreased cardiac output. Left ventricular myocardial infarction, hypertension, and aortic and mitral valve stenosis or regurgitation are common causes. As the decreased pumping ability of the left ventricle persists, fluid accumulates, backing up into the left atrium and then into the lungs. If this worsens, pulmonary edema and right-sided heart failure may also result.

SYSTOLIC OR DIASTOLIC
In patients with systolic heart failure, the left ventricle can't pump enough blood out to the systemic circulation during systole and the ejection fraction falls. Consequently, blood backs up into the pulmonary circulation, pressure rises in the pulmonary venous system, and cardiac output falls.

In patients with diastolic heart failure, the left ventricle can't relax and fill properly during diastole, and the stroke volume falls. Therefore, larger ventricular volumes are needed to maintain cardiac output.

ACUTE OR CHRONIC
Acute refers to the timing of the onset of symptoms and whether compensatory mechanisms kick in. Typically, fluid status is normal or low, and sodium and water retention don't occur.

In patients with chronic heart failure, signs and symptoms have been present for some time, compensatory mechanisms have taken effect, and fluid volume overload persists. Drug therapy, diet changes, and activity restrictions usually help control symptoms.

---

cough, cyanosis or pallor, palpitations, arrhythmias, elevated blood pressure, and pulsus alternans.

Clinical signs of right-sided heart failure include dependent peripheral edema, hepatomegaly, splenomegaly, jugular vein distention, ascites, slow weight gain, arrhythmias, positive hepatojugular reflex, abdominal distention, nausea, vomiting, anorexia, weakness, fatigue, dizziness, and syncope. (See *Classifying heart failure*.)

Complications
▶ Pulmonary edema (see *Pulmonary edema: How to intervene,* page 28)
▶ Venostasis, with predisposition to thromboembolism (associated primarily with prolonged bed rest)
▶ Cerebral insufficiency

▶ Renal insufficiency, with severe electrolyte imbalance
▶ Excessive fluid accumulating in the pericardium, requiring removal through pericardiocentesis

Diagnosis
▶ Electrocardiography may reflect heart strain or enlargement, ischemia, or an old MI. It may also reveal atrial enlargement, tachycardia, and extrasystoles.
▶ Chest X-ray shows increased pulmonary vascular markings, interstitial edema, or pleural effusion and cardiomegaly.
▶ Pulmonary artery monitoring typically demonstrates elevated pulmonary artery and pulmonary artery wedge pressures, left ventricular end-diastolic pressure in left-sided heart failure, and elevated right atrial pres-

Pulmonary edema: How to intervene

Obtain the patient history, assist with diagnostic tests, and assess respiratory, mental, and cardio-vascular status.

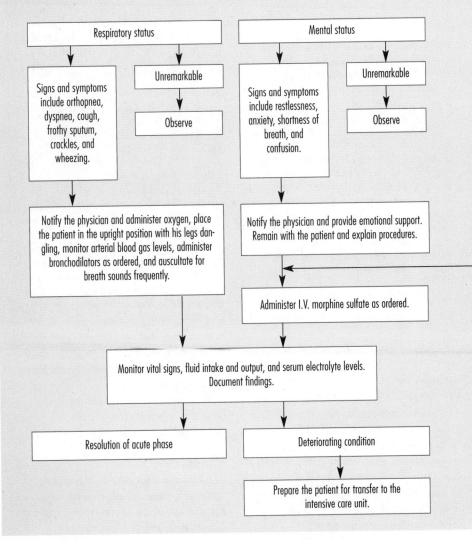

sure or central venous pressure in right-sided heart failure.

▶ Echocardiogram may demonstrate wall motion abnormalities and chamber dilation.

▶ Laboratory tests such as the B-type natri-uretic peptide are used to help diagnose heart failure and also patients at risk for sudden death from heart failure. (See *BNP and sudden death*.)

Other tests that may also demonstrate en-largement of the heart or decreased function-ing include chest computed tomography scan, cardiac magnetic resonance imaging, or nuclear scans, such as multiple-gated ac-

HEALTH & SAFETY

BNP and sudden death

Patients with heart failure have a high incidence of sudden death, and researchers have sought to develop a test to help indicate which patients are at higher risk for sudden death. B-type natriuretic peptide (BNP) has been shown to have diagnostic significance in heart failure. BNP levels were drawn for 452 patients with heart failure and analyzed over 3 years. In the end, it was determined that BNP levels could be used as predictors of sudden death in patients with heart failure.[7]

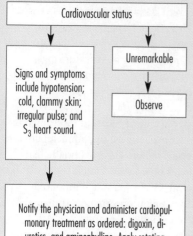

Cardiovascular status

Signs and symptoms include hypotension; cold, clammy skin; irregular pulse; and S₃ heart sound.

Unremarkable

Observe

Notify the physician and administer cardiopulmonary treatment as ordered: digoxin, diuretics, and aminophylline. Apply rotating tourniquets as ordered.

quisition scanning and radionuclide ventriculography.

Treatment

The goal of therapy is to improve pump function by reversing the compensatory mechanisms producing the clinical effects, underlying disorders, and precipitating factors. The ACC/AHA 2005 Guideline update makes therapy recommendations based on each stage of heart failure.[7]

Stage A treatment consists of:
▶ treating hypertension
▶ controlling metabolic syndrome
▶ treating lipid disorders
▶ treating diabetes
▶ treating thyroid disorders
▶ encouraging the cessation of smoking and regular exercise
▶ eliminating use of illicit drugs and alcohol.

In addition:
▶ Angiotensin-converting enzyme (ACE) inhibitors can be used to prevent heart failure in patients at high risk for developing heart failure who have a history of atherosclerotic vascular disease, diabetes mellitus, or hypertension with associated cardiovascular risk factors.
▶ Angiotensin II receptor blockers can be used to prevent heart failure in patients at high risk for developing heart failure who have a history of atherosclerotic vascular disease, diabetes mellitus, or hypertension with associated cardiovascular risk factors.

Stage B treatment includes the treatment for Stage A, plus:

▶ treating with ACE inhibitors or beta-adrenergic blockers to delay the onset of symptoms and decrease the risk of death and hospitalization.

Stage C treatment includes the treatment for Stages A and B, along with:

▶ restricting dietary salt

▶ diuresis with diuretics to reduce fluid retention, total blood volume, and circulatory congestion

▶ using other drug therapies (aldosterone inhibitors, diuretics, and angiotensin receptor blockers) for patients who can't tolerate ACE inhibitors, digoxin, or vasodilators

▶ avoiding drugs that are known to cause adverse reactions in heart failure patients, such as nonsteroidal anti-inflammatories, antiarrhythmics, and calcium channel blockers

▶ treating with anticoagulation therapy in patients with increased risk of thromboembolism

▶ biventricular pacing

▶ implantable defibrillators.

Stage D treatment includes the treatment for Stages A, B, and C, plus:

▶ improving cardiac performance, promoting diuresis with multiple drug therapies, such as I.V. diuretic, inotropic support, or vasodilators

▶ left ventricular assist devices, experimental surgery or drugs, or a heart transplant, as necessary

▶ end-of-life or hospice care, if indicated.

Special considerations

During the acute phase of heart failure:

▶ Place the patient in Fowler's position, and give him supplemental oxygen to help him breathe more easily.

▶ Weigh the patient daily, and check for peripheral edema. Carefully monitor I.V. intake and urine output, vital signs, and mental status. Auscultate the heart for abnormal sounds (S_3 gallop) and the lungs for crackles or rhonchi. Report changes immediately.

▶ Frequently monitor blood urea nitrogen, creatinine, and serum potassium, sodium, chloride, and magnesium levels.

▶ Make sure the patient has continuous cardiac monitoring during acute and advanced stages to identify and treat arrhythmias promptly.

▶ To prevent deep vein thrombosis caused by vascular congestion, assist the patient with range-of-motion exercises. Enforce bed rest and apply antiembolism stockings. Check regularly for calf pain and tenderness.

▶ Allow adequate rest periods.

To prepare the patient for discharge:

▶ Advise the patient to avoid foods high in sodium, such as canned or commercially prepared foods, to curb fluid overload. Teach the patient how to read food labels.

▶ Encourage participation in an outpatient cardiac rehabilitation program and an abstinence from smoking program.[4]

▶ Explain to the patient that the potassium he loses through diuretic therapy may need to be replaced by taking a prescribed potassium supplement and eating high-potassium foods, such as bananas and apricots.

▶ Stress the need for regular checkups.

▶ Teach the patient about the different practitioners he will encounter in a multidisciplinary approach to the treatment of heart failure.[5]

▶ Teach the patient to weigh himself daily.

▶ Stress the importance of taking digoxin exactly as prescribed. Tell the patient to watch for and immediately report signs of toxicity, such as anorexia, vomiting, and yellow vision.

▶ Tell the patient to notify the physician promptly if his pulse is unusually irregular or slow; if he experiences dizziness, blurred vision, shortness of breath, a persistent dry cough, palpitations, increased fatigue, paroxysmal nocturnal dyspnea, swollen ankles, or decreased urine output; or if he notices rapid weight gain (3 to 5 lb [1.5 to 2.5 kg] in 1 week).

REFERENCES

1. American Heart Association (2006 December 28). "Heart Disease and Stroke Statistics-2007 Update" [Online]. Available at *http://circ.aha-journals.org/cgi/content/full/CIRCULATIONAHA.106.17991.*
2. Hunt, S.A., et al. "ACC/AHA 2005 Guideline Update for the Diagnosis and Management of Chronic Heart Failure in the Adult—Summary Article," *Circulation* 112(12):e154-235, September 2005.
3. The Merck Manuals Online Medical Library (2008 January). "Heart Failure" [Online]. Available at *www.merck.com/mmhe/sec03/ch025/ch025a.html.*
4. Albert, N.M. "Evidence-Based Nursing Care for Patients with Heart Failure," *AACN Advances in Critical Care* 17(2):170-83, April-June 2006.
5. Miranda, M.B., et al. "An Evidence-Based Approach to Improving Care of Patients with Heart Failure across the Continuum," *Journal of Nursing Care Quality* 17(1):1-14, October 2002.
6. Berger, R., et al. "B-Type Natriuretic Peptide Predicts Sudden Death in Patients with Chronic Heart Failure," *Circulation* 105(20):2392-97, May 2002.
7. Unless otherwise noted, all the recommendations in the treatment section above are drawn from two sources: Hunt, S.A., et al. "ACC/AHA 2005 Guideline Update for the Diagnosis and Management of Chronic Heart Failure in the Adult—Summary Article," e154-235, as cited in reference 2, and Chojnowski, D. "Protecting Patients from Harm: Taking Aim at Heart Failure," *Nursing* 37(11):50-55, November 2007.

HYPERTENSION

Hypertension, an intermittent or sustained elevation in diastolic or systolic blood pressure, occurs as two major types: primary (essential or idiopathic) hypertension, the most common, and secondary hypertension, which results from renal disease or another identifiable cause. Malignant hypertension is a severe, fulminant form of hypertension common to both types. The prognosis is good if this disorder is detected early and treatment begins before complications develop. Severely elevated blood pressure (hypertensive crisis) may be fatal. (See *What happens in hypertensive crisis,* pages 32 and 33.)

Causes and incidence

Hypertension affects nearly 1 in 3 adults in the United States.[1] If untreated, it carries a high mortality. Risk factors for hypertension include family history, race (most common in blacks), obesity, dyslipidemia, diabetes, albumin in the urine, tobacco use, sedentary lifestyle, and age (older than 55 for men and older than 65 for women).[2] (See *Hypertension and family history,* page 34.)

The majority of people with hypertension have primary hypertension (90% to 95%).[3] Cardiac output and peripheral vascular resistance determine blood pressure. Increased blood volume, cardiac rate, and stroke volume as well as arteriolar vasoconstriction can raise blood pressure. The link to sustained hypertension, however, is unclear. The cause of primary hypertension is unknown, but it may also result from failure of intrinsic regulatory mechanisms:

▶ Renal hypoperfusion causes release of renin, which is converted by angiotensinogen, a liver enzyme, to angiotensin I. Angiotensin I is converted to angiotensin II, a powerful vasoconstrictor. The resulting vasoconstriction increases afterload. Angiotensin II stimulates adrenal secretion of aldosterone, which increases sodium reabsorption. Hypertonic-stimulated release of antidiuretic hormone from the pituitary gland follows, increasing water reabsorption, plasma volume, cardiac output, and blood pressure.

▶ Autoregulation changes an artery's diameter to maintain perfusion despite fluctuations in systemic blood pressure. The intrinsic mechanisms responsible include stress relaxation (vessels gradually dilate when blood

What happens in hypertensive crisis

Hypertensive crisis is a severe rise in arterial blood pressure caused by a disturbance in one or more of the regulating mechanisms. If left untreated, hypertensive crisis may result in renal, cardiac, or cerebral complications and, possibly, death.

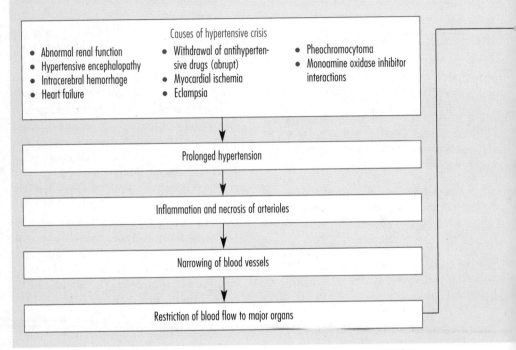

Causes of hypertensive crisis

- Abnormal renal function
- Hypertensive encephalopathy
- Intracerebral hemorrhage
- Heart failure

- Withdrawal of antihypertensive drugs (abrupt)
- Myocardial ischemia
- Eclampsia

- Pheochromocytoma
- Monoamine oxidase inhibitor interactions

↓

Prolonged hypertension

↓

Inflammation and necrosis of arterioles

↓

Narrowing of blood vessels

↓

Restriction of blood flow to major organs

pressure rises to reduce peripheral resistance) and capillary fluid shift (plasma moves between vessels and extravascular spaces to maintain intravascular volume).

▶ When the blood pressure drops, baroreceptors in the aortic arch and carotid sinuses decrease their inhibition of the medulla's vasomotor center, which increases sympathetic stimulation of the heart by norepinephrine. This, in turn, increases cardiac output by strengthening the contractile force, increasing the heart rate, and augmenting peripheral resistance by vasoconstriction. Stress can also stimulate the sympathetic nervous system to increase cardiac output and peripheral vascular resistance.

Secondary hypertension may result from renal vascular disease; pheochromocytoma; primary hyperaldosteronism; Cushing's syndrome; thyroid, pituitary, or parathyroid dysfunction; coarctation of the aorta; pregnancy; and neurologic disorders. The use of hormonal contraceptives or other drugs, such as cocaine or amphetamines, nonsteroidal anti-inflammatory drugs (NSAIDs), sympathomimetics, adrenal steroids, erythropoietin, cyclosporine and tacrolimus, licorice, and some over-the-counter dietary supplements and medications such as ma huang and bitter orange also are identifiable causes of hypertension.[2]

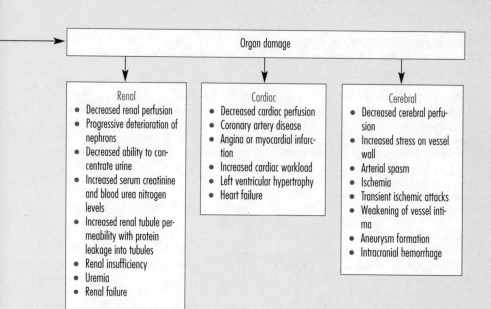

Organ damage

Renal
- Decreased renal perfusion
- Progressive deterioration of nephrons
- Decreased ability to concentrate urine
- Increased serum creatinine and blood urea nitrogen levels
- Increased renal tubule permeability with protein leakage into tubules
- Renal insufficiency
- Uremia
- Renal failure

Cardiac
- Decreased cardiac perfusion
- Coronary artery disease
- Angina or myocardial infarction
- Increased cardiac workload
- Left ventricular hypertrophy
- Heart failure

Cerebral
- Decreased cerebral perfusion
- Increased stress on vessel wall
- Arterial spasm
- Ischemia
- Transient ischemic attacks
- Weakening of vessel intima
- Aneurysm formation
- Intracranial hemorrhage

Signs and symptoms

Hypertension usually doesn't produce clinical effects until vascular changes in the heart, brain, or kidneys occur. Severely elevated blood pressure damages the intima of small vessels, resulting in fibrin accumulation in the vessels, development of local edema and, possibly, intravascular clotting. Symptoms produced by this process depend on the location of the damaged vessels:
- brain—stroke
- retina—blindness
- heart—myocardial infarction
- kidneys—proteinuria, edema and, eventually, renal failure.

Hypertension increases the heart's workload, causing left ventricular hypertrophy and, later, left- and right-sided heart failure and pulmonary edema.

Complications
- Stroke
- Cardiac disease—coronary artery disease, angina, myocardial infarction, heart failure, arrhythmias, sudden death
- Renal failure
- Cerebral infarctions
- Hypertensive encephalopathy
- Hypertensive retinopathy, which can cause blindness

Diagnosis
Serial blood pressure measurements are obtained and compared with previous readings

Hypertension and family history

Question: *How significant is family history in the development of hypertension?*

Research: Family history is important when determining hypertension risk for young adults as well as hypertension risk throughout adulthood. Particularly important is identifying whether the individual's parents have hypertension. To demonstrate the relationship between parental hypertension and blood pressure change and hypertension risk from young adulthood through the ninth decade of life, the researchers studied data obtained from 1,160 male former medical students who had been followed for 54 years. Several other factors were considered as contributing to increased risk, such as alcohol consumption, coffee drinking, physical activity, and cigarette smoking, and adjustments were made with respect to these factors.

Conclusion: The study demonstrated that participants with a history of parental hypertension had higher baseline mean systolic and diastolic blood pressure readings, as well as a higher rate of annual increase in systolic pressure, than participants without a parental history of hypertension. Although the study showed increased risk when only one parent had hypertension, the risk was significantly higher when both parents had hypertension. For example, a 35-year-old participant whose parents were both diagnosed with hypertension before age 55, had a 20.0-fold higher adjusted risk level.

Application: When performing a history and physical assessment it's important for the nurse to determine the patient's family history of hypertension. Young adults as well as older patients should be made aware that they're at increased risk for hypertension if either or both of their parents have hypertension. Teaching should focus on monitoring blood pressure, avoiding behaviors and substances that increase risk, and making healthy lifestyle choices.

Source: Wang, N.Y., et al. "Blood Pressure Change and Risk of Hypertension Associated with Parental Hypertension: The Johns Hopkins Precursors Study," *Archives of Internal Medicine* 168(6):643-48, March 24, 2008.

---

and trends to reveal an increase in diastolic and systolic pressures. (See *Classifying blood pressure readings.*)

Auscultation may reveal bruits over the abdominal aorta and the carotid, renal, and femoral arteries; ophthalmoscopy reveals arteriovenous nicking and, in hypertensive encephalopathy, papilledema. Patient history and the following additional tests may show predisposing factors and help identify an underlying cause such as renal disease:

▶ urinalysis—protein levels and red and white blood cell counts may indicate glomerulonephritis.

▶ excretory urography—renal atrophy indicates chronic renal disease; one kidney more than ⅝″ (1.5 cm) shorter than the other suggests unilateral renal disease.

▶ serum potassium—levels less than 3.5 mEq/L may indicate adrenal dysfunction (primary hyperaldosteronism).

▶ blood urea nitrogen (BUN) and serum creatinine—BUN level that's normal or elevated to more than 20 mg/dl and serum creatinine level that's normal or elevated to more than 1.5 mg/dl suggest renal disease.

Other tests help detect cardiovascular damage and other complications:

▶ Electrocardiography may show left ventricular hypertrophy or ischemia.

▶ Chest X-ray may show cardiomegaly.

▶ Echocardiography may show left ventricular hypertrophy.

Classifying blood pressure readings

The National Institutes of Health, which used to classify blood pressure according to severity categories—mild, moderate, severe, and very severe—has replaced this classification system with a system based on stages.

The following revised categories are based on the average of two or more readings taken on separate visits after an initial screening. They apply to adults age 18 and older who aren't taking antihypertensives, aren't acutely ill, and don't have other health conditions, such as diabetes and kidney disease. (If the systolic and diastolic pressures fall into different categories, use the higher of the two pressures to classify the reading. For example, a reading of 160/92 mm Hg should be classified as stage 2.)

Normal blood pressure with respect to cardiovascular risk is a systolic reading below 120 mm Hg and a diastolic reading below 80 mm Hg. In general, hypertension is defined as a systolic blood pressure of 140 mm Hg or higher or a diastolic pressure above 90 mm Hg. (For patients with diabetes or chronic kidney disease, hypertension is defined as a reading of 130/80 mm Hg or higher.)

In addition to classifying stages of hypertension based on average blood pressure readings, clinicians should also take note of target organ disease and any additional risk factors. For example, a patient with diabetes, left ventricular hypertrophy, and a blood pressure reading of 144/98 mm Hg would be classified as "stage I hypertension with target-organ disease (left ventricular hypertrophy) and another major risk factor (diabetes)." This additional information is important to obtain a true picture of the patient's cardiovascular health.

CATEGORY	SYSTOLIC		DIASTOLIC
Normal	<120 mm Hg	and	< 80 mm Hg
Pre-hypertension	120 to 139 mm Hg	or	80 to 89 mm Hg
Hypertension			
Stage 1	140 to 159 mm Hg	or	90 to 99 mm Hg
Stage 2	≥160 mm Hg	or	≥ 100 mm Hg

Treatment

The National Institutes of Health recommends the following approach for treating primary hypertension:[3]

▶ First, help the patient initiate necessary lifestyle modifications, including weight reduction, moderation of alcohol intake, regular physical exercise, reduction of sodium intake, and smoking cessation.

▶ If the patient fails to achieve the desired blood pressure or make significant progress, continue lifestyle modifications and begin drug therapy.

▶ For stage 1 hypertension (systolic blood pressure [SBP] 140 to 159 mm Hg, or diastolic blood pressure [DBP] 90 to 99 mm Hg) in the absence of compelling indications (heart failure, postmyocardial infarction, high coronary disease risk, diabetes, chronic kidney disease, or recurrent stroke prevention), give most patients thiazide-type diuretics. Also consider using an angiotensin-converting enzyme (ACE) inhibitor, beta-adrenergic blocker, calcium channel blocker (CCB), angiotensin-receptor blocker (ARB), or a combination.

▶ For stage 2 hypertension (SBP greater than 160 mm Hg, or DBP greater than 100 mm Hg) in the absence of compelling indications, give most patients a two-drug

combination (usually a thiazide-type diuretic and an ACE inhibitor, ARB, CCB, or beta-adrenergic blocker).

▶ If the patient has one or more compelling indications, base drug treatment on benefits from outcome studies or existing clinical guidelines. Treatment may include the following, depending on indication:
– heart failure—diuretic, beta-adrenergic blocker, ACE inhibitor, ARB, or aldosterone antagonist
– high coronary disease risk—diuretic, beta-adrenergic blocker, ACE inhibitor, or CCB
–diabetes—diuretic, beta-adrenergic blocker, ACE inhibitor, or CCB
–chronic kidney disease—ACE inhibitor or ARB
– postmyocardial failure—ACE inhibitor, beta-adrenergic blocker, or aldosterone antagonist
–recurrent stroke prevention—diuretic or ACE inhibitor.

Give other antihypertensive drugs as needed.

▶ If the patient fails to achieve the desired blood pressure, continue lifestyle modifications and optimize drug dosages or add additional drugs until the goal blood pressure is achieved. Also, consider consultation with a hypertension specialist.

Treatment of secondary hypertension focuses on correcting the underlying cause and controlling hypertensive effects.

Typically, hypertensive emergencies require parenteral administration of a vasodilator or an adrenergic inhibitor or oral administration of a selected drug, such as nifedipine, captopril, clonidine, or labetalol, to rapidly reduce blood pressure. The initial goal is to reduce mean arterial blood pressure by no more than 25% (within minutes to hours) then to 160/110 within 2 hours while avoiding excessive drops in blood pressure that can precipitate renal, cerebral, or myocardial ischemia.

Examples of hypertensive emergencies include hypertensive encephalopathy, intracra-nial hemorrhage, acute left-sided heart failure with pulmonary edema, and dissecting aortic aneurysm. Hypertensive emergencies are also associated with eclampsia or severe gestational hypertension, unstable angina, and acute myocardial infarction.

Hypertension without accompanying symptoms or target-organ disease seldom requires emergency drug therapy.

Special considerations

▶ To encourage adherence to antihypertensive therapy, suggest that the patient establish a daily routine for taking his medication. Warn that uncontrolled hypertension may cause stroke, heart attack, and heart failure. Tell him to report adverse drug effects. Also, advise him to avoid high-sodium antacids, NSAIDs, and over-the-counter cold and sinus medications, which contain harmful vasoconstrictors.

▶ Encourage a change in dietary habits. Help the obese patient plan a weight-reduction diet; tell him to avoid high-sodium foods (pickles, potato chips, canned soups, and cold cuts) and table salt.

▶ Help the patient examine and modify his lifestyle (for example, by reducing stress and exercising regularly).

▶ If a patient is hospitalized with hypertension, find out if he was taking his prescribed medication. If he wasn't, ask why. If he can't afford the medication, refer him to appropriate social service agencies. Tell the patient and his family to keep a record of drugs used in the past, noting which ones were effective and which weren't. Suggest recording this information on a card so that the patient can show it to his physician.

▶ When routine blood pressure screening reveals elevated pressure, first make sure the cuff size is appropriate for the patient's upper arm circumference. A narrow cuff may cause a falsely high reading.[2] Take the pressure in both arms in lying, sitting, and standing positions. Ask the patient if he smoked, drank a beverage containing caffeine, or was

emotionally upset before the test. Advise him to return for blood pressure testing at frequent, regular intervals.

▶ Six percent of hypertensive patients have a pressure difference of more than 10 mm Hg between arms, therefore measure blood pressure in both arms at the initial assessment, and in the arm with the higher pressure during subsequent assessments.[4]

▶ To help identify hypertension and prevent untreated hypertension in your patient population, participate in public education programs on hypertension, and explain what can be done to reduce risk factors. Encourage participation in blood pressure screening programs. Routinely screen all patients, especially those at risk (blacks and people with family histories of hypertension, stroke, or heart attack).[5]

REFERENCES

1. American Heart Association (2008 January 25). "High Blood Pressure Statistics" [Online]. Available at *www.americanheart.org/ presenter.jhtml?identifier=4621.*
2. *The Seventh Report of the Joint National Committee on Prevention, Detection, Evaluation, and Treatment of High Blood Pressure.* Bethesda, Md.: U.S. Department of Health and Human Services, National Institutes of Health, National Heart, Lung and Blood Institute, May 2003. Available at *www.nhlbi.nih.gov/guidelines/hypertension/.*
3. Woods, A. "Loosening the Grip of Hypertension," *Nursing* 34(12):36-43, December 2004.
4. Beevers, G., et al. "ABC of Hypertension. Blood Pressure Measurement. Conventional Sphygmomanometry: Technique of Auscultatory Blood Pressure Measurement," *British Medical Journal* 322(7293):1043-47, April 2001.
5. Haskell, W.L. "Cardiovascular Disease Prevention and Lifestyle Interventions: Effectiveness and Efficacy," *Journal of Cardiovascular Nursing* 18(4):245-55, September-October 2003.

HYPERTROPHIC CARDIOMYOPATHY

This primary disease of cardiac muscle, also called idiopathic hypertrophic subaortic stenosis, is characterized by disproportionate, asymmetrical thickening of the interventricular septum, particularly in the left ventricle's free wall. In hypertrophic cardiomyopathy, cardiac output may be low, normal, or high, depending on whether stenosis is obstructive or nonobstructive. If cardiac output is normal or high, the disorder may go undetected for years; but low cardiac output may lead to potentially fatal heart failure. The disease course varies; some patients progressively deteriorate; others remain stable for years.

Causes and incidence

Despite being designated as idiopathic, in almost all cases, hypertrophic cardiomyopathy is inherited as a non–sex-linked autosomal dominant trait.[1] Most patients have obstructive disease, resulting from effects of ventricular septal hypertrophy and the movement of the anterior mitral valve leaflet into the outflow tract during systole. Eventually, left ventricular dysfunction, from rigidity and decreased compliance, causes pump failure.

This disorder affects 1 in 500 people.[2] It affects males and females equally and has been reported in many races.[1] It's also the leading cause of sudden cardiac death in young athletes.[3] Genetic factors are being researched as a possible cause.[4] (See *Hypertrophic cardiomyopathy in athletes,* page 38.)

Signs and symptoms

Clinical features of the disorder may not appear until it's well advanced, when atrial dilation and, possibly, atrial fibrillation abruptly reduce blood flow to the left ventricle. Reduced inflow and subsequent low output may produce angina pectoris, arrhythmias, dyspnea, orthopnea, syncope, heart

Hypertrophic cardiomyopathy in atheletes

Question: *Is hypertrophic cardiomyopathy a common finding in highly-trained atheletes?*

Research: Hypertrophic cardiomyopathy (HCM) causes exercise-related sudden death in young athletes. Researchers conducted studies on 3,500 asymptomatic highly-trained athletes during a 10-year period to determine how frequently the disorder occurs and identify important factors related to screenings performed before participation in the exercise or sport. The athletes studied were between ages 14 and 35, 75% of them were male, and none had a known family history of HCM. Screenings consisted of 12-lead electrocardiograms (ECGs) and 2-dimensional echocardiograms.

Conclusion: Left ventricular hypertrophy was identified in 53 athletes, with 3 of these having a nondilated left ventricular cavity and associated deep T-wave inversion, which could indicate HCM. Resolution of the diagnostic abnormalities was shown in one of the 3 athletes who agreed to stop training for 12 weeks, with an echocardiogram confirming physiologic left ventricular hypertrophy. Researchers concluded that because of the low incidence of athletes

identified with HCM during the study, structural and functional changes associated with the disorder most likely keep those affected by HCM from participation in competitive sports. They also determined that electrocardiography should be used for screening, with echocardiography performed only on those with ECG findings that may indicate pathologic left ventricular hypertrophy.

Application: Although HCM is an uncommon condition, it remains a risk factor for exercise-related sudden death in young athletes. Screening programs for the disorder, performed before participation in sports or extreme exercise programs, should include an ECG, with echocardiography as indicated.

Source: Basavarajaiah, S., et al. "Prevalence of Hypertrophic Cardiomyopathy in Highly Trained Athletes: Relevance to Pre-participation Screening," *Journal of the American College of Cardiology* 51(10):1033-39, March 11, 2008.

---

failure, and death. Auscultation reveals a medium-pitched systolic ejection murmur along the left sternal border and at the apex; palpation reveals a peripheral pulse with a characteristic double impulse (pulsus biferiens) and, with atrial fibrillation, an irregular pulse.

Complications
▶ Pulmonary hypertension
▶ Heart failure
▶ Sudden death from ventricular arrhythmias

Diagnosis
Diagnosis depends on typical clinical findings and these test results:
▶ Echocardiogram (most useful) shows increased thickness of the intra-ventricular septum and abnormal motion of the anterior mitral leaflet during systole, occluding left ventricular outflow in obstructive disease.
▶ Cardiac catheterization reveals elevated left ventricular end-diastolic pressure and, possibly, mitral insufficiency.
▶ Electrocardiography usually shows left ventricular hypertrophy, T-wave inversion, left anterior hemiblock, Q waves in precordial and inferior leads, ventricular arrhythmias and, possibly, atrial fibrillation.

▶ Auscultation confirms an early systolic murmur.

Treatment

The goals of treatment are to relax the ventricle and to relieve outflow tract obstruction. Agents such as propranolol, a beta-adrenergic blocker, slow heart rate and increase ventricular filling by relaxing the obstructing muscle, thereby reducing angina, syncope, dyspnea, and arrhythmias. However, propranolol may aggravate symptoms of cardiac decompensation.

Atrial fibrillation necessitates both cardioversion to treat the arrhythmia and anticoagulant therapy until fibrillation subsides—because of the high risk of systemic embolism.

Vasodilators such as nitroglycerin are contraindicated in patients with hypertrophic cardiomyopathy because they reduce venous return by permitting pooling of blood in the periphery, decreasing ventricular volume and chamber size, so they may cause further obstruction. Also contraindicated are sympathetic stimulators such as isoproterenol, which enhance cardiac contractility and myocardial demands for oxygen, intensifying the obstruction.

Although quinidine is used to suppress ventricular arrhythmia, disopyramide is preferred because of its negative inotropic properties. For patients with potentially lethal arrhythmias, an implantable-cardioverter defibrillator is the most effective treatment to prevent sudden death.[1]

If drug therapy fails, surgery is indicated. Ventricular myotomy (resection of the hypertrophied septum) or ventricular myectomy (removal of the hypertrophied septum) alone—or combined with mitral valve replacement—may ease outflow tract obstruction and relieve symptoms. However, ventricular myotomy may cause complications, such as complete heart block and ventricular septal defect.

Special considerations

▶ Because syncope or sudden death may follow well-tolerated exercise, warn such patients against strenuous physical activity such as running.

▶ Administer medications as prescribed. Caution: Avoid nitroglycerin, digoxin, and diuretics because they can make the obstruction worse. Warn the patient not to stop taking propranolol abruptly, because doing so may increase myocardial demands. To determine the patient's tolerance for an increased dosage of propranolol, take his pulse to check for bradycardia. Also take his blood pressure while he's supine and standing. (A drop in blood pressure of more than 10 mm Hg when standing may indicate orthostatic hypotension.)

▶ Before dental work or surgery, tell the patient to discuss prophylaxis for subacute infective endocarditis with his health care provider.

▶ Provide psychological support. If the patient is hospitalized for a long time, be flexible with visiting hours. Encourage occasional weekends away from the hospital, if possible. Refer the patient for psychosocial counseling to help him and his family accept his restricted lifestyle and poor prognosis.

▶ If the patient is a child, have his parents arrange for him to continue his studies in the health care facility.

▶ Because sudden cardiac arrest is possible, urge the patient's family to learn cardiopulmonary resuscitation.

▶ Discuss screening options for family. Although hypertrophy usually begins in adolescence, it may not begin until middle age. Therefore, you may want to recommend that some relatives be checked for hypertrophic cardiomyopathy with an echocardiogram periodically into adulthood.[1]

REFERENCES

1. Maron, B.J. "Hypertrophic Cardiomyopathy," *Circulation* 106(19):2419-21, November 2002.

2. Cleveland Clinic, Heart and Vascular Institute (2006 May). "Hypertrophic Cardiomyopathy" [Online]. Available at *www.clevelandclinic.org/heartcenter/pub/guide/disease/hcm/default.htm#affected.*

3. Maron, B.J. et al. "Cardiovascular Preparticipation Screening of Competitive Athletes: A Statement for Health Professions from the Sudden Death Committee (Clinical Cardiology) and Congenital Cardiac Defects Committee (Cardiovascular Disease in the Young), American Heart Association," *Circulation* 94(4):850-56, August 1996.

4. Lashey, F.R. "Genetic Testing, Screening, and Counseling Issues in Cardiovascular Disease," *Journal of Cardiovascular Nursing* 13(4):110-26, July 1999.

MYOCARDIAL INFARCTION

Myocardial infarction (MI), more commonly known as a *heart attack*, results from prolonged myocardial ischemia due to reduced blood flow through one of the coronary arteries. It's part of a broader category of disease known as acute coronary syndrome. In cardiovascular disease, the leading cause of death in the United States,[1] death usually results from the cardiac damage or complications of MI. (See *Complications of myocardial infarction.*)

HEALTH & SAFETY *Mortality is high when treatment is delayed; almost one-half of sudden deaths due to an MI occur before hospitalization, within 1 hour of the onset of symptoms. The prognosis improves if vigorous treatment begins immediately.*[1]

Causes and incidence

Predisposing factors include:[2]
- aging
- diabetes mellitus
- elevated serum triglyceride, low-density lipoprotein, and cholesterol levels, and decreased serum high-density lipoprotein levels

- hypertension
- obesity or excessive intake of saturated fats, carbohydrates, or salt
- positive family history of coronary artery disease
- sedentary lifestyle
- smoking
- individual response to stress.

The site of the MI depends on the vessels involved. Occlusion of the circumflex branch of the left coronary artery causes a lateral wall infarction; occlusion of the anterior descending branch of the left coronary artery, an anterior wall infarction. True posterior or inferior wall infarctions generally result from occlusion of the right coronary artery or one of its branches. Right ventricular infarctions can also result from right coronary artery occlusion, can accompany inferior infarctions, and may cause right-sided heart failure.

Incidence is high: It's estimated that there are 565,000 new heart attacks and 300,000 recurrent heart attacks each year.[1] Males and postmenopausal females are more susceptible to MI than premenopausal females, although incidence is rising among females, especially those who smoke and take hormonal contraceptives. Females account for nearly one-half of deaths from heart attacks.[3] The average age of females having their first MI is 70.4; the average age for males is 65.8.[1]

Signs and symptoms

The cardinal symptom of MI is persistent, crushing substernal pain that may radiate to the left arm, jaw, neck, or shoulder blades. Such pain is usually described as heavy, squeezing, or crushing, and may persist for 12 hours or more. However, in some MI patients—particularly elderly people or those with diabetes—pain may not occur at all; in others, it may be mild and confused with indigestion. In females, pain or discomfort may be in the center of the chest or other areas of the upper body including arms, back,

Complications of myocardial infarction

COMPLICATION	DIAGNOSIS	TREATMENT
Arrhythmias	• Electrocardiogram (ECG) shows premature ventricular contractions, ventricular tachycardia, or ventricular fibrillation; in inferior wall myocardial infarction (MI), bradycardia and junctional rhythms or atrioventricular block; in anterior wall MI, tachycardia or heart block.	• Antiarrhythmics, atropine, and pacemaker; cardioversion for tachycardia
Heart failure	• In left-sided heart failure, chest X-rays show venous congestion, cardiomegaly, and Kerley's B lines. • Catheterization shows increased pulmonary artery pressure (PAP) and central venous pressure.	• Diuretics, angiotensin-converting enzyme inhibitors, vasodilators, inotropic agents, cardiac glycosides, and beta-adrenergic blockers
Cardiogenic shock	• Catheterization shows decreased cardiac output and increased PAP and pulmonary artery wedge pressure (PAWP). • Signs include hypertension, tachycardia, S_3, S_4, decreased levels of consciousness, decreased urine output, jugular vein distention, and cool, pale skin.	• I.V. fluids, vasodilators, diuretics, cardiac glycosides, intra-aortic balloon pump (IABP), and beta-adrenergic stimulants
Rupture of left ventricular papillary muscle	• Auscultation reveals an apical holosystolic murmur. Inspection of jugular vein pulse or hemodynamic monitoring shows increased v waves. • Dyspnea is prominent. • Color-flow and Doppler ECG show mitral insufficiency. Pulmonary artery catheterization shows increased PAP and PAWP.	• Nitroprusside • IABP • Surgical replacement of the mitral valve with possible concomitant myocardial revascularization (in patients with significant coronary artery disease)
Ventricular septal rupture	• In left-to-right shunt, auscultation reveals a holosystolic murmur and thrill. • Catheterization shows increased PAP and PAWP. • Confirmation by increased oxygen saturation of the right ventricle and pulmonary artery.	• Surgical correction, IABP, nitroglycerin, nitroprusside, low-dose inotropic agents, or pacemaker
Pericarditis or Dressler's syndrome	• Auscultation reveals a friction rub. • Chest pain is relieved by sitting up.	• Aspirin
Ventricular aneurysm	• Chest X-ray may show cardiomegaly. • ECG may show arrhythmias and persistent ST-segment elevation. • Left ventriculography shows altered or paradoxical left ventricular motion.	• Cardioversion, defibrillation, antiarrhythmics, vasodilators, anticoagulants, cardiac glycosides, and diuretics (If conservative treatment fails, surgical resection is necessary.)
Thromboembolism	• Patient may have severe dyspnea and chest pain or neurologic changes. • Nuclear scan shows ventilation-perfusion mismatch. • Angiography shows arterial blockage.	• Oxygen and heparin

Thrombus formation after stenting

Question: *Is left ventricular thrombus formation a common complication in patients with acute MI treated with stenting?*

Research: The current treatment of choice in patients with acute myocardial infarction (MI) is primary percutaneous coronary intervention (PCI) with stenting. The study was conducted to determine the incidence of left ventricular thrombus formation after the procedure. To form their conclusions, the researchers performed a retrospective study of 2,911 patients who met the diagnostic criteria and had undergone successful PCI with stenting. Left ventricular thrombi were diagnosed by echocardiography, performed between 3 and 5 days after the procedure. Patient characteristics that might predict thrombus formation were also analyzed.

Conclusion: The study identified 73 patients (2.5%) who met the criteria and developed left ventricular thrombi after the procedure, identifying this as a low-incidence complication. Predictive factors for thrombus formation, such as age, diabetes mellitus, prior MI, coronary artery disease, and hyperlipidemia, in addition to antiplatelet treatment, were similar in those with thrombus formation and those without. Further analysis of their results showed that the location (anterior MI) and size of the myocardial damage, an ejection fraction less than 40%, and

previous hypertension were factors that were strongly associated with thrombus formation after successful stenting.

Application: It's essential for the nurse to be aware of the possible complications associated with PCI with stenting, including thrombus formation, bleeding, inflammatory reactions, restenosis, and endothelial dysfunction. A patient who has had PCI with stenting is commonly discharged home within 1 or 2 days of the procedure. If complications develop, the patient may present at his doctor's office or the emergency room with initially vague symptoms that appear to be unrelated to the PCI. Although this study indicates that left ventricular thrombi are uncommon, the nurse should consider this complication a possibility in any patient who has had PCI with stenting.

Source: Zielinska, M., et al. "Predictors of Left Ventricular Thrombus Formation in Acute Myocardial Infarction Treated with Successful Primary Angioplasty with Stenting," *American Journal of Medical Sciences* 335(3):171-76, March 2008.

---

neck, jaw, or stomach.[3] In patients with coronary artery disease, angina of increasing frequency, severity, or duration (especially if not provoked by exertion, a heavy meal, or cold and wind) may signal impending infarction.

Other clinical effects include a feeling of impending doom, fatigue, nausea, vomiting, and shortness of breath. Females are more likely than males to feel these effects.[3] Some patients may have no symptoms. The patient may experience catecholamine responses, such as coolness in extremities, perspiration, anxiety, and restlessness. Fever is unusual at the onset of an MI, but a low-grade temper-

ature elevation may develop during the next few days. Blood pressure varies; hypotension or hypertension may be present.

Also, it has been found that most females have prodromal symptoms including unusual fatigue, sleep disturbance, shortness of breath, indigestion, and anxiety.[4]

Complications
▶ Recurrent or persistent chest pain, arrhythmias
▶ Left-sided heart failure (resulting in heart failure or acute pulmonary edema)
▶ Cardiogenic shock

▶ Thromboembolism (See *Thrombus formation after stenting.*)
▶ Papillary muscle dysfunction or rupture, causing mitral insufficiency
▶ Rupture of the ventricular septum, causing ventricular septal defect
▶ Rupture of the myocardium
▶ Ventricular aneurysm
▶ Up to several months after infarction, Dressler's syndrome is possible; symptoms include pericarditis, pericardial friction rub, chest pain, fever, leukocytosis and, possibly, pleurisy or pneumonitis

Diagnosis

Troponin I is used to definitively diagnose MI because it's specific to cardiac necrosis. Levels can be found in serum 3 to 6 hours after onset of chest pain; they remain elevated for 14 days.[5] Persistent chest pain, elevated ST segment on electrocardiogram (ECG), and elevated total creatine kinase (CK) and CK-MB levels over a 72-hour period also help confirm MI.

Auscultation may reveal diminished heart sounds, gallops and, in papillary dysfunction, the apical systolic murmur of mitral insufficiency over the mitral valve area.

When clinical features are equivocal, assume that the patient had an MI until tests rule it out. Diagnostic laboratory results include:
▶ serial 12-lead ECG—ECG abnormalities may be absent or inconclusive during the first few hours after an MI. When present, characteristic abnormalities include serial ST-segment depression in subendocardial MI and ST-segment elevation in transmural MI.
▶ serial serum enzyme levels—CK levels, specifically, levels of the CK-MB isoenzyme, are elevated.
▶ echocardiography—may show ventricular wall motion abnormalities in patients with a transmural MI.
▶ nuclear ventriculography scans (multiple-gated acquisition or radionuclide ventriculography)—using I.V. radioactive substance, can identify acutely damaged muscle by picking up radioactive nucleotide, which appears as a "hot spot" on the film; useful in localizing a recent MI.

Treatment

The goals of treatment are to relieve chest pain, stabilize heart rhythm, reduce cardiac workload, revascularize the coronary artery, and preserve myocardial tissue. Arrhythmias, the predominant problem during the first 48 hours after the infarction, may require antiarrhythmics, possibly a pacemaker and, rarely, cardioversion. Arrhythmias are best detected using a 12-lead ECG.

To preserve myocardial tissue in ST elevation MI, thrombolytic therapy should be started via I.V. within 30 minutes of arrival in the emergency department, if not contraindicated.[6] Thrombolytic therapy includes a choice of streptokinase, alteplase, urokinase, tenecteplase, or reteplase. (*See Comparing thrombolytics, page 44.*)

Primary percutaneous transluminal coronary angioplasty is a Class I recommendation for an alternative to thrombolytic therapy, but only if performed in a timely manner in high-volume centers by physicians skilled in the procedure and supported by experienced personnel.

Other treatments to consider include:
▶ lidocaine, vasopressin, or amiodarone for ventricular arrhythmias; or other drugs, such as procainamide, quinidine, or disopyramide
▶ antiplatelet therapy with glycoprotein IIb-IIIa inhibitors, such as ticlopidine and clopidogrel for non-ST-elevation MI
▶ atropine I.V. or a temporary pacemaker for heart block or bradycardia
▶ nitroglycerin (sublingual, topical, transdermal, or I.V.); calcium channel blockers, such as nifedipine, verapamil, or diltiazem (sublingual, oral, or I.V.); or isosorbide dinitrate (sublingual, oral, or I.V.) to relieve pain by redistributing blood to ischemic areas of the myocardium, increasing cardiac output, and reducing myocardial workload

Comparing thrombolytics

If your patient has suffered a myocardial infarction (MI), you must intervene promptly to minimize cardiac damage and avert death. If appropriate, prepare the patient for thrombolytic therapy as ordered.

Thrombolytic drugs enhance the body's natural ability to dispose of blood clots. To lyse (dissolve) fibrin—the essential component of a clot—tissue activators convert plasminogen to plasmin. A nonspecific protease, plasmin degrades fibrin, fibrinogen, and procoagulant factors (such as factors V, VII, and XII).

Candidates for thrombolytic therapy include patients with acute ST-segment elevation and chest pain that has lasted no more than 6 hours. Timely use of thrombolytic agents can restore myocardial perfusion and prevent further injury. When effective, thrombolytic agents relieve chest pain, restore the ST segment to baseline, and induce reperfusion arrhythmias within 30 to 45 minutes.

Contraindications to thrombolytic therapy include surgery within the past 2 months, active bleeding, history of stroke, intracranial neoplasm, arteriovenous malformation, aneurysm, or uncontrolled hypertension.

Here's how selected thrombolytics open occluded coronary arteries in patients with an acute MI.

ALTEPLASE

Alteplase is a naturally occurring enzyme that has been cloned and produced as a drug, alteplase (tissue plasminogen activator). Binding to plasminogen, it catalyzes the conversion of plasminogen to plasmin in the presence of fibrin. Because of its strong affinity for fibrin, alteplase concentrates at the clot site, resulting in a minimal decrease in the fibrinogen level.

This thrombolytic has a half-life of 5 minutes, so maintaining coronary artery patency depends on continued anticoagulation with heparin. Alteplase doesn't induce antigenic responses; doses may be repeated at any time.

RETEPLASE

Reteplase, recombinant plasminogen activator, has a half-life of 13 to 16 minutes. Its longer half-life allows it to be administered as a bolus. Two boluses are required.

ANISTREPLASE

Anistreplase is a partially synthetic thrombolytic drug that's composed of a complex of streptokinase bound to human plasminogen.

This complex binds to fibrin and promotes plasminogen conversion to plasmin. But the dose needed to lyse coronary artery clots can cause systemic clot lysis, characterized by fibrinogen depletion. This results in bleeding complications.

Anistreplase has the longest half-life (90 minutes). Because it's partially composed of streptokinase, a foreign protein, anistreplase is antigenic and may cause an allergic reaction. The per-dose cost is less than that for alteplase.

This drug's main advantage is ease of administration: Only a single bolus is required.

STREPTOKINASE

Streptokinase, a thrombolytic, is a bacterial protein that binds to circulating plasminogen and catalyzes plasmin formation. Its low specificity for fibrin induces a systemic lytic state and increases the risk of bleeding.

The half-life is approximately 20 minutes. Like anistreplase, streptokinase is antigenic.

TENECTEPLASE

Tenecteplase is a modified form of human tissue plasminogen activator that binds to fibrin and converts plasminogen to plasmin. It's given as a single bolus dose.

UROKINASE

Naturally produced by the human kidney, urokinase promotes thrombolysis by directly activating the conversion of plasminogen to plasmin.

With a serum half-life of 10 to 20 minutes, urokinase is rapidly cleared by the kidneys and liver. Unlike anistreplase and streptokinase, it doesn't induce an antigenic response. Urokinase isn't given through a peripheral I.V. line to treat an acute MI, but patients who undergo cardiac catheterization may receive it directly in a coronary artery.

▶ heparin I.V. (usually follows thrombolytic therapy)
▶ morphine I.V. for pain and sedation
▶ bed rest with bedside commode to decrease cardiac workload
▶ oxygen administration at a modest flow rate for 2 to 3 hours (a lower concentration is necessary if the patient has chronic obstructive pulmonary disease)
▶ angiotensin-converting enzyme inhibitors for patients with large anterior wall MIs and for those with an MI and a left ventricular ejection fraction less than 40%
▶ drugs to increase myocardial contractility or blood pressure
▶ beta-adrenergic blockers, such as propranolol or atenolol, after acute MI to help prevent reinfarction by reducing the heart's workload
▶ aspirin to inhibit platelet aggregation (initiated immediately and continued for years)
▶ pulmonary artery catheterization to detect left- or right-sided heart failure and to monitor the patient's response to treatment.

Special considerations

Care for patients who have suffered an MI is directed toward detecting complications, preventing further myocardial damage, and promoting comfort, rest, and emotional well-being. Most MI patients receive treatment in the intensive care unit (ICU), where they're under constant observation for complications.
▶ When the patient is first admitted to the ICU, monitor and record his ECG, blood pressure, temperature, and heart and breath sounds.
▶ Assess and record the severity and duration of the patient's pain, and administer analgesics. Avoid I.M. injections; absorption from the muscle is unpredictable and bleeding is likely if the patient is receiving thrombolytic therapy.
▶ Check the patient's blood pressure after giving nitroglycerin, especially the first dose.

▶ Frequently monitor the ECG to detect rate changes or arrhythmias. Place rhythm strips in the patient's chart periodically for evaluation.
▶ During episodes of chest pain, obtain 12-lead ECG (before and after nitroglycerin therapy as well), blood pressure, and pulmonary artery catheter measurements, and monitor them for changes.
▶ Watch for signs and symptoms of fluid retention (crackles, cough, tachypnea, and edema), which may indicate impending heart failure. Carefully monitor daily weight, intake and output, respirations, serum enzyme levels, and blood pressure. Auscultate for S_3 or S_4 gallops, new-onset heart murmurs, and adventitious breath sounds periodically (patients on bed rest frequently have atelectatic crackles, which disappear after coughing).
▶ Organize patient care and activities to maximize periods of uninterrupted rest.
▶ Initiate a cardiac rehabilitation program. This usually includes education regarding heart disease, exercise, and emotional support for the patient and his family.
▶ Ask the dietary department to provide a clear liquid diet until nausea subsides. A low-cholesterol, low-sodium, low-fat, high-fiber diet may be prescribed.
▶ Provide a stool softener to prevent straining during defecation, which causes vagal stimulation and may slow the heart rate. Allow use of a bedside commode, and provide as much privacy as possible.
▶ Assist with range-of-motion exercises. If the patient is completely immobilized by a severe MI, turn him often. Antiembolism stockings help prevent venostasis and thrombophlebitis.
▶ Provide emotional support and help reduce stress and anxiety; administer tranquilizers as needed. Explain procedures and answer questions. Explaining the ICU environment and routine can ease anxiety. Involve the patient's family in his care as much as possible.

To prepare the patient for discharge:

▶ Thoroughly explain dosages and therapy to promote compliance with the prescribed medication regimen and other treatment measures. Warn about adverse drug effects, and advise the patient to watch for and report signs of toxicity (anorexia, nausea, vomiting, and yellow vision, for example, if the patient is receiving digoxin).

▶ Review dietary restrictions with the patient. If he must follow a low-sodium or low-fat and low-cholesterol diet, provide a list of foods that he should avoid. Ask the dietitian to speak to the patient and his family.[7]

▶ Counsel the patient to resume sexual activity progressively.

▶ Advise the patient to report typical or atypical chest pain. Postinfarction syndrome may develop, producing chest pain that must be differentiated from recurrent MI, pulmonary infarct, or heart failure.

▶ If the patient has a Holter monitor in place, explain its purpose and use.

▶ Stress the need to stop smoking.

▶ Encourage participation in a cardiac rehabilitation program.

▶ Review follow-up procedures, such as office visits and treadmill testing, with the patient.

REFERENCES

1. American Heart Association. "2005 American Heart Association Guidelines for Cardiopulmonary Resuscitation and Emergency Cardiovascular Care: International Consensus on Science," *Circulation* 112(22Suppl):IV-1-IV-221, November 2005.
2. American Heart Association (2006 December 28). "Heart Disease and Stroke Statistics-2007 Update" [Online]. Available at *http://circ.ahajournals.org/cgi/content/full/CIRCULATIONAHA.106.179918.*
3. American Heart Association (2008 January 25). "Risk Factors and Coronary Heart Disease, AHA Scientific Position" [Online]. Available at *www.americanheart.org/presenter.jhtml?identifier=4726.*
4. National Heart, Lung, and Blood Institute. "Women and Heart Attack" [Online]. Available at *www.nhlbi.nih.gov/actintime/haws/women.htm.*
5. McSweeney, J.C., et al. "Women's Early Warning Symptoms of Acute Myocardial Infarction," *Circulation* 108(21):2619-23, November 2003.
6. Fenton, D.E. eMedicine from Web MD (2007 September 10). "Myocardial Infarction" [Online]. Available at *www.emedicine.com/emerg/topic327.htm.*
7. Menon, V., et al. "Thrombolysis and Adjunctive Therapy in Acute Myocardial Infarction: The Seventh ACCP Conference on Antithrombotic and Thrombolytic Therapy," *Chest* 126 (3Suppl):549S-75S, September 2004.
8. Cobb, S.L., et al. "Effective interventions for Lifestyle Change after Myocardial Infarction or Coronary Artery Revascularization," *Journal of the American Academy of Nurse Practitioners* 18(1):31-39, January 2006.

MYOCARDITIS

Myocarditis is focal or diffuse inflammation of the cardiac muscle (myocardium). It may be acute or chronic and can occur at any age. In many cases, myocarditis fails to produce specific cardiovascular symptoms or electrocardiogram (ECG) abnormalities, and recovery is usually spontaneous, without residual defects. Occasionally, myocarditis is complicated by heart failure; in rare cases, it leads to cardiomyopathy.

Causes and incidence

Myocarditis may result from:

▶ bacterial infections—diphtheria; tuberculosis; typhoid fever; tetanus; and staphylococcal, pneumococcal, and gonococcal infections

▶ chemical poisons—such as chronic alcoholism

▶ helminthic infections—such as trichinosis

▶ hypersensitive immune reactions—acute rheumatic fever and postcardiotomy syndrome

▶ parasitic infections—especially South American trypanosomiasis (Chagas' disease) in infants and immunosuppressed adults; also toxoplasmosis

▶ radiation therapy—large doses of radiation to the chest in treating lung or breast cancer

▶ viral infections (most common cause in the United States and western Europe)—coxsackievirus A and B strains and, possibly, poliomyelitis, influenza, rubeola, rubella, and adenoviruses and echoviruses

▶ human immunodeficiency virus.[1]

Myocarditis occurs in 1 to 10 of every 100,000 people in the United States. The average age for this disorder is 42, and incidence is 1.5 to 1 between males and females.[2] Children, especially neonates, and persons who are immunocompromised or pregnant (especially pregnant black women) are at higher risk for developing this disorder.

Up to 20% of sudden death in young adults may be due to myocarditis.[3]

Signs and symptoms

Myocarditis usually causes nonspecific symptoms—such as fatigue, dyspnea, palpitations, and fever—that reflect the accompanying systemic infection. Occasionally, it may produce mild, continuous pressure or soreness in the chest (unlike the recurring, stress-related pain of angina pectoris). Although myocarditis is usually self-limiting, it may induce myofibril degeneration that results in right- and left-sided heart failure, with cardiomegaly, jugular vein distention, dyspnea, persistent fever with resting or exertional tachycardia disproportionate to the degree of fever, and supraventricular and ventricular arrhythmias. Sometimes myocarditis recurs or produces chronic valvulitis (when it results from rheumatic fever), cardiomyopathy, arrhythmias, and thromboembolism.

Complications

▶ Arrhythmia
▶ Thromboembolism
▶ Valvulitis (when disease results from rheumatic fever)
▶ Recurrence of disease
▶ Left-sided heart failure (occasional)
▶ Cardiomyopathy (rare)

Diagnosis

Patient history commonly reveals recent febrile upper respiratory tract infection, viral pharyngitis, or tonsillitis. Physical examination shows supraventricular and ventricular arrhythmias, S_3 and S_4 gallops, a faint S_1, possibly a murmur of mitral insufficiency (from papillary muscle dysfunction) and, if pericarditis is present, a pericardial friction rub.

Laboratory tests can't unequivocally confirm myocarditis, but the following findings support this diagnosis:

▶ cardiac enzymes—elevated creatine kinase (CK), CK-MB, aspartate aminotransferase, and lactate dehydrogenase levels

▶ troponin T and troponin I (can show myocardial cell damage)[4]

▶ increased white blood cell count and erythrocyte sedimentation rate

▶ elevated antibody titers (such as antistreptolysin-O titer in rheumatic fever).

Endomyocardial biopsy is rarely performed to diagnose myocarditis; the procedure is invasive and costly. A negative biopsy doesn't exclude the diagnosis, and a repeat biopsy may be needed.

ECG typically shows diffuse ST-segment and T-wave abnormalities as in pericarditis, conduction defects (prolonged PR interval), and other supraventricular arrhythmias. Echocardiography demonstrates some degree of left ventricular dysfunction, and radionuclide scanning may identify inflammatory

and necrotic changes characteristic of myocarditis.

Stool and throat cultures may identify bacteria.

Treatment

Treatment includes antibiotics for bacterial infection, modified bed rest to decrease heart workload, and careful management of complications. Inotropic support of cardiac function with amrinone, dopamine, or dobutamine may be needed. Heart failure requires restriction of activity to minimize myocardial oxygen consumption, supplemental oxygen therapy, sodium restriction, diuretics to decrease fluid retention, and cardiac glycosides to increase myocardial contractility. However, cardiac glycosides should be administered cautiously because some patients with myocarditis may show a paradoxical sensitivity to even small doses. Arrhythmias necessitate prompt but cautious administration of antiarrhythmics because these drugs depress myocardial contractility.

Thromboembolism requires anticoagulation therapy. Treatment with corticosteroids or other immunosuppressants may be used to reduce inflammation, but they haven't been shown to change the progression of myocarditis infections. Nonsteroidal antiinflammatory drugs are contraindicated during the acute phase (first 2 weeks) because they increase myocardial damage.

Surgical treatment may include left ventricular assistive devices and extra corporeal membrane oxygenation for support of cardiogenic shock. Cardiac transplantation has been beneficial for giant cell myocarditis.

Special considerations

▶ Assess cardiovascular status frequently, watching for signs of heart failure, such as dyspnea, hypotension, and tachycardia. Check for changes in cardiac rhythm or conduction.
▶ Observe for signs of digoxin toxicity (anorexia, nausea, vomiting, blurred vision,

and cardiac arrhythmias) and for complicating factors that may potentiate toxicity, such as electrolyte imbalance or hypoxia.
▶ Stress the importance of bed rest. Assist with bathing, as necessary; provide a bedside commode because this stresses the heart less than using a bedpan. Reassure the patient that activity limitations are temporary. Offer diversional activities that are physically undemanding.
▶ During recovery, recommend that the patient resume normal activities slowly and avoid competitive sports.

REFERENCES

1. Mayoclinic.com (2006 March 15). "Myocarditis" [Online]. Available at *www.mayoclinic.com/health/myocarditis/ DS00521/DESECTION=3.*
2. Howes, D.S., and Booker E.A. eMedicine from WebMD (2005 April 14). "Myocarditis" [Online]. Available at *www.emedicine. com/emerg/topic.326htm.*
3. Myocarditis Foundation (2007). "About Myocarditis" [Online]. Available at *http:// myocarditisfoundation.org/ aboutMyocarditis.htm.*
4. Feldman, A.M., and McNamara, D. "Myocarditis," *New England Journal of Medicine* 343(19):1388-98, November 2000.

PERICARDITIS

Pericarditis is an inflammation of the pericardium, the fibroserous sac that envelops, supports, and protects the heart. It occurs in both acute and chronic forms. Acute pericarditis can be fibrinous or effusive, with purulent serous or hemorrhagic exudate; chronic constrictive pericarditis is characterized by dense fibrous pericardial thickening. (See *Understanding pericarditis.*)

The prognosis depends on the underlying cause but is generally good in acute pericarditis, unless constriction occurs.

Understanding pericarditis

Pericarditis occurs when a pathogen or other substance attacks the pericardium, leading to the following events:

INFLAMMATION

Pericardial tissue damaged by bacteria or other substances releases chemical mediators of inflammation (such as prostaglandins, histamines, bradykinins, and serotonins) into the surrounding tissue, starting the inflammatory process. Friction occurs as the inflamed pericardial layers rub against each other.

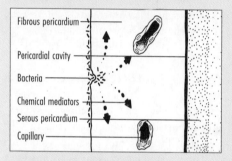

VASODILATION AND CLOTTING

Histamines and other chemical mediators cause vasodilation and increased vessel permeability. Local blood flow (hyperemia) increases. Vessel walls leak fluids and proteins (including fibrinogen) into tissues, causing extracellular edema. Clots of fibrinogen and tissue fluid form a wall, blocking tissue spaces and lymph vessels in the injured area. This wall prevents the spread of bacteria and toxins to adjoining healthy tissues.

INITIAL PHAGOCYTOSIS

Macrophages already present in the tissues begin to phagocytize the invading bacteria but usually fail to stop the infection.

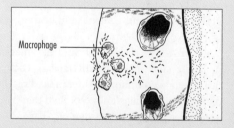

ENHANCED PHAGOCYTOSIS

Substances released by the injured tissue stimulate neutrophil production in the bone marrow. Neutrophils then travel to the injury site through the bloodstream and join macrophages in destroying pathogens. Meanwhile, additional macrophages and monocytes migrate to the injured area and continue phagocytosis.

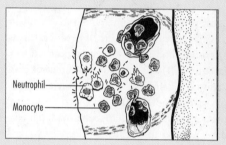

EXUDATION

After several days, the infected area fills with an exudate composed of necrotic tissue and dead and dying bacteria, neutrophils, and macrophages. This exudate, which is thinner than pus, forms until all infection ceases, creating a cavity that remains until tissue destruction stops. The contents of the cavity autolyze and are gradually reabsorbed into healthy tissue.

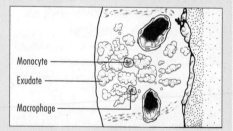

FIBROSIS AND SCARRING

As the end products of the infection slowly disappear, fibrosis and scar tissue may form. Scarring, which can be extensive, can ultimately cause heart failure if it restricts movement.

Causes and incidence

In up to 50% of patients, the cause of pericarditis is unknown.[1]

Common causes of this disease include:
▶ bacterial, fungal, or viral infection (infectious pericarditis)
▶ neoplasms (primary or metastatic from lungs, breasts, or other organs)
▶ high-dose radiation to the chest
▶ uremia
▶ hypersensitivity or autoimmune disease, such as acute rheumatic fever (most common cause of pericarditis in children), systemic lupus erythematosus, and rheumatoid arthritis
▶ postcardiac injury from a myocardial infarction (MI) can cause an autoimmune reaction (Dressler's syndrome) in the pericardium several months after an MI or an early form of pericarditis that occurs within a few days in 10 to 15% of MIs[2]
▶ trauma; or surgery that leaves the pericardium intact but causes blood to leak into the pericardial cavity
▶ drugs, such as hydralazine or procainamide
▶ idiopathic factors (most common in acute pericarditis).

Less common causes include aortic aneurysm with pericardial leakage, and myxedema with cholesterol deposits in the pericardium.

Pericarditis most commonly affects males ages 20 to 50, but it can also occur in children following infection with an adenovirus or coxsackievirus.

Signs and symptoms

Acute pericarditis typically produces a sharp and often sudden pain that usually starts over the sternum and radiates to the neck, shoulders, back, and arms. However, unlike the pain of MI, pericardial pain is often pleuritic, increasing with deep inspiration and decreasing when the patient sits up and leans forward, pulling the heart away from the diaphragmatic pleurae of the lungs.

Complications

▶ Pericardial effusion may produce effects of heart failure (such as dyspnea, orthopnea, and tachycardia), ill-defined substernal chest pain, and a feeling of fullness in the chest. (See *Patterns of cardiac pain*.)
▶ Cardiac tamponade may occur, resulting in pallor, clammy skin, hypotension, pulsus paradoxus (a decrease in systolic blood pressure of 15 mm Hg or more during slow inspiration), jugular vein distention and, eventually, cardiovascular collapse and death.
▶ Chronic constrictive pericarditis causes a gradual increase in systemic venous pressure and produces symptoms similar to those of chronic right-sided heart failure (fluid retention, ascites, and hepatomegaly).

Diagnosis

Because pericarditis commonly coexists with other conditions, diagnosis of acute pericarditis depends on typical clinical features and elimination of other possible causes. The pericardial friction rub, a classic symptom, is a grating sound heard as the heart moves. It can usually be auscultated best during forced expiration, while the patient leans forward or is on his hands and knees in bed. It may have up to three components, corresponding to the timing of atrial systole, ventricular systole, and the rapid-filling phase of ventricular diastole. Occasionally, this friction rub is heard only briefly or not at all. Nevertheless, its presence, together with other characteristic features, is diagnostic of acute pericarditis. In addition, if acute pericarditis has caused very large pericardial effusions, physical examination reveals increased cardiac dullness and diminished or absent apical impulse and distant heart sounds.[2]

Chest X-ray, echocardiogram, chest magnetic resonance imaging (MRI), heart MRI, heart computed tomography scan, and radionuclide scanning can detect fluid that has accumulated in the pericardial sac. They may also show enlargement of the heart and

Patterns of cardiac pain

PERICARDITIS

Onset and duration
- Sudden onset; continuous pain lasting for days; residual soreness

Location and radiation
- Substernal pain to left of midline; radiation to back or subclavicular area

Quality and intensity
- Mild ache to severe pain, deep or superficial; "stabbing," "knifelike"

Signs and symptoms
- Precordial friction rub; increased pain with movement, inspiration, laughing, coughing; decreased pain with sitting or leaning forward (sitting up pulls heart away from diaphragm)

Precipitating factors
- Myocardial infarction or upper respiratory tract infection; invasive cardiac trauma

ANGINA

Onset and duration
- Gradual or sudden onset; pain usually lasts less than 15 minutes and not more than 30 minutes (average: 3 minutes)

Location and radiation
- Substernal or anterior chest pain, not sharply localized; radiation to back, neck, arms, jaws, even upper abdomen or fingers

Quality and intensity
- Mild-to-moderate pressure; deep sensation; varied pattern of attacks; "tightness," "squeezing," "crushing," "pressure"

Signs and symptoms
- Dyspnea, diaphoresis, nausea, desire to void, belching, apprehension

Precipitating factors
- Exertion, stress, eating, cold or hot and humid weather

MYOCARDIAL INFARCTION

Onset and duration
- Sudden onset; pain lasts 30 minutes to 2 hours; waxes and wanes; residual soreness 1 to 3 days

Location and radiation
- Substernal, midline, or anterior chest pain; radiation to jaws, neck, back, shoulders, or one or both arms

Quality and intensity
- Persistent, severe pressure; deep sensation; "crushing," "squeezing," "heavy," "oppressive"

Signs and symptoms
- Nausea, vomiting, apprehension, dyspnea, diaphoresis, increased or decreased blood pressure; gallop heart sound, "sensation of impending doom"

Precipitating factors
- Occurrence at rest or during physical exertion or emotional stress

signs of inflammation or scarring, depending on the cause of pericarditis.

In patients with chronic pericarditis, acute inflammation or effusions don't occur—only restricted cardiac filling.

Laboratory results reflect inflammation and may identify its cause, which may be:
▶ normal or elevated white blood cell count, especially in infectious pericarditis.
▶ elevated erythrocyte sedimentation rate, C-reactive protein, and leukocyte count.[2]
▶ slightly elevated cardiac enzyme levels with associated myocarditis.

▶ culture of pericardial fluid obtained by open surgical drainage or cardiocentesis (sometimes identifies a causative organism in bacterial or fungal pericarditis).
▶ electrocardiography showing the following changes in acute pericarditis: elevation of ST segments in the standard limb leads and most precordial leads without significant changes in QRS morphology that occur with MI, atrial ectopic rhythms such as atrial fibrillation and, in pericardial effusion, diminished QRS voltage. Electrocardiograms are

abnormal in 90% of patients with pericarditis.[2]

Other pertinent laboratory data include blood urea nitrogen levels to check for uremia, antistreptolysin-O titers to detect rheumatic fever, and a purified protein derivative skin test to check for tuberculosis. In pericardial effusion, echocardiography is diagnostic when it shows an echo-free space between the ventricular wall and the pericardium.

Treatment

The goal of treatment is to relieve symptoms and manage the underlying systemic disease. In acute idiopathic pericarditis and postthoracotomy pericarditis, treatment consists of bed rest as long as fever and pain persist, and nonsteroidal drugs, such as aspirin and indomethacin, to relieve pain and reduce inflammation.[3] Post-MI patients should avoid nonsteroidal anti-inflammatory drugs (NSAIDs) and steroids because they may interfere with myocardial scar formation. If these drugs fail to relieve symptoms, corticosteroids may be used. Although corticosteroids produce rapid and effective relief, they should be used only in patients who don't respond to NSAID therapy.[3]

Infectious pericarditis that results from disease of the left pleural space, mediastinal abscesses, or septicemia requires antibiotics (possibly by direct pericardial injection), surgical drainage, or both. Cardiac tamponade may require pericardiocentesis. Signs of tamponade include pulsus paradoxus, jugular vein distention, dyspnea, and shock.

Recurrent pericarditis may necessitate partial pericardectomy, which creates a "window" that allows fluid to drain into the pleural space. In constrictive pericarditis, total pericardectomy to permit adequate filling and contraction of the heart may be necessary. Treatment must also include management of rheumatic fever, uremia, tuberculosis, and other underlying disorders.

Special considerations

A patient with pericarditis needs complete bed rest. In addition, health care includes:
▶ assessing pain in relation to respiration and body position to distinguish pericardial pain from myocardial ischemic pain
▶ placing the patient in an upright position to relieve dyspnea and chest pain; providing analgesics and oxygen; and reassuring the patient with acute pericarditis that his condition is temporary and treatable
▶ monitoring for signs of cardiac compression or cardiac tamponade, possible complications of pericardial effusion (Signs include decreased blood pressure, increased central venous pressure, and pulsus paradoxus. Because cardiac tamponade requires immediate treatment, keep a pericardiocentesis set handy whenever pericardial effusion is suspected.)
▶ explaining tests and treatments to the patient. If surgery is necessary, he should learn deep-breathing and coughing exercises beforehand. Postoperative care is similar to that given after cardiothoracic surgery.

REFERENCES
1. Holcomb, S.S. "Recognizing and Managing Pericarditis," *Nursing* 34(3):32cc1-32cc5, March 2004.
2. Humphreys, M. "Pericardial Conditions: Signs, Symptoms, and Electrocardiogram Changes," *Emergency Nurse* 14(1):30-36, April 2006.
3. Ross, A.M., and Grauer, S.E. "Acute Pericarditis," *Postgraduate Medicine* 115(3):67-74, March 2004.

RHEUMATIC FEVER AND RHEUMATIC HEART DISEASE

Acute rheumatic fever is a systemic—and in many case, recurrent—inflammatory disease of childhood, that follows a group A beta-hemolytic streptococcal infection. Rheumatic heart disease refers to the cardiac manifestations of rheu-

matic fever and includes pancarditis (myocarditis, pericarditis, and endocarditis) during the early acute phase and chronic valvular disease later. Long-term antibiotic therapy can minimize the recurrence of rheumatic fever, reducing the risk of permanent cardiac damage and eventual valvular deformity. However, severe pancarditis occasionally produces fatal heart failure during the acute phase. Of the patients who survive this complication, about 20% die within 10 years.

Causes and incidence

Rheumatic fever appears to be a hypersensitivity reaction to a group A beta-hemolytic streptococcal infection, in which antibodies manufactured to combat streptococci react and produce characteristic lesions at specific tissue sites, especially in the heart and joints. Because few persons (3%) with streptococcal infections ever contract rheumatic fever, altered host resistance must be involved in its development or recurrence. Although rheumatic fever tends to be familial, this may merely reflect contributing environmental factors. For example, in lower socioeconomic groups, incidence is highest in children ages 5 to 15, probably as a result of malnutrition and crowded living conditions. This disease strikes generally during cool, damp weather in the winter and early spring. In the United States, it's most common in the northern states. The prevalence of rheumatic heart disease peaks in adults ages 25 to 34.[1]

Signs and symptoms

In 95% of patients, rheumatic fever characteristically follows a streptococcal infection that appeared a few days to 6 weeks earlier. A temperature of at least 100.4° F (38° C) occurs, and most patients complain of migratory joint pain or polyarthritis. Swelling, redness, and signs of effusion usually accompany such pain, which most commonly affects the knees, ankles, elbows, or hips. In 5% of patients (generally those with carditis), rheumatic fever causes skin lesions such as erythema marginatum, a nonpruritic, macular, transient rash that gives rise to red lesions with blanched centers. Rheumatic fever may also produce firm, movable, nontender, subcutaneous nodules about 3 mm to 2 cm in diameter, usually near tendons or bony prominences of joints (especially the elbows, knuckles, wrists, and knees) and less commonly on the scalp and backs of the hands. These nodules persist for a few days to several weeks and, like erythema marginatum, often accompany carditis.

Later, rheumatic fever may cause transient chorea, which develops up to 6 months after the original streptococcal infection. Mild chorea may produce hyperirritability, deterioration in handwriting, or an inability to concentrate. Severe chorea (Sydenham's chorea) causes purposeless, nonrepetitive, involuntary muscle spasms; poor muscle coordination; and weakness. Chorea always resolves without residual neurologic damage.

The most destructive effect of rheumatic fever is carditis, which develops in up to 50% of patients and may affect the endocardium, myocardium, pericardium, or the heart valves. Pericarditis causes a pericardial friction rub and, occasionally, pain and effusion. Myocarditis produces characteristic lesions called Aschoff's bodies (in the acute stages) and cellular swelling and fragmentation of interstitial collagen, leading to formation of a progressively fibrotic nodule and interstitial scars. Endocarditis causes valve leaflet swelling, erosion along the lines of leaflet closure, and blood, platelet, and fibrin deposits, which form beadlike vegetations. Endocarditis affects the mitral valve most often in females; the aortic, most often in males. In both females and males, endocarditis affects the tricuspid valves occasionally and the pulmonic only rarely.

Severe rheumatic carditis may cause heart failure with dyspnea; right upper quadrant pain; tachycardia; tachypnea; a hacking, nonproductive cough; edema; and significant

mitral and aortic murmurs. The most common of such murmurs include:
▶ a systolic murmur of mitral insufficiency (high-pitched, blowing, holosystolic, loudest at apex, possibly radiating to the anterior axillary line)
▶ a midsystolic murmur due to stiffening and swelling of the mitral leaflet
▶ occasionally, a diastolic murmur of aortic insufficiency (low-pitched, rumbling, almost inaudible). Valvular disease may eventually result in chronic valvular stenosis and insufficiency, including mitral stenosis and insufficiency, and aortic insufficiency. In children, mitral insufficiency remains the major sequela of rheumatic heart disease.

Complications
▶ Pancarditis
▶ Pericardial effusion
▶ Fatal heart failure

Diagnosis
Diagnosis depends on recognition of one or more of the classic symptoms (carditis, rheumatic fever without carditis, polyarthritis, chorea, erythema marginatum, or subcutaneous nodules) and a detailed patient history. Laboratory data support the diagnosis:
▶ White blood cell count and erythrocyte sedimentation rate may be elevated (during the acute phase); blood studies show slight anemia due to suppressed erythropoiesis during inflammation.
▶ C-reactive protein is positive (especially during acute phase).
▶ Cardiac enzyme levels may be increased in severe carditis.
▶ Antistreptolysin-O titer is elevated in 95% of patients within 2 months of onset.
▶ Electrocardiogram changes aren't diagnostic; but the PR interval is prolonged in 20% of patients.
▶ Chest X-rays show normal heart size (except with myocarditis, heart failure, or pericardial effusion).

▶ Echocardiography helps evaluate valvular damage, chamber size, and ventricular function.
▶ Cardiac catheterization evaluates valvular damage and left ventricular function in severe cardiac dysfunction.

Treatment
Effective management eradicates the streptococcal infection, relieves symptoms, and prevents recurrence, reducing the chance of permanent cardiac damage. During the acute phase, treatment includes penicillin, sulfadiazine, or erythromycin. Salicylates such as aspirin relieve fever and minimize joint swelling and pain; if carditis is present or salicylates fail to relieve pain and inflammation, corticosteroids may be used. Supportive treatment requires strict bed rest for about 5 weeks during the acute phase with active carditis, followed by a progressive increase in physical activity, depending on clinical and laboratory findings and the response to treatment.

After the acute phase subsides, low-dose antibiotics may be used to prevent recurrence. Such preventive treatment usually continues for 5 years.[2] Heart failure necessitates continued bed rest and diuretics. Severe mitral or aortic valve dysfunction that causes persistent heart failure requires corrective valvular surgery, including commissurotomy (separation of the adherent, thickened leaflets of the mitral valve), valvuloplasty (inflation of a balloon within a valve), or valve replacement (with prosthetic valve). Such surgery is seldom necessary before late adolescence.

Special considerations
HEALTH & SAFETY *Because rheumatic fever and rheumatic heart disease require prolonged treatment, the care plan should include comprehensive patient teaching to promote compliance with the prescribed therapy.*

▶ Before giving penicillin, ask the patient or his parents if he has ever had a hypersensitive reaction to it. If he hasn't, warn that such a reaction is possible. Tell them to stop the drug and call the physician immediately if he develops a rash, fever, chills, or other signs of allergy at any time during penicillin therapy.

▶ Instruct the patient and his family to watch for and report early signs of heart failure, such as dyspnea and a hacking, nonproductive cough.

▶ Stress the need for bed rest during the acute phase and suggest appropriate, physically undemanding diversions. After the acute phase, encourage his family and friends to spend as much time as possible with the patient to minimize boredom. Advise his parents to secure tutorial services to help the child keep up with schoolwork during the long convalescence.

▶ Help his parents overcome any guilt feelings they may have about their child's illness. Tell them that failure to seek treatment for streptococcal infection is common because this illness usually seems no worse than a cold. Encourage the child and his parents to vent their frustrations during the long, tedious recovery. If the child has severe carditis, help them prepare for permanent changes in his lifestyle.

▶ Teach the patient and his family about this disease and its treatment. Warn parents to watch for and immediately report signs of recurrent streptococcal infection—sudden sore throat, diffuse throat redness and oropharyngeal exudate, swollen and tender cervical lymph glands, pain on swallowing, temperature of 101° to 104° F (38.3° to 40° C), headache, and nausea. Urge them to keep the child away from people with respiratory tract infections.

▶ Promote good dental hygiene to prevent gingival infection. Make sure the patient and his family understands the need to comply with prolonged antibiotic therapy. Arrange for a home health nurse to oversee home care if necessary.

▶ Teach the patient to follow current recommendations of the American Heart Association for prevention of bacterial endocarditis. Prophylactic antibiotics prior to dental procedures is recommended if the patient has a high risk of an adverse reaction from endocarditis, such as patients with previous endocarditis, a prosthetic cardiac valve, or specific forms of congenital heart disease. Prophylactic antibiotics are no longer recommended for patients with rheumatic heart disease prior to procedures for the GI or genitourinary tract.[3]

REFERENCES

1. Carapetis, J.R., et al. "Acute Rheumatic Fever," *Lancet* 366(9480):155-68, July 2005.
2. Parrillo, S.J., and Parrillo, C.V. eMedicine from WebMD (2007 February 7). "Rheumatic Fever" [Online]. Available at *www.emedicine.com/emerg/topic509.htm*.
3. Wilson, W., et al. "Prevention of Infective Endocarditis: Guidelines from the American Heart Association," *Circulation* 116(15):1736-54, October 2007.

THORACIC AORTIC ANEURYSM

Thoracic aortic aneurysm is the abnormal widening of the ascending, transverse, or descending part of the aorta. Aneurysm of the ascending aorta is the most common type and has the highest mortality. Aneurysms may be *dissecting*, with a hemorrhagic separation in the aortic wall, usually within the medial layer; *saccular*, an outpouching of the arterial wall, with a narrow neck; or *fusiform*, a spindle-shaped enlargement encompassing the entire aortic circumference. (See *Types of aortic aneurysms*, page 56.)

Types of aortic aneurysms

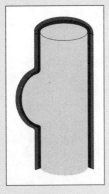

SACCULAR
Unilateral pouch-like bulge with a narrow neck

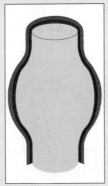

FUSIFORM
A spindle-shaped bulge encompassing the vessel's entire diameter

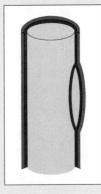

DISSECTING
A hemorrhagic separation of the medial layer of the vessel wall, which creates a false lumen

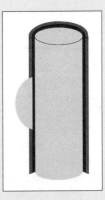

FALSE ANEURYSM
A pulsating hematoma resulting from trauma and often mistaken for an abdominal aneurysm

Causes and incidence

Thoracic aortic aneurysms commonly result from atherosclerosis, which weakens the aortic wall and gradually distends the lumen. An intimal tear in the ascending aorta initiates dissecting aneurysm in about 60% of the patients. Regardless of causation, these aneurysms affect about 15,000 people in the United States annually.[1]

Ascending aortic aneurysms, the most common type, are usually seen in hypertensive males younger than age 60. (See *A genetic link to thoracic aneurysms.*) Descending aortic aneurysms, usually found just below the origin of the subclavian artery, are most common in elderly males who are hypertensive.[2]

Descending aortic aneurysms are also seen in younger patients with a history of traumatic chest injury; less commonly in those with infection. Transverse aortic aneurysms are the least common type.

Other causes include:
▶ fungal infection (mycotic aneurysms) of the aortic arch and descending segments
▶ congenital disorders, such as coarctation of the aorta and Marfan syndrome
▶ trauma, usually of the descending thoracic aorta, from an accident that shears the aorta transversely (acceleration-deceleration injuries)
▶ syphilis, usually of the ascending aorta (uncommon because of antibiotics)
▶ hypertension in dissecting aneurysm (found in 70% to 80% of cases).[2]

Signs and symptoms

Only about one-half of the people with a thoracic aortic aneurysm note symptoms.[1]

The most common symptom of thoracic aortic aneurysm is pain. With ascending aneurysm, the pain is described as severe, boring, and ripping. It extends to the neck, shoulders, lower back, or abdomen but sel-

dom radiates to the jaw and arms. Pain is more severe on the right side.

Other signs of ascending aneurysm may include bradycardia, aortic insufficiency, pericardial friction rub caused by a hemo-pericardium, unequal intensities of the right carotid and left radial pulses, and a difference in blood pressure between the right and left arms. These signs are absent in descending aneurysm. If dissection involves the carotids, an abrupt onset of neurologic deficits may occur.

With descending aneurysm, pain usually starts suddenly between the shoulder blades and may radiate to the chest; it's described as sharp and tearing. Transverse aneurysm causes a sudden, sharp, tearing pain radiating to the shoulders. It may also cause hoarseness, dyspnea, dysphagia, and a dry cough because of compression of surrounding structures in this area. (See *Clinical characteristics of thoracic dissection*, page 58.)

Complications
▶ Rupture into the pericardium with resulting cardiac tamponade

Diagnosis
Diagnosis relies on patient history, clinical features, and appropriate tests. In an asymptomatic patient, diagnosis typically occurs accidentally when chest X-rays show widening of the mediastinum, enlargement of the aortic knob or tracheal displacement.[2] Other tests help confirm aneurysm:
▶ Aortography, the most definitive test, shows the lumen of the aneurysm, its size and location, and the false lumen in dissecting aneurysm.
▶ Electrocardiography helps distinguish thoracic aneurysm from myocardial infarction.
▶ Echocardiography may help identify dissecting aneurysm of the aortic root.
▶ Hemoglobin levels may be normal or low, due to blood loss from a leaking aneurysm.

IN THE NEWS

A genetic link to thoracic aneurysms

Researchers are currently studying a newly mapped gene that may increase a patient's likelihood of developing a thoracic aortic aneurysm and dissection. Families with a strong history of dissecting thoracic aortic aneurysms were found to have shared genetic markers on two subsets of genes. Researchers hope to use this information to monitor high-risk families and patients for signs of thoracic aortic aneurysms

▶ Computed tomography scan can confirm and locate the aneurysm and may be used to monitor its progression.
▶ Magnetic resonance imaging may aid diagnosis.
▶ Transesophageal echocardiography is used to diagnose and size an aneurysm in either the ascending or the descending aorta.

Treatment
Dissecting aortic aneurysm is an emergency that requires prompt surgery and stabilizing measures: antihypertensives such as nitroprusside; negative inotropic agents that decrease contractility force such as propranolol; oxygen for respiratory distress; opioids for pain; I.V. fluids and, possibly, whole blood transfusions.

Surgery consists of resecting the aneurysm, restoring normal blood flow through a Dacron or Teflon graft replacement and, with aortic valve insufficiency, replacing the aortic valve. Groin catheter placement may be used for aortic stenting. This procedure, which may be used for aneurysms of the descending aorta, eliminates the need for a chest incision.[3]

Postoperative measures include careful monitoring and continuous assessment in the intensive care unit, antibiotics, endotracheal

Clinical characteristics of thoracic dissection

ASCENDING AORTA	DESCENDING AORTA	TRANSVERSE AORTA
Character of pain		
Severe, boring, ripping, extending to neck, shoulders, lower back, or abdomen (rarely to jaw and arms); more severe on right side	Sudden onset, sharp, tearing, usually between the shoulder blades; may radiate to the chest; most diagnostic feature	Sudden onset, sharp, boring, tearing, radiates to shoulders
Other symptoms and effects		
If dissection involves carotids, abrupt onset of neurologic deficit (usually intermittent); bradycardia, aortic insufficiency, and hemopericardium detected by pericardial friction rub; unequal intensity of right and left carotid pulses and radial pulses; difference in blood pressure, especially systolic, between right and left arms	Aortic insufficiency without murmur, hemopericardium, or pleural friction rub; carotid and radial pulses and blood pressure in both arms tend to stay equal	Hoarseness, dyspnea, pain, dysphagia, and dry cough resulting from compression of surrounding structures
Diagnostic features		
Chest X-ray Best diagnostic tool; shows widening of mediastinum, enlargement of ascending aorta	Shows widening of mediastinum, descending aorta larger than ascending	Shows widening of mediastinum, descending aorta larger than ascending, widened transverse arch
Aortography Shows false lumen; narrowing of lumen of aorta in ascending section	Shows false lumen; narrowing of lumen of aorta in descending section	Shows false lumen, narrowing of lumen of aorta in transverse arch
Treatment		
This is a medical emergency requiring immediate, aggressive treatment to reduce blood pressure (usually with nitroprusside or trimethaphan). Surgical repair is also required.	Surgical repair is required but less urgent than for the ascending dissection. Nitroprusside and propranolol may be used to control hypertension if bradycardia and heart failure are absent.	Immediate surgical repair (mortality as high as 50%) and control of hypertension are required.

(ET) and chest tubes, electrocardiogram monitoring, and pulmonary artery catheterization.

Long-term management includes treatment of underlying conditions, such as heart disease and diabetes.

Special considerations

▶ Monitor blood pressure, pulmonary artery wedge pressure (PAWP), and central venous pressure (CVP). Assess pain, breathing, and carotid, radial, and femoral pulses.

▶ Make sure laboratory tests include complete blood count, differential, electrolyte

levels, type and crossmatching for whole blood, arterial blood gas studies, and urinalysis.

▸ Insert an indwelling urinary catheter. Administer dextrose 5% in water or lactated Ringer's solution, and antibiotics, as ordered. Carefully monitor nitroprusside I.V.; use a separate I.V. line for infusion. Titrate the infusion to control hypertension. Meanwhile, check blood pressure every 5 minutes until it stabilizes. With suspected bleeding from aneurysm, give whole blood transfusion.

▸ Explain diagnostic tests. If surgery is scheduled, explain the procedure and expected postoperative care (I.V. lines, ET and drainage tubes, cardiac monitoring, and ventilation).

After repair of thoracic aneurysm:

▸ Assess level of consciousness. Monitor vital signs; pulmonary artery pressure, PAWP, and CVP; pulse rate; urine output; and pain.

▸ Check respiratory function. Carefully observe and record type and amount of chest-tube drainage, and frequently assess heart and breath sounds.

▸ Monitor I.V. therapy.

▸ Give medications as appropriate.

▸ Watch for signs of infection, especially fever, and excessive wound drainage.

▸ Assist with range-of-motion exercises of legs to prevent thromboembolic phenomenon due to venostasis during prolonged bed rest.

▸ After stabilization of vital signs and respiration, encourage and assist the patient in turning, coughing, and deep breathing. Help the patient walk as soon as he's able.

▸ Before discharge, ensure compliance with antihypertensive therapy by explaining the need for such drugs and the expected adverse effects. Teach the patient how to monitor his blood pressure. Refer him to community agencies for continued support and assistance, as needed.

▸ Throughout hospitalization, offer the patient and his family psychological support.

Answer all of their questions honestly and provide reassurance.

REFERENCES

1. The Society for Vascular Surgery (2006 August 14). "Thoracic Aneurysms" [Online]. Available at *www.vascularweb.org/patients/NorthPoint/Thoracic_Aneurysm.html.*
2. Klein, D.G. "Thoracic Aortic Aneurysms," *Journal of Cardiovascular Nursing* 20(4):245-50 July-August 2005.
3. Jones, L.E. "Endovascular Stent Grafting of Thoracic Aortic Aneurysms: Technological Advancements Provide an Alternative to Traditional Surgical Repair," *Journal of Cardiovascular Nursing* 20(6):376-84, November-December 2005.

THROMBOPHLEBITIS

This acute condition, characterized by inflammation and thrombus formation, may occur in deep or superficial veins. Deep vein thrombosis (DVT) or thrombophlebitis affects small veins, such as the soleal venous sinuses, or large veins, such as the vena cava and the femoral, iliac, and subclavian veins, causing venous insufficiency. (See *Chronic venous insufficiency,* page 60.)

Superficial thrombophlebitis is usually self-limiting and seldom leads to pulmonary embolism. Thrombophlebitis commonly begins with localized inflammation alone (phlebitis), but such inflammation rapidly provokes thrombus formation. Rarely, venous thrombosis develops without associated inflammation of the vein (phlebothrombosis).

Causes and incidence

A thrombus occurs when an alteration in the epithelial lining causes platelet aggregation and consequent fibrin entrapment of red and white blood cells and additional platelets. Thrombus formation is more rapid in areas where blood flow is slower, due to greater

Chronic venous insufficiency

Chronic venous insufficiency results from the valvular destruction of deep vein thrombophlebitis, usually in the iliac and femoral veins, and occasionally the saphenous veins. It's often accompanied by incompetence of the communicating veins at the ankle, causing increased venous pressure and fluid migration into the interstitial tissue. Clinical effects include chronic swelling of the affected leg from edema, leading to tissue fibrosis, and induration; skin discoloration from extravasation of blood in subcutaneous tissue; and stasis ulcers around the ankle.

Treatment of small ulcers includes bed rest, elevation of the legs, warm soaks, and antimicrobial therapy for infection. Treatment to counteract increased venous pressure, the result of reflux from the deep venous system to surface veins, may include compression dressings, such as a sponge rubber pressure dressing or a zinc gelatin boot (Unna's boot). This therapy begins after massive swelling subsides with leg elevation and bed rest.

Large stasis ulcers unresponsive to conservative treatment may require excision and skin grafting. Patient care includes daily inspection to assess healing. Other care measures are the same as for varicose veins.

contact between platelet and thrombin accumulation. The rapidly expanding thrombus initiates a chemical inflammatory process in the vessel epithelium, which leads to fibrosis. The enlarging clot may occlude the vessel lumen partially or totally, or it may detach and embolize to lodge elsewhere in the systemic circulation.

DVT may be idiopathic, but it usually results from endothelial damage, accelerated blood clotting, and reduced blood flow. Predisposing factors are prolonged bed rest, trauma, surgery, childbirth, and use of hormonal contraceptives such as estrogens. It

occurs in about 80 of every 100,000 people; 1 of every 20 persons is affected at some point during his lifetime. Males are at slightly greater risk than females. People older than age 40 are also at increased risk.

Causes of superficial thrombophlebitis include trauma, infection, I.V. drug abuse, and chemical irritation due to extensive use of the I.V. route for medications and diagnostic tests.

Signs and symptoms
In both types of thrombophlebitis, clinical features vary with the site and length of the affected vein. In 50% to 80% of cases, DVT occurs without accompanying symptoms.[1] However, it may produce severe pain, fever, chills, malaise and, possibly, swelling and cyanosis of the affected arm or leg. Superficial thrombophlebitis produces visible and palpable signs, such as heat, pain, swelling, rubor, tenderness, and induration along the length of the affected vein. Varicose veins may also be present. (See *Varicose veins*.)

Extensive vein involvement may cause lymphadenitis.

Complications
▶ Pulmonary embolism
▶ Recurrent DVT
▶ Postthrombotic syndrome and possible lower extremity amputation[5]

Diagnosis
Some patients may display signs of inflammation and, possibly, a positive Homans' sign (pain on dorsiflexion of the foot) during physical examination; others are asymptomatic. Essential laboratory tests include:
▶ Duplex Doppler ultrasonography and impedance plethysmography make it possible to noninvasively examine the major veins (but not calf veins).
▶ Plethysmography shows decreased circulation distal to the affected area; this test is more sensitive than ultrasound in detecting DVT.

Varicose veins

Varicose veins are dilated, tortuous veins, usually affecting the subcutaneous leg veins—the saphenous veins and their branches. They can result from congenital weakness of the valves or venous wall, diseases of the venous system such as deep vein thrombophlebitis, conditions that produce prolonged venostasis such as pregnancy, or occupations that necessitate standing for an extended period.

Varicose veins may cause no symptoms or may produce mild to severe leg symptoms, including a feeling of heaviness; cramps at night; diffuse, dull aching after prolonged standing or walking; aching during menses; fatigability; palpable nodules and, with deep-vein incompetency, orthostatic edema and stasis pigmentation of the calves and ankles.

TREATMENT

In mild to moderate varicose veins, antiembolism stockings or elastic bandages counteract pedal and ankle swelling by supporting the veins and improving circulation. An exercise program such as walking promotes muscular contraction and forces blood through the veins, thereby minimizing venous pooling. Severe varicose veins may necessitate stripping and ligation or, as an alternative to surgery, injection of a sclerosing agent into small affected vein segments.

To promote comfort and minimize worsening of varicosities:

● Discourage the patient from wearing constrictive clothing.
● Advise the patient to elevate his legs above heart level whenever possible and to avoid prolonged standing or sitting.

After stripping and ligation or after injection of a sclerosing agent:

● To relieve pain, administer analgesics as ordered.
● Frequently check circulation in toes (color and temperature), and observe elastic bandages for bleeding. When ordered, rewrap bandages at least once a shift, wrapping from toe to thigh, with the leg elevated.
● Watch for signs of complications, such as sensory loss in the leg (which could indicate saphenous nerve damage), calf pain (thrombophlebitis), and fever (infection).

▶ Contrast venography, which shows filling defects, confirms the diagnosis.[2] Diagnosis must also rule out arterial occlusive disease, lymphangitis, cellulitis, and myositis. Diagnosis of superficial thrombophlebitis is based on physical examination (redness and warmth over the affected area, palpable vein, and pain during palpation or compression).

Treatment

The goals of treatment are to control thrombus development, prevent complications, relieve pain, and prevent recurrence of the disorder. Symptomatic measures include bed rest, with elevation of the affected arm or leg; warm, moist soaks to the affected area; and analgesics. After the acute episode of DVT subsides, the patient may resume activity while wearing antiembolism stockings that are applied before he gets out of bed.

Treatment also includes anticoagulants (initially, heparin; later, warfarin) to prolong clotting time. According to the 7th American College of Chest Physician Conference Guidelines, low-molecular-weight heparin (LMWH) has been shown to be effective in treating DVT.[3] I.V. or subcutaneous (subQ) unfractionated heparin may also be used, and a vitamin K antagonist should be used on the first day with LMWH or unfractionated heparin.[4] Full anticoagulant doses must be discontinued during any operative period because of the risk of hemorrhage. After some types of surgery, especially major abdominal or pelvic operations, prophylactic

doses of anticoagulants reduce the risk of DVT and pulmonary embolism.[2] For lysis of acute, extensive DVT, treatment should include streptokinase. Rarely, DVT may cause complete venous occlusion, which necessitates venous interruption through simple ligation to vein plication, or clipping. Embolectomy and insertion of a vena caval umbrella or filter may also be done.

To prevent postthrombotic syndrome, graduated elastic stockings are recommended for 2 years after the onset of DVT.[4]

Therapy for severe superficial thrombophlebitis may include an anti-inflammatory drug such as indomethacin, antiembolism stockings, warm soaks, and elevation of the leg.

Special considerations

Patient teaching, identification of high-risk patients, and measures to prevent venostasis can prevent DVT; close monitoring of anticoagulant therapy can prevent serious complications such as internal hemorrhage.

▶ Enforce bed rest as ordered, and elevate the patient's affected arm or leg. If you plan to use pillows for elevating the leg, place them so they support the entire length of the affected extremity to prevent possible compression of the popliteal space.

▶ Apply warm soaks to increase circulation to the affected area and to relieve pain and inflammation. Give analgesics to relieve pain, as ordered.

▶ Measure and record the affected arm or leg's circumference daily, and compare this measurement to the other arm or leg. To ensure accuracy and consistency of serial measurements, mark the skin over the area and measure at the same spot daily.

▶ Administer heparin I.V., as ordered, with an infusion monitor or pump to control the flow rate if necessary.

▶ Measure partial thromboplastin time regularly for the patient on heparin therapy; prothrombin time (PT) and international normalized ratio (INR) for the patient on

warfarin (therapeutic anticoagulation values are 1½ to 2 times control values for PT and an INR of 2 to 3). Watch for signs and symptoms of bleeding, such as dark, tarry stools; coffee-ground vomitus; and ecchymoses. Encourage the patient to use an electric razor and to avoid medications that contain aspirin.

▶ Be alert for signs of pulmonary emboli (crackles, dyspnea, hemoptysis, sudden changes in mental status, restlessness, and hypotension).

To prepare the patient with thrombophlebitis for discharge:

▶ Emphasize the importance of follow-up blood studies to monitor anticoagulant therapy.

▶ If the patient is being discharged on heparin therapy, teach him or his family how to give subQ injections. If he requires further assistance, arrange for a home health nurse.

▶ Tell the patient to avoid prolonged sitting or standing to help prevent recurrence.

▶ Teach the patient how to properly apply and use antiembolism stockings. Tell him to report any complications such as cold, blue toes.

▶ To prevent thrombophlebitis in high-risk patients, perform range-of-motion exercises while the patient is on bed rest, use intermittent pneumatic calf massage during lengthy surgical or diagnostic procedures, apply antiembolism stockings postoperatively, and encourage early ambulation.

REFERENCES

1. Nutescu, E.A. "Assessing, Preventing, and Treating Venous Thromboembolism: Evidence-Based Approaches," *American Journal of Health-System Pharmacists* 64(suppl.):S5-S13, June 2007.
2. Bartley, M.K. "Keep Venous Thromboembolism at Bay," *Nursing* 36(10):36-41, October 2006.
3. Schrieber, D. H., and Howard, A.D. "DVT: New Therapeutic Perspectives," *Practical*

Summaries in Acute Care 2(5):37-43, May 2007.

4. Buller H. R., et al. "Antithrombotic Therapy for Venous Thromboembolic Disease: The Seventh ACCP Conference on Antithrombotic and Thrombolytic Therapy," *Chest* 126(3 Suppl):401S-28S, September 2004.

5. The three items on this list are taken from Nutescu, E.A. "Assessing, Preventing, and Treating Venous Thromboembolism: Evidence-Based Approaches," cited in endnote 1 above.

VALVULAR HEART DISEASE

In valvular heart disease, three types of mechanical disruption can occur: stenosis, or narrowing, of the valve opening; incomplete closure of the valve; or prolapse of the valve—any one of which can lead to heart failure. The most likely causes: such disorders as endocarditis (most common), congenital defects, and inflammation.

Valvular heart disease occurs in varying forms, described below. (For additional information, see *Types of valvular heart disease,* pages 64 to 66.)

▶ *Mitral insufficiency:* In this form, blood from the left ventricle flows back into the left atrium during systole, causing the atrium to enlarge to accommodate the backflow. As a result, the left ventricle also dilates to accommodate the increased volume of blood from the atrium and to compensate for diminishing cardiac output. Ventricular hypertrophy and increased end-diastolic pressure result in increased pulmonary artery pressure, eventually leading to left- and right-sided heart failure.

▶ *Mitral stenosis:* Narrowing of the valve by valvular abnormalities, fibrosis, or calcification obstructs blood flow from the left atrium to the left ventricle. Consequently, left atrial volume and pressure rise, and the chamber dilates. Greater resistance to blood flow causes pulmonary hypertension, right ventricular hypertrophy, and right-sided

heart failure. Also, inadequate filling of the left ventricle produces low cardiac output.

▶ *Mitral valve prolapse (MVP):* One or both valve leaflets protrude into the left atrium causing incomplete closure of the valve and possible mitral regurgitation.[1]

▶ *Aortic insufficiency:* Blood flows back into the left ventricle during diastole, causing fluid overload in the ventricle, which dilates and hypertrophies. The excess volume causes fluid overload in the left atrium and, finally, the pulmonary system. Left-sided heart failure and pulmonary edema eventually result.

▶ *Aortic stenosis:* Increased left ventricular pressure tries to overcome the resistance of the narrowed valvular opening. The added workload increases the demand for oxygen, whereas diminished cardiac output causes poor coronary artery perfusion, ischemia of the left ventricle, and left-sided heart failure.

▶ *Pulmonic insufficiency:* Blood ejected into the pulmonary artery during systole flows back into the right ventricle during diastole, causing fluid overload in the ventricle, ventricular hypertrophy and, finally, right-sided heart failure.

▶ *Pulmonic stenosis:* Obstructed right ventricular outflow causes right ventricular hypertrophy, eventually resulting in right-sided heart failure.

▶ *Tricuspid insufficiency:* Blood flows back into the right atrium during systole, decreasing blood flow to the lungs and the left side of the heart. Cardiac output also lessens. Fluid overload in the right side of the heart can eventually lead to right-sided heart failure.

▶ *Tricuspid stenosis:* Obstructed blood flow from the right atrium to the right ventricle causes the right atrium to dilate and hypertrophy. Eventually, this leads to right-sided heart failure and increases pressure in the vena cava.

(Text continues on page 66.)

Types of valvular heart disease

CAUSES AND INCIDENCE	CLINICAL FEATURES	DIAGNOSTIC MEASURES
Aortic insufficiency • Results from rheumatic fever, syphilis, hypertension, endocarditis, or may be idiopathic • Associated with Marfan syndrome • Most common in males • Associated with ventricular septal defect, even after surgical closure	• Dyspnea, cough, fatigue, palpitations, angina, syncope • Pulmonary venous congestion, heart failure, pulmonary edema (left-sided heart failure), "pulsating" nail beds • Rapidly rising and collapsing pulses (pulsus biferiens), cardiac arrhythmias, wide pulse pressure in severe insufficiency • Auscultation reveals S_3 and diastolic blowing murmur at left sternal border • Palpation and visualization of apical impulse in chronic disease	• Cardiac catheterization: reduction in arterial diastolic pressures, aortic insufficiency, other valvular abnormalities, and increased left ventricular end-diastolic pressure • X-ray: left ventricular enlargement, pulmonary vein congestion • Echocardiography: left ventricular enlargement, alterations in mitral valve movement (indirect indication of aortic valve disease), and mitral thickening • Electrocardiogram (ECG): sinus tachycardia, left ventricular hypertrophy, and left atrial hypertrophy in severe disease
Aortic stenosis • Also results from congenital stenosis of valve cusps, rheumatic fever, or atherosclerosis in elderly persons • Most common in males • The two most common causes of calcification are tricuspid valves and congenital aortic bicuspid valve(s).	• Dyspnea on exertion, paroxysmal nocturnal dyspnea, fatigue, syncope, angina, palpitations • Pulmonary venous congestion, heart failure, pulmonary edema • Diminished carotid pulses, decreased cardiac output, cardiac arrhythmias; may have pulsus alternans • Auscultation reveals systolic murmur at base or in carotids and, possibly, S_4	• Cardiac catheterization: pressure gradient across valve (indicating obstruction), increased left ventricular end-diastolic pressures • X-ray: valvular calcification, left ventricular enlargement, and pulmonary venous congestion • ECG: thickened aortic valve and left ventricular wall • ECG: left ventricular hypertrophy
Mitral insufficiency • Results from rheumatic fever, hypertrophic cardiomyopathy, mitral valve prolapse, myocardial infarction, severe left-sided heart failure, or ruptured chordae tendineae • Associated with other congenital anomalies such as transposition of the great arteries • Rare in children without other congenital anomalies	• Orthopnea, dyspnea, fatigue, angina, palpitations • Peripheral edema, jugular vein distention (JVD), hepatomegaly (right-sided heart failure) • Tachycardia, crackles, pulmonary edema • Auscultation reveals holosystolic murmur at apex, possible split S_2, and S_3	• Cardiac catheterization: mitral insufficiency with increased left ventricular end-diastolic volume and pressure, increased atrial pressure and pulmonary artery wedge pressure (PAWP); and decreased cardiac output X-ray: left atrial and ventricular enlargement, pulmonary venous congestion • Echocardiography: abnormal valve leaflet motion, left atrial enlargement • ECG: left atrial and ventricular hypertrophy, sinus tachycardia, and atrial fibrillation

Types of valvular heart disease *(continued)*

CAUSES AND INCIDENCE	CLINICAL FEATURES	DIAGNOSTIC MEASURES
Mitral stenosis • Most common cause is rheumatic fever. Incidence has decreased with the decreased incidence of rheumatic fever.[3] • Most common in females • May be associated with other congenital anomalies	• Dyspnea on exertion, paroxysmal nocturnal dyspnea, orthopnea, weakness, fatigue, palpitations • Peripheral edema, JVD, ascites, hepatomegaly (right-sided heart failure in severe pulmonary hypertension) • Crackles, cardiac arrhythmias (atrial fibrillation), signs of systemic emboli • Auscultation reveals loud S_1 or opening snap and diastolic murmur at apex	• Echocardiography is study of choice to diagnose and assess severity: thickened mitral valve leaflets, left atrial enlargement[3] • Cardiac catheterization: diastolic pressure gradient across valve; elevated left atrial pressure and PAWP (> 15 mm Hg) with severe pulmonary hypertension and pulmonary artery pressures (PAPs); elevated right-sided heart pressure; decreased cardiac output; and abnormal contraction of the left ventricle • X-ray: left atrial and ventricular enlargement, enlarged pulmonary arteries, and mitral valve calcification • ECG: left atrial hypertrophy, atrial fibrillation, right ventricular hypertrophy, and right axis deviation
Mitral valve prolapse (MVP) syndrome • Cause unknown; researchers speculate that metabolic or neuroendocrine factors cause constellation of signs and symptoms. • MVP is most common valvular heart abnormality in the United States, affecting 2% to 6% of the population. It affects males and females and all ethnic groups equally.[1]	• May produce no signs • Chest pain, palpitations, headache, fatigue, exercise intolerance, dyspnea, lightheadedness, syncope, mood swings, anxiety, panic attacks[1] • Auscultation typically reveals mobile, midsystolic click, with or without mid-to-late systolic murmur	• Two-dimensional echocardiography and Doppler echocardiography: prolapse of mitral valve leaflets into left atrium • Stress echocardiography: may show exercise-induced mitral regurgitation or latent left ventricular function • Color-flow Doppler studies: mitral insufficiency • Resting ECG: ST-segment changes, biphasic or inverted T-waves in leads II, III, or AV • Exercise ECG: evaluates chest pain and arrhythmias
Pulmonic insufficiency • May be congenital or may result from pulmonary hypertension • May rarely result from prolonged use of pressure monitoring catheter in the pulmonary artery	• Dyspnea, weakness, fatigue, chest pain • Peripheral edema, JVD, hepatomegaly (right-sided heart failure) • Auscultation reveals diastolic murmur in pulmonic area	• Cardiac catheterization: pulmonic insufficiency, increased right ventricular pressure, and associated cardiac defects • X-ray: right ventricular and pulmonary arterial enlargement • ECG: right ventricular or right atrial enlargement

(continued)

Types of valvular heart disease *(continued)*

CAUSES AND INCIDENCE	CLINICAL FEATURES	DIAGNOSTIC MEASURES
Pulmonic stenosis • Results from congenital stenosis of valve cusp or rheumatic heart disease (infrequent) • Associated with other congenital heart defects such as tetralogy of Fallot	• May produce symptoms, such as dyspnea on exertion, fatigue, chest pain, syncope • May lead to peripheral edema, JVD, hepatomegaly (right-sided heart failure) • Auscultation reveals systolic murmur at left sternal border, split S_2 with delayed or absent pulmonic component	• Cardiac catheterization: increased right ventricular pressure, decreased PAP, and abnormal valve orifice • ECG: may show right ventricular hypertrophy, right axis deviation, right atrial hypertrophy, and atrial fibrillation
Tricuspid insufficiency • Results from right-sided heart failure, rheumatic fever and, rarely, trauma and endocarditis • Associated with congenital disorders	• Dyspnea and fatigue • May lead to peripheral edema, JVD, hepatomegaly, and ascites (right-sided heart failure) • Auscultation reveals possible S_3 and systolic murmur at lower left sternal border that increases with inspiration	• Right-sided heart catheterization: high atrial pressure, tricuspid insufficiency, decreased or normal cardiac output • X-ray: right atrial dilation, right ventricular enlargement • Echocardiography: systolic prolapse of tricuspid valve, right atrial enlargement • ECG: right atrial or right ventricular hypertrophy, atrial fibrillation
Tricuspid stenosis • Results from rheumatic fever • May be congenital • Associated with mitral or aortic valve disease • Most common in females	• May cause symptoms, such as dyspnea, fatigue, syncope • Possibly peripheral edema, JVD, hepatomegaly, and ascites (right-sided heart failure) • Auscultation reveals diastolic murmur at lower left sternal border that increases with inspiration	• Cardiac catheterization: increased pressure gradient across valve, increased right atrial pressure, decreased cardiac output • X-ray: right atrial enlargement • Echocardiography: leaflet abnormality, right atrial enlargement • ECG: right atrial hypertrophy, right or left ventricular hypertrophy, and atrial fibrillation

Treatment

Treatment depends on the nature and severity of associated symptoms. For example, heart failure requires digoxin, diuretics, a sodium-restricted diet and, in acute cases, oxygen. Other measures may include anticoagulant therapy or antiplatelet medications to prevent thrombus formation around diseased or replaced valves, prophylactic antibiotics before and after surgery or dental care, and valvuloplasty. An intra-aortic balloon pump may be used temporarily to reduce backflow by enhancing forward blood flow into the aorta.

If the patient has severe signs and symptoms that can't be managed medically, open heart surgery using cardiopulmonary bypass for valve replacement is indicated.

Special considerations

▶ Watch closely for signs of heart failure or pulmonary edema and for adverse effects of drug therapy.

▶ Teach the patient about diet restrictions, medications, and the importance of consistent follow-up care.

▶ If the patient has surgery, watch for hypotension, arrhythmias, and thrombus formation. Monitor vital signs, arterial blood gas values, intake, output, daily weight, blood chemistries, chest X-rays, and pulmonary artery catheter readings.

REFERENCES

1. Sims, J.M., and Miracle, V.A. "An Overview of Mitral Valve Prolapse," *Dimensions in Critical Care Nursing* 26(4):145-49, July-August 2007.
2. Phillips, D. "Aortic Stenosis: A Review," *AANA Journal* 74(4):309-15, August 2006.
3. Shipton, B., and Wahba, H. "Valvular Heart Disease: Review and Update," *American Family Physician* 63(11):2201-208, June 2001.

Respiratory disorders

ACUTE RESPIRATORY DISTRESS SYNDROME

Acute respiratory distress syndrome (ARDS) is a form of noncardiogenic pulmonary edema that causes acute respiratory failure. It results from an increased permeability of the alveolocapillary membrane. Fluid accumulates in the lung interstitium, alveolar spaces, and small airways, causing the lung to stiffen. Effective ventilation is thus impaired, prohibiting adequate oxygenation of pulmonary capillary blood. Severe ARDS can cause intractable and fatal hypoxemia. However, patients who recover may have little or no permanent lung damage. Acute lung injury (ALI) is sometimes grouped with ARDS as it's a milder form of ARDS.[1]

Causes and incidence

ARDS results from many respiratory and nonrespiratory insults, such as:

▶ aspiration of gastric contents
▶ sepsis (primarily gram-negative), or oxygen toxicity
▶ trauma
▶ viral, bacterial, or fungal pneumonia or microemboli (fat or air emboli or disseminated intravascular coagulation)
▶ drug overdose (barbiturates, glutethimide, or opioids) or blood transfusion

▶ smoke or chemical inhalation (nitrous oxide, chlorine, or ammonia)
▶ multiple blood transfusions
▶ pancreatitis, uremia, or miliary tuberculosis (rare)
▶ near drowning
▶ extensive burns
▶ pulmonary edema
▶ pulmonary contusion.[1]

Altered permeability of the alveolocapillary membrane causes fluid to accumulate in the interstitial space. If the pulmonary lymphatic glands can't remove this fluid, interstitial edema develops. The fluid collects in the peribronchial and peribronchiolar spaces, producing bronchiolar narrowing. Hypoxemia occurs as a result of fluid accumulation in alveoli and subsequent alveolar collapse, causing the shunting of blood through nonventilated lung regions. In addition, alveolar collapse causes a dramatic increase in lung compliance, which makes it more difficult to achieve adequate ventilation. (See *What happens in ARDS.*)

The incidence of ARDS is hard to pinpoint because different definitions of the disease are used in research, but it's thought to affect 150,000 to 200,000 people per year, with a mortality rate of 40% to 70%.

Signs and symptoms

ARDS initially produces rapid, shallow breathing and dyspnea within hours to days

What happens in ARDS

These illustrations depict the process and progress of acute respiratory distress syndrome (ARDS).

1. THE BODY RESPONDS TO INSULT

Injury reduces normal blood flow to the lungs, allowing platelets to aggregate. These platelets release such substances as serotonin (S), bradykinin (B) and, especially, histamine (H), which inflame and damage the alveolar membrane and later increase capillary permeability. At this early stage, signs and symptoms of ARDS are undetectable.

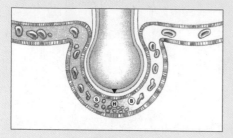

2. FLUID SHIFT CAUSES SYMPTOMS

Increased capillary permeability allows fluid to shift into the interstitial space. As a result, the patient may experience tachypnea, dyspnea, and tachycardia.

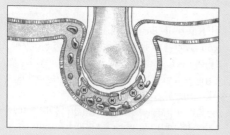

3. PULMONARY EDEMA RESULTS

As capillary permeability continues to increase, shifting of proteins and fluid increases interstitial osmotic pressure and causes pulmonary edema. At this stage, the patient may experience increased tachypnea, dyspnea, and cyanosis. Hypoxia (usually unresponsive to increased FIO_2), decreased pulmonary compliance, and crackles and rhonchi may also develop.

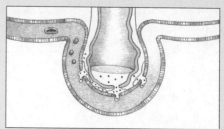

4. ALVEOLI COLLAPSE

Fluid in the alveoli and decreased blood flow damage surfactant in the alveoli, reducing the cells' ability to produce more surfactant. Without surfactant, alveoli collapse, impairing gas exchange. Look for thick, frothy sputum and marked hypoxemia with increased respiratory distress.

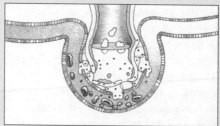

(continued)

What happens in ARDS *(continued)*

5. GAS EXCHANGE SLOWS
The patient breathes faster, but sufficient oxygen (O_2) can't cross the alveolocapillary membrane. Carbon dioxide (CO_2), however, crosses more easily and is lost with every exhalation. Both O_2 and CO_2 levels in the blood decrease. Look for increased tachypnea, hypoxemia, and hypocapnia.

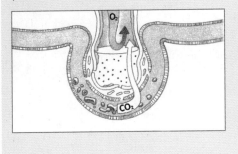

6. METABOLIC ACIDOSIS OCCURS
Pulmonary edema worsens. Meanwhile, inflammation leads to fibrosis, which further impedes gas exchange. The resulting hypoxemia leads to metabolic acidosis. At this stage, look for increased partial pressure of arterial carbon dioxide, decreased pH and partial pressure of arterial oxygen, decreased bicarbonate levels, and mental confusion.

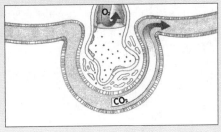

of the initial injury (sometimes after the patient's condition appears to have stabilized). Hypoxemia develops, causing an increased drive for ventilation. Because of the effort required to expand the stiff lung, intercostal and suprasternal retractions result. Fluid accumulation produces crackles and rhonchi; worsening hypoxemia causes restlessness, apprehension, mental sluggishness, motor dysfunction, and tachycardia (possibly with transient increased arterial blood pressure).

The older patient may appear to do well following an initial episode of ARDS. Symptoms commonly appear 2 to 3 days later.

Severe ARDS causes overwhelming hypoxemia. If uncorrected, this results in hypotension, decreasing urine output, respiratory and metabolic acidosis and, eventually, ventricular fibrillation or standstill.

Complications
▶ Metabolic and respiratory acidosis
▶ Cardiac arrest

Diagnosis
ARDS is diagnosed using the following criteria established by the North American-European Consensus Conference:
▶ The patient has an acute onset of lung injury.
▶ Chest X-ray shows diffuse bilateral infiltrates.
▶ Ratio of partial pressure of arterial oxygen (Pa_{O_2}) to fraction of inspired oxygen ($F_{I_{O_2}}$) is less than 200 mm Hg (in ALI, ratio is less than 300 mm Hg) (normal is 500 mm Hg).
▶ Pulmonary artery wedge pressure is less than 19 mm Hg with no clinical signs of heart failure.[1]

On room air, arterial blood gas (ABG) analysis initially shows decreased Pa_{O_2} (less than 60 mm Hg) and Pa_{CO_2} (less than 35 mm Hg). The resulting pH usually reflects respiratory alkalosis. As ARDS becomes more severe, ABG analysis shows respiratory acidosis (increasing Pa_{CO_2} [more than 45 mm Hg]), metabolic acidosis (decreasing

Are pulmonary artery catheters becoming outdated?

Studies have focused on the use of pulmonary artery catheters compared with central venous access devices to guide treatment of acute lung injuries. The studies have shown that pulmonary artery catheters don't improve the patient's survival, contrary to popular opinion. They have also shown that patients with central venous access devices actually had fewer complications than patients with pulmonary artery catheters.[3]

bicarbonate [less than 22 mEq/L]), and a decreasing PaO_2 despite oxygen therapy.

Here is other relevant information about diagnostic tests:

▶ Pulmonary artery catheterization helps identify the cause of pulmonary edema (cardiac versus noncardiac) by evaluating pulmonary artery wedge pressure; allows collection of pulmonary artery blood, which shows decreased oxygen saturation, reflecting tissue hypoxia; measures pulmonary artery pressure; measures cardiac output by thermodilution techniques; and provides information to allow calculation of the percentage of blood shunted through the lungs. (See *Are pulmonary artery catheters becoming outdated?*)

▶ Serial chest X-rays initially show bilateral infiltrates. In later stages, a ground-glass appearance and eventually (as hypoxemia becomes irreversible) "whiteouts" of both lung fields are apparent. Medical personnel can differentiate ARDS from heart failure by noting the following on serial chest X-rays:
– normal cardiac silhouette
– diffuse bilateral infiltrates that tend to be more peripheral and patchy, as opposed to the usual perihilar "bat wing" appearance of cardiogenic pulmonary edema
– fewer pleural effusions.

Differential diagnosis must rule out cardiogenic pulmonary edema, pulmonary vasculitis, and diffuse pulmonary hemorrhage. To establish the etiology, laboratory work should include sputum Gram stain, culture

and sensitivity tests, and blood cultures to detect infections; a toxicology screen for drug ingestion; and, when pancreatitis is a consideration, a serum amylase determination.

Treatment

When possible, treatment is designed to correct the underlying cause of ARDS as well as to prevent progression and the potentially fatal complications of hypoxemia and respiratory acidosis. Treatment of the underlying cause, such as infections like pneumonia or health care acquired infections, is important to decrease mortality.[2] Supportive medical care consists of administering humidified oxygen with continuous positive airway pressure. Hypoxemia that doesn't respond adequately to these measures requires ventilatory support with intubation, volume ventilation, and positive end-expiratory pressure (PEEP). Literature also suggests that the use of lung protective ventilation with small tidal volumes is beneficial.[2] Inhaled nitric oxide may be used to dilate pulmonary vessels and provide muscle relaxation.[1] Placing the patient in the prone position leads to substantial improvement in arterial oxygenation. However, there needs to be more research regarding this intervention because there's no agreement about how long the patient should be kept in a prone position.[4]

Other supportive measures include fluid restriction, nutrition support, diuretics, and

correction of electrolyte and acid-base abnormalities.

When ARDS requires mechanical ventilation, sedatives, opioids, or neuromuscular blocking agents may be ordered to optimize ventilation. Treatment to reverse severe metabolic acidosis with sodium bicarbonate may be necessary, although in severe cases, this may worsen the acidosis if carbon dioxide can't be cleared adequately. Use of fluids and vasopressors may be required to maintain blood pressure. Infections require appropriate anti-infective therapy.

Special considerations

ARDS requires careful monitoring and supportive care.

▶ Frequently assess the patient's respiratory status. Be alert for retractions on inspiration. Note the rate, rhythm, and depth of respirations; watch for dyspnea and the use of accessory muscles of respiration. On auscultation, listen for adventitious or diminished breath sounds. Check for clear, frothy sputum, which may indicate pulmonary edema.

▶ Observe and document the hypoxemic patient's neurologic status (level of consciousness and mental status).

▶ Maintain a patent airway by suctioning, using sterile, nontraumatic technique. Ensure adequate humidification to help liquefy tenacious secretions.

▶ Closely monitor heart rate and blood pressure. Watch for arrhythmias that may result from hypoxemia, acid-base disturbances, or electrolyte imbalance. With pulmonary artery catheterization, know the desired pressure levels. Check readings often, and watch for decreasing mixed venous oxygen saturation.

▶ Monitor serum electrolytes, and correct imbalances. Measure intake and output; weigh the patient daily.

▶ Check ventilator settings frequently, and empty condensate from tubing promptly to ensure maximum oxygen delivery. Monitor ABG studies and pulse oximetry. The patient with severe hypoxemia may need controlled mechanical ventilation with positive pressure. Give sedatives, as needed, to reduce restlessness.

▶ Because PEEP may decrease cardiac output, check for hypotension, tachycardia, and decreased urine output. Suction only as needed to maintain PEEP or use an in-line suctioning apparatus. Reposition the patient often, and record an increase in secretions, temperature, or hypotension that may indicate a deteriorating condition. Monitor peak pressures during ventilation. Because of stiff, noncompliant lungs, the patient is at high risk for barotrauma (pneumothorax), evidenced by increased peak pressures, decreased breath sounds on one side, and restlessness.[5]

▶ If the patient is placed in a prone position, monitor the patient and time carefully because turning the patient too early will interrupt the benefits of keeping the patient in the prone position.[1]

▶ Monitor nutrition, maintain joint mobility, and prevent skin breakdown. Accurately record calorie intake. Give tube feedings and parenteral nutrition, as ordered. Perform passive range-of-motion exercises or help the patient perform active exercises, if possible. Provide meticulous skin care. Plan patient care to allow periods of uninterrupted sleep.

▶ Provide emotional support to the patient and family. Warn them that recovering from ARDS will take some time and that the patient will feel weak for a while.

▶ Watch for and immediately report all respiratory changes in the patient with injuries that may adversely affect the lungs (especially during the 2- to 3-day period after the injury, when the patient may appear to be improving).

REFERENCES

1. Pruitt, B. "Take an Evidence-Based Approach to Treating Acute Lung Injury," *Critical Care Insider* 37(Supp.):14-18, May 2007.

2. Ware, L. B., and Matthay, M.A. "The Acute Respiratory Distress Syndrome," *New England Journal of Medicine* 342(18):1334-48, May 2000.

3. National Heart, Lung, and Blood Institute Acute Respiratory Distress Syndrome (ARDS) Clinical Trials Network, et al. "Pulmonary-Artery versus Central Venous Catheter to Guide Treatment of Acute Lung Injury," *New England Journal of Medicine* 354(21):2213-24, May 2006.

4. Vollman, K.M. "Prone Positioning in the Patient Who Has Acute Respiratory Distress Syndrome: The Art and Science," *Critical Care Nursing Clinics of North America* 16(3):319-36, September 2004.

5. Petty, T.L. "Tidal Volumes in ARDS and Meta-Analysis," *American Journal of Respiratory and Critical Care Medicine* 167(6):933, March 2003.

ATELECTASIS

Atelectasis is the incomplete expansion of lobules (clusters of alveoli) or lung segments, which may result in partial or complete lung collapse. Because parts of the lung are unavailable for gas exchange, unoxygenated blood passes through these areas unchanged, resulting in hypoxemia. Atelectasis may be chronic or acute. Many patients undergoing upper abdominal or thoracic surgery experience acute atelectasis to some degree.[1] The prognosis depends on prompt removal of any airway obstruction, relief of hypoxemia, and reexpansion of the collapsed lung.

Causes and incidence

Atelectasis commonly results from an occlusion of the large bronchus by a mucus plug or other obstruction.[1] It's present in many patients with chronic obstructive pulmonary disease, bronchiectasis, or cystic fibrosis and in those who smoke heavily. (Smoking increases mucus production and damages cilia.) Atelectasis may also result from occlu-

sion by foreign bodies, bronchogenic carcinoma, and inflammatory lung disease.

Other causes include respiratory distress syndrome of the neonate (hyaline membrane disease), oxygen toxicity, and pulmonary edema, in which alveolar surfactant changes increase surface tension and permit complete alveolar deflation.

External compression, which inhibits full lung expansion, or any condition that makes deep breathing painful, may also cause atelectasis. Such compression or pain may result from abdominal surgical incisions, rib fractures, pleuritic chest pain, tight dressings around the chest, stab wounds, impalement accidents, car accidents in which the driver slams into the steering column, or obesity (which elevates the diaphragm and reduces tidal volume).

Prolonged immobility may also cause atelectasis by producing preferential ventilation of one area of the lung over another. Mechanical ventilation using constant small tidal volumes without intermittent deep breaths may also result in atelectasis. Central nervous system depression (as in drug overdose) eliminates periodic sighing and is a predisposing factor of progressive atelectasis.

Atelectasis postoperatively is very common, with an incidence of 90% for patients who receive general anesthesia.[2]

Signs and symptoms

Clinical effects vary with the cause of collapse, the degree of hypoxemia, and any underlying disease but generally include some degree of dyspnea. Atelectasis of a small area of the lung may produce only minimal symptoms that subside without specific treatment. However, massive collapse can produce severe dyspnea, anxiety, cyanosis, diaphoresis, peripheral circulatory collapse, tachycardia, and substernal or intercostal retraction. Also, atelectasis may result in compensatory hyperinflation of unaffected areas of the lung, mediastinal shift to the affected side,

and elevation of the ipsilateral hemidiaphragm.

Complications
▶ Acute respiratory failure
▶ Pneumonia
▶ Bronchiectasis
▶ Sepsis
▶ Pleural effusion and empyema

Diagnosis
Diagnosis requires an accurate patient history, a physical examination, and a chest X-ray. Auscultation reveals diminished or bronchial breath sounds. When much of the lung is collapsed, percussion reveals dullness. However, extensive areas of "microatelectasis" may exist without abnormalities on the chest X-ray. In widespread atelectasis, the chest X-ray shows characteristic horizontal lines in the lower lung zones. With segmental or lobar collapse, characteristic dense shadows commonly associated with hyperinflation of neighboring lung zones are also apparent. If the cause is unknown, diagnostic procedures may include bronchoscopy to rule out an obstructing neoplasm or a foreign body.

Treatment
Treatment includes incentive spirometry, frequent coughing, and deep-breathing exercises. If atelectasis is secondary to mucus plugging, mucolytics, chest percussion, and postural drainage may be used. If these measures fail, bronchoscopy may be helpful in removing secretions. Humidity and bronchodilators can improve mucociliary clearance and dilate airways.

Atelectasis secondary to an obstructing neoplasm may require surgery or radiation therapy. Postoperative thoracic and abdominal surgery patients require analgesics to facilitate deep breathing, which minimizes the risk of atelectasis.

Special considerations
▶ To prevent atelectasis, encourage the postoperative or other high-risk patient to cough and deep-breathe every hour while awake.[3] To minimize pain during coughing exercises, splint the incision; teach the patient this technique as well. Gently reposition the patient often, and encourage ambulation as soon as possible. Administer adequate analgesics.
▶ If mechanical ventilation is used, tidal volume should be maintained at appropriate levels to ensure adequate expansion of the lungs. Use the sigh mechanism on the ventilator, if appropriate, to intermittently increase tidal volume at the rate of 10 to 15 sighs/hour.
▶ Use an incentive spirometer to encourage deep inspiration through positive reinforcement. Teach the patient how to use the spirometer, and encourage him to use it once every hour while awake.
▶ Humidify inspired air and encourage adequate fluid intake to mobilize secretions. To promote loosening and clearance of secretions, encourage deep-breathing and coughing exercises and use postural drainage and chest percussion.
▶ If the patient is intubated or uncooperative, provide suctioning, as needed. Use sedatives with discretion because they depress respirations and the cough reflex as well as suppress sighing. However, remember that the patient won't cooperate with treatment if he's in pain.
▶ Assess breath sounds and ventilatory status frequently; report changes at once.
▶ Teach the patient about respiratory care, including postural drainage, coughing, and deep breathing.[4]
▶ Encourage the patient to stop smoking and lose weight, as needed. Refer him to appropriate support groups for help.
▶ Provide reassurance and emotional support; the patient may be anxious due to hypoxia or respiratory distress.

REFERENCES

1. The Merck Manuals Online Medical Library (2003 February). "Atelectasis" [Online]. Available at *www.merck.com/mmhe/print/sec04/ch048/ch048a.html.*
2. Pruitt, B. "Help Your Patient Combat Postoperative Atelectasis," *Nursing* 36(5):64hn1-64hn6, May 2006.
3. Westerdahl, E., et al. "Deep-Breathing Exercises Reduce Atelectasis and Improve Pulmonary Function after Coronary Artery Bypass Surgery," *Chest* 128(5):3482-88, November 2005.
4. McCool, F.D., and Rosen, M.J. "Nonpharmacologic Airway Clearance Therapies: ACCP Evidence-Based Clinical Practice Guidelines," *Chest* 129(1 Suppl):250S-259S, January 2006.

CHRONIC OBSTRUCTIVE PULMONARY DISEASE

Chronic obstructive pulmonary disease (COPD) is chronic airway obstruction that results from emphysema or chronic bronchitis or both disorders together.[1] (See *Types of chronic obstructive pulmonary disease,* pages 76 and 77. Also see *Three types of emphysema,* page 78.) It doesn't always produce symptoms and causes only minimal disability in many patients. However, COPD tends to worsen over time.

Causes and incidence

Predisposing factors include cigarette smoking, recurrent or chronic respiratory infections, air pollution, secondhand smoke, occupational exposure to chemicals, and allergies. Smoking is by far the most important of these factors—it impairs ciliary action and macrophage function, inflames airways, increases mucus production, destroys alveolar septae, and causes peribronchiolar fibrosis. Early inflammatory changes may reverse if the patient stops smoking before lung destruction is extensive. Familial and hereditary factors (such as deficiency of alpha$_1$-antitrypsin) may also predispose a person to COPD.[1]

The most common chronic lung disease, COPD (also known as *chronic obstructive lung disease*) affects an estimated 11.4 million Americans, and its incidence is rising. It's the fourth leading cause of death in the United States with females dying more frequently than males. It affects more males than females, probably because until recently males were more likely to smoke heavily. Emphysema and chronic bronchitis occur mostly in people older than age 45, and chronic bronchitis is twice as likely to be diagnosed in females than males.

Signs and symptoms

The typical patient, a long-term cigarette smoker, has no symptoms until middle age. His ability to exercise or do strenuous work gradually starts to decline, and he begins to develop a productive cough. These signs are subtle at first, but become more pronounced as the patient gets older and the disease progresses. Eventually the patient may develop dyspnea on minimal exertion, frequent respiratory infections, intermittent or continuous hypoxemia, and grossly abnormal pulmonary function studies.

Complications

▶ Severe dyspnea
▶ Overwhelming disability
▶ Cor pulmonale
▶ Severe respiratory failure
▶ Death

Diagnosis

For specific diagnostic tests used to determine COPD, see *Types of chronic obstructive pulmonary disease,* pages 76 and 77.

Treatment

Treatment is designed to relieve symptoms and prevent complications. Because most patients with COPD receive outpatient treatment, they need comprehensive teaching to

Types of chronic obstructive pulmonary disease

DISEASE	CAUSES AND PATHOPHYSIOLOGY	CLINICAL FEATURES
Chronic bronchitis • Excessive mucus production with productive cough for at least 3 months per year for 2 successive years • Only a minority of patients with the clinical syndrome of chronic bronchitis develop significant airway obstruction.	• Severity of disease related to the amount and duration of smoking; respiratory infection exacerbates symptoms • Hypertrophy and hyperplasia of bronchial mucous glands, increased goblet cells, damage to cilia, squamous metaplasia of columnar epithelium, and chronic leukocytic and lymphocytic infiltration of bronchial walls; widespread inflammation, distortion, narrowing of airways, and mucus within the airways produce resistance in small airways and cause severe ventilation-perfusion imbalance	• Insidious onset, with productive cough and exertional dyspnea predominant symptoms • *Other signs and symptoms:* upper respiratory infections associated with increased sputum production and worsening dyspnea, which take progressively longer to resolve; copious sputum (gray, white, or yellow); weight gain due to edema; cyanosis; tachypnea; wheezing; prolonged expiratory time; and use of accessory muscles of respiration • Complications include recurrent respiratory tract infections, cor pulmonale, and polycythemia.
Emphysema • Abnormal, irreversible enlargement of air spaces distal to terminal bronchioles due to destruction of alveolar walls, resulting in decreased elastic recoil properties of lungs • Most common cause of death from respiratory disease in the United States	• Cigarette smoking and congenital deficiency of alpha-antitrypsin • Recurrent inflammation associated with release of proteolytic enzymes from cells in lungs causes bronchiolar and alveolar wall damage and, ultimately, destruction. Loss of lung supporting structure results in decreased elastic recoil and airway collapse on expiration. Destruction of alveolar walls decreases surface area for gas exchange.	• Insidious onset, with dyspnea the predominant symptom • *Other signs and symptoms of long-term disease:* anorexia, weight loss, malaise, barrel chest, use of accessory muscles of respiration, prolonged expiratory period with grunting, pursed-lip breathing, and tachypnea • *Complications* include recurrent respiratory tract infections, cor pulmonale, and respiratory failure.

help them comply with therapy and understand the nature of this chronic, progressive disease. If programs in pulmonary rehabilitation are available, encourage patients to enroll.[2]

Oxygen therapy is given to relieve hypoxia.[1,3]

Urge the patient to stop smoking. Provide smoking cessation counseling, or refer him to a program.[6] Avoid other respiratory irritants, such as secondhand smoke, aerosol spray products, and outdoor air pollution. An air conditioner with an air filter in his home may be helpful.

CONFIRMING DIAGNOSTIC MEASURES	MANAGEMENT
• *Physical examination:* barrel chest, rhonchi and wheezes on auscultation, prolonged expiration, jugular vein distention, and pedal edema • *Chest X-ray:* may show hyperinflation and increased bronchovascular markings • *PFTs:* increased residual volume, decreased vital capacity and forced expiratory volumes, and normal static compliance and diffusing capacity • *ABG analysis:* decreased partial pressure of arterial oxygen (Pao_2), normal or increased partial pressure of arterial carbon dioxide ($Paco_2$) • *Electrocardiogram (ECG):* may show atrial arrhythmias; peaked P waves in leads II, III, and aV_F; and, occasionally, right ventricular hypertrophy	• Antibiotics for infections • Avoidance of smoking and air pollutants • Bronchodilators to relieve bronchospasm and facilitate mucociliary clearance • Adequate fluid intake and chest physiotherapy to mobilize secretions • Ultrasonic or mechanical nebulizer treatments to loosen secretions and aid in mobilization • Occasionally, corticosteroids • Diuretics for edema • Oxygen for hypoxemia or cor pulmonale
• *Physical examination:* barrel chest, hyperresonance on percussion, decreased breath sounds, expiratory prolongation, and quiet heart sounds • *Chest X-ray:* in advanced disease, flattened diaphragm, reduced vascular markings at lung periphery, hyperexpansion of lungs, enlarged anteroposterior chest diameter, and large retrosternal air space • *Computed tomography scan:* may show emphysema • *PFTs:* increased residual volume, total lung capacity, and compliance; decreased vital capacity, diffusing capacity, and expiratory volumes • *ABG analysis:* reduced Pao_2 with normal $Paco_2$ until late in disease • *ECG:* tall, symmetrical P waves in leads II, III, and aV_F; vertical QRS axis; signs of right ventricular hypertrophy late in disease • *Red blood cell count:* increased hemoglobin late in disease when persistent severe hypoxia is present	• Oxygen at low-flow settings to treat hypoxia • Avoidance of smoking and air pollutants • Breathing techniques to control dyspnea • Treatment only slightly helpful for emphysema component of chronic obstructive pulmonary disease • Lung volume reduction surgery for selected patients

The patient is usually treated with beta-agonist bronchodilators (albuterol or salmeterol), anticholinergic bronchodilators (ipratropium), and corticosteroids (beclomethasone or triamcinolone).[3] These are usually given by metered-dose inhaler, requiring that the patient be taught the correct administration technique.

Antibiotics are used to treat respiratory infections. Stress the need to complete the prescribed course of antibiotic therapy.

Three types of emphysema

A Panacinar (panlobular): destroys alveoli and alveolar ducts; associated with aging and alpha$_1$-antitrypsin deficiency
B Paraseptal (distal acinar): commonly causes spontaneous pneumothorax in young adults
C Centriacinar (centrilobular): associated with chronic bronchitis and smoking; destroys respiratory bronchioles

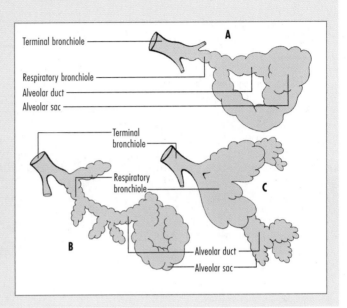

Special considerations

▶ Teach the patient and his family how to recognize early signs of infection; warn the patient to avoid contact with people with respiratory infections. Encourage good oral hygiene to help prevent infection. Pneumococcal vaccination and annual influenza vaccinations are important preventive measures.[6]
▶ To promote ventilation and reduce air trapping, teach the patient to breathe slowly, prolong expirations to two to three times the duration of inspiration, and to exhale through pursed lips.
▶ To help mobilize secretions, teach the patient how to cough effectively. If the patient with copious secretions has difficulty mobilizing secretions, teach his family how to perform postural drainage and chest physiotherapy. If secretions are thick, urge the patient to drink 12 to 15 glasses of fluid per day. A home humidifier may be beneficial, particularly in the winter.[4]

▶ Administer low concentrations of oxygen as ordered. Perform blood gas analysis to determine the patient's oxygen needs and to avoid carbon dioxide narcosis. If the patient is to continue oxygen therapy at home, teach him how to use the equipment correctly. The patient with COPD rarely requires more than 2 to 3 L/minute to maintain adequate oxygenation. Higher flow rates will further increase the partial pressure of arterial oxygen, but the patient whose ventilatory drive is largely based on hypoxemia commonly develops markedly increased partial pressure of arterial carbon dioxide tensions. In these cases, chemoreceptors in the brain are relatively insensitive to the increase in carbon dioxide. Teach the patient and his family that excessive oxygen therapy may eliminate the hypoxic respiratory drive, causing confusion and drowsiness, signs of carbon dioxide narcosis.
▶ Emphasize the importance of a balanced diet. Because the patient may tire easily when eating, suggest that he eat frequent,

small meals and consider using oxygen, administered by nasal cannula, during meals.

▶ Help the patient and his family adjust their lifestyles to accommodate the limitations imposed by this debilitating chronic disease. Instruct the patient to allow for daily rest periods and to exercise daily as his physician directs.[5]

▶ As COPD progresses, encourage the patient to discuss his fears.

▶ To help prevent COPD, advise all patients, especially those with a family history of COPD or those in its early stages, not to smoke.

▶ Assist in the early detection of COPD by urging persons to have periodic physical examinations, including spirometry and medical evaluation of a chronic cough, and to seek treatment for recurring respiratory infections promptly.[6]

▶ Lung volume reduction surgery is a new procedure for carefully selected patients with emphysema, primarily. Nonfunctional parts of the lung (tissue filled with disease and providing little ventilation or perfusion) are surgically removed. Removal allows more functional lung tissue to expand and the diaphragm to return to its normally elevated position.

REFERENCES

1. DeMeo, D.L. "Genetic Determinants of Emphysema Distribution in the National Emphysema Treatment Trial," *American Journal of Respiratory and Critical Care Medicine* 176(1):42-48, July 2007.
2. Ries, A.L., et al. "Pulmonary Rehabilitation: Joint ACCP/AACVPR Evidence-Based Clinical Practice Guidelines," *Chest* 131(5 Suppl):4S-42S, May 2007.
3. Qaseem, A., et al. "Diagnosis and Management of Stable Chronic Obstructive Pulmonary Disease: A Clinical Practice Guideline from the American College of Physicians," *Annals of Internal Medicine* 147(9):633-38, November 2007.
4. Braman, S.S. "Chronic Cough Due to Chronic Bronchitis: ACCP Evidence-Based Clinical Practice Guidelines," *Chest* 129(1 Suppl):104S-115S, January 2006.
5. McHugh, G. et al. "Caring for Patients with COPD and Their Families in the Community," *British Journal of Community Nursing* 12(5):219-22, May 2007.
6. Global Initiative for Chronic Constructive Lung Disease (2007 December). "Global Strategy for the Diagnosis, Management, and Prevention of Chronic Obstructive Pulmonary Disease" [Online]. Available at *www.goldcopd.com/Guidelineitem.asp?l1=2&l2=1&intId=989.*

COR PULMONALE

Cor pulmonale is right ventricular hypertrophy, dilation, or both as a result of pulmonary hypertension caused by pulmonary disorders.[1] Invariably, cor pulmonale follows some disorder of the lungs, pulmonary vessels, chest wall, or respiratory control center. For instance, chronic obstructive pulmonary disease (COPD) produces pulmonary hypertension, which leads to right ventricular hypertrophy and right-sided heart failure. Because cor pulmonale generally occurs late during the course of COPD and other irreversible diseases, the prognosis is generally poor.

Causes and incidence

Fifty percent of the cases of cor pulmonale are caused by COPD.[2]

Other respiratory disorders that produce cor pulmonale include:

▶ obstructive lung diseases—for example, bronchiectasis and cystic fibrosis

▶ restrictive lung diseases—for example, pneumoconiosis, interstitial pneumonitis, scleroderma, and sarcoidosis

▶ loss of lung tissue after extensive lung surgery

▶ congenital cardiac shunts—such as a ventricular septal defect

▶ pulmonary vascular diseases—for example, recurrent thromboembolism, primary

What happens in cor pulmonale

Although pulmonary restrictive disorders (such as fibrosis or obesity), obstructive disorders (such as bronchitis), or primary vascular disorders (such as recurrent pulmonary emboli) may cause cor pulmonale, these disorders share this common pathway.

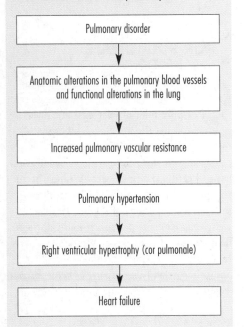

Pulmonary capillary destruction and pulmonary vasoconstriction (usually secondary to hypoxia) reduce the area of the pulmonary vascular bed. Thus, pulmonary vascular resistance is increased, causing pulmonary hypertension. To compensate for the extra work needed to force blood through the lungs, the right ventricle dilates and hypertrophies. In response to low oxygen content, the bone marrow produces more red blood cells (RBCs), causing erythrocytosis. When hematocrit (HCT) exceeds 55%, blood viscosity increases, which further aggravates pulmonary hypertension and increases the hemodynamic load on the right ventricle. Right-sided heart failure is the result. (See *What happens in cor pulmonale.*)

Cor pulmonale accounts for about 6% to 7% of all types of heart disease in the United States.[2] It's most common in areas of the world where the incidence of cigarette smoking and COPD is high; cor pulmonale affects middle-age to elderly males more often than females, but incidence in females is increasing. In children, cor pulmonale may be a complication of cystic fibrosis, hemosiderosis, upper airway obstruction, scleroderma, extensive bronchiectasis, neurologic diseases affecting respiratory muscles, or abnormalities of the respiratory control center.

Signs and symptoms

As long as the heart can compensate for the increased pulmonary vascular resistance, clinical features reflect the underlying disorder and occur mostly in the respiratory system. They include chronic productive cough, exertional dyspnea, wheezing respirations, fatigue, and weakness. Progression of cor pulmonale is associated with dyspnea (even at rest) that worsens on exertion, tachypnea, orthopnea, edema, weakness, and right upper quadrant discomfort. Chest examination reveals findings characteristic of the underlying lung disease.[3]

Signs of cor pulmonale and right-sided heart failure include dependent edema; dis-

pulmonary hypertension, schistosomiasis, and pulmonary vasculitis
▶ respiratory insufficiency without pulmonary disease—for example, in chest wall disorders such as kyphoscoliosis, neuromuscular incompetence due to muscular dystrophy and amyotrophic lateral sclerosis, polymyositis, and spinal cord lesions above C6
▶ obesity hypoventilation syndrome (pickwickian syndrome) and upper airway obstruction
▶ living at high altitudes (chronic mountain sickness).

tended jugular veins; prominent parasternal or epigastric cardiac impulse; hepatojugular reflux; an enlarged, tender liver; ascites; and tachycardia. Decreased cardiac output may cause a weak pulse and hypotension. Chest examination yields various findings, depending on the underlying cause of cor pulmonale.

In COPD, auscultation reveals wheezing, rhonchi, and diminished breath sounds. When the disease is secondary to upper airway obstruction or damage to central nervous system respiratory centers, chest findings may be normal, except for a right ventricular lift, gallop rhythm, and loud pulmonic component of S_2. Tricuspid insufficiency produces a pansystolic murmur heard at the lower left sternal border; its intensity increases on inspiration, distinguishing it from a murmur due to mitral valve disease. A right ventricular early murmur that increases on inspiration can be heard at the left sternal border or over the epigastrium. A systolic pulmonic ejection click may also be heard. Alterations in the patient's level of consciousness may occur.

Complications
▶ Right- and left-sided heart failure
▶ Hepatomegaly
▶ Edema
▶ Ascites
▶ Pleural effusion
▶ Thromboembolism due to polycythemia

Diagnosis
▶ Pulmonary artery pressure measurements show increased right ventricular and pulmonary artery pressures, stemming from increased pulmonary vascular resistance. Right ventricular systolic and pulmonary artery systolic pressures will exceed 30 mm Hg. Pulmonary artery diastolic pressure will exceed 15 mm Hg.
▶ Echocardiography or angiography indicates right ventricular enlargement; echocardiography can estimate pulmonary artery pressure while also ruling out structural and congenital lesions.[5]
▶ Chest X-ray shows large central pulmonary arteries and suggests right ventricular enlargement by rightward enlargement of the heart's silhouette on an anterior chest film.
▶ Arterial blood gas (ABG) analysis shows decreased partial pressure of arterial oxygen (Pao_2; typically less than 70 mm Hg and usually no more than 90 mm Hg on room air).
▶ Electrocardiogram frequently shows arrhythmias, such as premature atrial and ventricular contractions and atrial fibrillation during severe hypoxia; it may also show right bundle-branch block, right axis deviation, prominent P waves and inverted T wave in right precordial leads, and right ventricular hypertrophy.
▶ Pulmonary function tests show results consistent with the underlying pulmonary disease.
▶ HCT is typically greater than 50%.

Treatment
Treatment of cor pulmonale is designed to reduce hypoxemia, increase the patient's exercise tolerance and, when possible, correct the underlying condition.

In addition to bed rest, treatment may include administration of:
▶ a cardiac glycoside (digoxin)
▶ antibiotics when respiratory infection is present; culture and sensitivity of a sputum specimen helps select an antibiotic
▶ potent pulmonary artery vasodilators (such as diazoxide, nitroprusside, hydralazine, angiotensin-converting enzyme inhibitors, calcium channel blockers, or prostaglandins) in primary pulmonary hypertension
▶ nesiritide for patients with decompensated cor pulmonale to promote diuresis, dilation of systemic and pulmonary vessels, and decrease circulating levels of endothelin and aldosterone[4]

▶ a low-sodium diet, restricted fluid intake, and diuretics such as furosemide to reduce edema
▶ phlebotomy to reduce the RBC count
▶ anticoagulants to reduce the risk of thromboembolism
▶ oxygen by mask or cannula in concentrations ranging from 24% to 40%, depending on PaO_2, as necessary; in acute cases, therapy may also include mechanical ventilation.[2]

Depending on the underlying cause, some variations in treatment may be indicated. For example, a tracheotomy may be necessary if the patient has an upper airway obstruction. Steroids may be used in the patient with a vasculitis autoimmune phenomenon or acute exacerbations of COPD.

Special considerations

▶ Plan diet carefully with the patient and staff dietitian. Because the patient may lack energy and tire easily when eating, provide small, frequent feedings rather than three heavy meals.
▶ Prevent fluid retention by limiting the patient's fluid intake to 1 to 2 qt (1 to 2 L)/day and providing a low-sodium diet.
▶ Monitor serum potassium levels closely if the patient is receiving diuretics. Low serum potassium levels can increase the risk of arrhythmias associated with digoxin.
▶ Watch the patient for signs of digoxin toxicity, such as complaints of anorexia, nausea, vomiting, halos around visual images, and color perception shifts. Monitor for cardiac arrhythmias. Teach the patient to check his radial pulse before taking digoxin or any cardiac glycoside. He should be instructed to notify the physician if he detects changes in pulse rate.
▶ Reposition the bedridden patient often to prevent atelectasis.
▶ Provide meticulous respiratory care, including oxygen therapy and, for the patient with COPD, pursed-lip breathing exercises. Periodically measure ABG levels, and watch for signs of respiratory failure: changes in pulse rate, labored respirations, changes in mental status, and increased fatigue after exertion.

Before discharge, maintain the following protocol:
▶ Make sure that the patient understands the importance of maintaining a low-salt diet, weighing himself daily, and watching for increased edema. Teach him to detect edema by pressing the skin over a shin with one finger, holding it for a second or two, then checking for a finger impression. Increased weight, increased edema, or respiratory difficulty should be reported to the health care provider.
▶ Instruct the patient to plan for frequent rest periods and to do breathing exercises regularly.
▶ If the patient needs supplemental oxygen therapy at home, refer him to an agency that can help obtain the required equipment and, as necessary, arrange for follow-up examinations.
▶ If the patient has been placed on anticoagulant therapy, emphasize the need to watch for bleeding (epistaxis, hematuria, bruising) and to report signs to the physician. Also encourage him to return for periodic laboratory tests to monitor partial thromboplastin time, fibrinogen level, platelet count, HCT, hemoglobin level, and prothrombin time.
▶ Because pulmonary infection commonly exacerbates COPD and cor pulmonale, tell the patient to watch for and immediately report early signs of infection, such as increased sputum production, change in sputum color, increased coughing or wheezing, chest pain, fever, and tightness in the chest. Tell the patient to avoid crowds and persons known to have pulmonary infections, especially during the flu season. The patient should receive pneumovax and annual influenza vaccines.
▶ Warn the patient to avoid substances that may depress the ventilatory drive, such as sedatives and alcohol.

REFERENCES

1. Budev, M.M., et al. "Cor Pulmonale: An Overview," *Seminars in Respiratory and Critical Care Medicine* 24(3): 233-43, July, 2003. Available at *www.medscape.com/viewarticle/458659.*

2. Sovari, A.A. eMedicine from Web MD (2006 July 10). "Cor Pulmonale" [Online]. Available at *www.emedicine.com/med/topic449.htm.*

3. Voelkel, N.F., et al. "Right Ventricular Function and Failure: Report of a National Heart, Lung, and Blood Institute Working Group on Cellular and Molecular Mechanisms of Right Heart Failure," *Circulation* 114(17):1883-91, October 2006.

4. Kingman, M.S., et al. "Nesiritide for Pulmonary Arterial Hypertension with Decompensated Cor Pulmonale," *Progress in Cardiovascular Nursing* 20(4):168-72, Fall 2005.

5. Vieillard-Baron, A., et al. "Echo-Doppler Demonstration of Acute Cor Pulmonale at the Bedside in the Medical Intensive Care Unit," *American Journal of Critical Care Medicine* 166(10):1310-19, November 2005.

CYSTIC FIBROSIS

Cystic fibrosis (CF) is a generalized dysfunction of the exocrine glands that affects multiple organ systems. Transmitted as an autosomal recessive trait, it's the most common fatal genetic disease in white children.

CF is a chronic disease. With improvements in treatment over the past decade, the average life expectancy has risen from age 16 to age 28 and more. The median age of survival is 37 years.[1]

Causes and incidence

The gene responsible for CF, CFTF—which is located on chromosome 7—encodes a member-associated protein that involves chloride transport across epithelial membranes. More than 1,000 specific mutations of the gene are known.[2] (See *Cystic fibrosis transmission risk,* page 84.) The immediate causes of symptoms in CF are increased viscosity of bronchial, pancreatic, and other mucous gland secretions, and consequent obstruction of glandular ducts. CF accounts for almost all cases of pancreatic enzyme deficiency in children. In the United States, about 30,000 children and adults have CF.[1] Incidence is highest in Whites of northern European ancestry (1 in 3,200 live births) and lowest in Blacks (1 in 15,000 live births), Hispanics (1 in 9,200), and people of Asian ancestry (1 in 31,000). The disease occurs equally in both sexes.

Signs and symptoms

The clinical effects of CF may become apparent soon after birth or may take years to develop. They include major aberrations in sweat gland, respiratory, and GI function. Sweat gland dysfunction is the most consistent abnormality. Increased concentrations of sodium and chloride in the sweat lead to hyponatremia and hypochloremia and can eventually induce fatal shock and arrhythmias, especially in hot weather.

Respiratory symptoms reflect obstructive changes in the lungs: wheezy respirations; a dry, nonproductive paroxysmal cough; dyspnea; and tachypnea. These changes stem from thick, tenacious secretions in the bronchioles and alveoli and eventually lead to severe atelectasis and emphysema. Children with CF display a barrel chest, cyanosis, and clubbing of the fingers and toes. They suffer recurring bronchitis and pneumonia as well as associated nasal polyps and sinusitis. Death typically results from pneumonia, emphysema, or atelectasis.

The GI effects of CF occur mainly in the intestines, pancreas, and liver. One early symptom is meconium ileus; the neonate with CF doesn't excrete meconium, a dark green mucilaginous material found in the intestine at birth. He develops symptoms of intestinal obstruction, such as abdominal distention, vomiting, constipation, dehydration,

Cystic fibrosis transmission risk

The chance that a relative of a person with cystic fibrosis or a person with no family history will carry the cystic fibrosis gene appears in the chart below.

RELATIVE OF AFFECTED PERSON	CARRIER CHANCE
Brother or sister	2 in 3 (67%)
Niece or nephew	1 in 2 (50%)
Aunt or uncle	1 in 3 (33%)
First cousin	1 in 4 (25%)

NO KNOWN FAMILY HISTORY	CARRIER CHANCE
Whites	1 in 25 (4%)
Blacks	1 in 65 (1.5%)
Asians	1 in 150 (0.67%)

and electrolyte imbalance. As the child gets older, obstruction of the pancreatic ducts and resulting deficiency of trypsin, amylase, and lipase prevent the conversion and absorption of fat and protein in the GI tract. The undigested food is then excreted in frequent, bulky, foul-smelling, pale stools with a high fat content. This malabsorption induces poor weight gain, poor growth, ravenous appetite, distended abdomen, thin extremities, and sallow skin with poor turgor. The inability to absorb fats results in a deficiency of fat-soluble vitamins (A, D, E, and K), leading to clotting problems, retarded bone growth, and delayed sexual development. Males may experience azoospermia and sterility; females may experience secondary amenorrhea but can reproduce. A common complication in infants and children is rectal prolapse secondary to malnutrition and wasting of perirectal supporting tissues.

In the pancreas, fibrotic tissue, multiple cysts, thick mucus, and eventually fat replace the acini (small, saclike swellings normally found in this gland), producing symptoms of pancreatic insufficiency: insufficient insulin production, abnormal glucose tolerance, and glycosuria. About 15% of patients have ade-quate pancreatic exocrine function for normal digestion and, therefore, have a better prognosis. Biliary obstruction and fibrosis may prolong neonatal jaundice. In some patients, cirrhosis and portal hypertension may lead to esophageal varices, episodes of hematemesis and, occasionally, hepatomegaly.

Complications
▶ Bronchiectasis
▶ Pneumonia
▶ Atelectasis
▶ Hemoptysis
▶ Dehydration
▶ Distal intestinal obstructive syndrome
▶ Malnutrition
▶ Deficiency of fat-soluble vitamins
▶ Gastroesophageal reflux
▶ Nasal polyps
▶ Rectal prolapse
▶ Cor pulmonale
▶ Hepatic disease
▶ Diabetes (see *Cystic fibrosis and diabetes*)
▶ Pneumothorax
▶ Arthritis
▶ Pancreatitis
▶ Cholecystitis
▶ Hypochloremia

Cystic fibrosis and diabetes

Question: *Is cystic fibrosis-related diabetes common?*

Research: Diabetes is extremely common in people with cystic fibrosis (CF), especially as they get older. Commonly called *cystic fibrosis-related diabetes* (CFRD), it has some features of both type 1 and type 2 diabetes. People with CFRD don't make insulin because of pancreatic scarring. They exhibit insulin resistance caused by chronic underlying infections and high levels of cortisol. The researchers studied 237 children with CF (109 boys and 128 girls) to determine the history, mechanisms, and consequences of CFRD, from childhood to early adulthood. In their research, they used the oral glucose tolerance test to estimate pancreatic beta-cell function and the homeostasis model assessment to calculate insulin sensitivity.

Conclusion: The study showed that CFRD was evident at an early age, with a positive diagnosis in 20% of participants at age 15, 45% at age 20, and 70% at age 30. Impaired glucose tolerance was identified at earlier ages, with 20% of participants at age 10, 50% at age 15,

75% at age 20, and 82% at age 30 showing impairment. Most cases of CFRD were attributed to beta-cell deficiency. When CFRD developed earlier in life, it resulted in impaired nutrition and growth, lower survival rates, higher rates of lung transplantation, and increased mortality.

Application: The nurse must be aware of the prevalence of CFRD to ensure that children and young adults with CF are routinely monitored for the disorder and receive appropriate treatment. Teaching the child and his parents how to recognize the signs and symptoms of the disorder and encouraging consistent follow-up with the doctor and dietary adherence, may help delay the complications associated with CFRD.

Source: Bismuth, E., et al. "Glucose Tolerance and Insulin Secretion, Morbidity, and Death in Patients with Cystic Fibrosis," *Journal of Pediatrics* 152(4):540, April 2008.

▶ Clotting problems
▶ Retarded bone growth
▶ Delayed sexual development

Diagnosis

The Cystic Fibrosis Foundation has developed certain criteria for a definitive diagnosis: Two sweat tests using a pilocarpine solution (a sweat inducer) and the presence of leither obstructive pulmonary disease, confirmed pancreatic insufficiency or failure to thrive, or a family history of CF.

The following test results may support the diagnosis:

▶ Chest X-rays indicate early signs of obstructive lung disease.

▶ Stool specimen analysis indicates the absence of trypsin, suggesting pancreatic insufficiency.

▶ Deoxyribonucleic acid testing can now locate the presence of the Delta F 508 deletion (found in about 70% of CF patients, although the disease can cause more than 1,000 other mutations). Delta F 508 is a deletion of 1 amino acid on the CFTR protein.[2] It allows prenatal diagnosis in families with a previously affected child.

▶ Pulmonary function tests reveal decreased vital capacity, elevated residual volume due to air entrapments, and decreased forced expiratory volume in 1 second. This test is used if pulmonary exacerbation already exists.

▶ Liver enzyme tests may reveal hepatic insufficiency.

▶ Sputum culture reveals organisms that CF patients typically and chronically colonize, such as *Haemophilus influenzae, Staphylo-*

coccus aureus, *Pseudomonas aeruginosa,*
Burkholderia cepacia, Escherichia coli, and
Klebsiella pneumoniae.

P. aeruginosa is the most common—it affects 80% of patients by age 25.[3]

▶ Serum albumin measurement helps assess nutritional status.

▶ Electrolyte analysis assesses hydration status.

Treatment

The aim of treatment is to help the child lead as normal a life as possible. The type of treatment depends on the organ systems involved.

To combat electrolyte losses in sweat, salt foods generously and, in hot weather, administer sodium supplements.

To offset pancreatic enzyme deficiencies, give oral pancreatic enzymes with meals and snacks, as ordered. Maintain a diet that's low in fat, but high in protein and calories, and provide supplements of water-miscible, fat-soluble vitamins (A, D, E, and K).

Management of pulmonary dysfunction includes chest physiotherapy, postural drainage, and breathing exercises several times daily to aid removal of secretions from lungs.[5] Antihistamines are contraindicated because they have a drying effect on mucous membranes, making expectoration of mucus difficult or impossible. Aerosol therapy includes intermittent nebulizer treatments before postural drainage to loosen secretions.

Dornase alfa or DNAse (recombinant human deoxyribonuclease), genetically engineered pulmonary enzymes given by aerosol nebulizer, helps thin airway mucus, improving lung function and reducing the risk of pulmonary infection.

Pulmonary infections occur more frequently as the patient ages. Adults with CF experience at least one exacerbation a year.[3,4]

Treatment of pulmonary infection requires:

▶ broad-spectrum antimicrobials

▶ oxygen therapy as needed

▶ loosening and removal of mucopurulent secretions, using an intermittent nebulizer and postural drainage to relieve obstruction. Use of a mist tent is controversial because mist particles may become trapped in the esophagus and stomach and never even reach the lungs.

Lung transplantation may be considered in some cases. Genetic research is ongoing, with researchers hoping to cure CF by artificially inserting a "healthy" gene into a person through gene therapy. The gene would be inserted by using an intranasal form. Research on correcting the disorder before birth is promising.

Special considerations

▶ Throughout this illness, teach the patient and his family about the disease and its treatment. The Cystic Fibrosis Foundation can provide educational and support services.

▶ Although many males with CF are infertile, females may become pregnant (due to increased life expectancies). As a result, more CF patients are now facing difficult reproductive decisions. Refer such patients (or the parents of an affected child) for genetic counseling so they can discuss family planning issues or prenatal diagnosis options if they're considering having more children.

▶ Be aware that some patients have recently undergone lung transplants to reduce the effects of the disease. Also, aerosol gene therapy shows promise in reducing pulmonary symptoms.

Research indicates that the genetic defect responsible for CF has also been identified in individuals experiencing some forms of unexplained pancreatitis.

REFERENCES

1. Cystic Fibrosis Foundation (2007 June 5). "About Cystic Fibrosis" [Online]. Available at *www.cff.org/AboutCF.*

2. U.S. National Library of Medicine (2006 September). "Genetics Home Reference," [Online.] Available at *http://ghr.nlm.nih.gov/gene=cftr.*

3. Elpern, E.H. "Antibiotic Therapy for Pulmonary Exacerbations in Adults with Cystic Fibrosis," *MEDSURG Nursing* 16(5):293-97, October 2007.

4. Saiman, L., et al. "Infection Control Recommendations for Patients with Cystic Fibrosis: Microbiology, Important Pathogens, and Infection Control Practices to Prevent Patient-to-Patient Transmission," *Infection Control and Hospital Epidemiology* 24(5 Suppl):S6-52, May 2003.

5. McCool, F.D., and Rosen, M.J. "Nonpharmacologic airway clearance therapies: ACCP evidence-based clinical practice guidelines," *Chest* 129(1 Suppl):250S-59S, January 2006.

IDIOPATHIC PULMONARY FIBROSIS

Idiopathic pulmonary fibrosis (IPF) is a chronic and usually fatal interstitial pulmonary disease. About 50% of patients with IPF die within 5 years of diagnosis. Once thought to be a rare condition, it's now diagnosed with much greater frequency. IPF has been known by several other names over the years, including *cryptogenic fibrosing alveolitis, Hamman-Rich syndrome, diffuse interstitial fibrosis* and *idiopathic interstitial pneumonitis.*

The American Thoracic Society/European Respiratory Society international multidisciplinary consensus committee has defined IPF as a condition characterized by dyspnea, chronic cough, restrictive lung disease, and the histopathologic pattern of usual interstitial pneumonia.[1]

Causes and incidence

It was previously thought that the cause of IPF was inflammatory, immune, and fibrotic processes in the lung. However, despite many studies, the stimulus that begins the progression remains unknown. Current information identifies epithelial injury as the cause.[1] Also, a mutation in the SP-C protein has been found in families of patient's with IPF.[2] According to the Pulmonary Fibrosis Foundation, the pulmonary fibrosis is associated with inhaled environmental and occupational pollutants; smoking; scleroderma, rheumatoid arthritis, lupus, and sarcoidosis; certain medications; and therapeutic radiation.[2]

IPF is slightly more common in males than in females and is more common in smokers than in nonsmokers. It usually affects people ages 50 to 70.

Signs and symptoms

The usual presenting symptoms of IPF are dyspnea and a dry, hacking, and typically paroxysmal cough. Most patients have had these symptoms for several months to 2 years before seeking medical help. End-expiratory crackles, especially in the bases of the lungs, are usually heard early in the disease. Bronchial breath sounds appear later, when airway consolidation develops. Rapid, shallow breathing occurs, especially with exertion, and clubbing has been noted in more than 40% of patients. Late in the disease, cyanosis and evidence of pulmonary hypertension (augmented S_2 and S_3 gallop) commonly occur. As the disease progresses, profound hypoxemia and severe, debilitating dyspnea are the hallmark signs.

Complications

▶ Cor pulmonale
▶ Pulmonary hypertension
▶ Respiratory failure
▶ Pneumonia

Diagnosis

Diagnosis begins with a thorough patient history to exclude a more common cause of interstitial lung disease. Lung biopsy is helpful in the diagnosis of IPF. Biopsies may be

done through a thoracoscope or broncho-scope.[3]

Histologic features of the biopsy tissue vary, depending on the stage of the disease and other factors that aren't yet completely understood. The alveolar walls are swollen with chronic inflammatory cellular infiltrate composed of mononuclear cells and poly-morphonuclear leukocytes. Intra-alveolar in-flammatory cells may be found in early stages. As the disease progresses, excessive collagen and fibroblasts fill the interstitium. In advanced stages, alveolar walls are de-stroyed and are replaced by honeycombing cysts.

Chest X-rays may show one of four dis-tinct patterns: interstitial, reticulonodular, ground-glass, or honeycomb. Although chest X-rays are helpful in identifying the presence of an abnormality, they don't correlate well with histologic findings or pulmonary func-tion tests (PFTs) in determining the severity of the disease. They also don't help distin-guish inflammation from fibrosis. However, serial X-rays may help track the progression of the disease.

High-resolution computed tomography scans provide superior views of the four pat-terns seen on routine X-ray film and are used routinely to help establish the diagnosis of IPF. Research is currently under way to determine whether the four patterns of ab-normality seen on these scans correlate with responsiveness to treatment.

PFTs show reductions in vital capacity and total lung capacity and impaired diffus-ing capacity for carbon monoxide. Arterial blood gas (ABG) analysis and pulse oximetry reveal hypoxemia, which may be mild when the patient is at rest early in the disease but may become severe later in the disease. Oxygenation will always deteriorate, usually to a severe level, with exertion. Serial PFTs (especially carbon monoxide diffusing capac-ity) and ABG values may help track the course of the disease and the patient's re-sponse to treatment.

Treatment

Although it can't change the pathology of IPF, oxygen therapy can prevent the prob-lems related to dyspnea and tissue hypoxia in the early stages of the disease process. The patient may require little or no supplemental oxygen while at rest initially, but he'll need more as the disease progresses and during exertion.

No known cure exists.[2] Corticosteroids and cytotoxic drugs may be given to sup-press inflammation but are usually unsuc-cessful. Recently, interferon-gamma-1B and the combination of steroids and azathioprine plus N-acetylcysteine has shown some prom-ise in treating the disease.[1] Research for fur-ther treatment options is ongoing.

Lung transplantation may be successful for younger, otherwise healthy individuals.

Special considerations

▶ Explain all diagnostic tests to the patient, who may experience anxiety and frustration about the many tests required to establish the diagnosis.
▶ Monitor oxygenation at rest and with ex-ertion. The physician may prescribe one oxy-gen flow rate for use when the patient is at rest and a higher one for use during exer-tion, to help the patient maintain adequate oxygenation. Instruct the patient to increase his oxygen flow rate to the appropriate level for exercise.
▶ As IPF progresses, the patient's oxygen re-quirements will increase. He may need a nonrebreathing mask to supply high oxygen percentages. Eventually, maintaining ade-quate oxygenation may become impossible despite maximum oxygen flow.
▶ Most patients will need oxygen at home. Make appropriate referrals to discharge planners, respiratory care practitioners, and home equipment vendors to ensure continu-ity of care.
▶ Teach breathing, relaxation, and energy conservation techniques to help the patient manage severe dyspnea.

▶ Encourage the patient to be as active as possible. Refer him to a pulmonary rehabilitation program.

▶ Monitor the patient for adverse reactions to drug therapy.

▶ Teach the patient about prescribed medications, especially adverse effects. Teach the patient and his family members infection prevention techniques.

▶ Encourage good nutritional habits. Small, frequent meals with high nutritional value may be necessary if dyspnea interferes with eating.

▶ Provide emotional support for the patient and his family as they deal with the patient's increasing disability, dyspnea, and probable death.

REFERENCES

1. Burns, S. M. "Ask the Experts," *Critical Care Nurse,* 26(6):65-74, December 2006.
2. Pulmonary Fibrosis Foundation (2007 May 25). "Pulmonary Fibrosis" [Online]. Available at *www.pulmonaryfibrosis.org/ipf.htm.*
3. The Merck Manuals Online Medical Library (2003 February). "Idiopathic Pulmonary Fibrosis" [Online]. Available at *www.merck.com/mmhe/sec04/ch050/ch050b.html.*

PLEURAL EFFUSION AND EMPYEMA

Pleural effusion is an excess of fluid in the pleural space. Normally, this space contains a small amount of extracellular fluid that lubricates the pleural surfaces. Increased production or inadequate removal of this fluid results in pleural effusion. Empyema is the accumulation of pus and necrotic tissue in the pleural space. Blood (hemothorax) and chyle (chylothorax) may also collect in this space.

Causes and incidence

The balance of osmotic and hydrostatic pressures in parietal pleural capillaries normally results in fluid movement into the pleural space. Balanced pressures in visceral pleural capillaries promote reabsorption of this fluid. Excessive hydrostatic pressure or decreased osmotic pressure can cause excessive amounts of fluid to pass across intact capillaries. The result is a transudative pleural effusion, an ultrafiltrate of plasma-containing low concentrations of protein. Such effusions frequently result from heart failure, hepatic disease with ascites, peritoneal dialysis, hypoalbuminemia, and disorders resulting in overexpanded intravascular volume.

Exudative pleural effusions result when capillaries exhibit increased permeability with or without changes in hydrostatic and colloid osmotic pressures, allowing protein-rich fluid to leak into the pleural space. Exudative pleural effusions occur with tuberculosis (TB), subphrenic abscess, pancreatitis, bacterial or fungal pneumonitis or empyema, malignancy, pulmonary embolism with or without infarction, collagen disease (lupus erythematosus [LE] and rheumatoid arthritis), myxedema, and chest trauma.

Empyema is usually associated with infection in the pleural space. Such infection may be idiopathic or may be related to pneumonitis, carcinoma, perforation, or esophageal rupture.[4]

The incidence of pleural effusion is about 1 million per year in the United States. Most are caused by congestive heart failure, malignancy, infections, and pulmonary emboli.[1]

Signs and symptoms

Patients with pleural effusion characteristically display symptoms relating to the underlying pathologic condition but common symptoms are dyspnea, cough, and pleuritic chest pain.[2] Most patients with large effusions, particularly those with underlying pulmonary disease, complain of dyspnea. Those with effusions associated with pleurisy complain of pleuritic chest pain. Other clinical features depend on the cause of the effusion.

For instance, patients with empyema also develop fever and malaise.

Complications
▶ Atelectasis
▶ Infections
▶ Hypoxemia

Diagnosis
Auscultation of the chest reveals decreased breath sounds; percussion detects dullness over the effused area, which doesn't change with breathing. Chest X-ray shows fluid in dependent regions. However, diagnosis also requires other tests to distinguish transudative from exudative effusions and to help pinpoint the underlying disorder.

The most useful test is thoracentesis, in which pleural fluid is analyzed in the laboratory to show components. Thoracentesis is performed for patients with a pleural effusion of larger than 1 cm in height on X-ray, ultrasound, or computed tomography and if it's of unknown origin.[2] Acute inflammatory white blood cells and microorganisms may be evident in empyema.

In addition, if a pleural effusion results from esophageal rupture or pancreatitis, fluid amylase levels are usually higher than serum levels. Aspirated fluid may be tested for LE cells, antinuclear antibodies, and neoplastic cells. It may also be analyzed for color and consistency; acid-fast bacillus, fungal, and bacterial cultures; and triglycerides (in chylothorax). Cell analysis shows leukocytosis in empyema. A negative tuberculin skin test strongly rules against TB as the cause. In exudative pleural effusions in which thoracentesis isn't definitive, pleural biopsy may be done. This is particularly useful for confirming TB or malignancy.

Treatment
Depending on the amount of fluid present, symptom-producing effusion may require thoracentesis to remove fluid, or careful monitoring of the patient's own reabsorption of the fluid. Hemothorax requires drainage to prevent fibrothorax formation. Pleural effusions associated with lung cancer commonly re-accumulate quickly. Agents including talc, doxycycline, bleomycin sulfate, zinc sulfate, or quinacrine hydrochloride can prevent recurrence.[1] If a chest tube is inserted to drain the fluid, a sclerosing agent, such as talc, may be injected through the tube to cause adhesions between the parietal and visceral pleura, thereby obliterating the potential space for fluid to re-collect (called *chemical pleurodesis*). Chest tube is clamped for 2 hours and then unclamped and attached to suction to allow fluid to drain.[3]

Treatment of empyema requires insertion of one or more chest tubes after thoracentesis to allow drainage of purulent material and, possibly, decortication (surgical removal of the thick coating over the lung) or rib resection to allow open drainage and lung expansion. Empyema also requires parenteral antibiotics. Associated hypoxia requires oxygen administration.

Special considerations
▶ Explain thoracentesis to the patient. Before the procedure, tell him to expect a stinging sensation from the local anesthetic and a feeling of pressure when the needle is inserted. Instruct him to tell you immediately if he feels uncomfortable or has difficulty breathing during the procedure.
▶ Reassure the patient during thoracentesis. Remind him to breathe normally and avoid sudden movements, such as coughing or sighing. Monitor his vital signs, and watch for syncope. If fluid is removed too quickly, the patient may suffer bradycardia, hypotension, pain, pulmonary edema, or even cardiac arrest. Watch for respiratory distress or pneumothorax (sudden onset of dyspnea and cyanosis) after thoracentesis.
▶ Administer oxygen and, in empyema, antibiotics, as ordered.
▶ Encourage the patient to perform deep-breathing exercises to promote lung expan-

sion. Use an incentive spirometer to promote deep breathing.

▶ If your patient is receiving chemical pleurodesis, after the tube is clamped, help reposition the patient frequently over the 2-hour period, to make sure that all pleural surfaces are covered. Monitor the patient's vital signs, and assess respirations every 30 minutes for 2 hours after the procedure. Note the color and amount of drainage after the chest tube is unclamped.[3]

▶ Provide meticulous chest tube care, and use sterile technique for changing dressings around the tube insertion site in empyema. Ensure tube patency by watching for fluctuations of fluid or air bubbling in the underwater seal chamber. Continuous bubbling may indicate an air leak. Record the amount, color, and consistency of any tube drainage.

▶ If the patient has open drainage through a rib resection or intercostal tube, use hand and dressing precautions. Because weeks of such drainage are usually necessary to obliterate the space, make visiting nurse referrals for the patient who will be discharged with the tube in place.

▶ If pleural effusion was a complication of pneumonia or influenza, advise prompt medical attention for upper respiratory infections.

REFERENCES

1. Rubins, J. eMedicine from Web MD (2007 February 15). "Pleural Effusion" [Online]. Available at *www.emedicine.com/med/topic1843.htm*.
2. Porcel, J.M., and Light, R.W. "Diagnostic Approach to Pleural Effusion in Adults," *American Family Physician* 73(7):1211-20, April 2006.
3. Coughlin, A.M., and Parchinsky, C. "Go with the Flow of Chest Tube Therapy," *Nursing* 36(3):37-42, March 2006.
4. Almoosa, K.F., et al. "Elevated Glucose in Pleural Effusion: An Early Clue to Esophageal Perforation," *Chest* 131(5):1567-69, May 2007.

PNEUMONIA

Pneumonia is an acute infection of the lung parenchyma that commonly impairs gas exchange. The prognosis is generally good for people who have normal lungs and adequate host defenses before the onset of pneumonia. However, pneumonia and influenza are ranked together as the seventh leading cause of death in the United States, with pneumonia being responsible for the majority of those deaths causing more than 60,000 deaths per year.[1]

Causes and incidence

Pneumonia can be classified in several ways:

▶ Microbiologic etiology—Pneumonia can be viral, bacterial, fungal, protozoan, mycobacterial, mycoplasmal, or rickettsial in origin. (See *Types of pneumonia*, pages 92 and 93.)

▶ Location—Bronchopneumonia involves distal airways and alveoli; lobular pneumonia, part of a lobe; and lobar pneumonia, an entire lobe.

▶ Type—Primary pneumonia results from inhalation or aspiration of a pathogen; it includes pneumococcal and viral pneumonia. Secondary pneumonia may follow initial lung damage from a noxious chemical or other insult (superinfection), or may result from hematogenous spread of bacteria from a distant focus.

Predisposing factors for bacterial and viral pneumonia include chronic illness and debilitation; cancer (particularly lung cancer); abdominal and thoracic surgery; atelectasis; common colds or other viral respiratory infections, such as acquired immunodeficiency syndrome, chronic respiratory disease (chronic obstructive pulmonary disease, asthma, bronchiectasis, and cystic fibrosis); influenza; smoking; malnutrition; alcoholism; sickle cell disease; tracheostomy; ex-

(*Text continues on page 94.*)

Types of pneumonia

TYPE	SIGNS AND SYMPTOMS	DIAGNOSIS
Aspiration		
Results from vomiting and aspiration of gastric or oropharyngeal contents into trachea and lungs	• Noncardiogenic pulmonary edema that may follow damage to respiratory epithelium from contact with stomach acid • Crackles, dyspnea, cyanosis, hypotension, and tachycardia • May be subacute pneumonia with cavity formation; lung abscess may occur if foreign body is present	• *Chest X-ray:* locates areas of infiltrates, which suggest diagnosis
Bacterial		
Klebsiella	• Fever and recurrent chills; cough producing rusty, bloody, viscous sputum (currant jelly); cyanosis of lips and nail beds due to hypoxemia; and shallow, grunting respirations • Common in patients with chronic alcoholism, pulmonary disease, diabetes, or those at risk for aspiration	• *Chest X-ray:* typically, but not always, consolidation in the upper lobe that causes bulging of fissures • *White blood cell (WBC) count:* elevated • *Sputum culture and Gram stain:* may show gram-negative *Klebsiella*
Staphylococcus	• Temperature of 102° to 104° F (38.9° to 40° C), recurrent shaking chills, bloody sputum, dyspnea, tachypnea, and hypoxemia • Should be suspected with viral illness, such as influenza or measles, and in patients with cystic fibrosis	• *Chest X-ray:* multiple abscesses and infiltrates; high incidence of empyema • *WBC count:* elevated • *Sputum culture and Gram stain:* may show gram-positive staphylococci
Streptococcus (Streptococcus pneumoniae)	• Sudden onset of single, shaking chills and a sustained temperature of 102° to 104° F (38.9° to 40° C); commonly preceded by upper respiratory tract infection • Other signs include pleuritic chest pain, productive cough, dyspnea, tachypnea, and hypoxia	• *Chest X-ray:* areas of consolidation, commonly lobar • *WBC count:* elevated • *Sputum culture:* may show gram-positive *S. pneumoniae*; this organism not always recovered
Protozoan		
Pneumocystis carinii	• Occurs in immunocompromised persons • Dyspnea and nonproductive cough • Anorexia, weight loss, and fatigue • Low-grade fever	• *Fiber-optic bronchoscopy:* obtains specimens for histologic studies • *Chest X-ray:* nonspecific infiltrates, nodular lesions, or spontaneous pneumothorax

Types of pneumonia *(continued)*

TYPE	SIGNS AND SYMPTOMS	DIAGNOSIS
Viral		
Adenovirus (insidious onset; generally affects young adults)	• Sore throat, fever, cough, chills, malaise, small amounts of mucoid sputum, retrosternal chest pain, anorexia, rhinitis, adenopathy, scattered crackles, and rhonchi	• *Chest X-ray:* patchy distribution of pneumonia, more severe than indicated by physical examination • *WBC count:* normal to slightly elevated
Chicken pox (varicella) (uncommon in children, but present in 30% of adults with varicella)	• Cough, dyspnea, cyanosis, tachypnea, pleuritic chest pain, hemoptysis, and rhonchi 1 to 6 days after onset of rash	• *Chest X-ray:* shows more extensive pneumonia than indicated by physical examination and bilateral, patchy, diffuse, nodular infiltrates • *Sputum analysis:* predominant mononuclear cells and characteristic intranuclear inclusion bodies, with characteristic skin rash, confirm diagnosis
Cytomegalovirus	• Difficult to distinguish from other nonbacterial pneumonias • Fever, cough, shaking chills, dyspnea, cyanosis, weakness, and diffuse crackles • Occurs in neonates as devastating multisystemic infection; in normal adults, resembles mononucleosis; in immunocompromised hosts, varies from clinically inapparent to devastating infection • Common type of pneumonia with transplant recipients due to immunosuppressive treatments	• *Chest X-ray:* in early stages, variable patchy infiltrates; later, bilateral, nodular, and more predominant in lower lobes • *Percutaneous aspiration of lung tissue, transbronchial biopsy, or open lung biopsy:* microscopic examination shows typical intranuclear and cytoplasmic inclusions; the virus can be cultured from lung tissue
Influenza (prognosis poor even with treatment; 30% mortality)	• Cough (initially nonproductive; later, purulent sputum), marked cyanosis, dyspnea, high fever, chills, substernal pain and discomfort, moist crackles, frontal headache, and myalgia • Death results from cardiopulmonary collapse	• *Chest X-ray:* diffuse bilateral bronchopneumonia radiating from hilus • *WBC count:* normal to slightly elevated • *Sputum smears:* no specific organisms
Measles (rubeola)	• Fever, dyspnea, cough, small amounts of sputum, coryza, rash, and cervical adenopathy	• *Chest X-ray:* reticular infiltrates, sometimes with hilar lymph node enlargement • *Lung tissue specimen:* characteristic giant cells
Respiratory syncytial virus (most prevalent in infants and children)	• Listlessness, irritability, tachypnea with retraction of intercostal muscles, wheezing, slight sputum production, fine moist crackles, fever, severe malaise, and cough	• *Chest X-ray:* patchy bilateral consolidation • *WBC count:* normal to slightly elevated

posure to noxious gases; aspiration; and immunosuppressive therapy.

Predisposing factors for aspiration pneumonia include old age, debilitation, artificial airway use, nasogastric (NG) tube feedings, impaired gag reflex, poor oral hygiene, and decreased level of consciousness.

In elderly patients and patients who are debilitated, bacterial pneumonia may follow influenza or a common cold. Respiratory viruses are the most common cause of pneumonia in children ages 2 to 3. In school-age children, mycoplasma pneumonia is more common.

Streptococcus pneumonia accounts for 25% to 35% of community-acquired pneumonia and about 40,000 deaths per year.[1] It also accounts for 50% of hospital-acquired pneumonia.[2]

Signs and symptoms

The main symptoms of pneumonia are coughing, sputum production, pleuritic chest pain, shaking chills, shortness of breath, rapid shallow breathing, and fever. Physical signs vary widely, ranging from diffuse, fine crackles to signs of localized or extensive consolidation and pleural effusion. There may also be associated symptoms of headache, sweating, loss of appetite, excess fatigue, and confusion (in older people).

Complications

▶ Hypoxemia
▶ Respiratory failure
▶ Pleural effusion
▶ Empyema
▶ Lung abscess
▶ Bacteremia, with spread of infection to other parts of the body, resulting in meningitis, endocarditis, and pericarditis

Diagnosis

Clinical features, chest X-ray showing infiltrates, and sputum smear demonstrating acute inflammatory cells support the diagnosis. Gram stain and sputum culture may identify the organism. Positive blood cultures in the patient with pulmonary infiltrates strongly suggest pneumonia produced by the organisms isolated from the blood cultures. Pleural effusions, if present, should be tapped and fluid analyzed for evidence of infection in the pleural space. Occasionally, a transtracheal aspirate of tracheobronchial secretions or bronchoscopy with brushings or washings may be done to obtain material for smear and culture. The patient's response to antimicrobial therapy also provides important evidence of the presence of pneumonia.

Treatment

Antimicrobial therapy varies with the causative agent. The drug of choice for community-acquired bacterial pneumonia is a macrolide such as azithromycin, clarithromycin, or erythromycin.[3,4] The Infectious Disease Society of America outlines initial therapy for suspected bacterial community-acquired pneumonia in the immunocompetent adult.[3,4] The organization recommends pathogen specific drugs. Therapy should be reevaluated early in the course of treatment.

Supportive measures include humidified oxygen therapy for hypoxemia, mechanical ventilation for respiratory failure, a high-calorie diet and adequate fluid intake, bed rest, and an analgesic to relieve pleuritic chest pain. Patients with severe pneumonia on mechanical ventilation may require positive end-expiratory pressure to facilitate adequate oxygenation.

Special considerations

Correct supportive care can increase patient comfort, prevent complications, and speed recovery.

The following protocol should be observed throughout the illness:

▶ Maintain a patent airway and adequate oxygenation. Monitor pulse oximetry. Measure arterial blood gas levels, especially

in hypoxemic patients. Administer supplemental oxygen if the partial pressure of arterial oxygen is less than 55 to 60 mm Hg. Patients with underlying chronic lung disease should be given oxygen cautiously.

▶ Teach the patient how to cough and perform deep-breathing exercises to clear secretions; encourage him to do so often. In severe pneumonia that requires endotracheal intubation or tracheostomy (with or without mechanical ventilation), provide thorough respiratory care. Suction often, using sterile technique, to remove secretions.

▶ Obtain sputum specimens as needed, by suction if the patient can't produce specimens independently. Collect specimens in a sterile container, and deliver them promptly to the microbiology laboratory.

▶ Administer antibiotics as ordered and pain medication as needed; record the patient's response to medications. Fever and dehydration may require I.V. fluids and electrolyte replacement.

▶ Maintain adequate nutrition to offset hypermetabolic state secondary to infection. Ask the dietary department to provide a high-calorie, high-protein diet consisting of soft, easy-to-eat foods. Encourage the patient to eat. As necessary, supplement oral feedings with NG tube feedings or parenteral nutrition. Monitor fluid intake and output. Consider limiting the use of milk products because they may increase sputum production.

▶ Oral therapy should be used as soon as the patient is able to ingest medications and have a normally functioning GI tract. [3,4]

▶ Provide a quiet, calm environment for the patient, with frequent rest periods.

▶ Give emotional support by explaining all procedures (especially intubation and suctioning) to the patient and his family. Encourage family visits. Provide diversionary activities appropriate to the patient's age.

▶ To control the spread of infection, dispose of secretions properly. Tell the patient to sneeze and cough into a disposable tissue; tape a lined bag to the side of the bed for used tissues.

Pneumonia can be prevented as follows:

▶ Advise the patient to avoid using antibiotics indiscriminately during minor viral infections because this may result in upper airway colonization with antibiotic-resistant bacteria. If the patient then develops pneumonia, the organisms producing the pneumonia may require treatment with more toxic antibiotics.

▶ Encourage the pneumonia vaccine and annual influenza vaccination for adults aged 65 or older, or anyone over age 2 in high-risk environmental settings, or with chronic illness, anatomic or functional asplenia, a compromised immune system, or human immunodeficiency virus infection. [2]

▶ Urge all bedridden and postoperative patients to perform deep-breathing and coughing exercises frequently. Reposition such patients often to promote full aeration and drainage of secretions. Encourage early ambulation in postoperative patients.

▶ To prevent aspiration during NG tube feedings, elevate the patient's head, check the tube's position, and administer the formula slowly. Don't give large volumes at one time; this could cause vomiting. Keep the patient's head elevated 30 to 45 degrees during the feeding and for 1 hour after feeding. Check for residual formula every 4 hours. [4]

▶ Provide good oral care on a regular basis to help decrease organisms in the patient's mouth that could be aspirated. [5]

REFERENCES

1. American Lung Association (2006 April). "Pneumonia Fact Sheet" [Online]. Available at *www.lungusa.org/site/ pp.asp?c=dvLUK9O0E&b=35692.*

2. Atkins, W. et al., eds. *Epidemiology and Prevention of Vaccine Preventable Diseases,* 10th ed. Washington, D.C.: Public Health Foundation, 2007.

3. Bernheisel, C.R., and Schlaudecker, J.D. "Managing CAP: An Evidence-Based

Algorithm," *Journal of Family Practice* 58(9):722-26, September 2007.

4. Mandell, L.A., et al. "Update of Practice Guidelines for the Management of Community-Acquired Pneumonia in Immunocompetent Adults," *Clinical Infectious Disease* 37(11):1405-33, December 2003.

5. Ross, A., and Crumpler, J. "The Impact of an Evidence-Based Practice Education Program on the Role of Oral Care in the Prevention of Ventilator-Associated Pneumonia," *Intensive and Critical Care Nursing* 23(3):132-36, June 2007.

PNEUMOTHORAX

Pneumothorax is an accumulation of air or gas between the parietal and visceral pleurae. The amount of air or gas trapped in the intrapleural space determines the degree of lung collapse. There may be partial or complete collapse of the lung. Pneumothorax can also be classified as open or closed. In open pneumothorax (usually the result of trauma), air flows between the pleural space and the outside of the body. In closed pneumothorax, air reaches the pleural space directly from the lung.

Causes and incidence

Primary spontaneous pneumothorax (PSP) usually occurs in otherwise healthy males with long, lean bodies, ages 20 to 40.[1,2] The ratio of males to females is 6:1, and patients with PSP are likely to have a history of smoking.[2] There is a 30% to 50% risk of recurrence.[3] It may be caused by air leakage from ruptured congenital blebs adjacent to the visceral pleural surface, near the apex of the lung.

Secondary spontaneous pneumothorax (SSP) is a complication of underlying lung disease, such as chronic obstructive pulmonary disease (COPD), asthma, cystic fibrosis, tuberculosis, and whooping cough.[1] COPD is the most common cause of SSP.[2] Spontaneous pneumothorax may also occur in interstitial lung disease, such as eosinophilic granuloma or lymphangiomyomatosis. SSP is more likely to occur in men.[2]

Traumatic pneumothorax may result from insertion of a central venous line, thoracic surgery, or a penetrating chest injury, such as a gunshot or knife wound. It may follow a transbronchial biopsy or mechanical ventilation, or it may occur during thoracentesis or a closed pleural biopsy. When traumatic pneumothorax follows a penetrating chest injury, it frequently coexists with hemothorax (blood in the pleural space). The incidence is higher in patients with underlying lung diseases.[2]

In tension pneumothorax, positive pleural pressure develops as a result of traumatic pneumothorax. When air enters the pleural space through a tear in lung tissue and is unable to leave by the same vent, each inspiration traps air in the pleural space, resulting in positive pleural pressure. This in turn causes collapse of the ipsilateral lung and marked impairment of venous return, which can severely compromise cardiac output and may cause a mediastinal shift. Decreased filling of the great veins of the chest results in diminished cardiac output and lowered blood pressure. In tension pneumothorax, the air in the pleural space is under higher pressure than air in adjacent lung and vascular structures. Without prompt treatment, tension or large pneumothorax results in fatal pulmonary and circulatory impairment. Tension pneumothorax occurs in 1% to 3% of spontaneous pneumothoraces.[2]

Signs and symptoms

The cardinal features of pneumothorax are sudden, sharp, pleuritic pain (exacerbated by movement of the chest, breathing, and coughing); asymmetrical chest wall movement; and shortness of breath. Additional signs of tension pneumothorax are weak and rapid pulse, pallor, jugular vein distention, and anxiety. Tracheal deviations may be present with mediastinal shift. Tension pneu-

mothorax produces the most severe respiratory symptoms; a spontaneous pneumothorax that releases only a small amount of air into the pleural space may cause no symptoms. In non-tension pneumothorax, the severity of symptoms is usually related to the size of the pneumothorax and the degree of preexisting respiratory disease.

Complications
▶ Fatal pulmonary and circulatory impairment

Diagnosis
Sudden, sharp chest pain and shortness of breath suggest pneumothorax.

A chest X-ray showing air in the pleural space and, possibly, mediastinal shift confirms this diagnosis.
In the absence of a definitive chest X-ray, the physical examination may reveal:
▶ on inspection—overexpansion and rigidity of the affected chest side; in tension pneumothorax, jugular vein distention with hypotension and tachycardia
▶ on palpation—crackling beneath the skin (crepitus), indicating subcutaneous emphysema (air in tissue) and decreased vocal fremitus
▶ on percussion—hyperresonance on the affected side
▶ on auscultation—decreased or absent breath sounds over the collapsed lung.

If the pneumothorax is significant, arterial blood gas findings include pH less than 7.35, partial pressure of arterial oxygen less than 80 mm Hg, and partial pressure of arterial carbon dioxide above 45 mm Hg.

Treatment
Treatment is conservative for spontaneous pneumothorax in which no signs of increased pleural pressure (indicating tension pneumothorax) appear, lung collapse is less than 30%, and the patient shows no signs of dyspnea or other indications of physiologic compromise. Such treatment consists of bed rest, careful monitoring of blood pressure and pulse and respiratory rates, oxygen administration and, possibly, needle aspiration of air with a large-bore needle attached to a syringe. If more than 30% of the lung is collapsed, treatment to reexpand the lung includes placing a thoracostomy tube in the second or third intercostal space in the midclavicular line (or in the fifth or sixth intercostal space in the midaxillary line), connected to an underwater seal or low suction pressures.

Recurring spontaneous pneumothorax requires thoracotomy and pleurectomy or pleurodesis; these procedures prevent recurrence by causing the lung to adhere to the parietal pleura.[3] Traumatic and tension pneumothoraces require chest tube drainage; traumatic pneumothorax may also require surgery.

Special considerations
▶ Watch for pallor, gasping respirations, and sudden chest pain. Carefully monitor the patient's vital signs at least every hour for indications of shock, increasing respiratory distress, or mediastinal shift. Listen for breath sounds over both lungs. Falling blood pressure and rising pulse and respiratory rates may indicate tension pneumothorax, which could be fatal without prompt treatment.
▶ After the chest tube is in place, encourage the patient to cough and breathe deeply (at least once an hour) to facilitate lung expansion.
▶ If the patient is undergoing chest tube drainage, watch for continuing air leakage (bubbling), indicating the lung defect has failed to close; this may require surgery. Also watch for increasing subcutaneous emphysema (crepitus) by checking around the neck or at the tube insertion site for crackling beneath the skin. If the patient is on a ventilator, watch for difficulty in breathing in time with the ventilator as well as pressure changes on ventilator gauges.

▶ Change dressings around the chest tube insertion site, as necessary and according to your facility's policy. Be careful not to reposition or dislodge the tube. If it dislodges, immediately place a petroleum gauze dressing over the opening to prevent rapid lung collapse.

▶ Secure the chest tube drainage apparatus appropriately. Tape connections securely.

▶ Monitor the patient's vital signs frequently after thoracotomy. Also, for the first 24 hours, assess respiratory status by checking breath sounds hourly. Observe the chest tube site for leakage, noting the amount and color of drainage. Help the patient walk, as ordered (usually on the first postoperative day), to facilitate deep inspiration and lung expansion.

▶ To reassure the patient, explain what pneumothorax is, what causes it, and all diagnostic tests and procedures. Make him as comfortable as possible. (The patient with pneumothorax is usually most comfortable sitting up.)

REFERENCES

1. American Lung Association (2005 June). "Spontaneous Pneumothorax Fact Sheet" [Online]. Available at *www.lungusa.org/site/pp.asp?c=dvLUK9O0E&b=35772*.
2. Ryan, B. "Pneumothorax Assessment and Diagnostic Testing," *Journal of Cardiovascular Nursing* 20(4):251-53, July-August 2005.
3. Santillan-Doherty, P. et al. "Thoracoscopic Management of Primary Spontaneous Pneumothorax," *American Surgeon* 72(2):145-49, February 2006.

PULMONARY EMBOLISM

The most common pulmonary complication in hospitalized patients, pulmonary embolism (PE) is an obstruction of the pulmonary arterial bed by a dislodged thrombus, heart valve vegetation, or foreign substance. Although pulmonary infarction that results from embolism may be so mild as to not cause symptoms, massive embolism (more than 50% obstruction of pulmonary arterial circulation) and the accompanying infarction can be rapidly fatal.

Causes and incidence

Pulmonary embolism generally results from dislodged thrombi originating in the leg veins. About 90% of such thrombi arise in the deep veins of the legs.[1] Other less-common sources of thrombi are the pelvic veins, renal veins, hepatic vein, right side of the heart, and upper extremities. Such thrombus formation results directly from vascular wall damage, venostasis, or hypercoagulability of the blood. Trauma, clot dissolution, sudden muscle spasm, intravascular pressure changes, or a change in peripheral blood flow can cause the thrombus to loosen or fragment. Then the thrombus—now called an embolus—floats to the heart's right side and enters the lung through the pulmonary artery. There, the embolus may dissolve, continue to fragment, or grow.

By occluding the pulmonary artery, the embolus prevents alveoli from producing enough surfactant to maintain alveolar integrity. As a result, alveoli collapse and atelectasis develops. If the embolus enlarges, it may clog most or all of the pulmonary vessels and cause death.

Rarely, the emboli contain air, fat, bacteria, amniotic fluid, talc (from drugs intended for oral administration, which are injected I.V. by addicts), or tumor cells.

The most frequent predisposing factor for PE is immobility.[1] Other predisposing factors include chronic pulmonary disease, heart failure or atrial fibrillation, thrombophlebitis, polycythemia vera, thrombocytosis, autoimmune hemolytic anemia, sickle cell disease, varicose veins, recent surgery, advanced age, pregnancy, lower-extremity fractures or surgery, burns, obesity, vascular injury, cancer, I.V. drug abuse, or hormonal contraceptives.

More than 200,000 cases of PE occur in the United States every year, and 80% of those are associated with deep vein thrombosis.[2]

Signs and symptoms

Total occlusion of the main pulmonary artery is rapidly fatal; smaller or fragmented emboli produce symptoms that vary with the size, number, and location of the emboli. Usually, the first symptom of pulmonary embolism is dyspnea, which may be accompanied by anginal or pleuritic chest pain. Other clinical features include tachycardia, productive cough (sputum may be blood-tinged), low-grade fever, and pleural effusion. Less-common signs include massive hemoptysis, chest splinting, leg edema and, with a large embolus, cyanosis, syncope, and distended jugular veins.

In addition, pulmonary embolism may cause pleural friction rub and signs of circulatory collapse (weak, rapid pulse and hypotension) and hypoxia (restlessness and anxiety).

Complications

- ▶ Pulmonary infarction
- ▶ Hepatic congestion and necrosis
- ▶ Pulmonary abscess
- ▶ Shock
- ▶ Acute respiratory distress syndrome
- ▶ Massive atelectasis
- ▶ Venous overload
- ▶ $\dot{V}/\dot{Q}$ mismatch
- ▶ Emboli extension
- ▶ Death (with massive embolism)

Diagnosis

The patient history should reveal predisposing conditions for pulmonary embolism. A triad of deep vein thrombosis (DVT) formation is stasis, endothelial injury, and hypercoagulability. Risk factors include long car or plane trips, cancer, pregnancy, hypercoagulability, prior DVT, and pulmonary emboli.

▶ Chest X-ray helps to rule out other pulmonary diseases; areas of atelectasis, an elevated diaphragm and pleural effusion, a prominent pulmonary artery and, occasionally, the characteristic wedge-shaped infiltrate suggestive of pulmonary infarction, or focal oligemia of blood vessels, are apparent.

▶ Computed tomography pulmonary angiography is the preferred diagnostic test to evaluate patients suspected of having a PE.[2] After injection of the contrast medium, the chest is scanned for abnormalities. Studies suggest that this test is as accurate as invasive pulmonary angiography.[1]

▶ Pulmonary angiography is the most definitive test for PE.[1] However, it requires a skilled angiographer and radiologic equipment; it also poses some risk to the patient. Its use depends on the uncertainty of the diagnosis and the need to avoid unnecessary anticoagulant therapy in a high-risk patient.

▶ Electrocardiography may show right axis deviation; right bundle-branch block; tall, peaked P waves; depression of ST segments and T-wave inversions (indicative of right-sided heart strain); and supraventricular tachyarrhythmias in extensive pulmonary embolism. A pattern sometimes observed is S_1, Q_3, and T_3 (S wave in lead I, Q wave in lead III, and inverted T wave in lead III).

▶ Auscultation occasionally reveals a right ventricular S_3 gallop and an increased intensity of a pulmonic component of S_2. Also, crackles and a pleural rub may be heard at the embolism site.

▶ Arterial blood gas (ABG) analysis showing a decreased partial pressure of arterial oxygen and partial pressure of arterial carbon dioxide are characteristic but don't always occur.

▶ Serum D-dimer testing may be done when PE is initially suspected but it isn't sensitive enough to give a definitive diagnosis. A positive test identifies high levels of fibrin degradation products in the blood. Almost all patients with PE will have a D-dimer level of greater than 500 ng/ml, and a normal D-

dimer can exclude PE in more than 90% of the cases.[1] Elevated D-dimer tests are found in many other types of patients.

If pleural effusion is present, thoracentesis may rule out empyema, which indicates pneumonia.

Treatment

Treatment is designed to maintain adequate cardiovascular and pulmonary function during resolution of the obstruction and to prevent recurrence of embolic episodes. Because most emboli resolve within 10 to 14 days, treatment consists of oxygen therapy as needed and anticoagulation with heparin to inhibit new thrombus formation, followed by oral warfarin. Heparin therapy is monitored by daily coagulation studies (partial thromboplastin time). Unfractionated heparin or low-molecular-weight heparin is recommended for initial treatment. [3,4]

Patients with massive pulmonary embolism and shock may need fibrinolytic therapy with thrombolytic therapy (streptokinase, urokinase, or tissue plasminogen activator) to enhance fibrinolysis of the pulmonary emboli and remaining thrombi. Emboli that cause hypotension may require the use of vasopressors. Treatment of septic emboli requires antibiotics—not anticoagulants—and evaluation for the infection's source, particularly endocarditis.

Compression stockings are used to limit or prevent extension of thrombus and should provide a 30 to 40 mm Hg compression gradient.

Surgery is performed on patients who can't take anticoagulants, who have recurrent emboli during anticoagulant therapy, or who have been treated with thrombolytic agents or pulmonary thromboendarterectomy. This procedure (which shouldn't be performed without angiographic evidence of pulmonary embolism) consists of vena caval ligation, plication, or insertion of an inferior vena cava device to filter blood returning to the heart and lungs.

Special considerations

▶ Give oxygen by nasal cannula or mask. Check ABG levels if the patient develops fresh emboli or worsening dyspnea. Be prepared to provide endotracheal intubation with assisted ventilation if breathing is severely compromised.

▶ Administer heparin, as ordered, through I.V. push or continuous drip. Monitor coagulation studies daily. Watch closely for nosebleeds, petechiae, and other signs of abnormal bleeding; check stools for occult blood. Patients should be protected from trauma and injury; avoid I.M. injections, and maintain pressure over venipuncture sites for 5 minutes, or until bleeding stops, to reduce hematoma.

▶ After the patient is stable, encourage him to move about often, and assist with isometric and range-of-motion exercises. Check pedal pulses, temperature, and color of feet to detect venostasis. Never massage the patient's legs. Offer diversional activities to promote rest and relieve restlessness.

▶ Help the patient walk as soon as possible after surgery to prevent venostasis.

▶ Maintain adequate nutrition and fluid balance to promote healing.

▶ Report frequent pleuritic chest pain, so that analgesics can be prescribed. Also, incentive spirometry can assist in deep breathing. Provide tissues and a bag for easy disposal of expectorations.

▶ Warn the patient not to cross his legs; this promotes thrombus formation.

▶ To relieve anxiety, explain procedures and treatments. Encourage the patient's family to participate in his care.

▶ Most patients need treatment with an oral anticoagulant for at least 6 months after a pulmonary embolism. Advise these patients to watch for signs of bleeding (bloody stools, blood in urine, and large ecchymoses), to take the prescribed medication exactly as ordered, not to change dosages without consulting their physician, and to avoid taking additional medication (includ-

Post-surgical pulmonary embolism

Question: *What factors affect the recovery of a patient who develops pulmonary emboli following noncardiac surgery?*

Research: The prophylactic use of pharmacologic agents and mechanical devices for the prevention of deep venous thrombosis and pulmonary emboli has become standard care for the perioperative patient. The researchers in this study searched the Mayo Clinic electronic medical records and Autopsy Registry, between January 1, 1998 and December 31, 2001, to determine 30-day mortality and predictors of mortality following perioperative pulmonary embolism. Patients selected for inclusion in the study had developed a pulmonary embolism within 30 days after noncardiac surgery that was performed under general or neuraxial anesthesia. Their medical records were reviewed, using standardized data collection forms.

Conclusion: The 30-day mortality rate was determined to be about 25%, as 40 of the 158 patients with probable or definite perioperative pulmonary emboli died. The most common predictors of mortality were hemodynamic instabili-

ty and hypotension requiring treatment. Patients who developed these complications had very low survival rates. Other factors that affected mortality included the need for mechanical ventilation, intensive care unit admission, prolonged length of surgery, central vein cannulation, and the intraoperative use of blood products.

Application: The nurse caring for a perioperative patient should make sure that measures to prevent pulmonary emboli have been ordered and instituted. If the patient develops pulmonary emboli with hemodynamic instability and severe hypotension, aggressive treatment should be instituted to prevent death.

Source: Comfere, T.B., et al. "Predictors of Mortality Following Symptomatic Pulmonary Embolism in Patients Undergoing Noncardiac Surgery," *Canadian Journal of Anaesthesia* 54(8):634-41, August 2007.

ing aspirin and vitamins). Stress the importance of follow-up laboratory tests (International Normalized Ratio) to monitor anticoagulant therapy.

▶ To prevent pulmonary emboli, encourage early ambulation in patients predisposed to this condition. With close medical supervision, low-dose heparin may be useful prophylactically. (See *Post-surgical pulmonary embolism.*)

▶ Low-molecular-weight heparin may be given to prevent pulmonary embolism in high-risk patients.

REFERENCES

1. Cloutier, L.M. "Diagnosis of Pulmonary Embolism," *Clinical Journal of Oncology Nursing* 11(3):343-48, June 2007.

2. American College of Radiology, (2006). "Guideline for Acute Chest Pain-Suspected Pulmonary Embolism" [Online]. Available at *www.guideline.gov/summary/summary.aspx? doc_id=10600&nbr=5542&ss=6&xl=999.*

3. Damlo, S. "AAFP and ACP Publish Recommendations on Diagnosis and Management of VTE," *American Family Physician* 76(8):1125-30, October 2007.

4. Bruller, H.R., et al. "Antithrombotic Therapy for Venous Thromboembolic Disease: The Seventh ACCP Conference on Antithrombotic and Thrombolytic Therapy," *Chest* 126(3 Suppl):401S-28S, September 2004.

PULMONARY HYPERTENSION

Pulmonary hypertension occurs when pulmonary artery pressure (PAP) rises above normal for reasons other than aging or altitude. The National Institutes of Health identifies primary pulmonary hypertension when the mean PAP is 25 mm Hg or more and pulmonary capillary wedge pressure is 15 mm Hg or more. In 2003, the World Health Organization further classified pulmonary hypertension into five categories that are helpful in describing its cause.[1] Pulmonary hypertension can also be classified as primary—occurring from an unknown cause, and secondary—occurring secondary to another disorder. The prognosis depends on the cause of the underlying disorder, but the long-term prognosis is poor. Within 5 years of diagnosis, only 25% of patients are still alive.

Causes and incidence

Pulmonary hypertension begins as hypertrophy of the small pulmonary arteries. The medial and intimal muscle layers of these vessels thicken, decreasing distensibility and increasing resistance. This disorder then progresses to vascular sclerosis and obliteration of small vessels.

In most cases, pulmonary hypertension occurs secondary to an underlying disease process, including:

▶ alveolar hypoventilation from chronic obstructive pulmonary disease (most common cause in the United States), sarcoidosis, diffuse interstitial disease, pulmonary metastasis, and certain diseases such as scleroderma. (In these disorders, pulmonary vascular resistance occurs secondary to hypoxemia and destruction of the alveolocapillary bed. Other disorders that cause alveolar hypoventilation without lung tissue damage include obesity, kyphoscoliosis, and obstructive sleep apnea.)

▶ vascular obstruction from pulmonary embolism, vasculitis, and disorders that cause obstruction of small or large pulmonary veins, such as left atrial myxoma, idiopathic veno-occlusive disease, fibrosing mediastinitis, and mediastinal neoplasm.

▶ primary cardiac disease, which may be congenital or acquired. Congenital defects that cause left-to-right shunting of blood—such as patent ductus arteriosus or atrial or ventricular septal defect—increase blood flow into the lungs and, consequently, raise pulmonary vascular pressure. Acquired cardiac diseases, such as rheumatic valvular disease and mitral stenosis, increase pulmonary venous pressure by restricting blood flow returning to the heart.

Primary (or idiopathic) pulmonary hypertension is rare, occurring most commonly—and with no known cause—in females ages 20 to 40.[2] Secondary pulmonary hypertension results from existing cardiac, pulmonary, thromboembolic, or collagen vascular diseases or from the use of certain drugs. About 300 cases of primary pulmonary hypertension are diagnosed each year.[3]

Signs and symptoms

Most patients complain of increasing dyspnea on exertion, weakness, syncope, and fatigability. Many also show signs of right-sided heart failure, including peripheral edema, ascites, jugular vein distention, and hepatomegaly. Other clinical effects vary with the underlying disorder.

Complications

▶ Cor pulmonale
▶ Cardiac failure
▶ Cardiac arrest

Diagnosis

Characteristic diagnostic findings:
▶ Auscultation reveals abnormalities associated with the underlying disorder.

▶ Arterial blood gas (ABG) analysis indicates hypoxemia (decreased partial pressure of arterial oxygen).

▶ Electrocardiography shows right axis deviation and tall or peaked P waves in inferior leads in the patient with right ventricular hypertrophy.

▶ Cardiac catheterization reveals pulmonary systolic pressure above 30 mm Hg as well as increased pulmonary artery wedge pressure (PAWP) if the underlying cause is left atrial myxoma, mitral stenosis, or left-sided heart failure (otherwise normal).

▶ Pulmonary angiography detects filling defects in pulmonary vasculature such as those that develop in patients with pulmonary emboli.

▶ Pulmonary function tests may show decreased flow rates and increased residual volume in underlying obstructive disease and decreased total lung capacity in underlying restrictive disease.

Treatment

Treatment usually includes oxygen therapy to decrease hypoxemia and resulting pulmonary vascular resistance. It may also include vasodilator therapy (nifedipine, diltiazem, or prostaglandin E). For patients with right-sided heart failure, treatment also includes fluid restriction, cardiac glycosides to increase cardiac output, and diuretics to decrease intravascular volume and extravascular fluid accumulation. Treatment aims to correct the underlying cause. Newer treatments include prostanoids, phosphodiesterase-5 inhibitors, and endothelin receptor antagonists. Prostanoids act as vasodilators and antiplatelet agents.[1] The phosphodiesterase inhibitor sildenafil has been approved for use as a vasorelaxing agent.[1] Antilipid agents such as bosentan help decrease pulmonary vascular resistance.[1] Also, anticoagulation with warfarin is recommended.[1]

Some patients with pulmonary hypertension may be candidates for heart-lung transplantation to improve their chances of survival.[4] Other surgical treatment options include pulmonary thromboendarterectomy and atrial septostomy.[5]

Special considerations

Pulmonary hypertension requires keen observation and careful monitoring as well as skilled supportive care.

▶ Administer oxygen therapy as ordered, and observe the patient's response. Report any signs of increasing dyspnea to the physician so that treatment can be adjusted accordingly.

▶ Monitor ABG levels for acidosis and hypoxemia. Report any change in the patient's level of consciousness at once.

▶ When caring for a patient with right-sided heart failure, especially one receiving diuretics, record his weight daily, carefully measure intake and output, and explain all medications and diet restrictions. Check for worsening jugular vein distention, which may indicate fluid overload.

▶ Monitor the patient's vital signs, especially blood pressure and heart rate. Watch for hypotension and tachycardia. If he has a pulmonary artery catheter, check PAP and PAWP, as ordered. Report any changes.

▶ Before discharge, help the patient adjust to the limitations imposed by this disorder. Advise against overexertion, and suggest frequent rest periods between activities. Refer the patient to the social services department if he'll need special equipment, such as oxygen equipment, for home use. Make sure that he understands the prescribed medications and diet and the need to weigh himself daily.

REFERENCES

1. LaRaia, A.V., and Waxman, A.B. "Pulmonary Arterial Hypertension: Evaluation and Management," *Southern Medical Journal* 100(4):393-98 April 2007.
2. American Heart Association (2008 January 28). "Primary or Unexplained Pulmonary

Hypertension" [Online]. Available at *www.americanheart.org/presenter.jhtml?identifier=4752.*

3. National Heart Lung and Blood Institute (2006 August). "What is Pulmonary Arterial Hypertension?" [Online]. Available at *www.nhlbi.nih.gov/health/dci/Diseases/pah/pah_what.html.*

4. Badesch, D.B., et al. "Medical Therapy for Pulmonary Arterial Hypertension: Updated ACCP Evidence-Based Clinical Practice Guidelines," *Chest* 131(6):1917-28, June 2007.

5. Doyle, R.L., et al. "Surgical Treatments/Interventions for Pulmonary Arterial Hypertension: ACCP Evidence-Based Clinical Practice Guidelines," *Chest* 126(1 Suppl):63S-71S, July 2004.

Emerging infection

SEVERE ACUTE RESPIRATORY SYNDROME

Severe acute respiratory syndrome (SARS) is a viral respiratory infection that can progress to pneumonia and, eventually, death. The disease was first recognized in 2003 with outbreaks in China, Canada, Singapore, Taiwan, and Vietnam. Other countries, including the United States, reported a smaller numbers of cases. There were more than 8,000 cases and 780 deaths worldwide.[1]

Causes and incidence

SARS is caused by the SARS-associated coronavirus (SARS-CoV). Coronaviruses are a common cause of mild respiratory illnesses in humans, but researchers believe that a virus may have mutated, allowing it to cause this potentially life-threatening disease.

Close contact with a person who's infected with SARS, including contact with infectious aerosolized droplets or body secretions, is the method of transmission. Most people who contracted the disease during the 2003 outbreak contracted it during travel to endemic areas. However, the virus has been found to live on hands, tissues, and other surfaces for up to 6 hours in its droplet form. It has also been found to live in the stool of people with SARS for up to 4 days. The virus may be able to live for months or years in below-freezing temperatures.

Signs and symptoms

The incubation period for SARS is typically 4 to 6 days, and most people show signs and symptoms within 2 to 10 days after exposure.[1] Initial signs and symptoms include fever, shortness of breath and other minor respiratory symptoms, general discomfort, headache, rigors, chills, myalgia, sore throat, and dry cough. Some individuals may develop diarrhea or a rash.

Complications

▶ Respiratory failure
▶ Liver failure
▶ Heart failure
▶ Myelodysplastic syndrome
▶ Death

Diagnosis

Diagnosis of severe respiratory illness is made when the patient has a fever greater than 100.4° F (38° C) or upon clinical findings of lower respiratory illness and a chest X-ray demonstrating pneumonia or acute respiratory distress syndrome.

Laboratory validation for the virus includes cell culture of SARS-CoV, detection of SARS-CoV ribonucleic acid by the reverse transcription polymerase chain reaction (PCR) test, or detection of serum antibodies to SARS-CoV.[2] Detectable levels of antibodies may not be present until 21 days after the onset of illness, but some individuals develop antibodies within 14 days. A negative PCR, antibody test, or cell culture doesn't rule out the diagnosis.

Treatment

Treatment is symptomatic and supportive and includes maintenance of a patent airway and adequate nutrition. Other treatment measures include supplemental oxygen, chest physiotherapy, or mechanical ventilation. In addition to standard precautions, recommended contact precautions include requiring the use of gowns and gloves, the use of a negative-pressure isolation room and, if patients are hospitalized, the use of properly fitted N-95 respirators. Quarantine may be used to prevent the spread of infection.[4]

Antibiotics may be given to treat bacterial causes of atypical pneumonia. Antiviral medications have also been used. High doses of corticosteroids have been used to reduce lung inflammation. In some serious cases, serum from individuals who have already recovered from SARS (convalescent serum) has been given. The general benefit of these treatments hasn't been determined conclusively.[3]

Special considerations

▶ Report suspected cases of SARS to local and national health organizations.[4]
▶ Frequently monitor the patient's vital signs and respiratory status.
▶ Maintain isolation as recommended. The patient will need emotional support to deal with anxiety and fear related to the diagnosis of SARS and as a result of isolation.[4]
▶ Provide teaching to both the patient and family, making sure to explain how important it is for the patient to wash his hands frequently, cover his mouth and nose when coughing or sneezing, and avoid close personal contact while infected or potentially infected. Make sure the patient and his family are aware that such items as eating utensils, towels, and bedding shouldn't be shared until they have been washed with soap and hot water, and that disposable gloves and household disinfectant should be used to clean any surface that may have been exposed to the patient's body fluids.

▶ Emphasize to the patient the importance of following his health care providers recommendations as they pertain to staying home from work or school and avoiding other public places while he's infected or potentially infected.[4]

REFERENCES

1. Department of Health and Human Services Center for Disease Control and Prevention (2005 May 3). "In the Absence of SARS-CoV Transmission Worldwide: Guidance for Surveillance, Clinical and Laboratory Evaluation, and Reporting Version 2" [Online]. Available at *www.cdc.gov/ncidod/sars/ absenceofsars.htm.*
2. Centers for Disease Control and Prevention. "Revised U.S. Surveillance Case Definition for Severe Acute Respiratory Syndrome (SARS) and Update on SARS Cases—United States and Worldwide, December 2003," *MMWR* 52(49):1202-206, December 2003. Also available at *www.cdc.gov/mmwr/preview/ mmwrhtml/mm5249a2.htm#box.*
3. Ong, K.C., et al. "1-year Pulmonary Function and Health Status in Survivors of Severe Acute Respiratory Syndrome," *Chest* 128(3):1393-400, September 2005.
4. Srinivasan, A., et al. "Foundations of the Severe Acute Respiratory Syndrome Preparedness and Response Plan for Healthcare Facilities," *Infection Control and Hospital Epidemiology* 25(12):1020-25, December 2004.

● TUBERCULOSIS

An acute or chronic infection caused by *Mycobacterium tuberculosis*, tuberculosis (TB) is characterized by pulmonary infiltrates, formation of granulomas with caseation, fibrosis, and cavitation. People who live in crowded, poorly ventilated conditions and those who are immunocompromised are most likely to become infected. In patients with strains that are sensitive to the usual antitubercular agents, the prognosis is excellent with correct treatment. However, in those with strains that are re-

sistant to two or more of the major antitubercular agents, mortality is 50%.

Causes and incidence

After exposure to *M. tuberculosis*, roughly 10% of infected people develop active TB at some time in their life; in the remainder, microorganisms cause a latent infection.[1] The host's immune system usually controls the tubercle bacillus by enclosing it in a tiny nodule (tubercle). The bacillus may lie dormant within the tubercle for years and later reactivate and spread. Activation of dormant bacteria occurs within the first 2 years in 50% of the cases.

Although the primary infection site is the lungs, mycobacteria commonly exist in other parts of the body. Several factors increase the risk of infection reactivation: gastrectomy, uncontrolled diabetes mellitus, Hodgkin's disease, leukemia, silicosis, acquired immunodeficiency syndrome, treatment with corticosteroids or immunosuppressants, and advanced age.

Transmission is by droplet nuclei produced when infected persons cough or sneeze. Persons with a cavitary lesion are particularly infectious because their sputum usually contains 1 to 100 million bacilli per milliliter. If an inhaled tubercle bacillus settles in an alveolus, infection occurs, with alveolocapillary dilation and endothelial cell swelling. Alveolitis results, with replication of tubercle bacilli and influx of polymorphonuclear leukocytes. These organisms spread through the lymph system to the circulatory system and then through the body.

Cell-mediated immunity to the mycobacteria, which develops 3 to 6 weeks later, usually contains the infection and arrests the disease. If the infection reactivates, the body's response characteristically leads to caseation—the conversion of necrotic tissue to a soft, cheese-like material. The caseum may localize, undergo fibrosis, or excavate and form cavities, the walls of which are studded with multiplying tubercle bacilli. If

this happens, infected caseous debris may spread throughout the lungs by the tracheobronchial tree. Sites of extrapulmonary TB include the pleurae, meninges, joints, lymph nodes, peritoneum, genitourinary tract, and bowel.

The incidence of TB has been increasing in the United States since 1992 and tends to be concentrated in urban areas, among patients with human immunodeficiency virus infection, and in minority and foreign born populations.[1] Globally, TB is the leading infectious cause of morbidity and mortality, generating 8 million new cases each year.

Signs and symptoms

After an incubation period of 4 to 8 weeks, TB usually doesn't produce symptoms in primary infection but may produce nonspecific symptoms, such as fatigue, weakness, anorexia, weight loss, night sweats, and low-grade fever. Fever and night sweats, the typical hallmarks of TB, may not be present in elderly patients, who instead may exhibit a change in activity or weight. Assess older patients carefully.

In reactivation, symptoms may include a cough that produces mucopurulent sputum, occasional hemoptysis, and chest pains.

Complications

▶ Massive pulmonary tissue damage leading to respiratory failure
▶ Bronchopleural fistulas resulting in pneumothorax
▶ Hemorrhage
▶ Pleural effusion
▶ Pneumonia
▶ Extrapulmonary TB
▶ Liver involvement from drug therapy

Diagnosis

Diagnostic tests include chest X-rays, a tuberculin skin test, and sputum smears and cultures to identify *M. tuberculosis*. The diagnosis must be precise because several other diseases (such as lung cancer, lung abscess,

EVIDENCE-BASED PRACTICE

Accuracy of new TB tests

Question: *Are new TB tests accurate for diagnosing active TB?*

Research: Tuberculin skin testing, when positive, shows only that the individual has been exposed to the mycobacterium tuberculosis, which causes most cases of tuberculosis (TB). Positive tests results require chest X-ray or sputum culture confirmation that the individual has TB. Researchers at two urban hospitals in the United Kingdom compared the sensitivity of tuberculin skin testing with two new blood tests, ELISpot and ELISpot-Plus, for diagnosing patients with suspected active TB. The participants in the study consisted of 389 adults who were mainly of South Asian and Black ethnicity.

Conclusion: Active TB was diagnosed in 194 of the study participants, with 79% of cases confirmed by sputum culture and the remainder classified as highly probable. The study showed that tuberculin skin testing was able to accurately determine TB infection in 79% of these cases, ELISpot in 85% of cases, and ELISpot-Plus in 89% of cases. However, when tuberculin skin testing and ELISpot-Plus were used together, the combined accuracy enabled the tests to rule out active TB infection with an accuracy of 99%. In addition, the ELISpot-Plus is able to distinguish TB infection from Bacille Calmette Guerin (BCG) vaccination, which the tuberculin skin test can't do.

Application: Using a combination of the ELISpot-Plus and tuberculin skin testing can enable the diagnosis of TB in a shorter time period, with less stress on the patient, and at a lower cost than current testing protocols. Patients who don't have TB can avoid being subjected to chest X-rays and sputum cultures, which may require hospitalization and isolation until the results are returned. Additionally, patients who have previously received the BCG vaccine can be tested with the ELISpot-Plus and don't have to be subjected to chest X-rays for screening purposes. The ELISpot-Plus is not yet licensed for use, but approval is expected to come very soon.

Source: Dosanjh, D.P., et al. "Improved Diagnostic Evaluation of Suspected Tuberculosis," *Annals of Internal Medicine* 148(5):325-36, March 4, 2008.

---

pneumoconiosis, and bronchiectasis) may mimic TB. (See *Accuracy of new TB tests*.)

These procedures aid in diagnosis:
▶ Auscultation detects crepitant crackles, bronchial breath sounds, wheezing, and whispered pectoriloquy.
▶ Chest percussion detects dullness over the affected area, indicating consolidation or pleural fluid.
▶ Chest X-ray shows nodular lesions, patchy infiltrates (mainly in upper lobes), cavity formation, scar tissue, and calcium deposits; however, it may not be able to distinguish active from inactive TB.
▶ Tuberculin skin test detects TB exposure. Five tuberculin units (0.1 ml) of intermediate-strength purified protein derivatives are injected intracutaneously on the forearm. The test results are read in 48 to 72 hours; a positive reaction (induration of 5 to 15 mm or more, depending on risk factors) develops 2 to 10 weeks after exposure in active and inactive TB. However, severely immunosuppressed patients may never develop a positive reaction.

Stains and cultures (of sputum, cerebrospinal fluid, urine, drainage from abscess, or pleural fluid) show heat-sensitive, nonmotile, aerobic, acid-fast bacilli.

Treatment

First-line agents for the treatment of TB are isoniazid (INH), rifampin (RIF), ethambutol

(EMB) or streptomycin, and pyrazinamide.[2] Latent TB is usually treated with daily INH for 9 months. RIF daily for 4 months may be used for people with latent TB whose contacts are INH resistant. For most adults with active TB, the recommended dosing includes the administration of all four drugs daily for 2 months, followed by 4 months of INH and RIF. Drug therapy must be selected according to patient condition and organism susceptibility. Another first-line drug used for TB is rifapentine. Second-line agents, such as cycloserine, ethionamide, p-Aminosalicylic acid, streptomycin, and capreomycin, are reserved for special circumstances or drug-resistant strains. Interruption of drug therapy may require initiation of therapy from the beginning of the regimen or additional treatment.

Directly observed therapy (DOT) may be selected or required. In this therapy, an assigned caregiver directly observes the administration of the drug. The goal of DOT is to monitor the treatment regimen and reduce the development of resistant organisms.[4]

Special considerations

▶ Initiate acid-fast bacillus (AFB) isolation precautions immediately for all patients suspected or confirmed to have TB. AFB isolation precautions include the use of a private room with negative pressure in relation to surrounding areas and a minimum of six air exchanges per hour (air exhausted should be exhausted directly to the outside).[3]
▶ Continue AFB isolation until there's clinical evidence of reduced infectiousness (substantially decreased cough, fewer organisms on sequential sputum smears).
▶ Teach the infectious patient to cough and sneeze into tissues and to dispose of all secretions properly. Place a covered trash can nearby, or tape a lined bag to the side of the bed to dispose of used tissues.
▶ Instruct the patient to wear a mask when outside his room.

▶ Visitors and staff members should wear particulate respirators that fit closely around the face when they're in the patient's room.
▶ Remind the patient to get plenty of rest. Stress the importance of eating balanced meals to promote recovery. If the patient is anorexic, urge him to eat small meals frequently. Record weight weekly.
▶ Be alert for adverse effects of medications. Because INH sometimes leads to hepatitis or peripheral neuritis, monitor aspartate aminotransferase and alanine aminotransferase levels. To prevent or treat peripheral neuritis, give pyridoxine (vitamin B_6), as ordered. If the patient receives EMB, watch for optic neuritis; if it develops, discontinue the drug. If he receives RIF, watch for hepatitis and purpura. Observe the patient for other complications such as hemoptysis.
▶ Before discharge, advise the patient to watch for adverse effects from the medication and report them immediately. Emphasize the importance of regular follow-up examinations. Instruct the patient and his family concerning the signs and symptoms of recurring TB. Stress the need to follow long-term treatment faithfully.
▶ Advise staff members and other persons who have been exposed to infected patients to receive tuberculin tests; chest X-rays and prophylactic INH may also be ordered.
▶ Emphasize to the patient the importance of taking the medications daily as prescribed. He may enroll in a supervised administration program to avoid the development of drug-resistant organisms.

REFERENCES

1. Rockwood, R.R. "Extrapulmonary TB: What You Need to Know," *Nurse Practitioner* 32(8):44-49, August 2007.
2. Herchline, T., and Amorosa, J.K. eMedicine from Web MD (2007 January 8). "Tuberculosis" [Online]. Available at *www.emedicine.com/MED/topic2324.htm*.
3. Rosen, M.J. "Chronic Cough Due to Tuberculosis and Other Infections: ACCP

Evidence-Based Clinical Practice Guidelines,"
Chest 129(1 Suppl):197S-201S, January 2006.

4. American Thoracic Society; Centers for Disease
Control and Prevention; Infectious Diseases
Society of America. "American Thoracic
Society/Centers for Disease Control and
Prevention/Infectious Diseases Society of
America: Controlling Tuberculosis in the
United States," *American Journal of
Respiratory and Critical Care Medicine*
172(9):1169-227, November 2005.

3

Neurologic disorders

ALZHEIMER'S DISEASE

Alzheimer's disease, also called *primary degenerative dementia*, accounts for more than half of all dementias. It results in memory loss, confusion, impaired judgment, personality changes, disorientation, and loss of language skills; it essentially steals the patient's mind. Because this is a primary progressive dementia, the prognosis for a patient with this disease is poor. It's the seventh leading cause of death in the United States.[1]

Causes and incidence

The cause of Alzheimer's disease is unknown. Several factors are thought to be implicated in this disease. These include *neurochemical factors,* such as deficiencies in the neurotransmitter acetylcholine, somatostatin, substance P, and norepinephrine; *environmental factors;* and *genetic immunologic factors.* Genetic studies show that an autosomal dominant form of Alzheimer's disease is associated with early onset and early death, accounting for about 100,000 deaths a year. A family history of Alzheimer's disease and the presence of Down syndrome are two established risk factors. Alzheimer's disease isn't exclusive to the elder population; its onset begins in middle age in 1% to 10% of cases.

The brain tissue of patients with Alzheimer's disease has three hallmark features: neurofibrillary tangles, neuritic plaques, and granulovacuolar degeneration. Examination of the brain after death also finds that it's atrophic, commonly weighing less than 1,000 g, compared with a normal brain weight of about 1,380 g.

About 360,000 new cases of Alzheimer's are diagnosed each year.

Signs and symptoms

Onset is insidious. Initially, the patient undergoes almost imperceptible changes, such as forgetfulness, recent memory loss, difficulty learning and remembering new information, deterioration in personal hygiene and appearance, and an inability to concentrate. Gradually, tasks that require abstract thinking and activities that require judgment become more difficult. Progressive difficulty in communication and severe deterioration in memory, language, and motor function result in a loss of coordination and an inability to write or speak. Personality changes (restlessness, irritability) and nocturnal awakenings are common.

Patients also exhibit loss of eye contact, a fearful look, wringing of the hands, and other signs of anxiety. When a patient with Alzheimer's disease is overwhelmed with anxiety, he becomes dysfunctional, acutely confused, agitated, compulsive, or fearful.

Organic brain syndrome

Although many behavioral disturbances are clearly linked to organic brain dysfunction, the clinical syndromes associated with this type of impairment are sometimes hard to detect because they aren't always determined by the affected area of the brain or even by the extent of tissue damage. Instead, the way the patient's personality interacts with the brain injury determines the specific clinical effects. General symptoms commonly include impairment of orientation, memory, and intellectual and emotional function. These primary cognitive deficits help to distinguish organic brain syndromes from neurosis and depression.

DIAGNOSIS
Diagnosis of an organic brain syndrome depends on a detailed history of the onset of cognitive and behavioral disturbances; a complete neurologic assessment; and such tests as EEG, computed tomography scans, brain X-rays, cerebrospinal fluid analysis, and psychological studies. Organic brain syndromes are classified by etiology and specific clinical effects. Causes include infection, brain trauma, nutritional deficiency, cerebrovascular disease, degenerative disease, tumor, toxins, and metabolic or endocrine disorders.

TREATMENT
Effective treatment requires correction of the underlying cause. Special considerations may include reality orientation, emotional support for the patient and his family, a safe environment, mat therapy for an agitated or aggressive patient, and referral for psychological counseling.

Eventually, the patient becomes disoriented, and emotional lability and physical and intellectual disability progress. The patient becomes susceptible to infection and accidents. Usually, death results from infection.

Complications
▶ Accidents and injury
▶ Pneumonia
▶ Malnutrition
▶ Aspiration

Diagnosis
Early diagnosis of Alzheimer's disease is difficult because the patient's signs and symptoms are subtle. (See *Organic brain syndrome*.) Diagnosis relies on an accurate history from a reliable family member, mental status and neurologic examinations, and psychometric testing. Currently, the disease is diagnosed by exclusion; that is, tests are performed to rule out other disorders. The presence of Alzheimer's can't be confirmed until death, when pathologic findings are revealed at autopsy.

Treatment
Therapy consists of attempts to slow disease progression, manage behavioral problems, modify the home environment, and elicit family support. Some medications have proven helpful. Cholinesterase inhibitors such as donepezil, rivastigmine, and galantamine are helpful for mild to moderate Alzheimer's disease.[2] Memantine has been approved for moderate to severe Alzheimer's. It works by delaying the worsening of symptoms.[3] Underlying disorders that contribute to the patient's confusion, such as hypoxia, are also identified and treated. (See *Does lowering cholesterol help Alzheimer's disease?* page 112.)

Special considerations
Overall care is focused on supporting the patient's remaining abilities and compensating for those he has lost.
▶ Establish an effective communication system with the patient and his family to help them adjust to the patient's altered cognitive abilities.

Does lowering cholesterol help Alzheimer's disease?

Research has found some evidence suggesting that lowering serum cholesterol may slow the pathogenesis of Alzheimer's disease.[4] Findings also suggest that there may be a relationship between the use of cholesterol-lowering drugs (also called *statins*) and a decrease in the development of Alzheimer's disease. Studies are ongoing to determine if there is indeed a link between these two and how to best benefit the patient.[6]

▶ Offer emotional support to the patient and his family members. Behavior problems may be made worse by excess stimulation or changes in established routines. Teach the patient and his family about the disease, and refer them to social service and community resources for legal and financial advice and support.

▶ Behavior modification, including prompt and scheduled toileting to reduce urinary incontinence, can improve functional performance.

▶ Anxiety may cause the patient to become agitated or fearful. Intervene by helping him focus on another activity.

▶ Provide the patient with a safe environment. Encourage him to exercise, as ordered, to help maintain mobility.

▶ Reminiscence therapy may have some benefit in treating mood and behavior in Alzheimer's patients; however, further research is necessary to identify significant benefits.[5]

REFERENCES

1. Alzheimer's Association (2007 November 21). "What is Alzheimer's?" [Online]. Available at *www.alz.org/alzheimers_disease_what_is_alszheimers.asp.*

2. Birks, J. "Cholinesterase Inhibitors for Alzheimer's Disease," *Cochrane Database of Systematic Reviews* (1):CD005593, 2006. Available at *www.cochrane.org/reviews/en/ab005593.html.*

3. Alzheimer's Association (2007 November 21). "Standard Treatment." [Online]. Available at *www.alz.org/alzheimers_disease_standard_prescriptions.asp.*

4. Scott, H.D., and Laake, K. "Statins for the Prevention of Alzheimer's Disease," *Cochrane Database of Systematic Reviews* (3):CD003160, 2001. Available at *www.cochrane.org/reviews/en/ab003160.html.*

5. Woods, B., et al. "Reminiscence Therapy for Dementia," *Cochrane Database of Systematic Reviews* (3):CD001120. Available at *www.cochrane.org/reviews/en/ab001120.html.*

6. Li, G., et al. "Statin Therapy is Associated with Reduced Neuropathologic Changes of Alzheimer Disease," *Neurology* 69(9):878-85, August 2007.

AMYOTROPHIC LATERAL SCLEROSIS

Amyotrophic lateral sclerosis (ALS), also called *Lou Gehrig disease,* is the most common of the motor neuron diseases that cause muscle atrophy. (See *Motor neuron disease.*) Other motor neuron diseases include progressive muscular atrophy and progressive bulbar palsy. Symptoms develop between the ages of 40 and 70.[1] A chronic, progressively debilitating disease, ALS may be fatal in less than 1 year or continue for 10 years or more, depending on the muscles it affects.

Causes and incidence

ALS affects about 5 in 100,000 people.[2] ALS is more common in males than females but with increasing age, the incidence is equal.[1]

The exact cause of ALS is unknown, but about 10% of cases have a genetic component. In these patients, it's an autosomal dominant trait and affects males and females equally.

Other than a family member affected with the hereditary form, there are no known risk factors.

Signs and symptoms

Progressive loss of muscle strength and coordination eventually interfere with everyday activities. Patients with ALS develop fasciculations, accompanied by atrophy and weakness, especially in the muscles of the feet and the hands. Other signs include impaired speech; difficulty chewing, swallowing, and breathing and, occasionally, choking and excessive drooling. Mental deterioration doesn't occur, but patients may become depressed as a reaction to the disease.

Complications

▸ Respiratory tract infections
▸ Respiratory failure
▸ Aspiration
▸ Physical immobility complications, such as pressure ulcers and contractures

Diagnosis

Characteristic clinical features indicate a combination of upper and lower motor neuron involvement without sensory impairment. Electromyography and muscle biopsy indicate that the motor nerves aren't functioning, yet sensory nerves are normal. Computed tomography scan and magnetic resonance imaging may help rule out other conditions, such as multiple sclerosis, spinal cord neoplasm, central nervous system syphilis, polyarteritis, syringomyelia, myasthenia gravis, progressive muscular dystrophy, and progressive strokes. Some patients with ALS have increased serum angiogenin levels, but research is still being done to determine the implications of this finding.[4]

Motor neuron disease

In its final stages, motor neuron disease affects both upper and lower motor neuron cells. However, the site of initial cell damage varies according to the specific disease:

• *progressive bulbar palsy:* degeneration of upper motor neurons in the medulla oblongata
• *progressive muscular atrophy:* degeneration of lower motor neurons in the spinal cord
• *amyotrophic lateral sclerosis:* degeneration of upper motor neurons in the medulla oblongata and lower motor neurons in the spinal cord.

Treatment

Management aims to control symptoms and provide emotional, psychological, and physical support. The drug riluzole may increase quality of life and survival but doesn't reverse or stop disease progression.

Baclofen or diazepam helps control spasticity that interferes with activities of daily living.[2] Glycopyrrolate, benztropine, transdermal hyoscine, atropine, trihexyphenidyl or amitriptyline may be used for impaired ability to swallow saliva.[3] Gastrostomy may be needed early to prevent choking; referral to an otolaryngologist is advised to evaluate the risk of choking. Physical therapy, rehabilitation, and use of appliances or orthopedic intervention may be required to maximize function. Devices to assist in breathing at night or mechanical ventilation should be discussed, but the patient's wishes need to be respected.

Special considerations

Because mental status remains intact while progressive physical degeneration takes place, the patient acutely perceives every change. This threatens the patient's relationships, career, income, muscle coordination, sexuality, and energy.

▶ Implement a rehabilitation program designed to maintain independence as long as possible.

▶ Help the patient obtain assistive equipment, such as a walker and a wheelchair. Arrange for a visiting nurse to oversee the patient's status, to provide support, and to teach the family about the illness.

▶ Depending on the patient's muscular capacity, assist with bathing, personal hygiene, and transfers from wheelchair to bed. Help establish a regular bowel and bladder routine.

▶ To help the patient handle increased accumulation of secretions and dysphagia, teach him to suction himself. He should have a suction machine handy at home to reduce the fear of choking.

▶ To prevent skin breakdown, provide good skin care when the patient is bedridden. Turn him often, keep his skin clean and dry, and use pressure-reducing devices such as an alternating air mattress.

▶ If the patient has difficulty swallowing, give him soft, solid foods, and position him upright during meals. Gastrostomy and nasogastric tube feedings may be necessary if he can no longer swallow. Teach the patient (if he's still able to feed himself) or his family how to administer gastrostomy feedings.

▶ Provide emotional support. Directives regarding health care decisions should be discussed before the patient becomes unable to communicate his wishes. Prepare the patient and his family members for his eventual death, and encourage the start of the grieving process. Patients with ALS may benefit from a hospice program or the local ALS support group chapter.[5]

REFERENCES

1. ALS Association. "Who Gets ALS?" [Online]. Available at *www.alsa.org/als/who.cfm.*
2. Clem, K. eMedicine from *WebMD* (2006 May 15). "Amyotrophic Lateral Sclerosis." [Online]. Available at *www.emedicine.com/emerg/topic24.htm.*
3. Miller, R.G., et al. "Practice Parameter: The Care of the Patient with Amyotrophic Lateral Sclerosis (An Evidence-Based Review)," *Muscle Nerve* 22(8):1104-118, August 1999.
4. Cronin, S., et al. "Elevated Serum Angiogenin Levels in ALS," *Neurology* 67(10):1833-36, November 2006.
5. Mitsumoto, H., and Rabkin, J.G. "Palliative Care for Patients with Amyotrophic Lateral Sclerosis: 'Prepare for the Worst and Hope for the Best,'" *JAMA* 298(2):207-16, July 2007.

ARTERIOVENOUS MALFORMATIONS

Cerebral arteriovenous malformation (AVM) is a disorder of the blood vessels characterized by an abnormal connection between the arteries and the veins in the brain. It's a congenital disorder that commonly results in tangled masses of thin-walled, dilated blood vessels between arteries and veins that aren't connected by capillaries. AVM primarily occurs in the posterior portion of the cerebral hemispheres. Adequate perfusion of brain tissue is prevented due to abnormal channels between the arterial and venous systems that allow mixing of oxygenated and unoxygenated blood. AVMs range in size from a few millimeters to large malformations that extend from the cerebral cortex to the ventricles. Patients typically present with multiple AVMs, and 38% to 70% of AVMs present with hemorrhage.[1]

Causes and incidence

Although some AVMs occur as a result of penetrating injuries such as trauma, most are present at birth. However, symptoms typically don't occur until between the ages of 10 and 20. Very large AVMs may short-circuit blood flow enough to cause cardiac decompensation, a condition in which the heart can't pump enough blood to compensate for bleeding in the brain. This typically occurs in infants and young children.

The vessels of an AVM are very thin, and one or more arteries feed into it, causing it to appear dilated and tortuous. Typically, high-pressured arterial flow moves into the venous system through the connecting channels to increase venous pressure, engorging and dilating the venous structures. If the AVM is large enough, the shunting can deprive the surrounding tissue of adequate blood flow. Thin-walled vessels may ooze small amounts of blood—they may even rupture—causing hemorrhage into the brain or subarachnoid space.

Cerebral arteriovenous malformations occur in approximately 3 out of 10,000 people. Only about 12% of the affected population (36,000 of an estimated 300,000 Americans with AVMs) actually have symptoms.[1] Although the lesion is present at birth, symptoms may occur at any time. Two-thirds of cases occur before age 40. Evidence suggests that some AVMs run in families, but the numbers are small. There have been no clearly identified risk factors. Males and females are affected equally.

Signs and symptoms

An AVM may be asymptomatic until complications occur; these may include rupture and a resulting sudden bleed in the brain, known as a hemorrhagic stroke. Arteriovenous malformations vary in size and location within the brain. Systolic bruit may be auscultated over the carotid artery, mastoid process, or orbit on examination.

Symptoms that occur prior to an AVM rupture are related to smaller and slower bleeding from the abnormal vessels, which are usually fragile because their structure is abnormal.

In more than half of patients with AVM, hemorrhage from the malformation is the first symptom. Depending on the location and the severity of the bleed, the hemorrhage can be profoundly disabling or fatal. The risk of bleeding from an AVM is approximately 2% to 4% per year.

The first symptoms often include headache, seizure, or other sudden neurological problems, such as vision problems, weakness, inability to move a limb or a side of the body, lack of sensation in part of the body, or abnormal sensations, such as ringing and numbness. Symptoms are the same as for stroke. The individual with an AVM may complain of chronic mild headache, a sudden and severe headache, or a localized or general headache. The headache may resemble a migraine, and vomiting may occur. Seizures may result from focal neurologic deficits (depending on the location of the AVM) resulting from compression and diminished perfusion. Symptoms of intracranial (intracerebral, subarachnoid, or subdural) hemorrhage result. Muscle weakness and decreased sensation can occur in any part of the body. Mental status change can occur where the individual appears sleepy, stuporous, lethargic, confused, disoriented, or irritable. Additional symptoms may include stiff neck, speech or sense of smell impairment, dysfunctional movement, fainting, facial paralysis, eyelid drooping, tinnitus, dizziness, and decreased level of consciousness (LOC).

If an AVM bleeds once, the risk is greater that it will bleed again in the future.[2] Intracerebral or subarachnoid hemorrhages are the most common first symptoms of cerebral arteriovenous malformation. In some cases, symptoms may also occur due to lack of blood flow to an area of the brain (ischemia), compression or distortion of brain tissue by large AVMs, or abnormal brain development in the area of the malformation. Progressive loss of nerve cells in the brain may occur, caused by mechanical (pressure) and ischemic (lack of blood supply) factors.

Complications

▶ Aneurysm and subsequent rupture

▶ Hemorrhage (intracerebral, subarachnoid, or subdural, depending on the location of the AVM)
▶ Hydrocephalus

Diagnosis

Cerebral angiography confirms the presence of AVMs and evaluates blood flow.[1] It is invasive and has a slight risk of stroke.[1] Other noninvasive tests used to diagnose AVM include head computed tomography scan, cranial magnetic resonance imaging, and magnetic resonance angiography. An EEG may also be performed if symptoms include seizures, but this test won't diagnose the specific area of the lesion.

Doppler ultrasonography of the cerebrovascular system indicates abnormal, turbulent blood flow.

Treatment

General support measures include aneurysm precautions to prevent possible rupture. This involves placing the patient on bed rest or with limited activity and maintaining a quiet atmosphere. Analgesics may be given for headache, and sedatives may be given to help calm the patient and prevent rupture. Stool softeners may be given to prevent straining, which increases intracranial pressure.

A bleeding AVM is a medical emergency that requires immediate hospitalization. The goal of treatment is to prevent further complications by limiting bleeding, controlling seizures and, if possible, removing the AVM. Corrective surgery may include block dissection, laser, or ligation to repair the communicating channels and remove the feeding vessels. Endovascular embolization or radiation therapy may be done, if surgery isn't possible, to close the communicating channels and feeder vessels, thereby reducing blood flow to the AVM. Open brain surgery, endovascular treatment, and radiosurgery may be used separately or in any combination, depending upon the physician and the patient's individual situation. Surgery is dependent upon the accessibility and size of the lesion and the patient's status. Open brain surgery involves the actual removal of the malformation in the brain through an opening made in the skull. This surgery is particularly risky because the surgery itself may cause the AVM to bleed uncontrollably.

Endovascular embolization (injecting a glue-like substance into the abnormal vessels to stop aberrant blood flow into the AVM) may be an alternative if surgery isn't feasible due to the size or location of the lesion. Stereotactic radiosurgery may also be an alternative for patients with inoperable arteriovenous malformation that are 3 cm in diameter or less. It's particularly useful for small, deep lesions that are difficult to remove by surgery. New techniques also include using real-time ultrasound angiography during surgery to help pinpoint the arteries feeding the AVM.[3]

Anticonvulsant medications such as phenytoin are usually prescribed if seizures occur.

Special considerations

▶ Patients who have had surgery or endovascular interventions will require intensive care monitoring.
▶ Monitor vital signs and titrate medications to control hypertension.
▶ Monitor neurologic status.
▶ Monitor for seizure activity, and institute seizure precautions.
▶ Maintain a quiet atmosphere, and provide relaxation techniques.
▶ Discuss the importance of reporting any signs of intracranial bleeding immediately (sudden severe headache, vision changes, decreased movement in extremities, and change in LOC).
▶ Administer narcotics or alternative treatments to decrease pain, which will assist in blood pressure reduction.

▶ Refer to social services for support services if neurological deficits have occurred from a ruptured AVM.

REFERENCES

1. National Institute of Neurological Disorders and Stroke. "Arteriovenous Malformations and Other Vascular Lesions of the Central Nervous System Fact Sheet," Last updated 12/11/07. Available at *www.ninds.nih.gov/disorders/avms/detail_avms.htm.*
2. Yamada, S., et al. "Risk Factors for Subsequent Hemorrhage in Patients with Cerebral Arteriovenous Malformations," *Journal of Neurosurgery* 107(5):965-72, November 2007.
3. Wang, Y., et al. "Intraoperative Real-Time Contrast-Enhanced Ultrasound Angiography: A New Adjunct in the Surgical Treatment of Arteriovenous Malformations," *Journal of Neurosurgery* 107(5):959-64, November 2007.

CEREBRAL ANEURYSM

Cerebral aneurysm is a localized dilation of a cerebral artery that typically results from a congenital weakness in the arterial wall. Its most common form is the saccular aneurysm (or berry aneurysm), a saclike outpouching in a cerebral artery. Cerebral aneurysms may arise at an arterial junction in the Circle of Willis, the circular anastomosis formed by the major cerebral arteries at the base of the brain. Cerebral aneurysms can rupture and cause subarachnoid hemorrhage. (See *Most common sites of cerebral aneurysm,* page 118.)

The prognosis is guarded: Forty percent of patients die from the effects of hemorrhage within the first 24 hours; another 25% die within 6 months from complications.[1]

Causes and incidence

Cerebral aneurysm may result from a congenital defect, a degenerative process, or a combination of both. For example, hypertension and atherosclerosis may disrupt blood flow and exert pressure against a congenitally weak arterial wall, stretching it like an over-filled balloon and making it likely to rupture. After such rupture, blood leaks into the space normally occupied by cerebrospinal fluid (CSF), resulting in subarachnoid hemorrhage. Blood may also leak into the brain tissue and form a clot, which can result in potentially fatal increased intracranial pressure (ICP) and brain-tissue damage.

HEALTH & SAFETY *The size of the aneurysm doesn't affect the patient's outcome; the more important factor in patient survival is the amount of blood that leaks into the brain tissue.[4]*

Incidence is slightly higher in females than in males, and in people ages 30 to 60 years, but cerebral aneurysm may occur at any age, in both females and males. Ruptured aneurysms occur in 10 out of 100,000 people per year.[1]

Signs and symptoms

Occasionally, rupture of a cerebral aneurysm causes premonitory symptoms, such as headache, blurred vision, cranial nerve palsy, or dilated pupils.[2] Usually, however, onset is abrupt and without warning, causing a sudden severe headache, nausea, vomiting and, depending on the severity and location of bleeding, altered consciousness (including deep coma).

Bleeding causes meningeal irritation, resulting in nuchal rigidity, back and leg pain, fever, restlessness, irritability, occasional seizures, and blurred vision. Bleeding into the brain tissues causes hemiparesis, hemisensory defects, dysphagia, and visual defects. If the aneurysm is near the internal carotid artery, it compresses the oculomotor nerve and causes diplopia, ptosis, dilated pupil, and inability to rotate the eye.

The severity of symptoms varies considerably from patient to patient, depending on the site and amount of bleeding. To better describe their conditions, patients with rup-

Most common sites of cerebral aneurysm

Cerebral aneurysms usually arise at arterial bifurcations in the Circle of Willis and its branches. The illustration below shows the most common aneurysm sites around this circle.

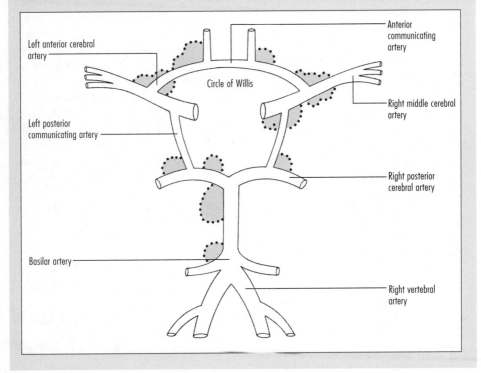

tured cerebral aneurysms are grouped as follows according to the Hunt and Hess Scale:
▶ *Grade I (minimal bleed):* Patient is alert with no neurologic deficit; he may have a slight headache and nuchal rigidity.
▶ *Grade II (mild bleed):* Patient is alert, with a mild to severe headache, nuchal rigidity and, possibly, third-nerve palsy.
▶ *Grade III (moderate bleed):* Patient is confused or drowsy, with nuchal rigidity and, possibly, a mild focal deficit.
▶ *Grade IV (severe bleed):* Patient is stuporous, with nuchal rigidity and, possibly, mild to severe hemiparesis.
▶ *Grade V (moribund; commonly fatal):* If nonfatal, patient is in deep coma or decerebrate.

Complications

Generally, cerebral aneurysm poses three major threats:
▶ *Death from increased ICP:* Increased ICP may push the brain downward, impair brain stem function, and cut off blood supply to the part of the brain that supports vital functions.[5]
▶ *Rebleed:* Generally, after the initial bleeding episode, a clot forms and seals the rupture, which reinforces the wall of the aneurysm for 7 to 10 days. However, after the seventh day, fibrinolysis begins to dissolve the clot and increases the risk of rebleeding. Signs and symptoms are similar to those accompanying the initial hemorrhage. Rebleeds during the first 24 hours after ini-

tial hemorrhage aren't uncommon, and they contribute to cerebral aneurysm's high mortality.

▶ *Vasospasm:* Why this occurs isn't clearly understood. Usually, vasospasm occurs in blood vessels adjacent to the cerebral aneurysm, but it may extend to major vessels of the brain, causing ischemia and altered brain function.

Other complications of cerebral aneurysm include pulmonary embolism (a possible adverse effect of deep vein thrombosis or aneurysm treatment) and acute hydrocephalus, occurring as CSF accumulates in the cranial cavity because of blockage by blood or adhesions.

Diagnosis

Diagnosis of cerebral aneurysm is based on the patient history and a neurologic examination; computed tomography scan, which reveals subarachnoid or ventricular blood; or magnetic resonance imaging, which can identify a cerebral aneurysm as a flow void.

Cerebral angiography remains the procedure of choice for diagnosing cerebral aneurysm.[3] Lumbar puncture may be used to identify blood in CSF if other studies are negative and the patient has no signs of increased ICP. Lumbar puncture should be performed if no contraindication is present and you strongly suspect a bleed, because imaging studies may miss a bleed.

Other baseline laboratory studies include complete blood count, urinalysis, arterial blood gas (ABG) analysis, coagulation studies, serum osmolality, and electrolyte and glucose levels.

Treatment

Treatment aims to reduce the risk of vasospasm and cerebral infarction by repairing the aneurysm. Endovascular coiling represents a significant advancement in care and is now used to treat most aneurysms. Endovascular coiling is a minimally invasive procedure that uses a catheter to insert plat-

Aneurysm clip

Clipping is a method of surgical repair for a cerebral aneurysm. The neurosurgeon grasps the clip, opens the jaw, and then slides the clip over the hemorrhaging blood vessel. He then closes the clip over the blood vessel, and the applied pressure stems the hemorrhaging without compromising vessel integrity.

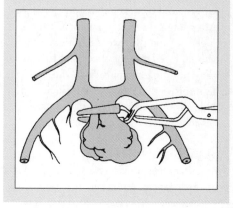

inum or titanium coils into the aneurysm, which causes thrombosis and prevents rupture.[2,3] Surgical repair by clipping (ligation, or wrapping the aneurysm neck with muscle) can also be done. The goal of surgical clipping is to deprive the aneurysm of circulation without blocking normal vessels. (See *Aneurysm clip.*) Several studies have compared coiling to surgical clipping. Coiling was found to be safer.[3] Both procedures continue to be used, however, depending on the patient and the specifics of the aneurysm. Clipping or coiling usually occurs within about 48 to 72 hours of the onset of symptoms, or after 10 to 14 days.

When the aneurysm is in a dangerous location, making surgery risky, or when surgery is delayed because of vasospasm, treatment includes:

▶ bed rest in a quiet, darkened room; if immediate surgery isn't possible, such bed rest may continue for 4 to 6 weeks

▶ avoidance of coffee, other stimulants, and aspirin

▶ codeine or another analgesic, as needed

▶ antihypertensive agents if the patient is hypertensive

▶ calcium channel blockers to decrease spasm

▶ corticosteroids to reduce edema

▶ phenytoin or another anticonvulsant

▶ sedatives

▶ a fibrinolytic inhibitor, to minimize the risk of rebleed by delaying blood clot lysis.

After surgical repair, the patient's condition depends on the extent of damage from the initial bleed and the success of treatment for any resulting complications. Surgery can't improve the patient's neurologic condition unless it removes a hematoma or reduces the compression effect.

Special considerations

An accurate neurologic assessment, good patient care, patient and family teaching, and psychological support can speed recovery and reduce complications.

▶ During initial treatment after hemorrhage, establish and maintain a patent airway if the patient needs supplementary oxygen. Position the patient to promote pulmonary drainage and prevent upper airway obstruction. If he's intubated, administering 100% oxygen before suctioning to remove secretions will prevent hypoxia and vasodilation from carbon dioxide accumulation. Suction no longer than 15 seconds to avoid increased ICP. Give frequent nose and mouth care.

▶ Impose aneurysm precautions to minimize the risk of rebleed and to avoid increased ICP. Such precautions include bed rest in a quiet, darkened room (keep the head of the bed flat or under 30 degrees, as ordered); limited visitors; restricted fluid intake; no straining during bowel movements; and no strenuous physical activity. In addition, warn the patient to avoid all unnecessary physical activity. Be sure to explain why these restrictive measures are necessary.

Preventive measures and good patient care can minimize other complications:

▶ Turn the patient often. Encourage occasional deep breathing and leg movement. Assist with active range-of-motion (ROM) exercises; if the patient is paralyzed, perform regular passive ROM exercises.

▶ Monitor ABG levels, LOC, and vital signs often, and accurately measure intake and output. Avoid taking the patient's temperature rectally because vagus nerve stimulation may cause cardiac arrest.

▶ Watch for these danger signals, which may indicate an enlarging aneurysm, rebleeding, intracranial clot, vasospasm, or other complication: decreased LOC, unilateral enlarged pupil, onset or worsening of hemiparesis or motor deficit, increased blood pressure, slowed pulse, worsening of headache or sudden onset of a headache, renewed or worsened nuchal rigidity, and renewed or persistent vomiting. Intermittent signs such as restlessness, extremity weakness, and speech alterations can also indicate increasing ICP.

▶ Give fluids as ordered, and monitor I.V. infusions to avoid increased ICP.

▶ If the patient has facial weakness, assess the gag reflex, and assist him during meals by placing food in the unaffected side of his mouth. If he can't swallow, insert a nasogastric tube as ordered, and give all tube feedings slowly. Prevent skin breakdown by taping the tube so it doesn't press against the nostril. If the patient can eat solid foods, provide a high-fiber diet to prevent straining at stool, which can increase ICP. Obtain an order for a stool softener such as dioctyl sodium sulfosuccinate, or a mild laxative, and administer as ordered. Don't force fluids. Implement a bowel program based on previous habits. If the patient is receiving steroids, check the stool for blood.

▶ With third or facial nerve palsy, administer artificial tears or ointment to the affected

eye, and tape the eye shut at night to prevent corneal damage.

▶ To minimize stress, encourage relaxation techniques. If possible, avoid using restraints because these can cause agitation and raise ICP.

▶ Administer antihypertensives as ordered. Carefully monitor blood pressure, and immediately report *any* significant change, but especially a rise in systolic pressure.

▶ Prevent deep vein thrombosis by applying antiembolism stockings or sequential compression sleeves.

▶ If the patient can't speak, establish a simple means of communication, or use cards or a notepad. Try to limit conversation to topics that won't frustrate the patient. Encourage his family to speak to him in a normal tone, even if he doesn't seem to respond.

▶ Provide emotional support, and include the patient's family in his care as much as possible. Encourage family members to adopt a realistic attitude, but don't discourage hope.

▶ Before discharge, make a referral to a visiting nurse or a rehabilitation center when necessary, and teach the patient and his family how to recognize signs of rebleeding.

REFERENCES

1. National Institute of Neurological Disorders and Stroke (2007 December 11). "Cerebral Aneurysm Fact Sheet." [Online]. Available at *www.ninds.nih.gov/disorders/cerebral_ aneurysm/detail_cerebral_aneurysm.htm.*
2. Olson, D., and Halley, N. "Cerebral Aneurysm Rupture: Are You Prepared?" *Nursing2007* 37(3):64cc1-64cc4. March 2007.
3. Brain Aneurysm Resources. "Treatment Options: Treatment of Brain Aneurysm." [Online]. Available at *www.brainaneurysm. com/aneurysm-treatment.html.*
4. Salary, M., et al. "Relation among Aneurysm Size, Amount of Subarachnoid Blood, and Clinical Outcome," *Journal of Neurosurgery* 107(1):13-17, July 2007.
5. Rosen, D.S., et al. "Intraventricular Hemorrhage from Ruptured Aneurysm: Clinical Characteristics, Complications, and Outcomes in a Large, Prospective, Multicenter Study Population," *Journal of Neurosurgery* 107(2):261-65, August 2007.

CREUTZFELDT-JAKOB DISEASE

Creutzfeldt-Jakob disease (CJD) is a rare, rapidly progressive viral disease that attacks the central nervous system, causing dementia and neurologic signs and symptoms, such as myoclonic jerking, ataxia, aphasia, visual disturbances, and paralysis. CJD is always fatal. A new variant of CJD (vCJD) emerged in Europe in 1996. (See *Understanding vCJD,* page 122.)

Causes and incidence

The causative organism is difficult to identify because no foreign ribonucleic acid or deoxyribonucleic acid has been linked to the disease. CJD is believed to be caused by a specific protein called a prion, which lacks nucleic acids, resists proteolytic digestion, and spontaneously aggregates in the brain. Most cases are sporadic; between 5% and 15% are familial, with an autosomal dominant pattern of inheritance. Although CJD isn't transmitted by normal casual contact, human-to-human transmission can occur as a result of certain medical procedures, such as corneal and cadaveric dura mater grafts. Isolated cases are attributed to treatment during childhood with human growth hormone and to improperly decontaminated neurosurgical instruments and brain electrodes. (See *Transmission of CJD variants,* page 123.)

CJD generally affects adults about 60 years old.[3] It occurs in more than 50 countries. Males and females are affected equally. Incidence is 1 in 1,000,000 worldwide, and there are about 200 diagnosed each year in the United States.[3]

Understanding vCJD

Like conventional Creutzfeldt-Jakob disease (CJD), this variant of the disease (vCJD) is a rare, fatal neurodegenerative disease. Most cases have been reported in the United Kingdom. The likeliest cause of vCJD is exposure to bovine spongiform encephalopathy (BSE)—a fatal brain disease in cattle also known as *mad cow disease*—via ingestion of beef products from cattle with BSE.

This variant, vCJD, affects patients at a much younger age (average age 29 years) than CJD. The duration of the illness is much longer (14 months).[1]

Regulations have been established in Europe to control outbreaks of BSE in cattle and to prevent contaminated meat from entering the food supply. The Centers for Disease Control and Prevention and the World Health Organization are still exploring vCJD and its relationship to BSE.

Researchers are looking into whether vCJD is transmitted via blood or blood components.[2]

New medications to treat CJD

Until recently, there was no thought of treating Creutzfeldt-Jakob disease (CJD) with medications. However, new research is underway that may change that. The most promising medication at this time is an antibody against prions, the cause of CJD. This research is extremely new, but very promising, and will continue in hopes of finding a treatment for CJD.[5]

Signs and symptoms

Early signs and symptoms of mental impairment may include slowness in thinking, difficulty concentrating, impaired judgment, and memory loss. Dementia is progressive and occurs early. Involuntary movements, such as muscle twitching, trembling, peculiar body movements, and visual disturbances, appear with disease progression and advancing mental deterioration. Hallucinations are also common. Duration of the typical illness is 4 months.

Complications

▶ Death from bronchopneumonia

Diagnosis

CJD must be considered for anyone experiencing signs of progressive dementia. Neurologic examination is the most effective tool in diagnosing CJD. Difficulty with rapid alternating movements and point-to-point movements are typically evident early in the disease.

An EEG may be performed to assess the patient for typical changes in brain wave activity. Computed tomography scan, magnetic resonance imaging of the brain, and lumbar puncture may be useful in ruling out other disorders that cause dementia.[4] Although not diagnostic, presence of the 14-3-3 protein in the spinal fluid is highly suggestive of the disease when it's accompanied by other characteristic symptoms. Definitive diagnosis usually isn't obtained until an autopsy is done and brain tissue is examined.

Treatment

There's no cure for CJD, and its progress can't be slowed. Palliative care is provided to make the patient comfortable and to ease symptoms. Medications may be needed to control aggressive behaviors. (See *New medications to treat CJD*.) These include sedatives and antipsychotics.

The need to provide a safe environment, control aggressive or agitated behavior, and meet physiologic needs may require monitor-

Transmisssion of CJD variants

Question: *Can variants of Creutzfeldt-Jakob disease be transmitted through blood transfusions?*

Research: Creutzfeldt-Jakob disease (CJD) is characterized by an abnormal prion protein that can replicate and replace nervous tissue. Other forms of the disease include sporadic CJD (sCJD), familial CJD (fCJD), and variant CJD (vCJD), found in lymphoid tissue. Researchers are involved in an ongoing study in the United Kingdom (UK) to determine whether CJD, vCJD, sCJD, and fCJD (all reportable diseases) are transmitted through blood transfusions. The study is being conducted through look-back investigations of the National CJD Surveillance Unit (NCJDSU) and the UK Blood Services, the reporting agencies. Cases of all types of CJD in blood donors are investigated, the blood product recipients are identified, and details of the identified recipients and donors are checked against the NCJDSU register to determine if there are any matches.

Conclusion: As of March 1, 2006—the last date on which the results below were compiled—no confirmed transmission through blood transfusion was reported for classic CJD. Although there aren't enough data to make a definitive determination, there was also no evidence of transmission of sCJD or fCJD by blood transfusion. However, vCJD appears to be transmissible through transfusion because the study

identified two confirmed cases in patients who had received blood from donors already on the NCJDSU register. A third person, who had received red blood cells from a donor before the donor developed clinical symptoms, was identified as having abnormal prion protein in his lymphoid tissue. The finding was made 5 years after the transfusion during a postmortem examination and was classified as a probable transmission. The study also demonstrated a significant incubation period for vCJD before the development of clinical symptoms, ranging from 18 months to 7 years.

Application: Nurses must be well informed about the necessary precautions and decontamination procedures required when caring for a patient with known CJD or a rapidly progressive unexplained dementia. Additionally, nurses play a major role in providing supportive care and educating patients, their families, and community organizations and agencies about CJD.

Source: Hewitt, P.E., et al. "Creutzfeldt-Jakob Disease and Blood Transfusion: Results of the UK Transfusion Medicine Epidemiological Review Study," *Vox Sanguinis* 91(3):221-30, October 2006.

ing and assistance in the home or in an institutionalized setting. Family counseling may help in coping with the changes required for home care.

Behavior modification may be helpful, in some cases, for controlling unacceptable or dangerous behaviors. Reality orientation, with repeated reinforcement of environmental and other cues, may help reduce disorientation.

Legal advice for the patient's family may be appropriate early in the course of the disorder, to form advance directives, power of

attorney, and other legal actions that may make it easier to make ethical decisions regarding the care of an individual with CJD.

Special considerations

▶ Offer emotional support to the patient and his family. Teach them about the disease, and assist them through the grieving process. Refer the patient and his family to CJD support groups, and encourage participation.

▶ Contact social services and hospice, as appropriate, to assist the family with their needs.

▶ Encourage the patient and his family to discuss and complete advance directives.

▶ To prevent disease transmission, use caution when handling body fluids and other materials from patients suspected of having CJD.

REFERENCES

1. World Health Organization (2002 November). "Variant Creutzfeldt-Jakob Disease." [Online]. Available at *www.who.int/mediacentre/ factsheets/fs180/en/*.

2. Ironside J.W. "Variant Creutzfeldt-Jakob Disease: Risk of Transmission by Blood Transfusion and Blood Therapies," *Haemophilia* 12(Suppl1):8-15, March 2006.

3. National Institute of Neurological Disorders and Stroke (2006 December 13). "Creutzfeldt-Jakob Disease Fact Sheet." [Online]. Available at *www.ninds.nih.gov/disorders/cjd/detail_cjd. htm*.

4. Tan, K.M., et al. "Creutzfeldt-Jakob Disease with Focal Electroencephalographic and Magnetic Resonance Imaging Findings," *Archives in Neurology* 64(4):600-601, April 2007.

5. Korth, C., and Peters, C.J. "Emerging Pharmacotherapies for Creutzfeldt-Jakob Disease," *Archives of Neurology* 63(4):497-501, April 2006.

ENCEPHALITIS

E ncephalitis is a severe inflammation of the brain, commonly caused by a mosquito-borne or, in some areas, a tick-borne virus. However, transmission by means other than arthropod bites may occur through ingestion of infected goat's milk and accidental injection or inhalation of the virus. Person to person, airborne transmission of viruses (such as measles or mumps) may also lead to encephalitis in nonimmunized populations. Eastern equine encephalitis may produce permanent neurologic damage and is commonly fatal. (See *Types of encephalitis*.)

In encephalitis, intense lymphocytic infiltration of brain tissues and the leptomeninges causes cerebral edema, degeneration of the brain's ganglion cells, and diffuse nerve cell destruction.

Causes and incidence

Encephalitis generally results from infection with arboviruses specific to rural areas. However, in urban areas, it's most frequently caused by enteroviruses (coxsackievirus, poliovirus, and echovirus). Other causes include herpesvirus, mumps virus, human immunodeficiency virus, adenoviruses, and demyelinating diseases after measles, varicella, rubella, or vaccination.

Between World War I and the Depression, a type of encephalitis known as *lethargic encephalitis, von Economo's disease,* or *sleeping sickness* occurred with some regularity. The causative virus was never clearly identified, and the disease is rare today. Even so, the term *sleeping sickness* persists and is commonly, although wrongly, used to describe other types of encephalitis as well.

Signs and symptoms

All viral forms of encephalitis have similar clinical features, although certain differences do occur. Usually, the acute illness begins with sudden onset of fever, headache, and vomiting and progresses to include signs and symptoms of meningeal irritation (stiff neck and back) and neuronal damage (drowsiness, coma, paralysis, seizures, ataxia, tremors, nausea, vomiting, and organic psychoses). After the acute phase of the illness, coma may persist for days or weeks.

The severity of arbovirus encephalitis may range from subclinical to rapidly fatal necrotizing disease. Herpes encephalitis also produces signs and symptoms that vary from subclinical to acute and commonly fatal ful-

(Text continues on page 127.)

Types of encephalitis

Four main viral agents cause most cases of encephalitis in the United States: eastern equine encephalitis (EEE), western equine encephalitis (WEE), St. Louis encephalitis (SLE), and La Crosse (LAC) encephalitis, all of which are transmitted by mosquitoes. Another virus, Powassan (POW), is a minor cause of encephalitis in the northern United States; this virus is transmitted by ticks. Most cases of arboviral encephalitis occur from June through September, when arthropods are most active. In milder parts of the country, where arthropods are active late into the year, cases can occur into the winter months.

No vaccines are available for these U.S.–based diseases. However, a Japanese encephalitis (JE) vaccine is available for those who will be traveling to Japan, a tick-borne encephalitis vaccine is available for those who will be traveling to Europe, and an equine vaccine is available for EEE, WEE, and Venezuelan equine encephalitis (VEE). Public health measures often require spraying of insecticides to kill larvae and adult mosquitoes as well as controlling standing water that can provide mosquito-breeding sites.

EASTERN EQUINE ENCEPHALITIS
• EEE is caused by an alphavirus transmitted to humans and equines by the bite of an infected mosquito.
• Incubation is 3 to 10 days.
• Symptoms begin with a sudden onset of fever, general muscle pains, and a headache of increasing severity; can progress to seizures and coma.
• One-third of those afflicted will die from the disease. Approximately one-half of those who survive will have mild to severe permanent neurologic damage.[1]
• Human cases are usually preceded by outbreaks in horses.
• The virus occurs in natural cycles involving birds in swampy areas nearly every year during the warm months. The virus doesn't escape from these areas, however, and this mosquito doesn't usually bite humans or other mammals.
• The incidence of human EEE averages five cases per year.[1]

WESTERN EQUINE ENCEPHALITIS
• The alphavirus WEE is the causative agent. The virus is closely related to the EEE and VEE viruses.
• The enzootic cycle of WEE involves passerine birds, in which the infection is inapparent, and culicine mosquitoes, principally Culex (Cx.) tarsalis, a species associated with irrigated agriculture and stream drainages.
• Human WEE cases are usually first seen in June or July.
• Most WEE infections are asymptomatic or present as mild, nonspecific illness. Patients with clinically apparent illness usually have a sudden onset with fever, headache, nausea, vomiting, anorexia, and malaise, followed by altered mental status, weakness, and signs of meningeal irritation.
• Children, especially those younger than age 1, are affected more severely than adults and may be left with permanent sequelae, which is seen in 5% to 30% of young patients.
• Mortality is about 3%.

ST. LOUIS ENCEPHALITIS
• The leading cause of SLE is flaviviral. SLE is the most common mosquito-transmitted human pathogen in the United States.
• Mosquitoes become infected by feeding on birds infected with the SLE virus. Infected mosquitoes then transmit the virus to humans and animals during the feeding process. The virus grows both in the infected mosquito and the infected bird, but doesn't make either one sick.
• Less than 1% of SLE viral infections are clinically apparent; the majority are undiagnosed.
• Illness ranges in severity from a simple febrile headache to meningoencephalitis, with an overall case-fatality ratio of 5% to 15%.
• The incubation period is 5 to 15 days.[2]
• Mild infections present with fever and headache. More severe infection is marked by headache, high fever, neck stiffness, stupor, disorientation, coma, tremors, occasional seizures (especially in infants), and spastic (but rarely flaccid) paralysis.
• The disease is generally milder in children than in adults, but in those children who

(continued)

Types of encephalitis *(continued)*

do have disease, there's a high rate of encephalitis.
- Elderly people are at highest risk for severe disease and death.
- During the summer season, SLE virus is maintained in a mosquito-bird-mosquito cycle, with periodic amplification by peridomestic birds and *Culex* mosquitoes.
- SLE occurs in 100 cases per year.[2]

LA CROSSE ENCEPHALITIS
- The LAC virus, a Bunyavirus, is a zoonotic pathogen cycled between the daytime-biting tree hole mosquito, *Aedes triseriatus*, and vertebrate amplifier hosts (chipmunks, tree squirrels) in deciduous forest habitats. The virus is maintained over the winter by transmission in mosquito eggs. If the female mosquito is infected, she may lay eggs that carry the virus. Vector uses artificial containers (tires, buckets, and so forth) in addition to tree holes.
- LAC encephalitis initially presents as a nonspecific summertime illness with fever, headache, nausea, vomiting, and lethargy.
- Severe disease occurs most commonly in children younger than age 16 and is characterized by seizures, coma, paralysis, and a variety of neurological sequelae after recovery.
- Death occurs in less than 1% of clinical cases.
- Cases are often reported as aseptic meningitis or viral encephalitis of unknown etiology.
- During an average year, about 70 cases of LAC encephalitis are reported to the Centers for Disease Control and Prevention.[3]

POWASSAN ENCEPHALITIS
- The POW virus is a flavivirus.
- Recently a Powassan-like virus was isolated from the deer tick, *Ixodes scapularis*. The virus has been recovered from ticks (*Ixodes marxi* and *Dermacentor andersoni*) and from the tissues of a skunk (*Spilogale putorius*).
- It's a rare cause of acute viral encephalitis.
- Patients who recover may have residual neurologic problems.

VENEZUELAN EQUINE ENCEPHALITIS
- Like EEE and WEE viruses, VEE is an alphavirus that causes encephalitis in horses and humans. VEE is a significant veterinary and public health problem in Central and South America.
- Infection of humans with the VEE virus is less severe than with EEE and WEE viruses, and fatalities are rare.
- Adults usually develop only an influenza-like illness; overt encephalitis is usually confined to children.
- Effective VEE virus vaccines are available for equines.

JAPANESE ENCEPHALITIS
- JE virus, which is related to SLE, is a flavivirus. It's widespread throughout Asia.
- Epidemics occur in late summer in temperate regions, but the infection is enzootic and occurs throughout the year in many tropical areas of Asia.
- The virus is maintained in a cycle involving culicine mosquitoes and water birds. It's transmitted to humans by Culex mosquitoes, primarily *Cx. tritaeniorhynchus*, which breed in rice fields.
- Mosquitoes become infected by feeding on domestic pigs and wild birds infected with the JE virus. Infected mosquitoes then transmit the virus to humans and animals during the feeding process. The virus is amplified in domestic pigs and wild birds.
- The incubation period is 5 to 14 days.
- Mild infections occur without apparent symptoms other than fever with headache. More severe infection is marked by quick onset, headache, high fever, neck stiffness, stupor, disorientation, coma, tremors, occasional seizures (especially in infants), and spastic (but rarely flaccid) paralysis.
- The illness resolves in 5 to 7 days if there's no central nervous system involvement.
- The mortality is less than 10%, but is higher in children and can exceed 30%. Neurologic sequelae in patients who recover are reported in up to 30% of cases.

Types of encephalitis *(continued)*

- A vaccine is currently available for human use in the United States for individuals who might be traveling to endemic countries.

TICK-BORNE ENCEPHALITIS
- Tick-borne encephalitis (TBE) is caused by two closely related flaviviruses. The eastern subtype causes Russian spring-summer encephalitis (RSSE) and is transmitted by *Ixodes persulcatus*, whereas the western subtype is transmitted by *I. ricinus* and causes Central European encephalitis (CEE).
- RSSE is the more severe infection, having a mortality of up to 25% in some outbreaks, whereas mortality in CEE seldom exceeds 5%.
- The incubation period is 7 to 14 days.
- Infection usually presents as a mild, influenza-type illness or as benign, aseptic meningitis, but may result in fatal meningoencephalitis.
- Fever is often biphasic, and there may be severe headache and neck rigidity, with transient paralysis of the limbs, shoulders or, less commonly, the respiratory musculature. A few patients are left with residual paralysis.
- Although the great majority of TBE infections follow exposure to ticks, infection has occurred through the ingestion of infected cows' or goats' milk.
- An inactivated TBE vaccine is currently available in Europe and Russia.

WEST NILE ENCEPHALITIS
- West Nile virus (WNV) is a flavivirus belonging to the Japanese encephalitis serocomplex that includes the closely related SLE virus, Kunjin, and Murray Valley encephalitis viruses, as well as others.
- SLE and WNV viruses are related.

- WNV can infect a wide range of vertebrates; in humans, it usually produces either asymptomatic infection or mild febrile disease, but can cause severe and fatal infection in a small percentage of patients.
- The incubation period is thought to range from 3 to 14 days.
- Symptoms generally last 3 to 6 days.
- Like SLE virus, WNV is transmitted principally by *Culex* species mosquitoes, but also can be transmitted by *Aedes*, *Anopheles*, and other species.
- The mild form of WNV infection has presented as a febrile illness of sudden onset, often accompanied by malaise, anorexia, nausea, vomiting, eye pain, headache, myalgia, rash, and lymphadenopathy.
- A minority of patients with severe disease develops a maculopapular or morbilliform rash involving the neck, trunk, arms, or legs. Some patients experience severe muscle weakness and flaccid paralysis. Neurological presentations include ataxia, cranial nerve abnormalities, myelitis, optic neuritis, polyradiculitis, and seizures. Although not observed in recent outbreaks, myocarditis, pancreatitis, and fulminant hepatitis have been described.

MURRAY VALLEY ENCEPHALITIS
- Murray Valley encephalitis is a zootic flavavirus and is closely-related to the Kunjin virus.
- Murray Valley encephalitis is endemic in New Guinea and in parts of Australia.
- It's related to the SLE, WN, and JE viruses.
- Infections are common, and the small number of fatalities have mostly been in children.

minating disease. Associated effects include disturbances of taste or smell.

Complications
▶ Bronchial pneumonia
▶ Urine retention
▶ Urinary tract infection
▶ Pressure ulcers
▶ Coma
▶ Epilepsy
▶ Parkinsonism
▶ Mental deterioration

Diagnosis
During an encephalitis epidemic, diagnosis is readily made on clinical findings and patient

history. However, sporadic cases are difficult to distinguish from other febrile illnesses, such as gastroenteritis or meningitis. Diagnosis may be assisted by serologic assays, such as immunoglobulin (Ig) M-capture ELISA (MAC-ELISA) and IgG ELISA. Early in infection, IgM antibody is more specific, whereas later, IgG is more reactive. Monoclonal antibody studies show promise in diagnosis. Polymerase chain reaction is also being investigated.

When possible, identification of the virus in cerebrospinal fluid (CSF) or blood confirms this diagnosis.[4] The common viruses that also cause herpes, measles, and mumps are easier to identify than arboviruses. Both herpesviruses and arboviruses can be isolated by inoculating young mice with a specimen taken from the patient. In herpes encephalitis, serologic studies may show rising titers of complement-fixing antibodies.

In all forms of encephalitis, CSF pressure is elevated and despite inflammation, the fluid is usually clear. White blood cell and protein levels in CSF are slightly elevated, but the glucose level remains normal. An EEG reveals abnormalities. Occasionally, a computed tomography scan or magnetic resonance imaging may be ordered to rule out cerebral hematoma.

Treatment

The antiviral agent acyclovir may be prescribed for herpes encephalitis.[4] Antibiotics may be prescribed if the infection is caused by bacteria. Treatment of all other forms of encephalitis is entirely supportive. Drug therapy includes phenytoin or another anticonvulsant, usually given I.V.; steroids such as dexamethasone may be used to reduce cerebral inflammation and edema; corticosteroids; mannitol to reduce cerebral swelling; sedatives for restlessness; and aspirin or acetaminophen to relieve headache and reduce fever. Ribavirin and interferon alpha-2b were found to have some effect on West Nile encephalitis. Other supportive measures include adequate fluid and electrolyte intake to prevent dehydration and antibiotics for an associated infection such as pneumonia. Isolation is unnecessary.

Special considerations

During the acute phase of the illness:
▶ Assess neurologic function often. Observe level of consciousness and signs of increased intracranial pressure (ICP). These include increasing restlessness, plucking at the bedcovers, vomiting, seizures, and changes in pupil size, motor function, and vital signs, such as rising blood pressure, widening pulse pressure, and slowly falling pulse. Watch for cranial nerve involvement (ptosis, strabismus, and diplopia), abnormal sleep patterns, and behavior changes.
▶ Maintain adequate fluid intake to prevent dehydration, but avoid fluid overload, which may increase cerebral edema. Measure and record intake and output accurately, and assess daily weights.
▶ Carefully position the patient to prevent joint stiffness and neck pain, and turn him often. Assist with range-of-motion exercises.
▶ Maintain adequate nutrition. It may be necessary to give the patient small, frequent meals or to supplement meals with nasogastric tube or parenteral feedings.
▶ To prevent constipation and minimize the risk of increased ICP resulting from straining at stool, give the patient a mild laxative or stool softener.
▶ Provide mouth care.
▶ Maintain a quiet environment. Darkening the room may decrease photophobia and headache. If the patient naps during the day and is restless at night, plan daytime activities to minimize napping and promote sleep at night.
▶ Provide emotional support and reassurance because the patient is apt to be frightened by the illness and frequent diagnostic tests.
▶ If the patient is delirious or confused, attempt to reorient him often. Providing a cal-

endar or a clock in the patient's room may be helpful.

▶ Reassure the patient and his family that behavior changes caused by encephalitis usually disappear. If a neurologic deficit is severe and appears permanent, refer the patient to a rehabilitation program as soon as the acute phase has passed.

▶ Discuss prevention through personal protective measures (proper clothing, insect repellent with N,N-diethyl-meta-toluamide [DEET]) and suggest reducing time outdoors in early evening hours.

REFERENCES

1. Centers for Disease Control and Prevention, Division of Vector-Borne Infectious Diseases (2006 July 12). "Eastern Equine Encephalitis Fact Sheet." [Online]. Available at *www.cdc.gov/ncidod/dvbid/arbor/eeefact.htm.*
2. Centers for Disease Control and Prevention (2006 June 11). "St. Louis Encephalitis Fact Sheet." Available at *www.cdc.gov/ncidod/dvbid/sle/Sle_FactSheet.htm.*
3. Centers for Disease Control and Prevention, Division of Vector-Borne Infectious Diseases (2005 November 7). "La Crosse Encephalitis Fact Sheet." [Online]. Available at *www.cdc.gov/ncidod/dvbid/arbor/lacfact.htm.*
4. Tyler, K.L., et al. "CSF Findings in 250 Patients with Serologically Confirmed West Nile Virus Meningitis and Encephalitis," *Neurology* 66(3):361-65, February 2006.

GUILLAIN-BARRÉ SYNDROME

Guillain-Barré syndrome is an acute, rapidly progressive, and potentially fatal form of polyneuritis that causes muscle weakness and mild distal sensory loss. Recovery is spontaneous and complete in about 95% of patients, although mild motor or reflex deficits in the feet and legs may persist. The prognosis is best when symptoms clear between 15 and 20 days after onset.

Causes and incidence

Precisely what causes Guillain-Barré syndrome is unknown, but it may be a cell-mediated immunologic attack on peripheral nerves in response to a virus. The major pathologic effect is segmental demyelination of the peripheral nerves. Because this syndrome causes inflammation and degenerative changes in both the posterior (sensory) and anterior (motor) nerve roots, signs of sensory and motor losses occur simultaneously.

This syndrome (also called *infectious polyneuritis, Landry-Guillain-Barré syndrome,* and *acute idiopathic polyneuritis*) can occur at any age but is most common between ages 30 and 50; it affects both sexes equally. In the United States, it has an incidence of 1 case per 100,000 people.[1]

Signs and symptoms

About 50% of patients with Guillain-Barré syndrome have a history of minor febrile illness (10 to 14 days before onset), usually an upper respiratory tract infection or, less commonly, gastroenteritis. When infection precedes onset of Guillain-Barré syndrome, signs of infection subside before neurologic features appear. Other possible precipitating factors include surgery, rabies or swine influenza vaccination, viral illness, Hodgkin's or other malignant disease, and lupus erythematosus.

Symmetrical muscle weakness, the major neurologic sign, usually appears in the legs first (ascending type) and then extends to the arms and facial nerves in 24 to 72 hours. Sometimes, muscle weakness develops in the arms first (descending type) or in the arms and legs simultaneously. (See *Testing for thoracic sensation,* page 130.) In milder forms of this disease, muscle weakness may affect only the cranial nerves or may not occur at all.

Another common neurologic sign is paresthesia, which sometimes precedes muscle weakness but tends to vanish quickly. However, some patients with this disorder

Testing for thoracic sensation

When Guillain-Barré syndrome progresses rapidly, test for ascending sensory loss by touching the patient or pressing his skin lightly with a pin every hour. Move systematically from the iliac crest (T12) to the scapula, occasionally substituting the blunt end of the pin to test the patient's ability to discriminate between sharp and dull.

Mark the level of diminished sensation to measure any change. If diminished sensation ascends to T8 or higher, the patient's intercostal muscle function (and consequently respiratory function) will probably be impaired. As Guillain-Barré syndrome subsides, sensory and motor weakness descends to the lower thoracic segments, heralding a return of intercostal and extremity muscle function.

SEGMENTAL DISTRIBUTION OF SPINAL NERVES TO BACK OF THE BODY

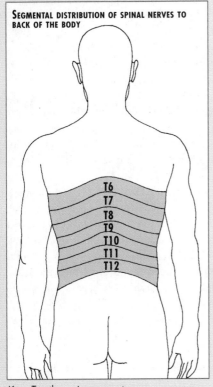

T6
T7
T8
T9
T10
T11
T12

Key: T = thoracic segments

never develop this symptom. Other clinical features may include facial diplegia (possibly with ophthalmoplegia), dysphagia or dysarthria and, less commonly, weakness of the muscles supplied by cranial nerve XI. Muscle weakness develops so quickly that muscle atrophy doesn't occur, but hypotonia and areflexia do. Stiffness and pain in the form of a severe "charley horse" commonly occur.

The clinical course of Guillain-Barré syndrome is divided into three phases. The initial phase begins when the first definitive symptom appears and ends 1 to 3 weeks later, when no further deterioration manifests. The plateau phase lasts several days to 2 weeks and is followed by the recovery phase, which is believed to coincide with remyelination and axonal process regrowth. The recovery phase extends over a period of 4 to 6 months; patients with severe disease may take up to 2 years to recover, and recovery may not be complete. (See *ICU complications in Guillain-Barré.*)

Complications
- ▶ Mechanical ventilatory failure
- ▶ Aspiration
- ▶ Pneumonia
- ▶ Sepsis
- ▶ Joint contractures
- ▶ Deep vein thrombosis
- ▶ Unexplained autonomic nervous system involvement may cause sinus tachycardia or bradycardia, hypertension, postural hypotension, or loss of bladder and bowel sphincter control.

Diagnosis
A history of preceding febrile illness (usually a respiratory tract infection) and typical clinical features suggest Guillain-Barré syndrome.

Several days after onset of signs and symptoms, cerebrospinal fluid (CSF) protein levels begin to rise, peaking in 4 to 6 weeks, probably as a result of widespread inflam-

ICU complications in Guillain-Barré

Question: *Does admission to the intensive care unit affect the recovery time of a patient with Guillain-Barré syndrome?*

Research: Guillain-Barré syndrome (GBS) is a rare neurologic disorder that requires admission to the intensive care unit (ICU) in one-third of the patients affected by the syndrome. The researchers studied 76 adult patients with GBS who had been admitted to a specific ICU over a 20-year period. Their goal was to determine the frequency, type, and predictors of complications experienced by these patients because ICU admission with GBS is linked to a significant risk of morbidity, mortality, and incomplete recovery. The information gathered for the study was extracted from longitudinal follow-up data.

Conclusion: The study found that 78% of patients with GBS admitted to the ICU required mechanical ventilation, two-thirds experienced at least one major complication (54% with pneumonia), and five patients died. Significant predictors of complications and factors that delayed recovery were identified as prolonged mechanical ventilation, male gender, advanced age, and early axonal abnormalities. Recovery of independent ambulation was seen in 75% of the patients with the median time to ambulation being 198 days; however, it was shown that recovery could take as long as 10 years.

Application: The nurse providing care to the patient with GBS in ICU should be aware of the predictors of complications and the long recovery period ahead of the patient. Although the time to ambulation may be significant, the patient should be provided with encouragement and supportive care because functional recovery occurs in a large percentage of patients.

Source: Dhar, R., et al. "The Morbidity and Outcome of Patients with Guillain-Barré Syndrome Admitted to the Intensive Care Unit," *Journal of the Neurological Sciences* 264(1-2):121-28, January 15, 2008.

matory disease of the nerve roots. Normal CSF protein levels occur in about 10% of patients. CSF white blood cell count remains normal, but in severe disease, CSF pressure may rise above normal. New research indicates finding a specific protein, the tau protein, in the CSF increases the likelihood of a Guillain-Barré diagnosis.[2] Protein 14-3-3 is also commonly seen in patients with Guillain-Barré syndrome.[4] Probably because of predisposing infection, complete blood count shows leukocytosis and a shift to immature forms early in the illness, but blood studies soon return to normal. Electromyography may show repeated firing of the same motor unit instead of widespread sectional stimulation. Nerve conduction velocities are slowed soon after paralysis develops and show demyelination. Diagnosis must rule out similar diseases such as acute poliomyelitis.

Treatment

Treatment is primarily supportive, including such measures as endotracheal (ET) intubation or tracheotomy if the patient has difficulty clearing secretions. Preventing complications is another goal of treatment.

Plasmapheresis is useful in decreasing severity of symptoms, thereby facilitating a more rapid recovery. I.V. immune globulin is equally effective in reducing the severity and duration of symptoms.[3]

Special considerations

Monitoring the patient for escalation of symptoms is of special concern.

▶ Watch for ascending sensory loss, which precedes motor loss. Also, monitor vital signs and level of consciousness.

▶ Assess and treat respiratory dysfunction. If respiratory muscles are weak, take serial vital capacity recordings. Use a respirometer with a mouthpiece or a face mask for bedside testing.

▶ Obtain arterial blood gas measurements. Because neuromuscular disease results in primary hypoventilation with hypoxemia and hypercapnia, watch for respiratory failure. Be alert for signs of rising partial pressure of carbon dioxide (such as confusion and tachypnea).

▶ Auscultate breath sounds, turn and position the patient, and encourage coughing and deep breathing. Begin respiratory support at the first sign of dyspnea or with decreasing partial pressure of arterial oxygen.

▶ If respiratory failure becomes imminent, establish an emergency airway with an ET tube.

▶ Give meticulous skin care to prevent skin breakdown. Establish a strict turning schedule; inspect the skin (especially sacrum, heels, and ankles) for breakdown, and reposition the patient every 2 hours. After each position change, stimulate circulation by carefully massaging pressure points. Also, use foam, gel, or alternating pressure pads at points of contact.[6]

▶ Perform passive range-of-motion exercises within the patient's pain limits to prevent contractures. Schedule throughout the day to prevent long periods of inactivity. When the patient's condition stabilizes, change to gentle stretching and active resistance exercises.

▶ To prevent aspiration, test the gag reflex, and elevate the head of the bed before giving the patient anything to eat. If the gag reflex is absent, give nasogastric feedings until this reflex returns. If the patient has severe paralysis and is expected to have a long recovery period, a gastrostomy tube may be necessary to provide adequate nourishment.

▶ As the patient regains strength and can tolerate a vertical position, be alert for postural hypotension. Monitor blood pressure and pulse during tilting periods and, if necessary, apply toe-to-groin elastic bandages to prevent postural hypotension.

▶ Inspect the patient's legs regularly for signs of thrombophlebitis (localized pain, tenderness, erythema, edema, and positive Homans' sign), a common complication of Guillain-Barré syndrome. To prevent thrombophlebitis, apply antiembolism stockings, and give prophylactic anticoagulants, as ordered.

▶ If the patient has facial paralysis, give eye and mouth care every 4 hours.

▶ Watch for urine retention. Measure and record intake and output every 8 hours, and offer the bedpan every 3 to 4 hours. Encourage adequate fluid intake of 2 qt [2 L] per day, unless contraindicated. If urine retention develops, begin intermittent catheterization as ordered. Because the abdominal muscles are weak, the patient may need manual pressure on the bladder (Credé's method) before he can urinate.

▶ To prevent or relieve constipation, offer the patient plenty of water, prune juice, and a high-bulk diet. If necessary, give daily or alternate-day suppositories (glycerin or bisacodyl) or enemas, as ordered.

▶ Before discharge, prepare a home care plan. Teach the patient how to transfer from the bed to a wheelchair, from a wheelchair to the toilet or tub, and how to walk short distances with a walker or a cane. Teach the family how to help him eat, compensating for facial weakness, and how to help him avoid skin breakdown. Stress the need for a regular bowel and bladder routine. Refer the patient for physical therapy as needed.

▶ Refer the patient's family to the Guillain-Barré Syndrome Foundation International, located in Narberth, PA. (The Foundation's Web site is *www.gbsfi.com/.*)

REFERENCES

1. National Institute of Neurological Disorders and Stroke (2007 December 11). "Guillain-Barré Syndrome Fact Sheet." [Online]. Available at *www.ninds.nih.gov/disorders/gbs/detail_gbs.htm.*
2. Asbury, A. "CSF Tau Protein: A New Prognostic Marker for Guillain-Barré Syndrome," *Neurology* 68(17):1438-39, April 2007.
3. Hughes, R.A., et al. "Immunotherapy for Guillain-Barré Syndrome: A Systematic Review," *Brain* 130(Pt 9):2245-57, September 2007.
4. Bersano, A., et al. "Detection of CSF 14-3-3 Protein in Guillain-Barré Syndrome," *Neurology* 67(12):2211-16, December 2006.
5. Atkinson, S.B., et al. "The Challenges of Managing and Treating Guillain-Barré Syndrome during the Acute Phase," *Dimensions in Critical Care Nursing* 25(6):256-63, November-December 2006.

HEADACHE

Headaches, a common patient complaint, can be divided into four classifications: vascular, muscle contraction (tension), traction, and inflammatory.[1] Vascular headaches include migraine headaches, toxic headaches caused by fever or diseases, and cluster headaches (intense pain that occurs in clusters, often at the same time of day for several days). Traction headaches and inflammatory headaches are symptoms of other disorders.[1] Ninety percent of all headaches are vascular, muscle contraction, or a combination; ten percent are due to underlying intracranial, systemic, or psychological disorders. Migraine headaches, probably the most intensively studied, are throbbing, vascular headaches that usually begin to appear in childhood or adolescence and recur throughout adulthood.

Causes and incidence

Most chronic headaches result from tension (muscle contraction), which may be caused by emotional stress, fatigue, menstruation, or environmental stimuli (noise, crowds, or bright lights). Other possible causes include glaucoma; inflammation of the eyes or mucosa of the nasal or paranasal sinuses; diseases of the scalp, teeth, extracranial arteries, or external or middle ear; muscle spasms of the face, neck, or shoulders; and cervical arthritis. In addition, headaches may be caused by vasodilators (nitrates, alcohol, and histamine), systemic disease, hypoxia, hypertension, head trauma and tumor, intracranial bleeding, abscess, or aneurysm.

The cause of migraine headache is unknown, but it's associated with constriction and dilation of intracranial and extracranial arteries. Certain biochemical abnormalities are thought to occur during a migraine attack. These include local leakage of a vasodilator polypeptide called neurokinin through the dilated arteries and a decrease in the plasma level of serotonin.

Headache pain may emanate from the pain-sensitive structures of the skin, scalp, muscles, arteries, and veins; cranial nerves V, VII, IX, and X; or cervical nerves 1, 2, and 3. Intracranial mechanisms of headaches include traction or displacement of arteries, venous sinuses, or venous tributaries, and inflammation or direct pressure on the cranial nerves with afferent pain fibers.

Affecting up to 10% of Americans, headaches are more common in females and have a strong familial incidence.

Signs and symptoms

Initially, migraine headaches usually produce unilateral, pulsating pain, which later becomes more generalized. They're commonly preceded by a scintillating scotoma, hemianopsia, unilateral paresthesia, or speech disorders. The patient may experience irritability, anorexia, nausea, vomiting, and

Clinical features of migraine headaches

TYPE	SIGNS AND SYMPTOMS
Common migraine Usually occurs on weekends and holidays	• Prodromal symptoms (fatigue, nausea, vomiting, and fluid imbalance) precede headache by about 1 day. • Sensitivity to light and noise (most prominent feature) • Headache pain (unilateral or bilateral, aching or throbbing)
Classic migraine Usually occurs in compulsive personalities and within families	• Prodromal symptoms include visual disturbances, such as zigzag lines and bright lights (most common), sensory disturbances (tingling of face, lips, and hands), or motor disturbances (staggering gait). • Recurrent and periodic headaches
Hemiplegic and ophthalmoplegic migraine (rare) Usually occurs in young adults	• Severe, unilateral pain • Extraocular muscle palsies (involving third cranial nerve) and ptosis • With repeated headaches, possible permanent third cranial nerve injury • In hemiplegic migraine, neurologic deficits (hemiparesis, hemiplegia) may persist after the headache subsides.
Basilar artery migraine Occurs in young females before their menstrual periods	Prodromal symptoms usually include partial vision loss followed by vertigo, ataxia, dysarthria, tinnitus and, sometimes, tingling of the fingers and toes, lasting from several minutes to almost an hour. • Headache pain, severe occipital throbbing, vomiting
Cluster headaches Occur in males more commonly than females and occur at all ages, but more commonly in adolescents and middle-age people.	• Episodic type (more common) and involves one to three short-lived attacks of periorbital pain per day over a 4-to 8-week period followed by a pain-free interval averaging 1 year. Chronic type occurs after an episodic pattern is established. • Unilateral pain occurs without warning, reaching a crescendo within 5 minutes. It is described as excruciating and deep, with attacks lasting from 30 minutes to 2 hours. • Associated symptoms may include tearing, reddening of the eye, nasal stuffiness, lid ptosis, and nausea.

photophobia. (See *Clinical features of migraine headaches*.)

Muscle contraction (tension) and traction headaches produce a dull, persistent ache, tender spots on the head and neck, and a feeling of tightness around the head, with a characteristic "hatband" distribution. The pain is usually severe and unrelenting. If caused by intracranial bleeding, these headaches may result in neurologic deficits, such as paresthesia and muscle weakness; narcotics may fail to relieve pain in these cases. If caused by a tumor, pain is most severe when the patient awakens.

Diagnosis

Diagnosis requires a history of recurrent headaches and physical examination of the

head and neck. Such examination includes percussion, auscultation for bruits, inspection for signs of infection, and palpation for defects, crepitus, or tender spots (especially after trauma). Firm diagnosis also requires a complete neurologic examination, assessment for other systemic diseases—such as hypertension—and a psychosocial evaluation, when such factors are suspected.

Diagnostic tests include cervical spine and sinus X-rays, EEG, computed tomography scan or magnetic resonance imaging. A lumbar puncture is indicated if the following diseases are suspected: viral or bacterial meningitis, subarachnoid hemorrhage, carcinomatous meningitis, pseudotumor cerebri, encephalitis, systemic diseases that affect the central nervous system.[2] A lumbar puncture isn't done if there's evidence of increased intracranial pressure or if a brain tumor is suspected because rapidly reducing pressure by removing spinal fluid can cause brain herniation.

Treatment

Depending on the type of headache, analgesics—ranging from aspirin to codeine or meperidine—may provide symptomatic relief. Other measures include identification and elimination of causative factors and, possibly, psychotherapy for headaches caused by emotional stress. Chronic tension headaches may also require muscle relaxants.

For migraine headaches, ergotamine alone or with caffeine may be an effective treatment. The Food and Drug Administration allows labeling of various analgesic preparations that include caffeine to state that they're for the treatment of migraine headaches. Remember that these medications can't be taken by pregnant women because they stimulate uterine contractions. These drugs and others, such as metoclopramide or naproxen, work best when taken early in the course of an attack. If nausea and vomiting make oral administration impossible, drugs may be given as rectal suppositories.

Drugs in the class of sumatriptan are considered by many clinicians to be the drug of choice for acute migraine attacks or cluster headaches. Ergotamine tartrate, a vasoconstrictor, is also used for migraines.[1] In addition, drugs that can help prevent migraine headaches include antidepressants (such as nortriptyline or fluoxetine), beta blockers (propranolol), and calcium-channel blockers (verapamil). Corticosteroids provide short-term relief for some patients with cluster headaches.

Special considerations

Headaches seldom require hospitalization unless caused by a serious disorder. If that's the case, direct your care to the underlying problem.

▶ Obtain a complete patient history: duration and location of the headache; time of day it usually begins; nature of the pain; concurrence with other symptoms such as blurred vision; precipitating factors, such as tension, menstruation, loud noises, menopause, or alcohol; medications taken such as oral contraceptives; or prolonged fasting. Exacerbating factors can also be assessed through ongoing observation of the patient's personality, habits, activities of daily living, family relationships, coping mechanisms, and relaxation activities.[3]

▶ Using the history as a guide, help the patient avoid exacerbating factors. Advise him to lie down in a dark, quiet room during an attack and to place ice packs on his forehead or a cold cloth over his eyes.

▶ Instruct the patient to take the prescribed medication at the onset of migraine symptoms, to prevent dehydration by drinking plenty of fluids after nausea and vomiting subside, and to use other headache relief measures.

▶ The patient with a migraine headache usually needs to be hospitalized only if nau-

sea and vomiting are severe enough to induce dehydration and possible shock.

▶ Avoid repeated use of narcotics if possible.

REFERENCES

1. National Institute of Neurological Disorders and Stroke (2007 November 13). "Headache: Hope Through Research." [Online]. Available at *www.ninds.nih.gov/disorders/headache/detail_headache.htm.*

2. Martin, V., and Elkind, A. "Diagnosis and Classification of Primary Headache Disorders," in *Standards of Care for Headache Diagnosis and Treatment.* Chicago, Ill.: National Headache Foundation, 2004. Available at *www.guideline.gov/summary/summary.aspx?ss =15&doc_id=6111&nbr=3966.*

3. Peters, M., et al. "Migraine and Chronic Daily Headache Management: Implications for Primary Care Practitioners," Journal of Clinical Nursing 16(7B):159-67, July 2007.

MENINGITIS

In meningitis, the brain and the spinal cord meninges become inflamed, usually as a result of a viral or, less commonly, a bacterial infection. Such inflammation may involve all three meningeal membranes—the dura mater, the arachnoid, and the pia mater. Viral meningitis is more common, and the illness is less severe.[1] In bacterial meningitis, the prognosis is good, and complications are rare—*if* the disease is recognized early and the infecting organism responds to antibiotics. Mortality in untreated meningitis, however, is 70% to 100%. The prognosis is worse for infants and elderly patients, particularly if antibiotic therapy isn't started within hours of symptom onset.

Causes and incidence

Meningitis is almost always a complication of another bacterial infection—sinusitis, otitis media, encephalitis, myelitis, brain abscess, or bacteremia (especially from pneumonia, empyema, osteomyelitis, or endocarditis). The most common cause of meningitis in infants and young children in the United States is *Streptococcus pneumoniae.*[1] Other causes are *Neisseria meningitidis,* which is highly contagious and is usually from an upper respiratory infection; *Haemophilus influenzae,* which is not so prevalent in the United States today because of immunizations; and *Listeria monocytogenes,* which is found in soil, dust, and foods.[1] In some cases, a virus is suspected. (See *Lymphocytic choriomeningitis.*) Meningitis may also follow skull fracture, a penetrating head wound, lumbar puncture, or ventricular shunting procedure. Aseptic meningitis may result from a virus or other organism. Sometimes, no causative organism can be found. Meningitis commonly begins as an inflammation of the pia-arachnoid, which may progress to congestion of adjacent tissues and destruction of some nerve cells.

Children younger than age 5, young adults ages 16 to 25, and people older than age 55 are more susceptible to meningitis.[2]

Signs and symptoms

The cardinal signs of meningitis are those of infection (fever, chills, and malaise) and of increased intracranial pressure (ICP); headache, vomiting and, rarely, papilledema. Signs of meningeal irritation include nuchal rigidity, positive Brudzinski's and Kernig's signs, exaggerated and symmetrical deep tendon reflexes, and opisthotonos (a spasm in which the back and extremities arch backward so that the body rests on the head and heels). (See *Two signs of meningitis,* page 138.) Other manifestations of meningitis are irritability; sinus arrhythmias; photophobia, diplopia, and other visual problems; and delirium, deep stupor, and coma.

An infant may not show clinical signs of infection, but may be fretful and refuse to eat. Such an infant may vomit a great deal, leading to dehydration. This prevents a

Lymphocytic choriomeningitis

Lymphocytic choriomeningitis (LCM) is a mild, biphasic, febrile illness lasting about 2 weeks. Human infection occurs through inhalation of the LCM virus or arenavirus from infectious aerosolized particles of the host (rodents such as mice or hamsters) or its excreta (urine, feces, or saliva) 1 to 3 weeks before the onset of symptoms. It can also result from contact with food contaminated with the virus or by contamination of mucous membranes, skin lesions, or cuts with infected body fluids. Handlers of infected animals or their excreta are at risk for this disease. Most cases occur in the northeast and eastern seaboard areas of the United States. LCM is more common during fall and winter.

The incubation period is 8 to 13 days after exposure. Early characteristics include fever, malaise, anorexia, weakness, muscle aches, retro-orbital headache, nausea, and vomiting. Sore throat, nonproductive cough, joint pain, chest pain, testicular pain, and parotid (salivary gland) pain may occur. Meningeal symptoms appear in 15 to 21 days, with signs and symptoms of meningitis (fever, increased headache, and stiff neck) or encephalitis (drowsiness, confusion, sensory disturbances, and motor abnormalities such as paralysis). Alopecia may also occur.

Complications include temporary or permanent neurologic damage, possible maternal transmission (pregnancy-related infection is associated with spontaneous abortion, congenital hydrocephalus, chorioretinitis, and mental retardation), myelitis, Guillain-Barré–type syndrome, orchitis or parotitis, myocarditis, psychosis, joint pain and arthritis, and prolonged convalescence with continuing dizziness, somnolence, and fatigue.

Diagnosis is made by detection of immunoglobulin M antibodies by enzyme-linked immunosorbent assay from serum or cerebrospinal fluid (CSF), which is the preferred diagnostic test. Lumbar-puncture CSF is typically abnormal and reveals increased opening pressure, increased protein levels, and a lymphocytic pleocytosis, usually in the range of several hundred white blood cells. Treatment is generally supportive and includes anti-inflammatory drugs, bed rest, and analgesics. Ribavirin has been shown to be effective against LCM in vitro. Acute hydrocephalus may require surgical shunting to relieve increased intracranial pressure.

Prevention involves teaching rodent control measures, basic hygiene practices, use of a personal respirator, importance of adequate ventilation, and use of a liquid disinfectant, such as a diluted household bleach solution, to clean areas with rodent droppings.

bulging fontanel and thus masks this important sign of increased ICP. As the illness progresses, twitching, seizures (in 30% of infants), or coma may develop. Most older children have the same symptoms as adults. In subacute meningitis, the onset may be insidious.

Complications
▶ Visual impairment
▶ Optic neuritis
▶ Cranial nerve palsies
▶ Deafness
▶ Personality change
▶ Headache
▶ Paresis or paralysis
▶ Endocarditis
▶ Coma
▶ Vasculitis
▶ Cerebral infarctions
▶ Children possibly developing sensory hearing loss, epilepsy, mental retardation, hydrocephalus, or subdural effusions

Diagnosis
Blood samples for culture and a lumbar puncture are performed immediately for rapid diagnosis.[3] A lumbar puncture showing

Two signs of meningitis

Brudzinski's sign: Place the patient in a dorsal recumbent position, put your hands behind her neck, and bend it forward. Pain and resistance may indicate meningeal inflammation, neck injury, or arthritis. If the patient also flexes her hips and knees in response to this manipulation, chances are she has meningitis.

Kernig's sign: Place the patient in a supine position. Flex her leg at the hip and knee and then straighten the knee. Pain or resistance points to meningitis.

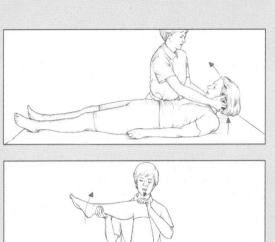

typical cerebrospinal fluid (CSF) findings, when accompanied by positive Brudzinski's and Kernig's signs, usually establishes a diagnosis. The following tests can uncover the primary sites of infection: cultures of blood, urine, and nose and throat secretions; chest X-ray; electrocardiogram; and a physical examination, with special attention to skin, ears, and sinuses. Lumbar puncture usually indicates elevated CSF pressure, from obstructed outflow at the arachnoid villi. The fluid may appear cloudy or milky white, depending on the number of white blood cells present. CSF protein levels tend to be high; glucose levels may be low. (In subacute meningitis, CSF findings may vary.) CSF culture and sensitivity tests usually identify the infecting organism, unless it's a virus. Leukocytosis and serum electrolyte abnormalities are also common. Computed tomography scan can rule out cerebral hematoma, hemorrhage, or tumor.

Treatment

Treatment of meningitis includes appropriate antibiotic therapy for bacterial meningitis and vigorous supportive care. Usually, I.V. antibiotics are given for at least 2 weeks, followed by oral antibiotics. Antibiotic treatment should be started as soon as possible after diagnosis to decrease morbidity and mortality.[3] Dexamethasone has been shown to be effective as adjunctive therapy in the treatment of pneumococcal meningitis if given before the first dose of antibiotic. [3] It has also been shown to reduce the incidence of deafness, a common complication of meningitis.

Other drugs include mannitol to decrease cerebral edema, an anticonvulsant (usually given by I.V.), or sedative to reduce restlessness, and aspirin or acetaminophen to relieve headache and fever. Supportive measures include bed rest, fever reduction, and measures to prevent dehydration. The patient's room is kept darkened and quiet because any increase in sensory stimulation may cause a

seizure. Isolation is necessary if nasal cultures are positive. Appropriate therapy for any coexisting conditions, such as endocarditis or pneumonia, is included as well. To prevent meningitis, prophylactic antibiotics are sometimes used after ventricular shunting procedures, skull fracture, or penetrating head wounds, but this use is controversial.

For viral meningitis, treatment is supportive.

Special considerations

Patients must be watched carefully for changes in neurologic function or other signs of worsening condition.

▶ Assess neurologic function often. Observe level of consciousness (LOC) and signs of increased ICP (restlessness, irritability, vomiting, seizures, and a change in motor function and vital signs). Watch for signs of cranial nerve involvement (ptosis, strabismus, and diplopia).

HEALTH & SAFETY *Be especially alert for a temperature increase up to 102° F (38.9° C), deteriorating LOC, onset of seizures, and altered respirations, all of which may signal an impending crisis.*

▶ Monitor fluid balance. Maintain adequate fluid intake to avoid dehydration, but avoid fluid overload because of the danger of cerebral edema. Measure central venous pressure and intake and output accurately.

▶ Watch for adverse effects of I.V. antibiotics and other drugs. To avoid infiltration and phlebitis, check the I.V. site often, and change the site according to your facility's policy.

▶ Position the patient carefully to prevent joint stiffness and neck pain. Turn him often, according to a planned positioning schedule. Assist with range-of-motion exercises.

▶ Maintain adequate nutrition and elimination. It may be necessary to provide small, frequent meals or to supplement meals with nasogastric tube or parenteral feedings. To prevent constipation and minimize the risk

of increased ICP resulting from straining at stool, give the patient a mild laxative or stool softener.

▶ Ensure the patient's comfort. Provide mouth care regularly. Maintain a quiet environment. Darkening the room may decrease photophobia. Relieve headache with a non-opioid analgesic, such as aspirin, acetaminophen, or ibuprofen as ordered. (Opioids interfere with accurate neurologic assessment.)

▶ Provide reassurance and support. The patient may be frightened by his illness and frequent lumbar punctures. If he's delirious or confused, attempt to reorient him often. Reassure his family that the delirium and behavior changes caused by meningitis usually disappear. However, if a severe neurologic deficit appears permanent, refer the patient to a rehabilitation program as soon as the acute phase of this illness has passed.

▶ To help prevent development of meningitis, teach patients with chronic sinusitis or other chronic infections the importance of proper medical treatment. Follow strict sterile technique when treating patients with head wounds or skull fractures.

REFERENCES

1. Mayoclinic.com (2007 September 14). "Meningitis." [Online]. Available at *www.mayoclinic.com/health/meningitis/DS00118/DSECTION=1*.
2. Meningitis Foundation of America (2008). "Top 20 Questions about Meningitis." [Online]. Available at *www.meningitisfoundationofamerica.org/templates/section-view/18/index.html*.
3. Tunkel, A.R., et al. "Practice Guidelines for the Management of Bacterial Meningitis," *Clinical Infectious Diseases* 39(9):1267-84, November 2004.

MULTIPLE SCLEROSIS

Multiple sclerosis (MS) is a progressive disease caused by demyelination of the white matter of the brain

Demyelination in multiple sclerosis

Transverse section of cervical spine shows partial loss of myelin, characteristic of multiple sclerosis (MS). This degenerative process is called demyelination.

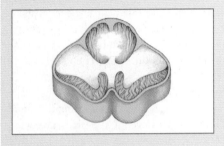

In this illustration, the loss of myelin is nearly complete. Clinical features of MS depend on the extent of demyelination.

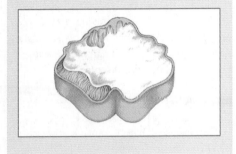

Causes and incidence

The exact cause of MS is unknown, but current theories suggest a slow-acting or latent viral infection and an autoimmune response. Other theories suggest that environmental and genetic factors may also be linked to MS. Emotional stress, overwork, fatigue, pregnancy, and acute respiratory tract infections have been known to precede the onset of this illness.

MS usually begins between ages 20 and 40. It affects twice as many females as males.[1] It affects 0.5 to 1 per 1,000 people in the United States. A family history of MS and living in a geographical area with higher incidence of MS (northern Europe, northern United States, southern Australia, and New Zealand) increase the risk.

Signs and symptoms

Clinical findings in MS depend on the extent and site of myelin destruction, the extent of remyelination, and the adequacy of subsequent restored synaptic transmission.

Signs and symptoms in MS may be transient, or they may last for hours or weeks. They may wax and wane with no predictable pattern, vary from day to day, and be bizarre and difficult for the patient to describe.

In most patients, visual problems and sensory impairment, such as numbness and tingling sensations (paresthesia), are the first signs that something may be wrong.

Other characteristic changes include:
▶ *ocular disturbances:* optic neuritis, diplopia, ophthalmoplegia, blurred vision, and nystagmus
▶ *muscle dysfunction:* weakness, paralysis ranging from monoplegia to quadriplegia, spasticity, hyperreflexia, intention tremor, and gait ataxia
▶ *urinary disturbances:* incontinence, frequency, urgency, and frequent infections
▶ *emotional lability:* characteristic mood swings, irritability, euphoria, and depression.

and spinal cord. (See *Demyelination in multiple sclerosis.*) In this disease, sporadic patches of demyelination throughout the central nervous system induce widely disseminated and varied neurologic dysfunction. Characterized by exacerbations and remissions, MS is a major cause of chronic disability in young adults.

The prognosis varies; MS may progress rapidly, disabling some patients by early adulthood or causing death within months of onset. However, 70% of patients lead active, productive lives with prolonged remissions. (See *MS and neurology access.*)

EVIDENCE-BASED PRACTICE

MS and neurology access

Question: *What percentage of people with multiple sclerosis see neurologists for their medical care?*

Research: Multiple sclerosis (MS) is a chronic disease that attacks the central nervous system. Researchers studied a broad sample of people with MS in the United States to determine what percentage of them had access to and use of neurologists; identify demographic, economic, and clinical factors associated with access and use; and examine differences in treatment and management of MS. They collected data from 2,156 people using computer-assisted telephone interviews.

Conclusion: The researchers determined that 72.2% of patients in the study regularly saw a neurologist for MS care. The participants' access to and use of neurologists were affected negatively by such factors as lower economic status, lack of health insurance, illness for more than 15 years, and limited mobility. Blacks were less likely than other races to see a neurol-

ogist; women significantly more likely than men. Patients who saw neurologists were more likely to receive treatment with disease-modifying agents, participate in outpatient rehabilitation programs, and see other specialists.

Application: Patients who aren't seeing neurologists may not be receiving the medications and other therapies that would improve their physical condition and quality of life. The nurse should explore the patient's reasons for not seeking the care of a neurologist and refer the patient, if appropriate, to social services or community agencies for assistance.

Source: Minden, S.L., et al. "Access to and Utilization of Neurologists by People with Multiple Sclerosis," *Neurology* 70(13 Pt 2): 1141-49, March 25, 2008.

Associated signs and symptoms include poorly articulated or scanning speech and dysphagia. Clinical effects may be so mild that the patient is unaware of them or so bizarre that he appears hysterical.

Complications
▶ Injuries from falls
▶ Urinary tract infections
▶ Constipation
▶ Joint contractures
▶ Pressure ulcers
▶ Rectal distention
▶ Pneumonia

Diagnosis
A misdiagnosis of psychiatric problems is common. Because early symptoms may be mild, years may elapse between onset of the

first signs and the diagnosis, which typically requires evidence of multiple neurologic attacks and characteristic remissions and exacerbations. Magnetic resonance imaging may detect MS lesions; however, diagnosis still remains difficult. Periodic testing and close observation of the patient are necessary, perhaps for years, depending on the course of the disease.

Abnormal EEG findings occur in one-third of patients. Lumbar puncture shows elevated gamma globulin fraction of immunoglobulin G, but normal total cerebrospinal fluid (CSF) protein levels. Elevated CSF gamma globulin is significant only when serum gamma globulin levels are normal because it reflects hyperactivity of the immune system due to chronic demyelination. Oligoclonal bands of immunoglobulin

can be detected when gamma globulin in CSF is examined by electrophoresis, and these bands are present in most patients, even when the percentage of gamma globulin in CSF is normal. In addition, the white blood cell count in CSF may rise. Differential diagnosis must rule out spinal cord compression, foramen magnum tumor (may mimic the exacerbations and remissions of MS), multiple small strokes, syphilis or other infection, and psychological disturbances.

Treatment

The aim of treatment is to shorten exacerbations and relieve neurologic deficits so that the patient can resume a normal lifestyle. Those with relapsing-remitting courses are placed on immune modulating therapy, with beta interferon, and glatiramer acetate.[2] A drug approved by the FDA in 2006, Natalizumab, is also available but at limited sites due to the risk of progressive multifocal leukoencephalopathy.[2] Mitoxantrone is an immunosuppressive drug that is also commonly used.[4] Steroids are used to reduce the associated edema of the myelin sheath during exacerbations.[3]

Other drugs include baclofen, tizanidine, or diazepam to relieve spasticity, cholinergic agents to relieve urine retention and minimize frequency and urgency, amantadine to relieve fatigue, and antidepressants to help with mood or behavioral symptoms.

HEALTH & SAFETY *The patient should continue to receive all appropriate vaccinations. This has been shown to help decrease the risk of infections, which may lead to acute exacerbations.*[5]

During acute exacerbations, supportive measures include bed rest, comfort measures such as massages, prevention of fatigue, prevention of pressure ulcers, bowel and bladder training (if necessary), administration of antibiotics for bladder infections, physical therapy, and counseling. Physical therapy, speech therapy, occupational therapy, and support groups are also useful. Planned exercise programs help with maintaining muscle tone.

Special considerations

Management considerations focus on educating the patient and his family.

▶ Assist with physical therapy. Increase patient comfort with massages and relaxing baths. Assist with active, resistive, and stretching exercises to maintain muscle tone and joint mobility, decrease spasticity, improve coordination, and boost morale.

▶ Educate the patient and his family concerning the chronic course of MS. Emphasize the need to avoid temperature extremes, stress, fatigue, and infections and other illnesses, all of which can trigger an MS attack. Advise him to maintain independence by developing new ways of performing daily activities.

▶ Stress the importance of eating a nutritious, well-balanced diet that contains sufficient roughage and adequate fluids to prevent constipation.

▶ Evaluate the need for bowel and bladder training during hospitalization. Encourage adequate fluid intake and regular urination. Eventually, the patient may require urinary drainage by self-catheterization or, in males, condom drainage. Teach the correct use of suppositories to help establish a regular bowel schedule.

▶ Promote emotional stability. Help the patient establish a daily routine to maintain optimal functioning. Activity level is regulated by tolerance level. Encourage daily physical exercise and regular rest periods to prevent fatigue.[4]

▶ Inform the patient that exacerbations are unpredictable, necessitating physical and emotional adjustments in lifestyle.

▶ For more information, refer him to the National Multiple Sclerosis Society.

REFERENCES

1. Mayoclinic.com (2006 December 6). "Multiple Sclerosis." [Online]. Available at *www.mayoclinic.com/health/multiplesclerosis/DS00118/DSECTION=1*.
2. National Multiple Sclerosis Society (2006 October 19). "Brochures: The Disease-Modifying Drugs." [Online]. Available at *www.nationalmssociety.org/site/PageServer?pagename=HOM_LIB_brochures_comparing*.
3. Martinelli Boneschi, F., et al. "Mitoxantrone for Multiple Sclerosis," *Cochrane Database of Systematic Review* (4):CD002127, 2005.
4. Walker, I.D., and Gonzalez, E.W. "Review of Intervention Studies on Depression in Persons with Multiple Sclerosis," *Issues in Mental Health Nursing* 28(5):511-31, May 2007.
5. Rutschmann, O.T., et al. "Immunization and MS: A Summary of Published Evidence and Recommendations," *Neurology* 59(12):1837-43, December 2002.

MYASTHENIA GRAVIS

Myasthenia gravis produces sporadic but progressive weakness and abnormal fatigability of striated (skeletal) muscles, exacerbated by exercise and repeated movement, but improved by anticholinesterase drugs. Usually, this disorder affects muscles innervated by the cranial nerves (face, lips, tongue, neck, and throat), but it can affect any muscle group. Myasthenia gravis follows an unpredictable course of recurring exacerbations and periodic remissions. There's no known cure. Drug treatment has improved prognosis and allows patients to lead relatively normal lives except during exacerbations. When the disease involves the respiratory system, it may be life-threatening.

Causes and incidence

Myasthenia gravis causes a failure in transmission of nerve impulses at the neuromuscular junction. Theoretically, such impairment may result from an autoimmune response, ineffective acetylcholine release, or inadequate muscle fiber response to acetylcholine. (See *Impaired transmission in myasthenia gravis*, page 144.)

Myasthenia gravis affects 20 of every 100,000 people at any age.[1] It's more common in young females (under 40) and older males (over 60).[2] About 20% of neonates born to mothers with myasthenia gravis have transient (or occasionally persistent) myasthenia. This disease may coexist with immunologic and thyroid disorders; about 15% of patients with myasthenia gravis have thymomas. Research is currently being done to identify the relationship between the thymus gland and myasthenia gravis.[1] Remissions occur in about 25% of patients.

Signs and symptoms

The dominant symptoms of myasthenia gravis are skeletal muscle weakness and fatigability. In the early stages, easy fatigability of certain muscles may appear with no other findings. Later, it may be severe enough to cause paralysis. Typically, myasthenic muscles are strongest in the morning but weaken throughout the day, especially after exercise. Short rest periods temporarily restore muscle function. Muscle weakness is progressive; more and more muscles become weak, and eventually some muscles may lose function entirely. Resulting symptoms depend on the muscle group affected; they become more intense during menses and after emotional stress, prolonged exposure to sunlight or cold, or infections.

Onset may be sudden or insidious. In many patients, weak eye closure, ptosis, and diplopia are the first signs that something is wrong. Patients with myasthenia gravis usually have blank, expressionless faces and nasal vocal tones. They experience frequent nasal regurgitation of fluids and have difficulty chewing and swallowing. Because of this, they usually worry about choking. Their eyelids droop (ptosis), and they may

Impaired transmission in myasthenia gravis

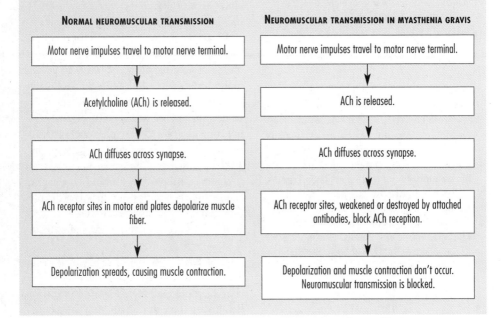

NORMAL NEUROMUSCULAR TRANSMISSION

Motor nerve impulses travel to motor nerve terminal.

↓

Acetylcholine (ACh) is released.

↓

ACh diffuses across synapse.

↓

ACh receptor sites in motor end plates depolarize muscle fiber.

↓

Depolarization spreads, causing muscle contraction.

NEUROMUSCULAR TRANSMISSION IN MYASTHENIA GRAVIS

Motor nerve impulses travel to motor nerve terminal.

↓

ACh is released.

↓

ACh diffuses across synapse.

↓

ACh receptor sites, weakened or destroyed by attached antibodies, block ACh reception.

↓

Depolarization and muscle contraction don't occur. Neuromuscular transmission is blocked.

have to tilt their heads back to see. Their neck muscles may become too weak to support their heads without bobbing.

In patients with weakened respiratory muscles, decreased tidal volume and vital capacity make breathing difficult and predispose to pneumonia and other respiratory tract infections. Respiratory muscle weakness (myasthenic crisis) may be severe enough to require an emergency airway and mechanical ventilation.

Complications
▶ Respiratory distress
▶ Pneumonia
▶ Chewing and swallowing difficulties leading to choking and food aspiration

Diagnosis
Repeated muscle use over a very short time that fatigues and then improves with rest suggests a diagnosis of myasthenia gravis.

Tests for this neurologic condition record the effect of exercise and subsequent rest on muscle weakness. Electromyography, with repeated neural stimulation, may help confirm this diagnosis. Acetylcholine receptor antibodies may be present in the blood.

The classic proof of myasthenia gravis is improved muscle function after an I.V. infection of edrophonium or neostigmine (anticholinesterase drugs).

In patients with myasthenia gravis, muscle function improves within 30 to 60 seconds and lasts up to 30 minutes. Long-standing ocular muscle dysfunction may fail to respond to such testing. This test can differentiate a myasthenic crisis from a cholinergic crisis (caused by acetylcholine overactivity at the neuromuscular junction). The acetylcholine receptor antibody titer may be elevated in generalized myasthenia. Evaluation should rule out thyroid disease and thymoma.

Treatment

Treatment is symptomatic. Anticholinesterase drugs, such as neostigmine and pyridostigmine, counteract fatigue and muscle weakness and allow about 80% of normal muscle function. However, these drugs become less effective as the disease worsens. Corticosteroids may relieve symptoms. Immunosuppressants are also used.[2] Plasmapheresis is used in severe myasthenic exacerbation. Immunoglobulin is also used, but more research is needed to determine its effectiveness.[3]

Patients with thymomas require thymectomy, which may cause remission in some cases of adult-onset myasthenia.[4] Acute exacerbations that cause severe respiratory distress necessitate emergency treatment. Tracheotomy, positive-pressure ventilation, and vigorous suctioning to remove secretions usually produce improvement in a few days. Because anticholinesterase drugs aren't effective in myasthenic crisis, they're stopped until respiratory function improves. Myasthenic crisis requires immediate hospitalization and vigorous respiratory support.

Special considerations

Careful baseline assessment, early recognition and treatment of potential crises, supportive measures, and thorough patient teaching can minimize exacerbations and complications. Continuity of care is essential.

▶ Establish an accurate neurologic and respiratory baseline. Thereafter, monitor tidal volume and vital capacity regularly. The patient may need a ventilator and frequent suctioning to remove accumulating secretions.

▶ Be alert for signs of an impending crisis (increased muscle weakness, respiratory distress, and difficulty in talking or chewing).

▶ To prevent relapses, adhere closely to the ordered drug administration schedule. Be prepared to give atropine for anticholinesterase overdose or toxicity.

▶ Plan exercise, meals, patient care, and activities to make the most of energy peaks. For example, give medication 20 to 30 minutes before meals to facilitate chewing or swallowing. Allow the patient to participate in his care.

▶ When swallowing is difficult, give soft, solid foods instead of liquids to lessen the risk of choking.

▶ Patient teaching is essential because myasthenia gravis is usually a lifelong condition. Help the patient plan daily activities to coincide with energy peaks. Stress the need for frequent rest periods throughout the day. Emphasize that periodic remissions, exacerbations, and day-to-day fluctuations are common.

▶ Teach the patient how to recognize adverse effects and signs of toxicity of anticholinesterase drugs (headaches, weakness, sweating, abdominal cramps, nausea, vomiting, diarrhea, excessive salivation, and bronchospasm) and corticosteroids (euphoria, insomnia, edema, and increased appetite).

▶ Warn the patient to avoid strenuous exercise, stress, infection, and needless exposure to the sun or cold. All of these things may worsen signs and symptoms. However, the patient should be encouraged to participate in a regular, gentle exercise routine or physical therapy.[5]

▶ For more information and an opportunity to meet other myasthenia gravis patients who lead full, productive lives, refer the patient to the Myasthenia Gravis Foundation.

REFERENCES

1. National Institute of Neurological Disorders and Stroke (2007 December 13). "Myasthenia Gravis Fact Sheet." [Online]. Available at *www.ninds.nih.gov/disorders/myasthenia_gravis/detail_myasthenia_gravis.htm#1051331 53*.
2. Myasthenia Gravis Foundation of America (2007 February 15). "What Is Myasthenia Gravis?" [Online]. Available at *www.myasthenia.org/amg_whatismg.cfm*.

3. Gajdos, P., et al. "Intravenous Immunoglobulin for Myasthenia Gravis," *Cochrane Database of Systematic Reviews* (2):CD002277, 2003.

4. Kim, H.K., et al. "Neurologic Outcomes of Thymectomy in Myasthenia Gravis: Comparative Analysis of the Effect of Thymoma," *Journal of Thoracic and Cardiovascular Surgery* 134(3):601-607, September 2007.

5. Cup, E.H., et al. "Exercise Therapy and Other Types of Physical Therapy for Patients with Neuromuscular Diseases: A Systematic Review," *Archives of Physical Medicine and Rehabilitation* 88(11):1452-64, November 2007.

PARKINSON'S DISEASE

Named for James Parkinson, the English physician who wrote the first accurate description of the disease in 1817, Parkinson's disease characteristically produces progressive muscle rigidity, akinesia, involuntary tremor, and dementia. Death may result from aspiration pneumonia or an infection.

Causes and incidence

Although the cause of Parkinson's disease is unknown, study of the extrapyramidal brain nuclei (corpus striatum, globus pallidus, and substantia nigra) has established that a dopamine deficiency prevents affected brain cells from performing their normal inhibitory function within the central nervous system. The symptoms of Parkinson's disease occur when 80% of dopamine-producing cells are damaged.[1] Parkinson's disease occurs in families in some cases, and several genes have been linked to Parkinson's.[2] It is also thought to be secondary to environmental factors and toxins.[2] Parkinson's disease, also called *parkinsonism, paralysis agitans,* and *shaking palsy*, is one of the most common crippling diseases in the United States. It strikes 2 in every 1,000 people, most often developing at the average age of 60; howev-

er, it also occurs in children and young adults. Because of increased longevity, this amounts to roughly 50,000 to 60,000 new cases diagnosed annually in the United States alone.[1,2] Incidence of the disease increases in persons with repeated brain injury, including professional athletes and persons using psychoactive substances, whether prescribed or illicit.

Signs and symptoms

The cardinal symptoms of Parkinson's disease are muscle rigidity, akinesia, and an insidious resting tremor that begins in the fingers (unilateral pill-roll tremor), increases during stress or anxiety, and decreases with purposeful movement and sleep. Muscle rigidity results in resistance to passive muscle stretching, which may be uniform (lead-pipe rigidity) or jerky (cogwheel rigidity). Akinesia causes the patient to walk with difficulty (gait lacks normal parallel motion and may be retropulsive or propulsive) and produces a high-pitched, monotone voice; drooling; a masklike facial expression; loss of posture control (the patient walks with body bent forward); and dysarthria, dysphagia, or both. Occasionally, akinesia may also cause oculogyric crises (eyes are fixed upward, with involuntary tonic movements) or blepharospasm (eyelids are completely closed). Parkinson's disease itself doesn't impair the intellect, but a coexisting disorder, such as arteriosclerosis, may do so.

Complications

▶ Injury from falls
▶ Food aspiration
▶ Urinary tract infections
▶ Skin breakdown

Diagnosis

Generally, laboratory data are of little value in identifying Parkinson's disease. Consequently, diagnosis is based on the patient's age, history, and characteristic clinical picture.

Conclusive diagnosis is possible only after ruling out other causes of tremor, involutional depression, cerebral arteriosclerosis and, in patients younger than age 30, intracranial tumors, Wilson's disease, or phenothiazine or other drug toxicity.

Treatment

Because Parkinson's disease has no cure, the primary aim of treatment is to relieve symptoms and keep the patient functional as long as possible. Treatment consists of drugs, physical therapy and—in severe disease states unresponsive to drugs—stereotactic neurosurgery, or a controversial treatment known as fetal cell transplantation. In this treatment, fetal brain tissue is injected into the patient's brain. If the injected cells grow within the recipient's brain, they allow the brain to process dopamine, thereby either halting or reversing disease progression. Neurotransplantation techniques, including the use of nerve cells from other parts of the patient's body, have been attempted with varying results.

Drug therapy usually includes levodopa, a dopamine replacement that's most effective during early stages. It's given in increasing doses until symptoms are relieved or adverse effects appear. Because adverse effects can be serious, levodopa is frequently given in combination with carbidopa (a decarboxylase inhibitor) to halt peripheral dopamine synthesis. Occasionally, levodopa proves ineffective, producing dangerous adverse effects that include postural hypotension, hallucinations, and increased libido, leading to inappropriate sexual behavior. In that case, alternative drug therapy includes anticholinergics such as trihexyphenidyl, antihistamines such as diphenhydramine, and amantadine, an antiviral agent.[4]

Research on the oxidative stress theory has caused a controversy in drug therapy for Parkinson's disease. Traditionally, levodopa-carbidopa has been a first-line drug in management; however, it has also been associated with an acceleration of disease process.[3] Inclusion of entacapone or tolcapone, (COMT inhibitor) potentiates the effects of levodopa-carbidopa treatment so that less frequent doses are required.[2]

Selegiline, an enzyme-inhibiting agent (MAO-B inhibitor), allows conservation of dopamine and enhances the therapeutic effect of levodopa. Selegiline used with tocopherols delays the time when the patient with Parkinson's disease becomes disabled.

HEALTH & SAFETY *Elderly patients may need smaller doses of antiparkinsonian drugs because of reduced tolerance. Be alert for and report orthostatic hypotension, irregular pulse, blepharospasm, and anxiety or confusion.*

When drug therapy fails, stereotactic neurosurgery, such as subthalamotomy and pallidotomy, may provide an alternative. In these procedures, electrical coagulation, freezing, radioactivity, or ultrasound destroy the ventrolateral nucleus of the thalamus to prevent involuntary movement. This is most effective in young, otherwise healthy people with unilateral tremor or muscle rigidity. Neurosurgery can only relieve symptoms. Brain stimulator implantation alters the activity of the area where Parkinson's disease symptoms originate.[5] A pacemaker is implanted into the chest wall, and the electrode is threaded (using magnetic resonance imaging for guidance) to the thalamus, pallidum, or subthalamic nucleus. A successful procedure reduces the need for medication, thus reducing the medication-related adverse effects experienced by the patient.

Individually planned physical therapy complements drug treatment and neurosurgery to maintain normal muscle tone and function. Appropriate physical therapy includes both active and passive range-of-motion exercises, routine daily activities, walking, and baths and massage to help relax muscles.

Special considerations

Effectively caring for the patient with Parkinson's disease requires careful monitoring of drug treatment, emphasis on teaching self-reliance, and generous psychological support.

▶ Monitor drug treatment and adjust dosage, if necessary, to minimize adverse effects.[4]

▶ If the patient has surgery, watch for signs of hemorrhage and increased intracranial pressure by frequently checking his level of consciousness and vital signs.

▶ Encourage independence. The patient with excessive tremor may achieve partial control of his body by sitting on a chair and using its arms to steady himself. Advise the patient to change position slowly and dangle his legs before getting out of bed. Remember that fatigue may cause him to depend more on others.

▶ Encourage the patient to start an exercise program. Research has shown that a regular exercise program may be useful in improving motor function.[3]

▶ Help the patient overcome problems related to eating and elimination. For example, if he has difficulty eating, offer supplementary or small, frequent meals to increase caloric intake. Help establish a regular bowel routine by encouraging him to drink at least 2 qt (2 L) of liquids daily and eat high-fiber foods. He may need an elevated toilet seat to assist him from a standing to a sitting position.

▶ Give the patient and his family emotional support. Teach them about the disease, its progressive stages, and the adverse effects of his prescription drugs. Show the family how to prevent pressure ulcers and contractures by proper positioning. Inform them of the dietary restrictions levodopa imposes, and explain household safety measures to prevent accidents. Help the patient and his family express their feelings and frustrations about the progressively debilitating effects of the disease. Establish long- and short-term treatment goals, and be aware of the patient's need for intellectual stimulation and diversion. Refer the patient and his family to the National Parkinson Foundation or the United Parkinson Foundation for more information. (The first has offices in Miami, Fla., the second, in Chicago, Ill.)

REFERENCES

1. National Parkinson Foundation. "About Parkinson Disease." [Online]. Available at *www.parkinson.org/NETCOMMUNITY/Page.aspx?pid=225&srcid=201.*
2. National Institute of Neurological Disorders and Stroke (2007 December 13). "Parkinson's Disease: Hope through Research." [Online]. Available at *www.ninds.nih.gov/disorders/parkinsons_disease/detail_parkinsons_disease.htm.*
3. Suchowersky, O., et al. "Practice Parameter: Neuroprotective Strategies and Alternative Therapies for Parkinson Disease (An Evidence-Based Review): Report of the Quality Standards Subcommittee of the American Academy of Neurology," *Neurology* 66(7):976-82, April 2006.
4. Miyasaki, J.M., et al. "Practice Parameter: Evaluation and Treatment of Depression, Psychosis, and Dementia in Parkinson Disease (An Evidence-Based Review): Report of the Quality Standards Subcommittee of the American Academy of Neurology," *Neurology* 66(7):996-1002, April 2006.
6. Pahwa, R., et al. "Practice Parameter: Treatment of Parkinson Disease with Motor Fluctuations and Dyskinesia (An Evidence-Based Review): Report of the Quality Standards Subcommittee of the American Academy of Neurology," *Neurology* 66(7):983-95, April 2006.

SEIZURE DISORDER

Seizure disorder, also called *epilepsy*, is a condition of the brain marked by a susceptibility to recurrent seizures—paroxysmal events associated with abnormal electrical discharges of neurons in the brain.

Causes and incidence

In about one-half of cases of epilepsy, the cause is unknown.[1] However, some possible causes of epilepsy include:

▶ birth trauma (inadequate oxygen supply to the brain, blood incompatibility, or hemorrhage)

▶ perinatal infection

▶ anoxia (after respiratory or cardiac arrest)

▶ infectious diseases (meningitis, encephalitis, or brain abscess)

▶ ingestion of toxins (mercury, lead, or carbon monoxide)

▶ tumors of the brain

▶ inherited disorders or degenerative disease, such as phenylketonuria or tuberous sclerosis

▶ head injury or trauma

▶ metabolic disorders, such as hypoglycemia or hypoparathyroidism

▶ stroke (hemorrhage, thrombosis, or embolism)

▶ alcohol withdrawal, which can cause nonepileptic seizures.

Epilepsy affects 1% to 2% of the population. However, 80% of patients have good seizure control if they strictly adhere to the prescribed treatment regimen.[1] Incidence is highest for children younger than age 2 and adults older than age 65. It's also higher in blacks and socially disadvantaged populations.[2]

Signs and symptoms

The hallmarks of epilepsy are recurring seizures, which can be classified as partial or generalized (some patients may be affected by more than one type).

Partial seizures arise from a localized area of the brain, causing specific symptoms. In some patients, partial seizure activity may spread to the entire brain, causing a generalized seizure. Partial seizures include simple partial (jacksonian) and complex partial seizures (psychomotor or temporal lobe).

A simple partial motor-type seizure begins as a localized motor seizure characterized by a spread of abnormal activity to adjacent areas of the brain. It typically produces stiffening or jerking in one extremity, accompanied by a tingling sensation in the same area. For example, it may start in the thumb and spread to the entire hand and arm. The patient seldom loses consciousness, although the seizure may progress to a generalized seizure.

A simple partial sensory-type seizure involves perceptual distortion, which can include hallucinations.

The symptoms of a complex partial seizure vary but usually include purposeless behavior. The patient experiences an aura immediately before the seizure. An aura represents the beginning of abnormal electrical discharges within a focal area of the brain and may include a pungent smell, GI distress (nausea or indigestion), a rising or sinking feeling in the stomach, a dreamy feeling, an unusual taste, or a visual disturbance. Overt signs of a complex partial seizure include a glassy stare, picking at one's clothes, aimless wandering, lip-smacking or chewing motions, and unintelligible speech; these signs may last for just a few seconds or as long as 20 minutes. Mental confusion may last several minutes after the seizure; as a result, an observer may mistakenly suspect intoxication with alcohol or drugs or psychosis.

Generalized seizures, as the term suggests, cause a generalized electrical abnormality within the brain and include several distinct types:

▶ Absence (petit mal) seizures occur most commonly in children, although they may affect adults as well. They usually begin with a brief change in level of consciousness, indicated by blinking or rolling of the eyes, a blank stare, and slight mouth movements. There's little or no tonic-clonic movement. The patient retains his posture and continues preseizure activity without difficulty. Typically, each seizure lasts from 1 to 10 seconds. If not properly treated, seizures can recur as often as 100 times per day. An ab-

sence seizure may progress to generalized tonic-clonic seizures.

▶ A myoclonic *(bilateral massive epileptic myoclonus)* seizure is characterized by brief, involuntary muscular jerks of the body or extremities, which may occur in a rhythmic fashion and may precede generalized tonic-clonic seizures by months or years.

▶ A generalized tonic-clonic *(grand mal)* seizure typically begins with a loud cry, precipitated by air rushing from the lungs through the vocal cords. The patient then falls to the ground, losing consciousness. The body stiffens (tonic phase) and then alternates between episodes of muscular spasm and relaxation (clonic phase). Tongue-biting, incontinence, labored breathing, apnea, and subsequent cyanosis may also occur. The seizure stops in 2 to 5 minutes, when abnormal electrical conduction of the neurons is completed. The patient then regains consciousness but is somewhat confused and may have difficulty talking. If he can talk, he may complain of drowsiness, fatigue, headache, muscle soreness, and arm or leg weakness. He may fall into deep sleep after the seizure. These seizures may start as facial seizures and spread to become generalized.

An akinetic seizure is characterized by a general loss of postural tone (the patient falls in a flaccid state) and a temporary loss of consciousness. It occurs in young children and is sometimes called a "drop attack" because it causes the child to fall.

Status epilepticus is a continuous seizure state that can occur in all seizure types. The most life-threatening example is generalized tonic-clonic status epilepticus, a continuous generalized tonic-clonic seizure without intervening return of consciousness. Status epilepticus is accompanied by respiratory distress. It can result from abrupt withdrawal of anticonvulsant medications, hypoxic encephalopathy, acute head trauma, metabolic encephalopathy, or septicemia secondary to encephalitis or meningitis.

Complications
▶ Anoxia
▶ Traumatic injury from a fall or rapid jerking movements

Diagnosis
Clinically, the diagnosis of epilepsy is based on the occurrence of one or more seizures and proof or the assumption that the condition that led to them is still present.

Diagnostic information is obtained from the patient's history and description of seizure activity and from family history, physical and neurologic examinations, EEG and computed tomography scan or magnetic resonance imaging.[2] These scans offer density readings of the brain and may indicate abnormalities in internal structures. Paroxysmal abnormalities on the EEG confirm the diagnosis by providing evidence of the continuing tendency to have seizures. A negative EEG doesn't rule out epilepsy because the paroxysmal abnormalities occur intermittently. Other tests may include serum glucose and calcium studies, skull X-rays, lumbar puncture, brain scan, and cerebral angiography.

Treatment
Generally, treatment of epilepsy consists of anticonvulsant therapy to reduce the number of future seizures. The most commonly prescribed drugs include phenytoin, carbamazepine, valproate, lamotrigine, or oxcarbazepine.[1] Other commonly prescribed drugs are clonazepam, phenobarbital, and primidone. Ethosuximide is commonly prescribed for absence seizures. Gabapentin, felbamate, tiagabine, topiramate, and levetiracetam are newer anticonvulsant drugs.[1] New research has shown that lamotrigine given once daily is also an effective medication that can be used to decrease seizures.[6] Up to 80% of seizures can be managed with one medication.[3]

A patient taking anticonvulsant medications requires monitoring for toxic signs:

nystagmus, ataxia, lethargy, dizziness, drowsiness, slurred speech, irritability, nausea, and vomiting.

If drug therapy fails, treatment may include surgical removal of a demonstrated focal lesion to attempt to stop seizures.[5] Emergency treatment of status epilepticus usually consists of diazepam (or lorazepam), phenytoin, or phenobarbital; dextrose 50% I.V. (when seizures are secondary to hypoglycemia); and thiamine I.V. (in chronic alcoholism or withdrawal).

Special considerations

A key to support is a true understanding of the nature of epilepsy and of the misconceptions that surround it.

▶ Encourage the patient and his family to express their feelings about the patient's condition. Answer their questions, and help them cope by dispelling some of the myths about epilepsy, for example, the myth that epilepsy is contagious. Assure them that epilepsy is controllable for most patients who follow a prescribed regimen of medication and that most patients maintain a normal lifestyle.

Because drug therapy is the treatment of choice for most people with epilepsy, information about medications is invaluable.

▶ Stress the need for compliance with the prescribed drug schedule. Reinforce dosage instructions, and stress the importance of taking medication regularly, at scheduled times. Caution the patient to monitor the quantity of medication he has so he doesn't run out of it.

▶ Warn against possible adverse effects—drowsiness, lethargy, hyperactivity, confusion, and visual and sleep disturbances—all of which indicate the need for dosage adjustment. Phenytoin therapy may lead to hyperplasia of the gums, which may be relieved by conscientious oral hygiene. Instruct the patient to report adverse effects immediately.

▶ Lifestyle considerations include driving limitations or restrictions around water,

avoiding heights, and caution when using power tools.

▶ When administering phenytoin I.V., use a large vein, and monitor vital signs frequently. Avoid I.M. administration and mixing with dextrose solutions.

▶ Emphasize the importance of having anticonvulsant blood levels checked at regular intervals, even if the seizures are under control.

▶ Warn the patient against drinking alcoholic beverages and other potential triggers.

▶ Know which social agencies in your community can help epileptic patients. Refer the patient to the Epilepsy Foundation of America for general information and to the state motor vehicle department for information about a driver's license. (The Epilepsy Foundation has offices in Landover, Md. Its Web site address is *www.epilepsy foundation.org.*)

▶ The primary goals of the health care professional and family members caring for a patient having a seizure are protection from injury, protection from aspiration, and observation of the seizure activity. Generalized tonic-clonic seizures may necessitate first aid. Show the patient's family members how to administer first aid correctly:

– Avoid restraining the patient during a seizure.[4]

– Help the patient to a lying position, loosen any tight clothing, and place something flat and soft, such as a pillow, jacket, or hand, under his head.

– Clear the area of hard objects.

– Don't force anything into the patient's mouth if his teeth are clenched—a tongue blade or spoon could lacerate a mouth and lips or displace teeth, precipitating respiratory distress. However, if the patient's mouth is open, protect his tongue by placing a soft object (such as a folded cloth) between his teeth.

– Turn his head to provide an open airway.

– After the seizure subsides, reassure the patient that he's all right, orient him to time and place, and inform him that he's had a seizure.[7]

▶ If the patient is experiencing a complex partial seizure, protect him from injury by gently calling his name and directing him away from the source of danger. And again, *don't* restrain the patient during the seizure. Clear the area of any hard objects. After the seizure passes, reassure him and tell him that he has just had a seizure.

REFERENCES

1. National Institute of Neurological Disorders and Stroke (2007 December 14). "Seizures and Epilepsy: Hope Through Research." [Online]. Available at *www.ninds.nih.gov/disorders/ epilepsy/detail_epilepsy.htm#107253109*.
2. Epilepsy Foundation. "About Epilepsy." [Online]. Available at *www.epilepsyfoundation. org/about/*.
3. Texas Tech University Managed Health Care Network Pharmacy & Therapeutic Committee. *Acute Seizures and Seizure Disorder.* Conroe, Tex.: University of Texas Medical Branch Correctional Managed Care, April 2003. Available at *www.guideline.gov/summary/ summary.aspx?ss=15&doc_id=4389&string=*.
4. "Managing Seizures," *Nurse Practitioner* 32(5):19-20, May 2007.
5. Téllez-Zenteno, J.F., et al. "Long-Term Outcomes in Epilepsy Surgery: Antiepileptic Drugs, Mortality, Cognitive and Psychosocial Aspects," *Brain* 130(Pt 2):334-45, February 2007.
6. Naritoku, D.K., et al. "Lamotrigine Extended-Release as Adjunctive Therapy for Partial Seizures," *Neurology* 69(16):1610-18, October 2007.
7. Fagley, M.U. "Taking Charge of Seizure Activity," *Nursing* 37(9):42-47, September 2007.

STROKE

A stroke, also called *cerebrovascular accident* or *brain attack,* is a sudden impairment of cerebral circulation in one or more of the blood vessels supplying the brain. A stroke interrupts or diminishes oxygen supply and commonly causes serious damage or necrosis in brain tissues. The sooner circulation returns to normal after a stroke, the better chances are for complete recovery. However, about half of those who survive a stroke remain permanently disabled and experience a recurrence within weeks, months, or years. Stroke is the number one cause of disability.[1]

Causes and incidence

A stroke results from obstruction of a blood vessel, typically in extracerebral vessels, but occasionally in intracerebral vessels. Factors that increase the risk of stroke include history of transient ischemic attacks (TIAs), atherosclerosis, hypertension, kidney disease, arrhythmias (specifically atrial fibrillation), electrocardiogram changes, rheumatic heart disease, diabetes mellitus, postural hypotension, cardiac or myocardial enlargement, high serum triglyceride levels, lack of exercise, use of oral contraceptives, cigarette smoking, and family history of stroke. Being Black, Hispanic, Asian/Pacific Islander, older than age 55, and being male also increase the risk of stroke.[1] (See *Transient ischemic attack.*)

Strokes are classified as hemorrhagic or ischemic. Eighty-five percent of strokes are ischemic. Ischemic strokes are caused by thrombosis or embolism. Thrombosis is the most common cause in middle-age and elderly people, who have a higher incidence of atherosclerosis, diabetes, and hypertension. Thrombosis causes ischemia in brain tissue supplied by the affected vessel as well as congestion and edema; the latter may produce more clinical effects than thrombosis itself, but these symptoms subside with the

edema. Thrombosis may develop while the patient sleeps or shortly after he awakens; it can also occur during surgery or after a myocardial infarction. The risk increases with obesity, smoking, or the use of oral contraceptives. Cocaine-induced ischemic stroke is now being seen in younger patients.

Embolism, the second most common cause of stroke, is an occlusion of a blood vessel caused by a fragmented clot, a tumor, fat, bacteria, or air. It can occur at any age, especially among patients with a history of rheumatic heart disease, endocarditis, posttraumatic valvular disease, myocardial fibrillation and other cardiac arrhythmias, or after open-heart surgery. It usually develops rapidly—in 10 to 20 seconds—with no warning. When an embolus reaches the cerebral vasculature, it cuts off circulation by lodging in a narrow portion of an artery, most commonly the middle cerebral artery, causing necrosis and edema. If the embolus is septic and infection extends beyond the vessel wall, encephalitis or an abscess may develop.

Hemorrhage, the third most common cause of stroke, may, like embolism, occur suddenly, at any age. It affects more females than males. Hemorrhage results from chronic hypertension or aneurysms, which cause sudden rupture of a cerebral artery, thereby diminishing blood supply to the area served by the artery. In addition, blood accumulates deep within the brain, further compressing neural tissue and causing even greater damage.

Strokes are classified according to their course of progression. The least severe is the TIA, or "little stroke," which results from a temporary interruption of blood flow, most commonly in the carotid and vertebrobasilar arteries. A progressive stroke, or stroke-in-evolution (thrombus-in-evolution), begins with slight neurologic deficit and worsens in a day or two. In a completed stroke, neurologic deficits are maximal at onset.

Transient ischemic attack

A transient ischemic attack (TIA) is a recurrent episode of neurologic deficit that lasts from seconds to hours, and clears within 12 to 24 hours. It's usually considered a warning sign of an impending thrombotic stroke. In fact, TIAs have been reported in 50% to 80% of patients who have had a cerebral infarction from such thrombosis. The age of onset varies. Incidence rises dramatically after age 50 and is highest among blacks and males.

CAUSES
In TIA, microemboli released from a thrombus probably temporarily interrupt blood flow, especially in the small distal branches of the arterial tree in the brain. Small spasms in those arterioles may impair blood flow and also precede TIA. Predisposing factors are the same as for thrombotic strokes. The most distinctive characteristics of TIAs are the transient duration of neurologic deficits and complete return of normal function. The symptoms of TIA easily correlate with the location of the affected artery. These symptoms include double vision, speech deficits (slurring or thickness), unilateral blindness, staggering or uncoordinated gait, unilateral weakness or numbness, falling because of weakness in the legs, and dizziness.

TREATMENT
During an active TIA, treatment aims to prevent a completed stroke and consists of aspirin or anticoagulants to minimize the risk of thrombosis. After or between attacks, preventive treatment includes carotid endartectomy or cerebral microvascular bypass.

Stroke is the third most common cause of death in the United States.[1] It occurs in 1 out of 15 deaths in the United States each year.

Signs and symptoms
Clinical features of stroke vary with the artery affected (and, consequently, the portion

of the brain it supplies), the severity of damage, and the extent of collateral circulation that develops to help the brain compensate for decreased blood supply. If the stroke occurs in the left hemisphere, it produces symptoms on the right side; if in the right hemisphere, symptoms are on the left side. However, a stroke that causes cranial nerve damage produces signs of cranial nerve dysfunction on the same side as the hemorrhage.

Symptoms are usually classified according to the artery affected:

▶ *Middle cerebral artery:* aphasia, dysphasia, visual field cuts, and hemiparesis on affected side (more severe in the face and arm than in the leg)

▶ *Carotid artery:* weakness, paralysis, numbness, sensory changes, and visual disturbances on affected side; altered level of consciousness (LOC), bruits, headaches, aphasia, and ptosis

▶ *Vertebrobasilar artery:* weakness on affected side, numbness around lips and mouth, visual field cuts, diplopia, poor coordination, dysphagia, slurred speech, dizziness, amnesia, and ataxia

▶ *Anterior cerebral artery:* confusion, weakness, and numbness (especially in the leg) on affected side, incontinence, loss of coordination, impaired motor and sensory functions, and personality changes

▶ *Posterior cerebral arteries:* visual field cuts, sensory impairment, dyslexia, coma, and cortical blindness; typically, paralysis is absent.

Symptoms can also be classified as premonitory, generalized, and focal. Premonitory symptoms, such as drowsiness, dizziness, headache, and mental confusion, are rare. Generalized symptoms, such as headache, vomiting, mental impairment, seizures, coma, nuchal rigidity, fever, and disorientation, are typical. Focal symptoms, such as sensory and reflex changes, reflect the site of hemorrhage or infarct and may worsen.

Complications
▶ Unstable blood pressure
▶ Fluid imbalance
▶ Infections such as pneumonia
▶ Sensory impairment
▶ Altered level of consciousness
▶ Aspiration
▶ Contractures
▶ Pulmonary emboli

Diagnosis
Diagnosis of stroke is based on observation of clinical features, a history of risk factors, and the results of diagnostic tests:

▶ Computed tomography scan shows evidence of hemorrhagic stroke immediately but may not show evidence of thrombotic infarction for 48 to 72 hours.[4]

▶ Magnetic resonance imaging may help identify ischemic or infarcted areas and cerebral swelling.

▶ Electrocardiogram can help diagnose underlying heart disorders.

▶ Carotid duplex may detect carotid artery stenosis.

▶ Angiography outlines blood vessels and pinpoints occlusion or rupture site. It's mainly used if surgery is considered.

▶ EEG helps to localize damaged area.

Other baseline laboratory studies may be done to exclude immune conditions or abnormal clotting that can lead to clot formation.

Treatment
Surgery performed to improve cerebral circulation for patients with thrombotic or embolic stroke includes endarterectomy (removal of atherosclerotic plaques from the inner arterial wall) and microvascular bypass (surgical anastomosis of an extracranial vessel to an intracranial vessel).

Medications useful in stroke include the following:

▶ Aspirin is given within 48 hours of symptoms for acute ischemic stroke.[2]

▶ Tissue plasminogen activator has been used successfully in clot dissolution when administered within 3 hours of the onset of symptoms. In other circumstances, heparin and warfarin may be used as well as antiplatelet drugs.[4]

▶ Ticlopidine, an antiplatelet drug, can be used for patients who have already had a stroke or TIA and can't take aspirin, for preventing stroke, and for reducing the risk of recurrent stroke after therapy has begun.[3]

▶ Anticonvulsants may be used to treat or prevent seizures.

▶ Stool softeners may be used to prevent straining, which increases intracranial pressure (ICP).

▶ Corticosteroids may be indicated to minimize associated cerebral edema.

▶ Analgesics may be used to relieve the headache that typically follows hemorrhagic stroke.

Special considerations

During the acute phase, focus on survival needs and prevention of further complications. Effective care emphasizes continuing neurologic assessment, support of respiration, continuous monitoring of vital signs, careful positioning to prevent aspiration and contractures, management of GI problems, and careful monitoring of fluid, electrolyte, and nutritional status. Patient care must also include measures to prevent complications such as infection.

▶ Maintain patent airway and oxygenation. Loosen constricting clothes. Watch for ballooning of the cheek with respiration. The side that balloons is the side affected by the stroke. If the patient is unconscious, he could aspirate saliva, so keep him in a lateral position to allow secretions to drain naturally or suction secretions, as needed. Insert an artificial airway, and start mechanical ventilation or supplemental oxygen, if necessary.

▶ Check vital signs and neurologic status, record observations, and report any significant changes to the physician. Monitor blood pressure, LOC, pupillary changes, motor function (voluntary and involuntary movements), sensory function, speech, skin color, temperature, signs of increased ICP, and nuchal rigidity or flaccidity. Remember, if stroke is impending, blood pressure rises suddenly, pulse is rapid and bounding, and the patient may complain of a headache. Also, watch for signs of pulmonary emboli, such as chest pains, shortness of breath, dusky color, tachycardia, fever, and changed sensorium. If the patient is unresponsive, monitor his blood gases often and alert the physician to increased partial pressure of carbon dioxide or decreased partial pressure of oxygen.

▶ Maintain fluid and electrolyte balance. If the patient can take liquids orally, offer them as often as fluid limitations permit. Administer I.V. fluids as ordered; never give too much too fast because this can increase ICP. Offer the urinal or bedpan every 2 hours. If the patient is incontinent, he may need an indwelling urinary catheter, but this should be avoided, if possible, because of the risk of infection.

▶ Ensure adequate nutrition. Check for gag reflex before offering small oral feedings of semisolid foods. Place the food tray within the patient's visual field because loss of peripheral vision is common. If oral feedings aren't possible, insert a nasogastric tube.

▶ Manage GI problems. Be alert for signs that the patient is straining at elimination because this increases ICP. Modify diet, administer stool softeners, as ordered, and give laxatives, if necessary. If the patient vomits (usually during the first few days), keep him positioned on his side to prevent aspiration.

▶ Provide careful mouth care. Clean and irrigate the patient's mouth to remove food particles. Care for his dentures as needed.

▶ Provide meticulous eye care. Remove secretions with a cotton ball and sterile normal saline solution. Instill eyedrops as ordered. Patch the patient's affected eye if he can't close the lid.

▶ Position the patient and align his extremities correctly. Use high-topped sneakers to prevent footdrop and contracture and convoluted foam, flotation, or pulsating mattresses, or sheepskin, to prevent pressure ulcers. To prevent pneumonia, turn the patient at least every 2 hours. Elevate the affected hand to control dependent edema, and place it in a functional position.

▶ Assist the patient with exercise. Perform range-of-motion exercises for both the affected and unaffected sides. Teach and encourage the patient to use his unaffected side to exercise his affected side.

▶ Give medications as ordered, and watch for and report adverse effects.

▶ Establish and maintain communication with the patient. If he is aphasic, set up a simple method of communicating basic needs. Then, remember to phrase your questions so he'll be able to answer using this system. Repeat yourself quietly and calmly, and use gestures if necessary to help him understand. Even an unresponsive patient may be able to hear, so don't say anything in his presence you wouldn't want him to hear and remember.

▶ Provide psychological support. Set realistic short-term goals. Involve the patient's family in his care when possible, and explain his deficits and strengths.

Begin your rehabilitation of the patient who has had a stroke on admission. The amount of teaching you'll have to do depends on the extent of neurologic deficit.

▶ If necessary, teach the patient to comb his hair, dress, and wash. With the aid of a physical therapist and an occupational therapist, obtain appliances, such as walking frames, hand bars by the toilet, and ramps, as needed. The patient may fail to recognize that he has a paralyzed side (called unilateral neglect) and must be taught to inspect that side of his body for injury and to protect it from harm. If speech therapy is indicated, encourage the patient to begin as soon as possible and follow through with the speech pathologist's suggestions. To reinforce teaching, involve the patient's family in all aspects of rehabilitation. With their cooperation and support, devise a realistic discharge plan, and let them help decide when the patient can return home.

▶ Before discharge, warn the patient or his family to report any premonitory signs of a stroke, such as severe headache, drowsiness, confusion, and dizziness. Emphasize the importance of regular follow-up visits.

▶ If aspirin has been prescribed to minimize the risk of embolic stroke, tell the patient to watch for possible GI bleeding. Make sure the patient and his family realize that acetaminophen isn't a substitute for aspirin.

To help prevent stroke:

▶ Stress the need to control diseases, such as diabetes or hypertension.

▶ Teach all patients (especially those at high risk) the importance of following a low-cholesterol, low-salt diet; watching their weight; increasing activity; avoiding smoking and prolonged bed rest; and minimizing stress.

▶ Ensure that the patient understands that if symptoms develop, he should go to the emergency department immediately.

REFERENCES

1. National Stroke Association Web Page. "What Is Stroke?" [Online]. Available at *www.stroke.org/site/PageServer?pagename=STROKE.*

2. Coull, B.M., et al. "Anticoagulants and Antiplatelet Agents in Acute Ischemic Stroke: Report of the Joint Stroke Guideline Development Committee of the American Academy of Neurology and The American Stroke Association," *Stroke* 33(7):1934-42, July 2002.

3. National Stroke Association. "Complete Guide to Stroke." [Online]. Available at *www.stroke.org/site/DocServer/NSA_complete_guide.pdf?docID=341.*

4. 2005 American Heart Association Guidelines for Cardiopulmonary Resuscitation and Emergency Cardiovascular Care, Part 9: Adult Stroke. *Circulation* 112 (Suppl IV):IV-111-IV-121, December 2005.

Gastrointestinal disorders

APPENDICITIS

Appendicitis is an inflammation of the vermiform appendix, resulting from an obstruction.

Causes and incidence

Appendicitis probably stems from an obstruction of the appendiceal lumen caused by a fecal mass, stricture, barium ingestion, or viral infection. This obstruction sets off an inflammatory process that can lead to infection, thrombosis, necrosis, and perforation. If the appendix ruptures or perforates, the infected contents spill into the abdominal cavity, causing peritonitis, the most common and perilous complication of appendicitis.

Appendicitis occurs more commonly in males than in females, with a peak incidence in the late teens and early 20s. About 1 case per 1,000 people is recorded annually. It's a common cause of emergency surgery in children, with 4 appendectomies per 1,000 admissions for appendicitis annually in the United States.

Signs and symptoms

Typically, appendicitis begins with generalized or localized abdominal pain in the right upper abdomen, followed by anorexia, nausea, and vomiting (rarely profuse). Pain eventually localizes in the right lower abdomen (McBurney's point) with abdominal "boardlike" rigidity, retractive respirations, increasing tenderness, increasingly severe abdominal spasms and, almost invariably, rebound tenderness. (Rebound tenderness on the opposite side of the abdomen suggests peritoneal inflammation.)

Later signs and symptoms include constipation or diarrhea, slight fever, and tachycardia. The patient may walk bent over or lie with his right knee flexed to reduce pain. Sudden cessation of abdominal pain indicates perforation or infarction of the appendix.

Complications

▶ Rupture of appendix

Diagnosis

Diagnosis of appendicitis is based on physical findings and characteristic clinical symptoms. Supportive findings include a temperature of 99° to 102° F (37.2° to 38.9° C) and a moderately elevated white blood cell count (12,000 to 15,000/μl), with increased immature cells.

Diagnosis must rule out illnesses with similar symptoms, such as gastritis, gastroenteritis, ileitis, colitis, diverticulitis, pancreatitis, renal colic, bladder infection, ovarian cyst, and uterine disease. It may be strongly suspected based on abdominal sonography or computed tomography scan. Appendicitis

157

can be confirmed by exploratory laparoscopy.

Treatment

Appendectomy can be done with a small standard incision or through laparoscopy.[1] Laparoscopic appendectomies decrease the recovery time and thus the hospital stay.[3] If peritonitis develops, treatment involves GI intubation, parenteral replacement of fluids and electrolytes, and administration of antibiotics. Appendectomy has been thought to be the only effective treatment for appendicitis, but researchers are looking at using antibiotics alone as an alternative treatment.[2]

Special considerations

If appendicitis is suspected, or during preparation for appendectomy:

▶ Administer I.V. fluids to prevent dehydration. *Never* administer cathartics or enemas, which may rupture the appendix. Give the patient nothing by mouth, and administer analgesics judiciously because they may mask symptoms.

▶ To lessen pain, place the patient in Fowler's position. *Never* apply heat to the right lower abdomen; this may cause the appendix to rupture. An ice bag may be used for pain relief.

After appendectomy:

▶ Monitor the patient's vital signs and intake and output. Administer analgesics as ordered.

▶ Encourage the patient to cough, breathe deeply, and turn frequently to prevent pulmonary complications.

▶ Document bowel sounds, passing of flatus, and bowel movements. In a patient whose nausea and abdominal rigidity have subsided, these signs indicate readiness to resume oral fluids.

▶ Watch closely for possible surgical complications. Continuing pain and fever may signal an abscess. The complaint that "something gave way" may mean wound rupture. If an abscess or peritonitis develops, incision

and drainage may be necessary. Frequently assess the dressing for wound drainage.

▶ Help the patient walk as soon as possible after surgery.

▶ In appendicitis complicated by peritonitis, a nasogastric tube may be needed to decompress the stomach and reduce nausea and vomiting. If so, record drainage and provide mouth and nose care.

REFERENCES

1. National Digestive Diseases Information Clearinghouse (June 2004). "Appendicitis." [Online]. Available at *www.digestive.niddk.nih. gov/ddiseases/pubs/appendicitis/#4.*
2. Liu, K., et al. "Can Acute Appendicitis Be Treated by Antibiotics Alone?" *American Surgeon* 73(11):1161-65, November 2007.
3. Yau, K.K., et al. "Laparoscopic versus Open Appendectomy for Complicated Appendicitis," *Journal of the American College of Surgeons* 205(1):60-65, July 2007.

CHOLELITHIASIS AND RELATED DISORDERS

Diseases of the gallbladder and biliary tract are common and, in many cases, painful conditions that may be life-threatening and usually require surgery. They are generally associated with deposition of calculi and inflammation. (See *Common sites of calculi formation.*)

Causes and incidence

Cholelithiasis, stones or calculi (gallstones) in the gallbladder, results from changes in bile components. Gallstones are made of cholesterol, calcium bilirubinate, or a mixture of cholesterol and bilirubin pigment. Cholesterol stones are most common, accounting for about 75% to 80% of cases in the United States.[1] They are created during periods of sluggishness in the gallbladder due to pregnancy, hormonal contraceptives, diabetes mellitus, celiac disease, cirrhosis of

Common sites of calculi formation

The illustration below shows sites where calculi typically collect. Calculi vary in size; small calculi may travel.

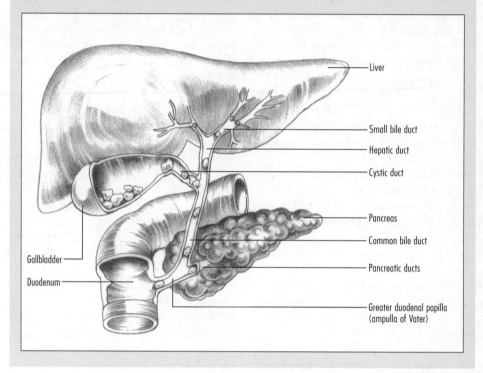

Liver

Small bile duct

Hepatic duct

Cystic duct

Pancreas

Common bile duct

Pancreatic ducts

Greater duodenal papilla (ampulla of Vater)

Gallbladder

Duodenum

the liver, and pancreatitis. Cholelithiasis is a common health problem, affecting about 10% to 20% of adults in the United States.[1] Prognosis is usually good with treatment unless infection occurs, in which case, the prognosis depends on its severity and response to antibiotics.

One out of every 10 patients with gallstones develops *choledocholithiasis*, or gallstones in the common bile duct (sometimes called "common duct stones"). This occurs when stones that passed out of the gallbladder lodge in the hepatic and common bile ducts and obstruct the flow of bile into the duodenum. Prognosis is good unless infection occurs.

Cholangitis, infection of the bile duct, is commonly associated with choledocholithiasis and may follow percutaneous transhepatic cholangiography or occlusion of endoscopic stents. Predisposing factors may include bacterial or metabolic alteration of bile acids. Widespread inflammation may cause fibrosis and stenosis of the common bile duct. The prognosis for this rare condition is poor without stenting or surgery.

Cholecystitis, acute or chronic inflammation of the gallbladder, is usually associated with a gallstone impacted in the cystic duct, causing painful distention of the gallbladder. Cholecystitis accounts for 10% to 25% of all surgeries in patients requiring gallbladder surgery. The acute form is most common

during middle age; the chronic form usually occurs among elderly patients. The prognosis is good with treatment.

Cholesterolosis, polyps or crystal deposits of cholesterol in the gallbladder's submucosa, may result from bile secretions containing high concentrations of cholesterol and insufficient bile salts. The polyps may be localized or speckle the entire gallbladder. Cholesterolosis, the most common pseudotumor, isn't related to widespread inflammation of the mucosa or lining of the gallbladder. Prognosis is good with surgery.

Biliary cirrhosis, ascending infection of the biliary system, sometimes follows viral destruction of liver and duct cells, but the primary cause is unknown. This condition usually leads to obstructive jaundice and involves the portal and periportal spaces of the liver. It's nine times more common among females ages 40 to 60 than among males. Prognosis is poor without liver transplantation.

Gallstone ileus results from a gallstone lodging at the terminal ileum; it's more common in the elderly. Prognosis is good with surgery.

Postcholecystectomy syndrome commonly results from residual gallstones or stricture of the common bile duct. It occurs in 1% to 5% of all patients whose gallbladders have been surgically removed. It may produce right upper quadrant abdominal pain, biliary colic, fatty food intolerance, dyspepsia, and indigestion. The prognosis is good with selected radiologic procedures, endoscopic procedures, or surgery.

Acalculous cholecystitis, which accounts for about 5% of cholecystitis cases, is more common in critically ill patients. It may result from primary infection with such organisms as *Salmonella typhi, Escherichia coli,* or *Clostridium* or from obstruction of the cystic duct due to lymphadenopathy or a tumor. It appears that ischemia, usually related to a low cardiac output, also has a role in the pathophysiology of this disease. Signs and symptoms of acalculous cholecystitis include unexplained sepsis, right upper quadrant pain, fever, leukocytosis, and a palpable gallbladder.

In most cases, gallbladder and bile duct diseases occur in people who are older than age 40 and are more prevalent in females and Native American, White, and Hispanic populations. Research shows that genetics may play a role in the development of gallstones.[1]

Signs and symptoms

Although gallbladder disease may produce no symptoms, acute cholelithiasis, acute cholecystitis, choledocholithiasis, and cholesterolosis produce the symptoms of a classic gallbladder attack. Attacks usually follow meals rich in fats or may occur at night, suddenly awakening the patient. They begin with acute abdominal pain in the right upper quadrant that may radiate to the back, between the shoulders, or to the front of the chest; the pain may be so severe that the patient seeks emergency department care. Other features may include recurring fat intolerance, biliary colic, belching, flatulence, indigestion, diaphoresis, nausea, vomiting, chills, low-grade fever, jaundice (if a stone obstructs the common bile duct), and clay-colored stools (with choledocholithiasis).

Clinical features of cholangitis include a rise in eosinophils, jaundice, abdominal pain, high fever, and chills; biliary cirrhosis may produce jaundice, related itching, weakness, fatigue, slight weight loss, and abdominal pain. Gallstone ileus produces signs and symptoms of small-bowel obstruction—nausea, vomiting, abdominal distention, and absent bowel sounds if the bowel is completely obstructed. Its most telling symptom is intermittent recurrence of colicky pain over several days.

Complications

Each of these disorders produces its own set of complications:

▶ Cholelithiasis may lead to cholangitis, cholecystitis, choledocholithiasis, and gallstone ileus.

▶ Cholecystitis may lead to gallbladder complications such as empyema, hydrops or mucocele, or gangrene.

▶ Gangrene may lead to perforation, resulting in peritonitis, fistula formation, pancreatitis, limy bile, and porcelain gallbladder.

▶ Other complications include chronic cholecystitis and cholangitis.

▶ Choledocholithiasis may lead to cholangitis, obstructive jaundice, pancreatitis, and secondary biliary cirrhosis.

▶ Cholangitis, especially in the suppurative form, may progress to septic shock and death.

▶ Gallstone ileus may cause bowel obstruction, which can lead to intestinal perforation, peritonitis, septicemia, secondary infection, and septic shock.

Diagnosis

Ultrasound is the procedure of choice to detect gallstones; it can detect gallstones larger than 2 mm.[1] X-rays also detect gallstones. Other tests may include the following:

▶ Abdominal computed tomography scan or ultrasound reflects stones in the gallbladder.

▶ Percutaneous transhepatic cholangiography, done under fluoroscopic control, distinguishes between gallbladder or bile duct disease and cancer of the pancreatic head in patients with jaundice.

▶ Endoscopic retrograde cholangiopancreatography visualizes the biliary tree after insertion of an endoscope down the esophagus into the duodenum, cannulation of the common bile and pancreatic ducts, and injection of contrast medium.[3]

▶ Hepatobiliary iminodiacetic acid scan of the gallbladder detects obstruction of the cystic duct.

▶ Oral cholecystography shows stones in the gallbladder and biliary duct obstruction.

An elevated icteric index and total bilirubin, urine bilirubin, and alkaline phosphatase levels support the diagnosis. The white blood cell count is slightly elevated during a cholecystitis attack. Differential diagnosis is essential because gallbladder disease can mimic other diseases (myocardial infarction, angina, pancreatitis, pancreatic head cancer, pneumonia, peptic ulcer, hiatal hernia, esophagitis, and gastritis). Serum amylase levels distinguish gallbladder disease from pancreatitis. With suspected heart disease, serial cardiac enzyme tests and electrocardiography should precede gallbladder and upper GI diagnostic tests.

Treatment

Surgery, usually elective, is the treatment of choice for gallbladder and bile duct diseases and may include open or laparoscopic cholecystectomy, cholecystectomy with operative cholangiography, and possibly exploration of the common bile duct. Early surgery helps decrease the risk of complications and shortens the hospital stay.[2] Electrohydraulic shock wave lithotripsy can be used to fragment gallstones if they're few in number; it may be used with ursodeoxycholic acid to improve dissolution. Other treatments include a low-fat diet to prevent attacks and vitamin K for itching, jaundice, and bleeding tendencies due to vitamin K deficiency. Treatment during an acute attack may include insertion of a nasogastric tube and an I.V. line and, possibly, antibiotic administration.

A nonsurgical treatment for choledocholithiasis involves placement of a catheter through the percutaneous transhepatic cholangiographic route. Guided by fluoroscopy, the catheter is directed toward the stone. A basket is threaded through the catheter, opened, twirled to entrap the stone, closed, and withdrawn. This procedure can be performed endoscopically.

Chenodeoxycholic acid, which dissolves radiolucent stones, provides an alternative for patients who are poor surgical risks or who refuse surgery.

Special considerations

Patient care for gallbladder and bile duct diseases focuses on supportive care and close postoperative observation.

▶ Before surgery, teach the patient to deep-breathe, cough, expectorate, and perform leg exercises that are necessary after surgery. Also teach splinting, repositioning, and ambulation techniques. Explain the procedures that will be performed before, during, and after surgery to help ease the patient's anxiety and to help ensure his cooperation.

▶ After surgery, monitor the patient's vital signs for signs of bleeding, infection, or atelectasis.

▶ Evaluate the incision site for bleeding. Serosanguineous drainage is common during the first 24 to 48 hours if the patient has a wound drain. If, after a choledochostomy, a T tube drain is placed in the duct and attached to a drainage bag, make sure that the drainage tube has no kinks. Also check that the connecting tubing from the T tube is well secured to the patient to prevent dislodgment.

▶ Measure and record T tube drainage daily (200 to 300 ml is normal).

▶ Teach patients who will be discharged with a T tube how to perform dressing changes and routine skin care.

▶ Monitor the patient's intake and output. Allow him nothing by mouth for 24 to 48 hours or until bowel sounds return and nausea and vomiting cease (postoperative nausea may indicate a full bladder).

▶ If the patient doesn't void within 8 hours (or if the amount voided is inadequate based on I.V. fluid intake), percuss over the symphysis pubis for bladder distention (especially in the patient receiving anticholinergics). The patient who has had a laparoscopic cholecystectomy may be discharged the same day or within 24 hours after surgery. He should have minimal pain, be able to tolerate a regular diet within 24 hours after surgery, and be able to return to normal activity within a few days to a week.

▶ Encourage deep-breathing and leg exercises every hour. The patient should ambulate after surgery. Provide elastic stockings to support the leg muscles and promote venous blood flow, thus preventing stasis and clot formation.

▶ Evaluate the location, duration, and character of any pain. Administer adequate medication to relieve pain, especially before such activities as deep breathing and ambulation, which increase pain.

▶ At discharge, advise the patient against heavy lifting or straining for 6 weeks. Urge him to walk daily. Tell him that food restrictions are unnecessary unless he has an intolerance to a specific food or some underlying condition (such as diabetes, atherosclerosis, or obesity) that requires such restriction.

▶ Instruct the patient to notify the surgeon if he has pain for more than 24 hours or notices any jaundice, anorexia, nausea or vomiting, fever, or tenderness in the abdominal area. These may indicate a biliary tract injury from cholecystectomy, requiring immediate attention.

REFERENCES

1. Lee, F.M., et al. eMedicine from *Web*MD (2006 June 12). "Cholelithiasis." [Online]. Available at *www.emedicine.com/emerg/topic97.htm*.
2. Rosing, D.K., et al. "Early Cholecystectomy for Mild to Moderate Gallstone Pancreatitis Shortens Hospital Stay," *Journal of the American College of Surgeons* 205(6):762-66, December 2007.
3. Sgouros, S.N., and Bergele, C. "Endoscopic Ultrasonography versus Other Diagnostic Modalities in the Diagnosis of Choledocholithiasis," Digestive Diseases and Science 51(12): 2280-86, December 2006.

CIRRHOSIS AND FIBROSIS

Cirrhosis is a chronic hepatic disease characterized by diffuse destruction and fibrotic regeneration of hepatic cells. As necrotic tissue yields to fibrosis, this

disease alters liver structure and normal vasculature, impairs blood and lymph flow, and ultimately causes hepatic insufficiency. The prognosis is better in noncirrhotic forms of hepatic fibrosis, which cause minimal hepatic dysfunction and don't destroy liver cells. Cirrhosis is the ninth leading cause of death in the United States.

Causes and incidence

Alcohol and hepatitis C are the most common causes of cirrhosis in the United States.[1] These clinical types of cirrhosis reflect its diverse etiology:

▶ Portal, nutritional, or alcoholic (Laennec's) cirrhosis, the most common type, occurs in 21% of cirrhotic patients. Liver damage results from malnutrition, especially of dietary protein, and chronic alcohol ingestion. Fibrous tissue forms in portal areas and around central veins.

▶ Chronic hepatitis C causes inflammation of the liver and causes 26% of cirrhosis.

Hepatitis C and alcoholic liver disease together cause 15% of cirrhosis.

▶ Hepatitis B and D cause inflammation in the liver. Hepatitis B causes 15% of cirrhosis.

▶ Biliary cirrhosis results from injury or prolonged obstruction.

▶ Postnecrotic (posthepatic) cirrhosis stems from various types of hepatitis.

▶ Pigment cirrhosis may result from disorders such as hemochromatosis.

▶ Cardiac cirrhosis (rare) refers to liver damage caused by right-sided heart failure.

▶ Idiopathic cirrhosis (18%) has no known cause.

Noncirrhotic fibrosis may result from schistosomiasis or congenital hepatic fibrosis or may be idiopathic.

Signs and symptoms

Clinical manifestations of cirrhosis and fibrosis are similar for all types, regardless of the cause. Early indications are vague, but usually include GI signs and symptoms (anorexia, indigestion, nausea, vomiting, constipation, or diarrhea) and a dull abdominal ache. Major and late signs and symptoms develop as a result of hepatic insufficiency and portal hypertension.

▶ Respiratory—pleural effusion and limited thoracic expansion due to abdominal ascites, interfering with efficient gas exchange and leading to hypoxia

▶ Central nervous system—progressive signs or symptoms of hepatic encephalopathy—lethargy, mental changes, slurred speech, asterixis (flapping tremor), peripheral neuritis, paranoia, hallucinations, extreme obtundation, and coma

▶ Hematologic—bleeding tendencies (nosebleeds, easy bruising, and bleeding gums) and anemia

▶ Endocrine—testicular atrophy, menstrual irregularities, gynecomastia, and loss of chest and axillary hair

▶ Skin—severe pruritus, extreme dryness, poor tissue turgor, abnormal pigmentation, spider angiomas, palmar erythema, and possibly jaundice

▶ Hepatic—jaundice, hepatomegaly, ascites, edema of the legs, hepatic encephalopathy, and hepatorenal syndrome comprise the other major effects of full-fledged cirrhosis

▶ Miscellaneous—musty breath, enlarged superficial abdominal veins, muscle atrophy, pain in the right upper abdominal quadrant that worsens when the patient sits up or leans forward, palpable liver or spleen, and temperature of 101° to 103° F (38.3° to 39.4° C). Bleeding from esophageal varices results from portal hypertension.

Complications

▶ Portal hypertension
▶ Bleeding esophageal varices
▶ Hepatic encephalopathy
▶ Hepatorenal syndrome
▶ Death

Diagnosis

Liver biopsy, the definitive test for cirrhosis, detects destruction and fibrosis of hepatic tissue.[2]

Liver scan shows abnormal thickening and a liver mass. Cholecystography and cholangiography visualize the gallbladder and the biliary duct system, respectively; splenoportal venography visualizes the portal venous system. Percutaneous transhepatic cholangiography differentiates extrahepatic from intrahepatic obstructive jaundice and discloses hepatic pathology and the presence of gallstones.

Laboratory findings that are characteristic of cirrhosis include:

▶ decreased white blood cell count, hemoglobin level and hematocrit, albumin, serum electrolyte levels (sodium, potassium, chloride, and magnesium), and cholinesterase
▶ elevated levels of globulin, serum ammonia, total bilirubin, alkaline phosphatase, serum aspartate aminotransferase, serum alanine aminotransferase, and lactate dehydrogenase and increased thymol turbidity
▶ anemia, neutropenia, and thrombocytopenia, characterized by prolonged prothrombin and partial thromboplastin times
▶ deficiencies of folic acid, iron, and vitamins A, B_{12}, C, and K.

Treatment

Treatment is designed to remove or alleviate the underlying cause of cirrhosis or fibrosis, prevent further liver damage, and prevent or treat complications. The patient may benefit from a high-calorie and moderate- to high-protein diet, but developing hepatic encephalopathy mandates restricted protein intake. In addition, sodium is usually restricted to 200 to 500 mg/day and fluids to 1 to 1½ qt (1 to 1.5 L)/day.

If the patient's condition continues to deteriorate, he may need tube feedings or total parenteral nutrition. He may also need supplemental vitamins—A, B complex, D, and K—to compensate for the liver's inability to store them and vitamin B_{12}, folic acid, and thiamine for deficiency anemia. Rest, moderate exercise, and avoidance of exposure to infections and toxic agents are essential.

Drug therapy requires special caution because the cirrhotic liver can't detoxify harmful substances efficiently. When absolutely necessary, vasopressin may be prescribed for esophageal varices, and diuretics may be given for edema. However, diuretics require careful monitoring because fluid and electrolyte imbalance may precipitate hepatic encephalopathy. Encephalopathy is treated with lactulose. Antibiotics are used to decrease intestinal bacteria and reduce ammonia production, which causes encephalopathy. Coagulopathy may be treated with blood products or vitamin K.

Low-protein diets are controversial. They aid in managing acute hepatic encephalopathy but are rarely necessary in chronic conditions because of the underlying protein-calorie malnutrition.

Paracentesis and infusions of salt-poor albumin, in addition to fluid and salt restriction, may alleviate ascites. Surgical procedures include treatment of varices by upper endoscopy with banding or sclerosis, splenectomy, esophagogastric resection, and splenorenal or portacaval anastomosis to relieve portal hypertension. (See *Portal hypertension and esophageal varices*. See also *Circulation in portal hypertension*, page 166.)

If cirrhosis progresses and becomes life-threatening, a liver transplant should be considered.

With advances in surgical procedures, organ preservation, and immunosuppression, liver transplantation has improved survival rates. Survival rates are 85% to 90% after 1 year and greater than 70% for 5 years.

Special considerations

The patient with cirrhosis needs close observation, first-rate supportive care, and sound nutritional counseling.

Portal hypertension and esophageal varices

Portal hypertension—elevated pressure in the portal vein—occurs when blood flow meets increased resistance. The disorder is a common result of cirrhosis, but may also stem from mechanical obstruction and occlusion of the hepatic veins (Budd-Chiari syndrome). As portal pressure rises, blood backs up into the spleen and flows through collateral channels to the venous system, bypassing the liver. Consequently, portal hypertension produces splenomegaly with thrombocytopenia, dilated collateral veins (esophageal varices, hemorrhoids, or prominent abdominal veins), and ascites. Nevertheless, in many patients, the first sign of portal hypertension is bleeding from esophageal varices—dilated tortuous veins in the submucosa of the lower esophagus. Bleeding esophageal varices commonly cause massive hematemesis, requiring emergency treatment to control hemorrhage and prevent hypovolemic shock.

DIAGNOSIS AND TREATMENT

These procedures help diagnose and correct esophageal varices.
• Endoscopy identifies the ruptured varix as the bleeding site and excludes other potential sources in the upper GI tract.
• Angiography may aid diagnosis, but is less precise than endoscopy.
• Vasopressin infused into the superior mesenteric artery may temporarily stop bleeding. When angiography is unavailable, vasopressin may be infused by I.V. drip or diluted with 5% dextrose in water (except in patients with coronary vascular disease), but this route is usually less effective.
• A Sengstaken-Blakemore or Minnesota tube may also help control hemorrhage by applying pressure on the bleeding site. Iced saline lavage through the tube may help control bleeding.
• The use of vasopressin or a Minnesota or Sengstaken-Blakemore tube is a temporary measure only, especially in the patient with a severely deteriorated liver. Fresh blood and

fresh frozen plasma, if available, are preferable for blood transfusions to replace clotting factors. Treatment with lactulose promotes elimination of old blood from the GI tract, which combats excessive ammonia production and accumulation.

Appropriate surgical bypass procedures include portosystemic anastomosis, splenorenal shunt, and mesocaval shunt. A portacaval or a mesocaval shunt decreases pressure within the liver and reduces ascites, plasma loss, and the risk of hemorrhage by directing blood from the liver into collateral vessels. Emergency shunts carry a mortality of 25% to 50%. Clinical evidence suggests that portosystemic bypass doesn't prolong the patient's survival time; however, he will eventually die of hepatic coma rather than of hemorrhage.

PATIENT CARE

Care for the patient who has portal hypertension with esophageal varices focuses on careful monitoring for signs and symptoms of hemorrhage and subsequent hypotension, compromised oxygen supply, and altered level of consciousness (LOC).
• Monitor the patient's vital signs, urine output, and central venous pressure to determine fluid volume status.
• Assess the patient's LOC often.
• Provide emotional support and reassurance in the wake of massive GI bleeding, which is always a frightening experience.
• Keep the patient as quiet and comfortable as possible, but remember that tolerance of sedatives and tranquilizers may be decreased because of liver damage.
• Clean the patient's mouth, which may be dry and flecked with dried blood.
• Carefully monitor the patient with a Minnesota or Sengstaken-Blakemore tube in place for persistent bleeding in gastric drainage, signs of asphyxiation from tube displacement, proper inflation of balloons, and correct traction to maintain tube placement.

Circulation in portal hypertension

As portal vein pressure rises, blood backs up into the spleen and flows through collateral channels to the venous system, bypassing the liver and resulting in esophageal varices.

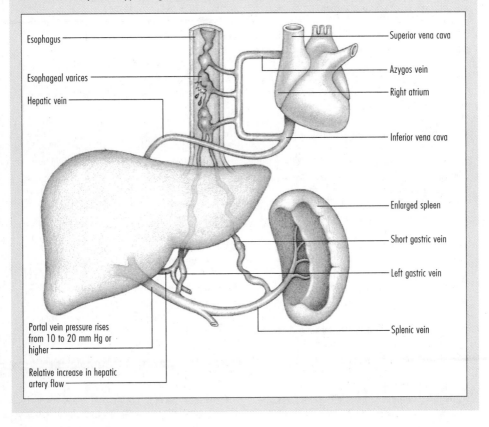

- Esophagus
- Esophageal varices
- Hepatic vein
- Portal vein pressure rises from 10 to 20 mm Hg or higher
- Relative increase in hepatic artery flow
- Superior vena cava
- Azygos vein
- Right atrium
- Inferior vena cava
- Enlarged spleen
- Short gastric vein
- Left gastric vein
- Splenic vein

▶ Check the patient's skin, gums, stools, and vomitus regularly for bleeding. Apply pressure to injection sites to prevent bleeding. Warn him against taking nonsteroidal anti-inflammatory drugs, straining at stool, and blowing his nose or sneezing too vigorously. Suggest using an electric razor and soft toothbrush.[3]

▶ Observe the patient closely for signs of behavioral or personality changes. Report increasing stupor, lethargy, hallucinations, or neuromuscular dysfunction. Awaken him periodically to determine his level of conscious-

ness. Watch for asterixis, a sign of developing hepatic encephalopathy.[3]

▶ To assess fluid retention, weigh the patient and measure abdominal girth at least daily, inspect his ankles and sacrum for dependent edema, and accurately record intake and output. Carefully evaluate the patient before, during, and after paracentesis; this drastic loss of fluid may induce shock.[4]

▶ To prevent skin breakdown associated with edema and pruritus, avoid using soap when you bathe the patient; instead, use lubricating lotion or moisturizing agents.

Handle him gently, and turn and reposition him often to keep his skin intact.

▶ Tell the patient that rest and good nutrition will conserve his energy and decrease metabolic demands on the liver. Urge him to eat frequent, small meals. Stress the need to avoid infections and abstain from alcohol. Refer him to Alcoholics Anonymous, if necessary.

REFERENCES

1. National Digestive Diseases Information Clearinghouse (2003 December). "Cirrhosis of the Liver," NIH Publication No. 04-1134. Available at *http://digestive.niddk.nih.gov/ddiseases/pubs/cirrhosis/*.
2. MayoClinic.com (2007 January 19). "Cirrhosis." [Online]. Available at *www.mayoclinic.com/health/cirrhosis/DS00373/DSECTION=6*.
3. Sargent, S. "Management of Patients with Advanced Liver Cirrhosis," *Nursing Standard* 21(11):48-56, November 2006.
4. Sargent, S. "The Management and Nursing Care of Cirrhotic Ascites," *Nursing Standard* 15(4):212-19, February-March 2006.

CROHN'S DISEASE

Crohn's disease, also known as *regional enteritis* and *granulomatous colitis,* is an inflammation of any part of the GI tract (usually the proximal portion of the colon or, less commonly, the terminal ileum) that extends through all layers of the intestinal wall. It may also involve regional lymph nodes and the mesentery. Granulomas are usually surrounded by normal mucosa; when these lesions are present in multiples, they're commonly referred to as *skip lesions.* The surface of the inflamed GI tract usually has a cobblestone appearance, which is different from alternating areas of inflammation and fissure crevices.

Causes and incidence

In Crohn's disease, lacteal blockage in the intestinal wall leads to edema and, eventually, inflammation, ulceration, and stenosis. Abscesses and fistulas may also occur.

Although the exact cause of Crohn's disease is unknown, autoimmune, genetic, and environmental factors are thought to play roles.[1] Researchers believe that an interaction with an environmental agent (maybe a virus) and the body's immune system may trigger the disease or cause damage to the intestinal wall, which initiates the disease process.[1] Researchers have found an abnormal mutation in a gene that occurs twice as often in patients with Crohn's.[1] Up to 25% of those with the disease may have one or more affected relatives with Crohn's disease or ulcerative colitis.[1] People of Jewish ancestry are more likely to get the disease, and blacks are less likely to develop the disease.[2] The incidence of Crohn's disease has risen steadily over the past 50 years; it is now estimated to affect half a million Americans, with males and females equally affected.[1] Crohn's disease is most prevalent in adults ages 15 to 35.[1]

Signs and symptoms

Clinical effects may be mild and nonspecific initially; they vary according to the location and extent of the lesion. Acute inflammatory signs and symptoms mimic appendicitis and include steady, colicky pain in the right lower quadrant, cramping, tenderness, flatulence, nausea, fever, and diarrhea. Bleeding may occur and, although usually mild, may be massive. Bloody stools may also occur.

Chronic symptoms, which are more typical of the disease, are more persistent and less severe; they include diarrhea (four to six stools per day) with pain in the right lower abdominal quadrant, steatorrhea (excess fat in feces), marked weight loss and, rarely, clubbing of fingers. The patient may complain of weakness and fatigue.

The "string sign"

The characteristic "string sign" (marked narrowing of the bowel), resulting from inflammatory disease and scarring, strengthens the diagnosis of Crohn's disease.

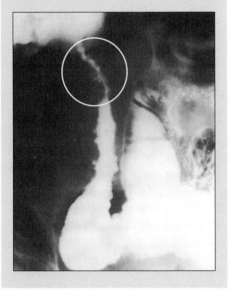

Complications

▶ Anal fistulas
▶ Perineal abscess
▶ Intestinal obstruction
▶ Nutritional deficiencies
▶ Peritonitis

Diagnosis

Barium enema showing the string sign (segments of stricture separated by normal bowel) supports a diagnosis of Crohn's disease. (See *The "string sign."*) Ultrasound shows areas of bowel wall thickening and reduced or absent peristalsis.[3]

Sigmoidoscopy and colonoscopy may show patchy areas of inflammation, thus helping to rule out ulcerative colitis. However, biopsy is required for a definitive diagnosis.[8] Computed tomography helps diagnose complications such as bowel obstruction, and magnetic resonance imaging scanning can identify bowel wall changes.[3]

Laboratory findings commonly indicate increased white blood cell count and erythrocyte sedimentation rate, hypokalemia, hypocalcemia, hypomagnesemia, and a decreased hemoglobin level. New research findings also indicate that newly discovered proteins that help protect the intestinal mucosa may be deficient in patients with Crohn's disease.[5]

Treatment

To control the inflammatory process, medications, such as 5-aminosalicylate, may be prescribed. Corticosteroids and immunomodulators (methotrexate, azathioprine and 6-MP) may be prescribed if 5-aminosalicylate isn't effective or in patients with severe Crohn's disease.[6] In debilitated patients, therapy includes total parenteral nutrition to maintain nutritional status while resting the bowel. If abscesses or fistulas occur, antibiotics may be prescribed. Infliximab (an antibody to tumor necrosis factor-alpha, an immune chemical that promotes inflammation) may be prescribed for patients who have not responded to corticosteroids or immunomodulators.[4]

Effective treatment requires important changes in lifestyle: physical rest, restricted diet (specific foods vary from person to person), and elimination of dairy products for lactose intolerance.

Surgery may be necessary to correct bowel perforation, massive hemorrhage, fistulas, or acute intestinal obstruction. Colectomy with ileostomy is necessary in many patients with extensive disease of the large intestine and rectum.[7] (See *Surgery rate and immunosuppressants.*)

Special considerations

Although treatment is based largely on symptoms, you should monitor the patient's status carefully for signs of worsening.

EVIDENCE-BASED PRACTICE

Surgery rate and immunosuppressants

Question: *Does the increased use of immunosuppressants in Crohn's Disease decrease the need for intestinal surgery?*

Research: Immunosuppressant drugs are used with Crohn's disease to block the immune reaction that contributes to inflammation, maintain remission, and to heal fistulas and intestinal ulcers caused by this disease. The study was performed to determine if the use of these drugs had decreased the need for intestinal surgery in patients with Crohn's disease during the previous 25 years, from 1978 to 2002. A retrospective review was performed on the medical records of 2,573 patients to determine the use of immunosuppressants, the need for intestinal resection, and the occurrence of intestinal complications.

Conclusion: The researchers found that the probability of immunosuppressant use increased from 0 in 1978 to 0.56 in the time period between 1998 and 2002. Throughout the 25-year period, there was no significant decrease in the need for intestinal resection or in the occurrence of intestinal complications of the disease.

Application: When providing care for the patient with Crohn's disease who's taking immunosuppressant drugs, the nurse needs to be aware of the possible complications that can occur with these drugs, such as the patient's increased risk of infection. The study indicates that the patient's risk of complications caused by Crohn's disease remains unchanged; therefore, the nurse must continue to assess for signs of bowel obstruction, fistulas, and nutritional deficiencies.

Source: Cosnes, J., et al. "Impact of the Increasing Use of Immunosuppressants in Crohn's Disease on the Need for Intestinal Surgery," *Gut* 54(2): 237-41, February 2005.

▶ Record fluid intake and output (including the amount of stool), and weigh the patient daily. Watch for dehydration, and maintain fluid and electrolyte balance. Be alert for signs of intestinal bleeding (bloody stools); check stools daily for occult blood.

▶ Check hemoglobin level and hematocrit regularly. Give iron supplements and blood transfusions, as ordered.

▶ Provide good patient hygiene and mouth care if the patient is restricted and may not take anything by mouth. After each of the patient's bowel movements, make sure surrounding skin is clean. Always keep a clean, covered bedpan within the patient's reach. Ventilate the room to eliminate odors.

▶ Observe the patient for fever and pain or pneumaturia, which may signal bladder fistula. Abdominal pain and distention and fever may indicate intestinal obstruction.

Watch for stools from the vagina and an enterovaginal fistula.

▶ Before ileostomy, arrange for a visit by an enterostomal therapist.

▶ After surgery, frequently check the patient's I.V. and nasogastric tube for proper functioning. Monitor his vital signs and fluid intake and output. Watch for wound infection. Provide meticulous stoma care, and teach it to the patient and his family. Realize that ileostomy changes the patient's body image, so offer reassurance and emotional support.

▶ Stress the need for a severely restricted diet and bed rest, which may be trying, particularly for the young patient. Encourage him to try to reduce tension. If stress is clearly an aggravating factor, refer him for counseling.

▶ Refer the patient to a support group such as the Crohn's and Colitis Foundation of America.

REFERENCES

1. Crohn's & Colitis Foundation of America. "About Crohn's Disease." [Online]: Available at *www.ccfa.org/info/about/crohns.*
2. National Digestive Diseases Information Clearinghouse (2006 February). "Crohn's Disease," NIH Publication No. 06-3410 [Online]. Available at *http://digestive.niddk.nih. gov/ddiseases/pubs/crohns/index.htm.*
3. Huprich J.E., et al. "Expert Panel on Gastrointestinal Imaging. Crohn's Disease," Reston, Va.: *American College of Radiology*; 2005. Available at *www.guideline.gov.*
4. Lichtenstein, G.R., et al. "American Gastroenterological Association Institute Medical Position Statement on Corticosteroids, Immunomodulators, and Infliximab in Inflammatory Bowel Disease," *Gastroenterology* 130(3):935-939 March 2006. Available at *www.guideline.gov.*
5. Renner, M., et al. "DMBT1 Confers Mucosal Protection in Vivo and a Deletion Variant Is Associated with Crohn's Disease," *Gastroenterology* 133(5):1499-509, November 2007.
6. Baumgart, D.C., and Sandborn, W.J. "Inflammatory Bowel Disease: Clinical Aspects and Established and Evolving Therapies," *Lancet* 369(9573):1641-57, May 2007.
7. Travis, S.P., et al. "European Evidence Based Consensus on the Diagnosis and Management of Crohn's Disease: Current Management," *Gut* 55(Suppl 1):i16-35, March 2006.
8. Stange, E.F., et al. "European Evidence Based Consensus on the Diagnosis and Management of Crohn's Disease: Definitions and Diagnosis," *Gut* 55(Suppl 1):i1-15, March 2006.

ESOPHAGEAL DIVERTICULA

Esophageal diverticula are hollow out-pouchings of one or more layers of the esophageal wall. They occur in three main areas: just above the upper esophageal sphincter (Zenker's, or pulsion diverticulum, the most common type); near the midpoint of the esophagus (traction); and just above the lower esophageal sphincter (epiphrenic). Generally, esophageal diverticula occur later in life—although they can affect infants and children—and are three times more common in males than in females. Epiphrenic diverticula usually occur in middle-age males, whereas Zenker's diverticula typically affect males older than age 60.

Causes and incidence

Esophageal diverticula are due to primary muscular abnormalities that may be congenital or to inflammatory processes adjacent to the esophagus. Zenker's diverticulum occurs when the pouch results from increased intraesophageal pressure; traction diverticulum occurs when the pouch is pulled out by adjacent inflamed tissue or lymph nodes. Some authorities classify all diverticula as traction diverticula.

Zenker's diverticulum results from developmental muscular weakness of the posterior pharynx above the border of the cricopharyngeal muscle. The pressure of swallowing aggravates this weakness, as does contraction of the pharynx before relaxation of the sphincter. A midesophageal (traction) diverticulum is a response to scarring and pulling on esophageal walls by an external inflammatory process such as tuberculosis. An epiphrenic diverticulum (rare) is generally right-sided and usually accompanies an esophageal motor disturbance, such as esophageal spasm or achalasia. It's thought to be caused by traction and pulsation.

Most diverticula occur in middle-age and elderly patients. Zenker's diverticula are most common in patients older than age 50 and are especially prevalent in patients in their 70s and 80s.[1]

Signs and symptoms

Midesophageal and epiphrenic diverticula with an associated motor disturbance (achalasia or spasm) seldom produce symptoms, although the patient may experience dysphagia and heartburn. Zenker's diverticulum, however, produces distinctly staged symptoms, beginning with initial throat irritation, followed by dysphagia and near-complete obstruction. In early stages, regurgitation occurs soon after eating; in later stages, regurgitation after eating is delayed and may even occur during sleep, leading to food aspiration and pulmonary infection.

HEALTH & SAFETY *Hoarseness, asthma, and pneumonitis may be the only signs of esophageal diverticula in elderly patients.*

Other signs and symptoms include noise when liquids are swallowed, chronic cough, hoarseness, a bad taste in the mouth or foul breath and, rarely, bleeding.

Complications

▶ Aspiration pneumonia[1]

Diagnosis

X-rays taken following a barium swallow usually confirm the diagnosis by showing characteristic outpouching.[2]

Esophagoscopy can rule out another lesion; however, the procedure risks rupturing the diverticulum by passing the scope into it rather than into the lumen of the esophagus, a special danger with Zenker's diverticulum.

Treatment

Treatment of Zenker's diverticulum is usually palliative and includes a bland diet, thorough chewing, and drinking water after eating to flush out the sac. However, severe symptoms or a large diverticulum necessitates surgery to remove the sac or facilitate drainage. An esophagomyotomy with cricopharyngeal myotomy, diverticular suspension with cricopharyngeal myotomy or cricopharyngeal myotomy alone may be necessary to prevent recurrence. This treatment is gaining use as it is proven to be increasingly safe for the patient.[3]

A midesophageal diverticulum seldom requires therapy except when esophagitis aggravates the risk of rupture, in which case, treatment includes antacids and an antireflux regimen: keeping the head elevated, maintaining an upright position for 2 hours after eating, eating small meals, controlling chronic coughing, and avoiding constrictive clothing.

Epiphrenic diverticulum requires treatment of accompanying motor disorders. Achalasia is treated by repeated dilations of the esophagus; acute spasm is controlled by anticholinergic administration and diverticulum excision; and dysphagia or severe pain are relieved by surgical excision or suspending the diverticulum to promote drainage. Treatment may also include parenteral feeding to improve the patient's nutritional status.

Special considerations

Care includes documenting the patient's symptoms and nutritional status and educating him about the disorder.

▶ Regularly assess the patient's nutritional status (weight, calorie intake, and appearance).

▶ If the patient regurgitates food and mucus, protect against aspiration by positioning him carefully (head elevated or turned to one side). To prevent aspiration, tell the patient to empty any visible outpouching in the neck by massage or postural drainage before retiring.

▶ If the patient has dysphagia, record well-tolerated foods and what circumstances ease swallowing. Provide a pureed diet, with vitamin or protein supplements, and encourage thorough chewing.

▶ Teach the patient about this disorder. Explain treatment instructions and diagnostic procedures.

REFERENCES

1. Bragg, J., et al. eMedicine from *WebMD* (2006 November 16). "Esophageal Diverticula." [Online]. Available at *www.emedicine.com/med/topic736.htm*.
2. Tsikoudas, A., et al. "Correlation of Radiologic Findings and Clinical Outcome in Pharyngeal Pouch Stapling," *Annals of Otolaryngology, Rhinology, and Laryngology* 115(10):721-26, October 2006.
3. McLean, T.R., and Haller, C.C. "Stapled Diverticulectomy and Myotomy for Symptomatic Zenker's Diverticulum," *American Journal of Surgery* 192(5):e28-31, November 2006.

GASTROENTERITIS

A self-limiting disorder, gastroenteritis is characterized by diarrhea, nausea, vomiting, and acute or chronic abdominal cramping. Also called *intestinal flu, traveler's diarrhea, viral enteritis,* or *food poisoning,* it occurs in persons of all ages and is a major cause of morbidity and mortality in underdeveloped nations. In the United States, gastroenteritis ranks second to the common cold as a leading cause of lost work time, and fifth as the leading cause of death among young children. It also can be life-threatening in elderly or debilitated people.

Causes and incidence

Gastroenteritis has many possible causes, including:

▶ bacteria (responsible for acute food poisoning), such as *Staphylococcus aureus, Salmonella, Shigella, Clostridium botulinum, C. perfringens,* and *Escherichia coli*
▶ amebae, especially *Entamoeba histolytica*
▶ parasites, such as *Ascaris, Enterobius,* and *Trichinella spiralis*
▶ viruses (may be responsible for traveler's diarrhea) such as adenoviruses, echoviruses, or coxsackie viruses
▶ ingestion of toxins, including plants or toadstools
▶ drug reactions; for example, to antibiotics
▶ enzyme deficiencies
▶ food allergens.

The bowel reacts to any of these enterotoxins with hypermotility, producing severe diarrhea and secondary depletion of intracellular fluid. Chronic gastroenteritis is usually the result of another GI disorder such as ulcerative colitis.

Diarrhea accounts for as many as 3% of pediatric office visits and 10% of hospitalizations for patients younger than age 5. Incidence is hard to determine due to underreporting, but the Centers for Disease Control and Prevention reports 3.5 million cases of acute diarrhea from rotavirus and 90,000 cases of food poisoning each year.[1] Traveler's diarrhea affects 20% to 50% of people traveling to developing countries each year.[2]

Signs and symptoms

Clinical manifestations vary depending on the pathologic organism and the level of GI tract involved. However, gastroenteritis in adults is usually an acute, self-limiting, nonfatal disease producing diarrhea, abdominal discomfort (ranging from cramping to pain), nausea, and vomiting. Other possible signs and symptoms include fever, malaise, and borborygmi. In children, elderly people, and the debilitated, gastroenteritis produces the same symptoms, but these patients' intolerance to electrolyte and fluid losses leads to a higher mortality.

Complications

▶ Severe dehydration and loss of electrolytes
▶ Shock
▶ Vascular collapse
▶ Renal failure

Diagnosis

Patient history can aid in the diagnosis of gastroenteritis. Stool culture (by direct rectal

swab) or blood culture identifies the causative bacteria or parasites.

Treatment

Treatment is usually supportive and consists of bed rest, nutritional support, and increased fluid intake. When gastroenteritis is severe or affects a young child or an elderly or debilitated person, treatment may necessitate hospitalization, specific antimicrobials, I.V. fluid and electrolyte replacement and, possibly, antiemetics (given orally, I.M., or by rectal suppository).

Special considerations

Patient care includes education, administering medications, and assessing symptoms for signs of improvement or worsening.

▶ Encourage parents of infants to have their child receive the rotavirus vaccine approved by the Food and Drug Administration in February 2006. It is given by mouth in three doses between 6 and 32 weeks.[3]

▶ Administer medications as ordered; correlate dosage, routes, and times appropriately with the patient's meals and activities (for example, give antiemetics 30 to 60 minutes before meals).

▶ If the patient can eat, replace lost fluids and electrolytes with broth, ginger ale, and lemonade, as tolerated. Vary the diet to make it more enjoyable, and allow some choice of foods. Warn the patient to avoid milk and milk products, which may provoke recurrence.

▶ Record intake and output carefully, and obtain serial weight measurements. Watch for signs of dehydration, such as dry skin and mucous membranes, fever, and sunken eyes.

▶ Wash your hands thoroughly after giving care to avoid spreading infection.

▶ To ease anal irritation, provide warm sitz baths or apply witch hazel compresses.

▶ If food poisoning is the likely cause of gastroenteritis, contact public health authorities so they can interview patients and food handlers, and take samples of the suspected contaminated food.

▶ Teach good hygiene to prevent recurrence. Instruct patients to cook foods—especially pork—thoroughly; to refrigerate perishable foods, such as milk, mayonnaise, potato salad, and cream-filled pastry; to always wash hands with warm water and soap before handling food, especially after using the bathroom; to clean utensils thoroughly; to avoid drinking water or eating raw fruit or vegetables when visiting a foreign country; and to eliminate flies and roaches in the home.

REFERENCES

1. Diskin, A. eMedicine from *WebMD* (2007 April 10). "Gastroenteritis." [Online]. Available at *www.emedicine.com/EMERG/topic213.htm.*
2. Centers for Disease Control and Prevention, Division of Bacterial and Mycotic Diseases (2006 November 21). "Traveler's Diarrhea." [Online]. Available at *www.cdc.gov/ncidod/dbmb/diseaseinfo/travelersdiarrhea_g.htm.*
3. "New Vaccine for Infants," *FDA Consumer* 40(3):3 May-June 2006.

GASTROESOPHAGEAL REFLUX

Gastroesophageal reflux, also called *gastroesophageal reflux disease* (GERD), is the backflow of gastric or duodenal contents, or both, into the esophagus and past the lower esophageal sphincter (LES) without associated belching or vomiting. Reflux may cause symptoms or pathologic changes. Persistent reflux may cause reflux esophagitis (inflammation of the esophageal mucosa). Prognosis varies with the underlying cause.

Causes and incidence

The function of the LES—a high-pressure area in the lower esophagus, just above the

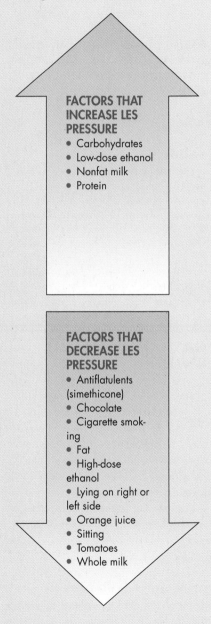

Influences on LES pressure

Several factors can influence lower esophageal sphincter (LES) pressure, thereby affecting reflux, as noted here.

FACTORS THAT INCREASE LES PRESSURE
- Carbohydrates
- Low-dose ethanol
- Nonfat milk
- Protein

FACTORS THAT DECREASE LES PRESSURE
- Antiflatulents (simethicone)
- Chocolate
- Cigarette smoking
- Fat
- High-dose ethanol
- Lying on right or left side
- Orange juice
- Sitting
- Tomatoes
- Whole milk

stomach—is to prevent gastric contents from backing up into the esophagus. Normally, the LES creates pressure, closing the lower end of the esophagus, but relaxes after each swallow to allow food into the stomach. Reflux occurs when LES pressure is deficient or when pressure within the stomach exceeds LES pressure. (See *Influences on LES pressure*.)

Studies have shown that a patient with symptom-producing reflux can't swallow often enough to create sufficient peristaltic amplitude to clear gastric acid from the lower esophagus. This results in prolonged periods of acidity in the esophagus when reflux occurs.

Predisposing factors include:
▶ pyloric surgery (alteration or removal of the pylorus), which allows reflux of bile or pancreatic juice
▶ long-term nasogastric (NG) intubation (more than 4 days)
▶ any agent that lowers LES pressure, such as food, alcohol, cigarettes; anticholinergics (atropine, belladonna, and propantheline); or other drugs (morphine, diazepam, calcium channel blockers, and meperidine)
▶ hiatal hernia with an incompetent sphincter
▶ any condition or position that increases intra-abdominal pressure, such as straining, bending, coughing, pregnancy, obesity, and recurrent or persistent vomiting.

About 25% to 40% of U.S. residents experience symptomatic GERD at some point in their lives, and 7% of U.S. residents experience heartburn symptoms on a daily basis.[1] True incidence figures may be even higher because many people with GERD take over-the-counter remedies without reporting their symptoms. Males experience episodes of esophagitis more frequently than females—the ratio is 2-3:1.

Signs and symptoms

GERD doesn't always cause symptoms, and in patients showing clinical effects, it isn't al-

ways possible to confirm physiologic reflux. The most common feature of GERD is heartburn, which may become more severe with vigorous exercise, bending, or lying down, and may be relieved by antacids or sitting upright. The pain of esophageal spasm resulting from reflux esophagitis tends to be chronic and may mimic angina pectoris, radiating to the neck, jaws, and arms.

Other symptoms include odynophagia, which may be followed by a dull substernal ache from severe, long-term reflux; dysphagia from esophageal spasm, stricture, or esophagitis; and bleeding (bright red or dark brown). Rarely, nocturnal regurgitation wakens the patient with coughing, choking, and a mouthful of saliva. Reflux may be associated with hiatal hernia. Direct hiatal hernia becomes clinically significant only when reflux is confirmed.

Pulmonary symptoms result from reflux of gastric contents into the throat and subsequent aspiration; they include chronic pulmonary disease or nocturnal wheezing, bronchitis, asthma, morning hoarseness, and cough. In children, other signs consist of failure to thrive and forceful vomiting from esophageal irritation. Such vomiting sometimes causes aspiration pneumonia. Other signs in children are nausea, coughing, wheezing, and asthma. Infants may demonstrate arching of the back during or after feedings and irritability.[2]

Complications

▶ Reflux esophagitis
▶ Esophageal stricture
▶ Esophageal ulcer
▶ Replacement of normal squamous epithelium with columnar epithelium
▶ Anemia
▶ Aspiration
▶ Chronic pulmonary disease

Diagnosis

After a careful history and physical examination, tests to confirm GERD include barium swallow fluoroscopy, esophageal pH probe, esophageal manometry, and esophagoscopy. In children, barium esophagography under fluoroscopic control can show reflux.

Ambulatory pH monitoring for 24 hours is the gold-standard diagnostic tool for detection of GERD.

Recurrent reflux after age 6 weeks is abnormal. An acid perfusion (Bernstein) test can show that reflux is the cause of symptoms. Finally, endoscopy and biopsy allow visualization and confirmation of any pathologic changes in the mucosa.

Treatment

Effective management begins by teaching the patient to avoid factors that decrease LES pressure or cause esophageal irritation. The patient should eat a low-fat, high-fiber diet and avoid caffeine, tobacco, and carbonated beverages. He shouldn't eat for 2 to 3 hours before going to bed and should avoid tight clothing, elevate the head of the bed 6" (15.2 cm), and maintain a normal body weight.[1] Promotility agents help increase LES sphincter tone and stimulate upper GI motility. Proton pump inhibitors (omeprazole) and histamine-2 (H_2) receptor antagonists (ranitidine) help reduce gastric acidity. If possible, NG intubation shouldn't be continued for more than 5 days because the tube interferes with sphincter integrity and allows reflux, especially when the patient lies flat.

Positional therapy is especially useful in infants and children who experience GERD without complications.

Surgery may be necessary to control severe and refractory symptoms, such as pulmonary aspiration, hemorrhage, obstruction, severe pain, perforation, an incompetent LES, or associated hiatal hernia. Surgical procedures that create an artificial closure at the gastroesophageal junction may be needed in some patients. These include a proce-

dure that invaginates the esophagus into the stomach and procedures that create a gastric wraparound with or without fixation. The fundoplication procedure can be performed endoscopically. Also, vagotomy or pyloroplasty may be combined with an antireflux regimen to modify gastric contents.

Special considerations

Teach the patient what causes reflux, how to avoid reflux with an antireflux regimen (medication, diet, and positional therapy), and what symptoms to watch for and report.[4]

▶ Instruct the patient to avoid circumstances that increase intra-abdominal pressure (such as bending, coughing, vigorous exercise, tight clothing, constipation, and obesity) as well as substances that reduce sphincter control (cigarettes, alcohol, fatty foods, and caffeine).

▶ Advise the patient to sit upright, particularly after meals, and to eat small, frequent meals.[1] Tell him to avoid highly seasoned food, acidic juices, alcoholic drinks, bedtime snacks, and foods high in fat or carbohydrates, which reduce LES pressure. He should eat meals at least 3 hours before lying down.[3]

▶ Tell the patient to take antacids, as ordered (usually 1 hour before or 3 hours after meals and at bedtime).

▶ Teach the patient correct preparation for diagnostic testing. For example, he shouldn't eat for 6 to 8 hours before a barium swallow or endoscopy.

▶ After surgery using a thoracic approach, carefully watch and record chest tube drainage and the patient's respiratory status. If needed, give chest physiotherapy and oxygen. Position the patient with an NG tube in semi-Fowler's position to help prevent reflux. Offer reassurance and emotional support.

REFERENCES

1. Liu, J.J., and Saltzman, J.R. "Management of Gastroesophageal Reflux Disease," *Southern Medical Journal* 99(7):735-41, July 2006.
2. National Digestive Diseases Information Clearinghouse. "Heartburn, Gastroesophageal Reflux (GER), and Gastroesophageal Reflux Disease (GERD)," NIH Publication No. 07-0882, May 2007. Available at *http://digestive.niddk.gov/ddiseases/pubs/gerd/*.
3. Scott, M., and Gelhot, A.R. "Gastroesophageal Reflux Disease: Diagnosis and Management," *American Family Physician* 59(5):1161-69, March 1999.
4. Kaltenbach, T. "Are Lifestyle Measures Effective in Patients with Gastroesophageal Reflux Disease? An Evidence-Based Approach," Archives of Internal Medicine 166(9):965-71, May 2006.

HEPATIC ENCEPHALOPATHY

Hepatic encephalopathy, also known as *portosystemic encephalopathy* or *hepatic coma,* is a neurologic syndrome that develops as a complication of chronic liver disease.[1] It may be acute and self-limiting or chronic and progressive. Treatment requires correction of the precipitating cause and reduction of blood ammonia levels. In advanced stages, the prognosis is extremely poor despite vigorous treatment.

Causes and incidence

The exact cause of hepatic encephalopathy isn't known.[1] Hepatic encephalopathy may follow rising blood ammonia and manganese levels. Ammonia is particularly harmful to the central nervous system. Normally, the ammonia produced by protein breakdown in the bowel is metabolized to urea in the liver. When portal blood shunts past the liver, ammonia directly enters the systemic circulation and is carried to the brain. Such shunting may result from the collateral venous circulation that develops in portal hypertension

or from surgically created portosystemic shunts. Other factors that predispose rising ammonia levels include excessive protein intake, sepsis, excessive accumulation of nitrogenous body wastes (from constipation or GI hemorrhage), and bacterial action on protein and urea to form ammonia. Certain other factors heighten the brain's sensitivity to ammonia intoxication: hypoxia, azotemia, impaired glucose metabolism, infection, and administration of sedatives, narcotics, and general anesthetics. Depletion of the intravascular volume, from bleeding or diuresis, reduces hepatic and renal perfusion and leads to contraction alkalosis. In turn, hypokalemia and alkalosis increase ammonia production and impair its excretion.[3]

Alkalosis, low oxygen levels, and the use of medications that suppress the central nervous system such as barbiturates or benzodiazepines, also may cause hepatic encephalopathy.[1]

Hepatic encephalopathy is found in about 70% of cirrhosis patients. The ammonia levels of 10% of patients with hepatic encephalopathy are normal. Researchers are still looking for the exact cause of this disease.

Signs and symptoms

Clinical manifestations of hepatic encephalopathy vary (depending on the severity of neurologic involvement) and develop in four stages:

▶ In the *prodromal* stage, early signs and symptoms are commonly overlooked because they're so subtle: slight personality changes (disorientation, forgetfulness, and slurred speech) and a slight tremor.

▶ During the *impending* stage, tremor progresses into asterixis (liver flap and flapping tremor), the hallmark of hepatic encephalopathy. Asterixis is characterized by quick, irregular extensions and flexions of the wrists and fingers, when the wrists are held out straight and the hands flexed upward.

Lethargy, aberrant behavior, and apraxia also occur.

▶ At the *stuporous* stage, hyperventilation occurs; the patient is typically stuporous, but becomes noisy and abusive when aroused.

▶ In the *comatose* stage, the patient has hyperactive reflexes, a positive Babinski's sign, fetor hepaticus (musty, sweet odor to the breath), and coma.

Complications

▶ Irreversible coma and death

Diagnosis

Diagnosis of hepatic encephalopathy is made by clinical features, a history of liver disease, and elevated serum ammonia levels in venous and arterial samples confirm hepatic encephalopathy.

Other supportive laboratory values include an EEG that slows as the disease progresses, an increase in spinal fluid glutamine, elevated bilirubin, and prolonged prothrombin time. Recently, evoked potential testing has been advocated as a more specific indicator of encephalopathy, but its benefit over an EEG isn't yet clear.

Treatment

Effective treatment stops progression of encephalopathy by reducing blood ammonia levels. Treatment includes eliminating ammonia-producing substances from the GI tract by administering neomycin to suppress bacterial flora (preventing them from converting amino acids into ammonia), performing sorbitol-induced catharsis to produce osmotic diarrhea and continuous aspiration of blood from the stomach, and reducing dietary protein intake.[3]

Lactulose, which traps ammonia in the bowel and promotes its excretion, is administered to reduce blood ammonia levels. Bacterial enzymes change lactulose to lactic acid, thereby rendering the colon too acidic for bacterial growth. At the same time, the resulting increase in free hydrogen ions pre-

vents diffusion of ammonia through the mucosa; lactulose promotes conversion of systemically absorbable ammonia to ammonium, which is poorly absorbed and can be excreted. It's usually given orally. However, if the patient is in a coma, it may be administered by retention enema.

Treatment may also include potassium supplements to correct alkalosis due to increased ammonia levels, especially if the patient is taking diuretics. Hemodialysis may sometimes be used to clear toxic blood temporarily.[4] Salt-poor albumin may be used to maintain fluid and electrolyte balance, replace depleted albumin levels, and restore plasma. Sedatives, tranquilizers, and other medications metabolized or excreted by the liver should be avoided if possible. Medications containing ammonium (including certain antacids) should also be avoided.

Special considerations

Patient care includes monitoring symptoms and support.

▶ Assess and record the patient's level of consciousness frequently. Continually orient him to place and time. Keep a daily record of his handwriting to monitor the progression of neurologic involvement.

▶ Monitor the patient's intake, output, and fluid and electrolyte balance. Check daily weight, and measure abdominal girth. Watch for, and immediately report, signs of anemia (decreased hemoglobin level), infection, alkalosis (increased serum bicarbonate), and GI bleeding (melena and hematemesis).

▶ If the encephalopathy is acute, ask the dietary department to provide the specified low-protein diet, with carbohydrates supplying most of the calories.

▶ Promote rest, comfort, and a quiet atmosphere. Discourage stressful exercise.[2]

▶ Use restraints, if necessary, but avoid sedatives. Protect the comatose patient's eyes from corneal injury by using artificial tears or eye patches.

▶ Provide emotional support for the patient's family in the terminal stage of encephalopathy.

REFERENCES

1. University of Pennsylvania Health System Encyclopedia (2006 October 13). "Hepatic Encephalopathy." [Online]. Available at *http://pennhealth.com/ency/article/000302.htm.*
2. McGuinness, A. "Role of the Nurse in Managing Patients with Hepatic Cerebral Edema," British Journal of Nursing 16(6):340-43, March-April 2007.
3. Sargent, S. "Pathophysiology and Management of Hepatic Encephalopathy," British Journal of Nursing 16(6):335-39, March-April 2006.
4. Han, M.K., and Hyzy, R. "Advances in Critical Care Management of Hepatic Failure and Insufficiency," Critical Care Medicine 34(9 Suppl):S225-31, September 2006.

HIATAL HERNIA

Hiatal hernia, also called *hiatus hernia,* is a defect in the diaphragm that permits a portion of the stomach to pass through the diaphragmatic opening into the chest. Hiatal hernia is the most common problem of the diaphragm affecting the alimentary canal. Two types of hiatal hernia can occur: sliding hernia and paraesophageal hernia. (See *Types of hiatal hernia.*) In a sliding hernia, the stomach and the gastroesophageal junction slip up into the chest, so the gastroesophageal junction is above the diaphragmatic hiatus. In paraesophageal hernia, a part of the greater curvature of the stomach rolls through the diaphragmatic defect. Treatment can prevent complications such as strangulation of the herniated intrathoracic portion of the stomach.

Causes and incidence

Hiatal hernia typically results from muscle weakening that's common with aging and may be secondary to esophageal carcinoma, kyphoscoliosis, trauma, or certain surgical

procedures. It may also result from certain diaphragmatic malformations that may cause congenital weakness. Obesity and smoking are common risk factors.

In hiatal hernia, the muscular collar around the esophageal and diaphragmatic junction loosens, permitting the lower portion of the esophagus and the stomach to rise into the chest when intra-abdominal pressure increases (possibly causing gastroesophageal reflux). Such increased intra-abdominal pressure may result from ascites, pregnancy, obesity, constrictive clothing, bending, straining, coughing, Valsalva's maneuver, or extreme physical exertion.

Sliding hernias are more common than paraesophageal hernias. The incidence of hiatal hernia increases with age; 10% of cases occur in people under age 40, and 70%, in people over age of 70.[1] Prevalence is higher in females than in males (especially the paraesophageal type).[1] Contributing factors include obesity and trauma. No racial predilection exists.

Signs and symptoms

Typically, a paraesophageal hernia produces no symptoms; it's usually an incidental finding during a barium swallow or when testing for occult blood. Because this type of hernia leaves the closing mechanism of the cardiac sphincter unchanged, it rarely causes acid reflux or reflux esophagitis. Symptoms result from displacement or stretching of the stomach and may include a feeling of fullness in the chest or pain resembling angina pectoris. Even if it produces no symptoms, this type of hernia needs surgical treatment because there's a high risk of strangulation if a large portion of stomach becomes caught above the diaphragm.

A sliding hernia without an incompetent sphincter produces no reflux or symptoms and, consequently, doesn't require treatment. When a sliding hernia causes symptoms, they are typical of gastric reflux, resulting from the incompetent lower esophageal

Types of hiatal hernia

A hiatal hernia is a displacement of the normal anatomy, as shown in the illustrations below.

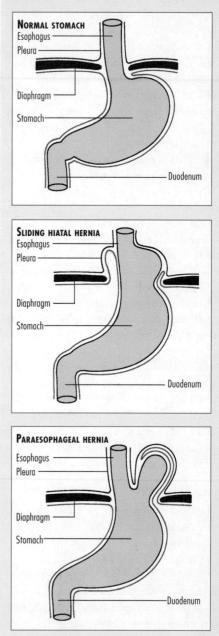

sphincter (LES). These may include the following:

▶ Pyrosis (heartburn) occurs 1 to 4 hours after eating (especially overeating) and is aggravated by reclining, belching, and increased intra-abdominal pressure. It may be accompanied by regurgitation or vomiting.

▶ Retrosternal or substernal chest pain results from reflux of gastric contents, stomach distention, and spasm or altered motor activity. Chest pain usually occurs after meals or at bedtime and is aggravated by reclining, belching, and increased intra-abdominal pressure.

Complications

Gastroesophageal reflux disease is a common complication of hiatal hernia.[2]

Other common symptoms reflect possible complications:

▶ Dysphagia occurs when the hernia produces esophagitis, esophageal ulceration, or stricture, especially with ingestion of very hot or cold foods, alcoholic beverages, or a large amount of food.

▶ Bleeding may be mild or massive, frank or occult; the source may be esophagitis or erosions of the gastric pouch.

▶ Severe pain and shock result from incarceration, in which a large portion of the stomach is caught above the diaphragm (which usually occurs with paraesophageal hernia). Incarceration may lead to perforation of the gastric ulcer, and strangulation and gangrene of the herniated portion of the stomach. It requires immediate surgery.

Diagnosis

Diagnosis of hiatal hernia is based on typical clinical features and on the results of these laboratory studies and procedures:

▶ In barium study, hernia may appear as an outpouching containing barium at the lower end of the esophagus. Small hernias, however, are difficult to recognize. This study also shows diaphragmatic abnormalities.

▶ Endoscopy (esophagogastroduodenoscopy) and biopsy differentiate among hiatal hernia, varices, and other small gastroesophageal lesions. They identify the mucosal junction and the edge of the diaphragm indenting the esophagus and can rule out malignancy that otherwise may be difficult to detect.

▶ Esophageal motility studies assess the presence of esophageal motor abnormalities before surgical repair of the hernia.

▶ Last but not least, pH studies assess for reflux of gastric contents.

Treatment

The primary goals of treatment are to manage and prevent complications and relieve symptoms by minimizing or correcting the incompetent cardia. Medical therapy is used first because symptoms usually respond and because hiatal hernia tends to recur after surgery. Such therapy attempts to modify or reduce reflux by changing the quantity or quality of refluxed gastric contents, by strengthening the LES muscle pharmacologically, or by decreasing the amount of reflux through gravity. These measures include restricting any activity that raises intra-abdominal pressure (coughing, straining, or bending), giving antiemetics, avoiding constrictive clothing, modifying diet, giving stool softeners or laxatives to prevent straining at stool, and discouraging smoking because it stimulates gastric acid production.

Modifying the diet means eating small, frequent, bland meals at least 2 hours before lying down (no bedtime snack), eating slowly, and avoiding spicy foods, fruit juices, alcoholic beverages, and coffee. Antacids also modify the fluid refluxed into the esophagus and are probably the best treatment for intermittent reflux.

To reduce the amount of reflux, the overweight patient should lose weight to decrease intra-abdominal pressure. Elevating the head of the bed 6" (15.2 cm) reduces gastric reflux by gravity.

Drug therapy to treat symptoms of GERD include histamine-2 blockers, such as famotidine and cimetidine, which are used to decrease the amount of acid secreted by the stomach and antacids.[2]

Surgical repair is necessary when symptoms can't be controlled medically, or at the onset of complications, such as stricture, bleeding, pulmonary aspiration, strangulation, or incarceration.

Surgery typically involves creating an artificial closing mechanism at the gastroesophageal junction to strengthen the LES's barrier function. The surgeon may use an abdominal or a thoracic approach, or he may repair the hernia by laparoscopic surgery, which allows for less dependence on a nasogastric (NG) tube and a shorter hospital stay.[3]

Special considerations

To enhance compliance with treatment, teach the patient about this disorder. Explain treatments, diagnostic tests, and significant symptoms.

▶ Prepare the patient for diagnostic tests as needed. After endoscopy, watch for signs of perforation (falling blood pressure, rapid pulse, shock, and sudden pain).

▶ If surgery is scheduled, review preoperative and postoperative considerations with the patient.

▶ After surgery, carefully record intake and output, including NG tube and wound drainage.

▶ While the NG tube is in place, provide meticulous mouth and nose care, but don't manipulate the tube. Give ice chips, if permitted, to moisten oral mucous membranes.

▶ If the surgeon used a thoracic approach, the patient may have chest tubes in place. Carefully observe chest tube drainage and the patient's respiratory status, and perform pulmonary physiotherapy.

▶ Before discharge, tell the patient what foods he can eat. Recommend small, frequent meals. Warn against activities that

cause increased intra-abdominal pressure, and advise a slow return to normal functions (within 6 to 8 weeks).

REFERENCES

1. Qureshi, W.A. eMedicine from *WebMD* (2006 February 28). "Hiatal Hernia." [Online]. Available at *www.emedicine.com/med/topic1012.htm*.
2. MayoClinic.com (2007 November 16). "Hiatal Hernia." [Online]. Available at *www.mayo clinic.com/health/hiatal-hernia/Ks00099/DSECTION=1*.
3. Wijnhoven, B.P., et al. "Laparoscopic Nissen Fundoplication with Anterior Versus Posterior Hiatal Repair: Long-Term Results of a Randomized Trial," *American Journal of Surgery* 195(1):61-65, January 2008.

IRRITABLE BOWEL SYNDROME

Irritable bowel syndrome (IBS), also called *spastic colon* and *spastic colitis,* is a common condition marked by chronic or periodic diarrhea alternating with constipation. It is accompanied by straining and abdominal cramps. The prognosis is good. Supportive treatment or avoidance of a known irritant usually relieves symptoms.

Causes and incidence

The specific cause of IBS in unknown.[1] It may be associated with psychological stress; however, it may result from a sensitivity to certain foods, abnormal motility in the colon (too fast or too slow or spastic), a bacterial infection, or mild celiac disease.[1] Some patients may experience a disturbance in the movement of the intestine or a lower tolerance for stretching and movement of the intestine.

IBS affects 20% of U.S. residents or 1 in 5. The condition occurs more commonly in females, and it occurs before the age of 35 in 50% of the cases.[1]

Signs and symptoms

IBS characteristically produces lower abdominal pain (usually relieved by defecation or passage of gas) and diarrhea that typically occurs during the day. These symptoms alternate with constipation or normal bowel function. Stools are commonly small and contain visible mucus. Dyspepsia and abdominal distention may occur. Some patients experience the feeling of needing to have a bowel movement after they've just had one.[2]

Complications

▶ Higher than normal incidence of diverticulitis and colon cancer

▶ Rarely, chronic inflammatory bowel disease

Diagnosis

Diagnosis of IBS requires a careful history to determine contributing psychological factors such as a recent stressful life change(s).[6] Diagnosis must also rule out other disorders, such as amebiasis, diverticulitis, colon cancer, and lactose intolerance. Appropriate diagnostic procedures include sigmoidoscopy, colonoscopy, barium enema, rectal biopsy, and stool examination for blood, parasites, and bacteria.[7]

Treatment

Therapy aims to relieve symptoms and includes counseling to help the patient understand the relationship between stress and his illness. Strict dietary restrictions aren't beneficial, but food irritants should be investigated, and the patient should be instructed to avoid them. Rest and heat applied to the abdomen are helpful, as is judicious use of sedatives and antispasmodics. However, with chronic use, the patient may become dependent on these drugs. An increase in *soluble* fiber helps diarrhea and constipation, and *insoluble* fiber helps relieve constipation.[2] Tegaserod helps patients with constipation-predominant IBS to increase the number of bowel movements they have each day and decrease the number of days without a bowel movement.[3] Researchers have found that some herbal therapies may improve symptoms of IBS, but additional study is needed.[4,5]

Special considerations

Because the patient with IBS isn't hospitalized, focus your care on patient teaching.

▶ Tell the patient to avoid irritating foods, and encourage him to develop regular bowel habits.

▶ Help the patient deal with stress, and warn against dependence on sedatives or antispasmodics.

▶ Encourage regular checkups because IBS is associated with a higher-than-normal incidence of diverticulitis and colon cancer. For patients older than age 40, emphasize the need for an annual sigmoidoscopy and rectal examination.[8]

REFERENCES

1. National Digestive Diseases Information Clearing House (2007 September). "Irritable Bowel Syndrome," NIH Publication No. 07-693 September 2007 [Online]. Available at *www.digestive.niddk.nih.gov/ddiseases/pubs/ibs/*.
2. Familydoctor.org (2006 December). "Irritable Bowel Syndrome: Tips on Controlling Your Symptoms." [Online]. Available at *www.familydoctor.org/online/famdocen/home/common/digestive/disorders/112.html*.
3. Evans, B.W. "Tegaserod for the Treatment of Irritable Bowel Syndrome," *Cochrane Database of Systematic Reviews* (1):CD003960, 2004. Available at *www.cochrane.org/reviews/en/ab003960.html*.
4. Lui, J.P., et al. "Herbal Medicines for Treatment of Irritable Bowel Syndrome," *Cochrane Database of Systematic Reviews* (1):CD004116, 2006. Available at *www.cochrane.org/reviews/en/ab004116.html*.
5. Lichtenstein, G.R., et al. "American Gastroenterological Association Institute Medical Position Statement on Corticosteroids, Immunomodulators, and Infliximab in Inflammatory Bowel Disease,"

Gastroenterology 130(3): 935-939, March 2006. Available at *www.guideline.gov.*

6. Baumgart, D.C., and Sandborn, W.J. "Inflammatory Bowel Disease: Clinical Aspects and Established and Evolving Therapies," *Lancet* 369(9573):1641-57, May 2007.

7. Travis, S.P., et al. "European Evidence Based Consensus on the Diagnosis and Management of Crohn's Disease: Current Management," *Gut* 55(Suppl 1):i16-35, March 2006.

8. Stange, E.F., et al. "European Evidence Based Consensus on the Diagnosis and Management of Crohn's Disease: Definitions and Diagnosis," *Gut* 55(Suppl 1):i1-15, March 2006.

LIVER ABSCESS

A liver abscess occurs when bacteria or protozoa destroy hepatic tissue, producing a cavity that fills with infectious organisms, liquefied liver cells, and leukocytes. Necrotic tissue then walls off the cavity from the rest of the liver.

Liver abscess is relatively uncommon. It carries a mortality rate of 30%.

Causes and incidence

In pyogenic liver abscesses, the common infecting organisms are *Escherichia coli, Klebsiella, Staphylococcus, Streptococcus, Bacteroides,* and enterococcus. The infecting organisms may invade the liver directly after a liver wound, or they may spread from the lungs, skin, or other organs by the hepatic artery, portal vein, or biliary tract. Pyogenic abscesses are generally multiple and commonly follow cholecystitis, peritonitis, pneumonia, and bacterial endocarditis.[4]

An amebic abscess results from infection with the protozoa *Entamoeba histolytica,* the organism that causes amebic dysentery. Amebic liver abscesses usually occur singly, in the right lobe.[2]

In the United States, pyogenic abscess accounts for 80% of liver abscesses, amebic abscess accounts for 10%, and fungal abscess accounts for less than 10%.[1] There are 8 to 16 cases of liver abscess for every 100,000 people hospitalized, and there's a 5% to 30% mortality rate.[1] Most cases occur in people in their 60s and 70s.

Signs and symptoms

The clinical manifestations of a liver abscess depend on the degree of involvement. Some patients are acutely ill; in others, the abscess is recognized only at autopsy, after death from another illness. The onset of symptoms of a pyogenic abscess is usually sudden; in an amebic abscess, the onset is more insidious. Common signs and symptoms include right abdominal and shoulder pain, weight loss, fever, chills, diaphoresis, nausea, vomiting, and anemia. Signs of right pleural effusion, such as dyspnea and pleural pain, develop if the abscess extends through the diaphragm. Liver damage may cause jaundice.

Complications

▶ Death without treatment
▶ Abscess ruptures into peritoneum, pleura, or pericardium

Diagnosis

A liver scan showing filling defects (at the area of the abscess) more than 2 cm in diameter, together with characteristic clinical features, confirms the diagnosis. A computed tomography scan also confirms the diagnosis.

A liver ultrasound may indicate defects caused by the abscess, but it's less definitive than a liver scan. Relevant laboratory values include elevated serum aspartate aminotransferase, alanine aminotransferase, alkaline phosphatase, and bilirubin levels; increased white blood cell count; and decreased serum albumin levels. In pyogenic abscess, a blood culture can identify the bacterial agent; in amebic abscess, a stool culture and serologic and hemagglutination tests can assist in diagnosis.

Treatment

If the organism causing the liver abscess is unknown, long-term antibiotic therapy begins immediately. When culture results are obtained, antibiotics that treat the specific organism are prescribed. Image-guided percutaneous drainage and aspiration are the standard of care and are combined with antibiotic therapy.[3] Surgery is usually avoided, but it may be done for a single pyogenic abscess or for an amebic abscess that fails to respond to antibiotics.

Special considerations

▶ Provide supportive care, monitor the patient's vital signs (especially temperature), and maintain fluid and nutritional intake.

▶ Administer anti-infectives and antibiotics as ordered, and watch for possible adverse effects. Stress the importance of compliance with therapy.

▶ Explain diagnostic and surgical procedures.

▶ Watch carefully for complications of abdominal surgery, such as hemorrhage or sepsis.

REFERENCES

1 Peralta, R., et al. eMedicine from *Web*MD (2006 November 6). "Liver Abscess." [Online]. Available at *www.emedicine.com/med/topic1316.htm.*
2. Krige, J.E., and Beckingham, I.J. "ABC of Diseases of Liver, Pancreas, and Biliary System," *British Medical Journal* 322(7285):537-540, March 2001.
3. Zerem, E., and Hadzic, A. "Sonographically Guided Percutaneous Catheter Drainage versus Needle Aspiration in the Management of Pyogenic Liver Abscess," *American Journal of Roentgenology* 189(3):W138-42, September 2007.
4. Hui, J.Y., et al. "Pyogenic Liver Abscesses Caused by Klebsiella Pneumoniae: U.S. Appearance and Aspiration Findings," *Radiology* 242(3):769-76, March 2007.

MALLORY-WEISS SYNDROME

Mallory-Weiss syndrome is mild to massive, usually painless bleeding due to a tear in the mucosa or submucosa of the cardia or lower esophagus. Such a tear, usually singular and longitudinal, results from prolonged or forceful vomiting. Sixty percent of these tears involve the cardia; 15%, the terminal esophagus; and 25%, the region across the esophagogastric junction.

Causes and incidence

Forceful or prolonged vomiting can cause esophageal tearing when the upper esophageal sphincter fails to relax during vomiting; this lack of sphincter coordination seems more common after excessive alcohol intake. Other factors that can increase intra-abdominal pressure and predispose a person to this type of tear include coughing, straining during bowel movements, traumatic injury, seizures, childbirth, hiatal hernia, esophagitis, gastritis, and atrophic gastric mucosa.

Mallory-Weiss syndrome accounts for 5% to 15% of all cases of upper GI bleeding. It's two to four times more common in males than in females. There's no racial predilection. Patients usually present with symptoms during their 50s and 60s, but it can affect people of all ages.[1]

Signs and symptoms

Mallory-Weiss syndrome typically begins with vomiting of blood or passing large amounts of blood rectally a few hours to several days after forceful vomiting. The bleeding, which may be accompanied by epigastric or back pain, may range from mild to massive, but is usually more profuse than in esophageal rupture. In Mallory-Weiss syndrome, the blood vessels are only partially severed, preventing retraction and closure of the lumen.

Endoscopic band ligation in Mallory-Weiss syndrome

Question: *Is endoscopic band ligation effective for patients with active bleeding caused by Mallory-Weiss syndrome?*

Research: Mallory-Weiss syndrome is characterized by lacerations in the distal esophagus and proximal stomach, which commonly lead to bleeding from submucosal arteries. To determine the effectiveness and safety of endoscopic band ligation therapy for this condition, researchers conducted a 7-year study of 37 patients with Mallory-Weiss syndrome who had active bleeding, exposed vessels, or both. The patients received treatment using endoscopic band ligation and were followed for a period between 1 and 24 months after the procedure.

Conclusion: The researchers determined that there was no recurrent bleeding, perforation, or other complications in 36 of the 37 participants in the study. One patient with the additional complications of severe liver failure and disseminated intravascular coagulation experienced rebleeding 12 hours after the procedure and died. The study results suggest that endoscopic band ligation is effective and safe for treating upper gastrointestinal bleeding related to Mallory-Weiss syndrome.

Application: When providing care for a patient with Mallory-Weiss syndrome, the nurse should closely monitor the patient for signs of bleeding from esophageal and stomach lacerations. Improvement in the patient's condition should be expected if he receives endoscopic band ligation. Keep in mind that the patient with multiple complications caused by Mallory-Weiss syndrome or other disorders may not benefit from endoscopic band ligation.

Source: Higuchi, N., et al. "Endoscopic Band Ligation Therapy for Upper Gastrointestinal Bleeding Related to Mallory-Weiss Syndrome," *Surgical Endoscopy* 20(9):1431-34, September 2006.

Complications

▶ Hypovolemia
▶ Massive bleeding—most likely when the tear is on the gastric side, near the cardia—may quickly lead to fatal shock.[2]

Diagnosis

Fiber-optic esophagogastroduodenoscopy confirms Mallory-Weiss syndrome by identifying esophageal tears.[1] Recent tears appear as erythematous longitudinal cracks in the mucosa; older tears appear as raised white streaks surrounded by erythema.

Treatment

Treatment varies with the severity of bleeding. GI bleeding usually stops spontaneously. After it stops, provide supportive measures and careful observation. There's no defini-tive treatment. However, if bleeding continues, treatment may include:

▶ proton pump inhibitors or histamine-2 receptor antagonists to help decrease acidity[3]
▶ blood transfusions if blood loss is great
▶ endoscopy with electrocoagulation or heater probe for hemostasis
▶ transcatheter embolization or thrombus formation with an autologous blood clot or other hemostatic material (such as a shredded adsorbable gelatin sponge)
▶ surgery to suture each esophageal laceration. (See *Endoscopic band ligation in Mallory-Weiss syndrome.*)

Special considerations

Observation is necessary to determine whether bleeding is transitory or ongoing.

▶ Evaluate the patient's respiratory status, monitor arterial blood gas values, and administer oxygen as necessary.

▶ Assess the amount of blood lost, and record the color, amount, consistency, and frequency of hematemesis and melena.

▶ Draw blood for coagulation studies (prothrombin time, partial thromboplastin time, and platelet count), and type and crossmatch.

▶ Try to keep three units of blood available at all times. Insert a 14G to 18G I.V. catheter, and start an infusion of I.V. solution as ordered. (If the I.V. infusion is for blood transfusion, use normal saline solution; if the infusion is for fluid replacement, use lactated Ringer's solution or another appropriate solution, depending on the results of laboratory tests.)

▶ Monitor the patient's vital signs, central venous pressure, urine output, neurologic status, and overall clinical status.

▶ Explain diagnostic tests to the patient.

▶ Keep the patient warm, and maintain a safe environment.

▶ Obtain a detailed history of recent medications taken, dietary habits, and alcohol ingestion.

▶ Administer antiemetics, as ordered, to prevent postoperative retching and vomiting.

▶ Advise the patient to avoid aspirin, alcohol, and other irritating substances.

REFERENCES

1. Liacouras, C. eMedicine from *Web*MD (2005 May 4). "Mallory-Weiss Syndrome." [Online]. Available at *www.emedicine.com/ped/ topic1359.htm.*

2. Imperiale, T.F., et al. "Predicting Poor Outcome from Acute Upper Gastrointestinal Hemorrhage," *Archives of Internal Medicine* 167(12):1291-96, June 2007.

3. Bajaj, B.S., et al. "Prospective, Randomized Trial Comparing Effect of Oral versus Intravenous Pantoprazole on Rebleeding after Nonvariceal Upper Gastrointestinal Bleeding: A Pilot Study," *Digestive Diseases and Sciences* 52(9):2190-94, September 2007.

NONVIRAL HEPATITIS

Nonviral inflammation of the liver (toxic or drug-induced hepatitis) is a form of hepatitis that usually results from exposure to certain chemicals or drugs. Most patients recover from this illness, although a few develop fulminating hepatitis or cirrhosis.

Causes and incidence

Various hepatotoxins—carbon tetrachloride, acetaminophen, trichloroethylene, poisonous mushrooms, and vinyl chloride—can cause the toxic form of this disease. Following exposure to these agents, liver damage usually occurs within 24 to 48 hours, depending on the size of the dose or degree of exposure. Alcohol, anoxia, and preexisting liver disease exacerbate the toxic effects of some of these agents.

Drug-induced (idiosyncratic) hepatitis may stem from a hypersensitivity reaction unique to the affected individual, unlike toxic hepatitis, which appears to affect all people indiscriminately. Among the drugs that may cause this type of hepatitis are niacin, halothane, sulfonamides, isoniazid, methyldopa, and phenothiazines (cholestasis-induced hepatitis). In hypersensitive people, symptoms of hepatic dysfunction may appear at any time during or after exposure to these drugs but usually emerge after 2 to 5 weeks of therapy. Not all adverse drug reactions are toxic. Hormonal contraceptives, for example, may impair liver function and produce jaundice without causing necrosis, fatty infiltration of liver cells, or hypersensitivity. Some herbs can cause liver damage including cascara, chaparral, comfrey, kava, and ma huang.[1]

Hepatic drug reactions are more common in females and in alcoholics. The elderly, persons with acquired immunodeficiency syndrome, and those who are malnourished also may be more susceptible to reactions.[2]

Signs and symptoms

Clinical features of toxic and drug-induced hepatitis vary with the severity of the liver damage and the causative agent. In most patients, signs and symptoms resemble those of viral hepatitis: anorexia, nausea, vomiting, jaundice, dark urine, hepatomegaly, possible abdominal pain (with acute onset and massive necrosis), and clay-colored stools or pruritus with the cholestatic form of hepatitis. Carbon tetrachloride poisoning also produces headache, dizziness, drowsiness, and vasomotor collapse; halothane-related hepatitis produces fever, moderate leukocytosis, and eosinophilia; chlorpromazine toxicity produces abrupt fever, rash, arthralgia, lymphadenopathy, and epigastric or right upper quadrant pain.

Complications

▶ Cirrhosis
▶ Hepatitis
▶ Liver failure

Diagnosis

Diagnostic findings include elevations in serum aspartate aminotransferase and alanine aminotransferase, total and direct bilirubin (with cholestasis), alkaline phosphatase, white blood cell (WBC) count, and eosinophil count (possible in drug-induced type). Liver biopsy may help identify the underlying pathology, especially infiltration with WBCs and eosinophils. Liver function tests have limited value in distinguishing between nonviral and viral hepatitis.

Treatment

Effective treatment must remove the causative agent by lavage, catharsis, or hyperventilation, depending on the route of exposure. Acetylcysteine may serve as an antidote for toxic hepatitis caused by acetaminophen poisoning but doesn't prevent drug-induced hepatitis caused by other substances. Corticosteroids may be ordered for patients with the drug-induced type.

Special considerations

▶ Monitor laboratory studies and note trends.
▶ Monitor the patient's vital signs, and provide support to maintain vital functioning, depending on the severity of his symptoms.
▶ Preventive measures should include instructing the patient about the proper use of drugs and the proper handling of cleaning agents and solvents.

REFERENCES

1. Mayoclinic.com (2006 October 5). "Toxic Hepatitis." [Online]. Available at *www.mayoclinic.com/health/toxic-hepatitis/DS00811/DSECTION=3*.
2. Mehta, N. eMedicine from *Web*MD. "Drug-Induced Hepatotoxicity" (2007 February 13). Available at *www.emedicine.com/med/topic3718.htm*.

PANCREATITIS

Pancreatitis, inflammation of the pancreas, occurs in acute and chronic forms and may be due to edema, necrosis, or hemorrhage. In males, this disease is commonly associated with alcoholism, trauma, or peptic ulcer; in females, it's linked to biliary tract disease. The prognosis is good when pancreatitis follows biliary tract disease, but poor when it follows alcoholism. For acute pancreatitis, the mortality rate in the United States is 9%, but the rate rises as high as 50% when pancreatitis is associated with necrosis and hemorrhage.[1] (See *Chronic pancreatitis,* page 188.)

Causes and incidence

The most common causes of pancreatitis are biliary tract disease and alcoholism, but it can also result from pancreatic cancer, trauma, or use of certain drugs, such as glucocorticoids, sulfonamides, chlorothiazide, and azathioprine. This disease also may develop as a complication of peptic ulcer, mumps, or

Chronic pancreatitis

Chronic pancreatitis is associated with alcoholism in more than 50% of patients, but can also follow hyperparathyroidism (causing hypercalcemia), hyperlipidemia or, infrequently, gallstones, trauma, or peptic ulcer. Inflammation and fibrosis cause progressive pancreatic insufficiency and eventually destroy the pancreas.

Symptoms of chronic pancreatitis include constant dull pain with occasional exacerbations, malabsorption, severe weight loss, and hyperglycemia (leading to diabetic symptoms). Diagnosis is based on the patient history, X-rays showing pancreatic calcification, an elevated erythrocyte sedimentation rate, and examination of stool for steatorrhea.

In many cases, the severe pain of chronic pancreatitis requires large doses of analgesics or opioids, making addiction a serious problem. Treatment also includes a low-fat diet and oral administration of pancreatic enzymes, such as pancreatin or pancrelipase, to control steatorrhea; insulin or oral hypoglycemics to curb hyperglycemia; and, occasionally, surgical repair of biliary or pancreatic ducts or the sphincter of Oddi to reduce pressure and promote the flow of pancreatic juice. The prognosis is good if the patient can avoid alcohol, but poor if he can't.

hypothermia. Rarer causes are stenosis or obstruction of the sphincter of Oddi, hyperlipidemia, metabolic endocrine disorders (hyperparathyroidism and hemochromatosis), vasculitis or vascular disease, viral infections, mycoplasmal pneumonia, and pregnancy.

Diabetes, pancreatic insufficiency, and calcification occur in young people, probably from malnutrition and alcoholism, and lead to pancreatic atrophy. Regardless of the cause, pancreatitis involves autodigestion: The enzymes normally excreted by the pancreas digest pancreatic tissue. (See *Anatomy of the pancreas.*) Chronic pancreatitis is a re-

sult of alcohol abuse in 70% of the cases.[2] Alcoholic chronic pancreatitis is more common in males between ages 30 and 40.[2]

In the United States, acute pancreatitis affects about 40 of every 100,000 people. It's uncommon in children. Blacks have a higher incidence; Blacks ages 35 to 64 have a 10 time higher risk than Whites in the same age-group. Males and females are affected equally. Among people with acquired immunodeficiency syndrome, it affects 4 to 22 people out of every 100.

Signs and symptoms

In many patients, the first and only symptom of mild pancreatitis is steady epigastric pain centered close to the umbilicus, radiating between the 10th thoracic and 6th lumbar vertebrae, and unrelieved by vomiting. However, a severe attack causes extreme pain, persistent vomiting, abdominal rigidity, diminished bowel activity (suggesting peritonitis), crackles at lung bases, and left pleural effusion. Progression produces extreme malaise and restlessness, with mottled skin, tachycardia, low-grade fever (100° to 102° F [37.7° to 38.8° C]), and cold, sweaty extremities. The proximity of the inflamed pancreas to the bowel may cause ileus.

Complications

▶ If pancreatitis damages the islets of Langerhans, complications may include diabetes mellitus.

▶ Fulminant pancreatitis causes massive hemorrhage and total destruction of the pancreas, resulting in diabetic acidosis, shock, or coma.

Diagnosis

A thorough patient history (especially for alcoholism) and physical examination are the first steps in diagnosis, but the retroperitoneal position of the pancreas makes physical assessment difficult.

Dramatically elevated serum amylase levels—in many cases, more than 500 units/L—

Anatomy of the pancreas

Pancreatitis is an inflammation of the pancreas, involving irritation and infection of the organ. Obstruction or overdistention of the pancreatic duct can initiate the inflammation that occurs with pancreatitis. Exposure to toxins and other underlying causes can also initiate it. The overall effect is a release of activated pancreatic destructive enzymes into the pancreas and surrounding tissue.

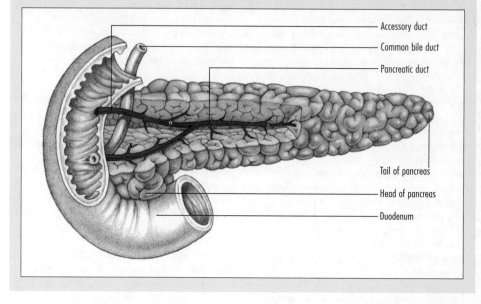

Accessory duct
Common bile duct
Pancreatic duct
Tail of pancreas
Head of pancreas
Duodenum

confirm pancreatitis and rule out perforated peptic ulcer, acute cholecystitis, appendicitis, and bowel infarction or obstruction. Similarly, dramatic elevations of amylase also occur in urine, ascites, or pleural fluid. Characteristically, amylase levels return to normal 48 hours after the onset of pancreatitis, despite continuing symptoms.

Supportive laboratory values include:
▶ increased serum lipase levels, which rise more slowly than serum amylase
▶ low serum calcium levels (hypocalcemia) from fat necrosis and formation of calcium soaps
▶ white blood cell counts ranging from 8,000 to 20,000/μl, with increased polymorphonuclear leukocytes
▶ elevated glucose levels—as high as 500 to 900 mg/dl, indicating hyperglycemia.

Tests used to diagnose pancreatitis may include the following:
▶ Abdominal X-rays or computed tomography (CT) scans show dilation of the small or large bowel or calcification of the pancreas.
▶ Ultrasound or CT scans reveal an increased pancreatic diameter and help distinguish acute cholecystitis from acute pancreatitis.

Treatment

The goal of therapy is to maintain circulation and fluid volume. Treatment measures must also relieve pain and decrease pancreatic secretions.

Emergency treatment of shock (which is the most common cause of death in early-stage pancreatitis) consists of vigorous I.V. replacement of electrolytes and proteins. Metabolic acidosis that develops secondary

Nutrition and pancreatitis

Question: *Are dietary supplements more beneficial than homemade food for patients with chronic pancreatitis?*

Research: Nutritional status is a major concern in patients with chronic pancreatitis, because as many as 50% of these patients are malnourished. Medium chain triglyceride (MCT)-enriched commercial dietary supplements are commonly prescribed for such patients to correct this condition. To determine whether the use of dietary supplements was more beneficial than dietary counseling that covers how to prepare a balanced diet of homemade food, the researchers studied 60 malnourished patients with chronic pancreatitis. The study participants received either dietary counseling about how to prepare a balanced diet at home or commercial MCT-enriched dietary supplements for a period of 3 months. The patients in both groups also received standard treatment measures for chronic pancreatitis and were given pancreatic enzyme supplements. Improvement in body mass index (BMI) was used as the outcome measurement.

Conclusion: At the end of the 3-month-period, the BMI as well as the triceps skinfold thickness,

dietary intake, fecal fat, and pain score of the patients in both groups had improved almost equally. The study demonstrated that dietary counseling for a balanced homemade diet provides the same benefits as commercial dietary supplements in improving malnutrition in patients with chronic pancreatitis.

Application: When counseling patients with chronic pancreatitis, the nurse should provide teaching and written instructions about the preparation of a nutritionally balanced homemade diet to prevent malnutrition. This is especially important with patients who are financially challenged and may not be able to afford the high cost of dietary supplements. The nurse should also provide a referral to a nutrition specialist, if possible.

Source: Singh, S., et al. "Dietary Counseling versus Dietary Supplements for Malnutrition in Chronic Pancreatitis: A Randomized Controlled Trial," *Clinical Gastroenterology and Hepatology* 6(3):353-59, March 2008.

to hypovolemia and impaired cellular perfusion requires vigorous fluid volume replacement.

Drug treatment may include opioids for pain, diazepam for restlessness and agitation, and antibiotics for bacterial infections.[4] Morphine and codeine are usually avoided as pain medications because of their effect on the sphincter of Oddi. If the patient has hypocalcemia, he'll need an infusion of 10% calcium gluconate; if he has elevated serum glucose levels, he may require insulin therapy.

After the emergency phase, continuing I.V. therapy should provide adequate electrolytes and protein solutions that don't stimulate the pancreas for 5 to 7 days. If the patient

isn't ready to resume oral feedings by then, total parenteral nutrition (TPN) may be necessary. Nonstimulating elemental gavage feedings may be safer because of the decreased risk of infection and overinfusion. In extreme cases, laparotomy to debride the pancreatic bed, partial pancreatectomy, or a combination of both and feeding jejunostomy may be necessary.[3]

Special considerations

Acute pancreatitis is a life-threatening emergency, requiring meticulous supportive care and continuous monitoring of vital systems.
▶ Monitor the patient's vital signs and pulmonary artery pressure or central venous pressure closely. Give plasma or albumin, if

ordered, to maintain blood pressure. Record fluid intake and output; check urine output hourly, and monitor electrolyte levels. Assess for crackles, rhonchi, or decreased breath sounds.

▶ For bowel decompression, maintain constant nasogastric suctioning, and give nothing by mouth. Provide good mouth and nose care.

▶ Watch for signs and symptoms of calcium deficiency—tetany, cramps, carpopedal spasm, and seizures. If you suspect hypocalcemia, keep airway and suction apparatus handy, and pad side rails. (See *Nutrition and pancreatitis.*)

▶ Administer analgesics as needed to relieve the patient's pain and anxiety. Remember that anticholinergics reduce salivary and sweat gland secretions. Warn the patient that he may experience dry mouth and facial flushing. *Caution:* Narrow-angle glaucoma contraindicates the use of atropine or its derivatives.

▶ Monitor glucose levels.

▶ Watch for complications due to TPN, such as sepsis, hypokalemia, overhydration, and metabolic acidosis. Watch for fever, cardiac irregularities, changes in arterial blood gas measurements, and deep respirations. Use strict aseptic technique when caring for the catheter insertion site.

REFERENCES

1. Holcomb, S.S. "Stopping the Destruction of Acute Pancreatitis," *Nursing* 37(6):42-47, June 2007.
2. National Digestive Diseases Information Clearinghouse (2004 February). "Pancreatitis," NIH Publication No. 04-1596 [Online]. Available at *www.digestive.niddk.nih.gov/d 0diseases/pubs/pancreatitis/.*
3. Besselink, M.G., et al. "Timing of Surgical Intervention in Necrotizing Pancreatitis," *Archives of Surgery* 142(12):1194-201, December 2007.
4. Besselink, M.G., et al. "Evidence-Based Treatment of Acute Pancreatitis: Antibiotic Prophylaxis in Necrotizing Pancreatitis,"

Annals of Surgery 244(4):637-38, October 2006.

PEPTIC ULCERS

Peptic ulcers—circumscribed lesions in the mucosal membrane—can develop in the lower esophagus, stomach, pylorus, duodenum, or jejunum. About 80% of all peptic ulcers are duodenal ulcers, which affect the proximal part of the small intestine.

Gastric ulcers, which affect the stomach mucosa, are most common in middle-age and elderly males, especially in chronic users of nonsteroidal anti-inflammatory drugs (NSAIDs), alcohol, or tobacco. Duodenal ulcers usually follow a chronic course, with remissions and exacerbations; 5% to 10% of patients develop complications that necessitate surgery.

Causes and incidence

Researchers recognize three major causes of peptic ulcer disease: infection with *Helicobacter pylori*, use of NSAIDs, and pathologic hypersecretory disorders such as Zollinger-Ellison syndrome. (See *How peptic ulcers develop,* page 192.)

H. pylori is the leading cause of peptic ulcers.[1] How *H. pylori* produces an ulcer isn't clear. Gastric acid, which was considered a primary cause, now appears mainly to contribute to the consequences of infection. Ongoing studies should soon unveil the full mechanism of ulcer formation.

Salicylates and other NSAIDs encourage ulcer formation by inhibiting the secretion of prostaglandins (the substances that suppress ulceration). Certain illnesses, such as pancreatitis, hepatic disease, Crohn's disease, preexisting gastritis, and Zollinger-Ellison syndrome, are also known causes.

Besides peptic ulcer's main causes, several predisposing factors are acknowledged. They include blood type (gastric ulcers tend to

How peptic ulcers develop

Peptic ulcers can result from factors that increase gastric acid production or from factors that impair mucosal barrier protection.

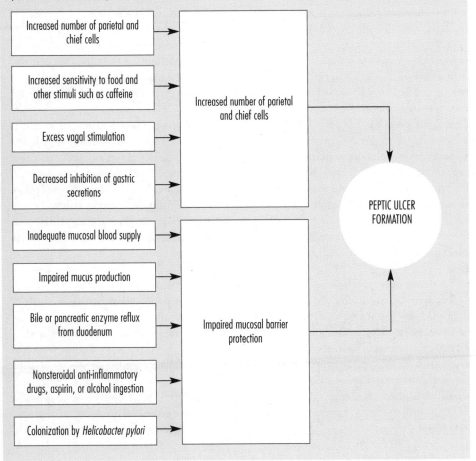

strike people with type A blood; duodenal ulcers tend to afflict people with type O blood) and other genetic factors. Exposure to irritants, such as alcohol, coffee, and tobacco, may contribute by accelerating gastric acid emptying and promoting mucosal breakdown. Ulceration occurs when the acid secretion exceeds the buffering factors. Physical trauma, emotional stress, and normal aging are additional predisposing conditions.

About 10% of people living in the United States develop peptic ulcers, with males developing them at twice the rate of females. A higher percentage of *H. pylori* infection occurs in people older than age 60. Duodenal ulcers occur more frequently in people ages 25 to 75, and gastric ulcers occur more frequently in people 55 to 65.[1]

Signs and symptoms

Heartburn and indigestion usually signal the beginning of a gastric ulcer attack. Eating stretches the gastric wall and may cause or, in some cases, relieve pain and feelings of fullness and distention. Other typical effects include weight loss and repeated episodes of massive GI bleeding.

Duodenal ulcers produce heartburn, well-localized midepigastric pain (relieved by food), weight gain (because the patient eats to relieve discomfort), and a peculiar sensation of hot water bubbling in the back of the throat. Attacks usually occur about 2 hours after meals, whenever the stomach is empty, or after consumption of orange juice, coffee, aspirin, or alcohol. Exacerbations tend to recur several times per year and then fade into remission. Vomiting and other digestive disturbances are rare.

Ulcers may penetrate the pancreas and cause severe back pain. Ulcers may, on occasion, produce no symptoms.

Complications

▶ GI hemorrhage leading to hypovolemic shock, perforation, and obstruction
▶ Abdominal or intestinal infarction
▶ Penetration of the ulcer to attached structures occurs in duodenal ulcer

Diagnosis

Esophagogastroduodenoscopy confirms the presence of an ulcer and permits cytologic studies and biopsy to rule out *H. pylori* or cancer.

Diagnosis may be confirmed by the following tests:
▶ Barium swallow or upper GI and small-bowel series may reveal the presence of the ulcer. This is the initial test performed on a patient whose symptoms aren't severe.
▶ Laboratory analysis may detect occult blood in stools.
▶ Serologic testing may disclose clinical signs of infection such as an elevated white blood cell count.

▶ Carbon 13 (^{13}C) urea breath test results reflect activity of *H. pylori*. [4]

Treatment

Experts recommend treating the patient with antibiotics to eradicate *H. pylori*. The patient taking NSAIDs may take a prostaglandin analog (misoprostol) to suppress ulceration, or the patient may take the analog with NSAIDs to prevent ulceration. Histamine-2 (H_2) receptor antagonists or proton pump inhibitors may reduce acid secretion.[3] A coating agent or bismuth may be administered to the patient with a duodenal ulcer to protect the lining.

If GI bleeding occurs, emergency treatment begins with passage of a nasogastric (NG) tube to allow for iced saline lavage, possibly containing norepinephrine. Gastroscopy allows visualization of the bleeding site and coagulation by laser or cautery to control bleeding. This type of therapy allows postponement of surgery until the patient's condition stabilizes. Surgery is indicated for perforation, unresponsiveness to conservative treatment, and suspected malignancy. Surgery for peptic ulcers may include:
▶ vagotomy and pyloroplasty—the severing of one or more branches of the vagus nerve to reduce hydrochloric acid secretion and refashioning the pylorus to create a larger lumen and facilitate gastric emptying
▶ distal subtotal gastrectomy (with or without vagotomy)—excising the antrum of the stomach, thereby removing the hormonal stimulus of the parietal cells, followed by anastomosis of the rest of the stomach to the duodenum or the jejunum
▶ pyloroplasty—surgical enlargement of the pylorus to provide drainage of gastric secretions.

Special considerations

Management of peptic ulcers requires careful administration of medications, thorough pa-

tient teaching, and skillful postoperative care.

▶ Watch for adverse reactions to H_2-receptor antagonists and omeprazole (dizziness, fatigue, rash, and mild diarrhea).

▶ Advise any patient who uses antacids, has a history of cardiac disease, or follows a sodium-restricted diet to take only antacids that contain low amounts of sodium.

▶ Warn the patient to avoid NSAIDs because they irritate the gastric mucosa. For the same reason, advise the patient to stop smoking.[2] Also advise them to avoid stressful situations, excessive intake of coffee, and drinking alcoholic beverages during exacerbations of peptic ulcer disease.

After gastric surgery:

▶ Keep the NG tube patent. If the tube isn't functioning, don't reposition it; you might damage the suture line or anastomosis. Notify the surgeon promptly.

▶ Monitor intake and output, including NG tube drainage. Check for bowel sounds, and allow the patient nothing by mouth until peristalsis resumes and the NG tube is removed or clamped.

▶ Replace fluids and electrolytes. Assess the patient for signs of dehydration, sodium deficiency, and metabolic alkalosis, which may occur secondary to gastric suction.

▶ Monitor the patient for possible complications: hemorrhage, shock, iron, folate, or vitamin B_{12} deficiency anemia from malabsorption (pernicious anemia) due to lack of intrinsic factor causing malabsorption of vitamin B_{12}; and dumping syndrome (a rapid gastric emptying, causing distention of the duodenum or jejunum produced by a bolus of food). Signs and symptoms of dumping syndrome include diaphoresis, weakness, nausea, flatulence, explosive diarrhea, distention, and palpitations within 30 minutes after a meal.

▶ To avoid dumping syndrome, advise the patient to lie down after meals, to drink fluids *between* meals rather than with meals, to avoid eating large amounts of carbohy-

drates, and to eat four to six small, high-protein, low-carbohydrate meals during the day.

REFERENCES

1. Shayne, P. eMedicine from *WebMD* (2006 May 10). "Gastritis and Peptic Ulcer Disease." [Online]. Available at *www.emedicine.com/ EMERG/topic820.htm.*
2. National Digestive Diseases Information Clearinghouse. "Peptic Ulcer," NIH Publication No. 05-5042, October 2004. Available at *www.digestive.niddk.nih.gov/ddiseases/pubs/ pepticulcers_ez/index.htm.*
3. Vaira, D., et al. "Sequential Therapy versus Standard Triple-Drug Therapy for Helicobacter Pylori Eradication: A Randomized Trial," *Annals of Internal Medicine* 146(8):556-63, April 2007.
4. Gatta, L., et al. "Accuracy of Breath Tests Using Low Doses of 13C-Urea to Diagnose Helicobacter Pylori Infection: A Randomized Controlled Trial," *Gut* 55(4):457-62, April 2006.

PERITONITIS

P eritonitis is an acute or chronic inflammation of the peritoneum, the membrane that lines the abdominal cavity and covers the visceral organs. Inflammation may extend throughout the peritoneum or may be localized as an abscess. Peritonitis commonly decreases intestinal motility and causes intestinal distention with gas. Mortality, which was much higher before the introduction of antibiotics, is 10%. Death is usually a result of bowel obstruction.

Causes and incidence

Although the GI tract normally contains bacteria, the peritoneum is sterile. When bacteria invade the peritoneum due to inflammation and perforation of the GI tract, peritonitis results. Bacterial invasion of the peritoneum typically results from appendici-

tis, diverticulitis, peptic ulcer, ulcerative colitis, volvulus, strangulated obstruction, abdominal neoplasm, or a stab wound. Peritonitis may also occur following chemical inflammation, as in the rupture of a fallopian or ovarian tube or the bladder, perforation of a gastric ulcer, or released pancreatic enzymes. It may also be associated with peritoneal dialysis.

In chemical and bacterial inflammation, accumulated fluids containing protein and electrolytes make the transparent peritoneum opaque, red, inflamed, and edematous. Because the peritoneal cavity is so resistant to contamination, infection is commonly localized as an abscess instead of disseminated as a generalized infection.

Overall incidence hasn't been established but about 10% to 30% of patients with liver cirrhosis and ascites develop bacterial peritonitis over time.[1]

Signs and symptoms
The key symptom of peritonitis is sudden, severe, and diffuse abdominal pain that tends to intensify and localize in the area of the underlying disorder. For instance, if appendicitis causes the rupture, pain eventually localizes in the right lower quadrant. Many patients display weakness, pallor, excessive sweating, and cold skin as a result of excessive loss of fluid, electrolytes, and protein into the abdominal cavity. Decreased intestinal motility and paralytic ileus result from the effect of bacterial toxins on the intestinal muscles. Intestinal obstruction causes nausea, vomiting, and abdominal rigidity.

Other clinical characteristics include hypotension, tachycardia, signs and symptoms of dehydration (oliguria, thirst, dry swollen tongue, and pinched skin), an acutely tender abdomen associated with rebound tenderness, temperature of 103° F (39.4° C) or higher, and hypokalemia. Inflammation of the diaphragmatic peritoneum may cause shoulder pain and hiccups. Abdominal distention and resulting upward displacement of the diaphragm may decrease respiratory capacity. Typically, the patient with peritonitis tends to breathe shallowly and move as little as possible to minimize pain. He may lie on his back, with his knees flexed, to relax abdominal muscles.

Complications
▶ Abscess
▶ Septicemia
▶ Respiratory compromise
▶ Bowel obstruction
▶ Shock
▶ Peritonitis

Diagnosis
Severe abdominal pain in a person with direct or rebound tenderness suggests peritonitis. Abdominal X-rays or computed tomography scan showing edematous and gaseous distention of the small and large bowel support the diagnosis. In the case of perforation of a visceral organ, the X-ray shows air lying under the diaphragm in the abdominal cavity. Other appropriate tests include:
▶ Chest X-ray may show elevation of the diaphragm and air in the abdomen.[2]
▶ Blood studies show leukocytosis (more than 20,000/μl).
▶ Paracentesis reveals bacteria, exudate, blood, pus, or urine.
▶ Laparotomy may be necessary to identify the underlying cause.

Treatment
Early treatment of GI inflammatory conditions and preoperative and postoperative antibiotic therapy help prevent peritonitis. After peritonitis develops, emergency treatment must combat infection, restore intestinal motility, and replace fluids and electrolytes.

Antibiotic therapy depends on the infecting organisms. If peritonitis is associated with peritoneal dialysis, antibiotics may be infused through the dialysis catheter; however, if the infection is severe, the catheter must

be removed. To decrease peristalsis and prevent perforation, the patient should receive nothing by mouth; he should receive supportive fluids and electrolytes parenterally.

Other supplementary treatment measures include preoperative and postoperative administration of an analgesic, nasogastric (NG) intubation to decompress the bowel and, possibly, using a rectal tube to facilitate passage of flatus. When peritonitis results from perforation, surgery is necessary as soon as possible. Surgery aims to eliminate the source of infection by evacuating the spilled contents and inserting drains.[2]

Special considerations
Patient care includes monitoring and measures to prevent complications and the spread of infection.
▶ Monitor the patient's vital signs, fluid intake and output, and amount of NG drainage or vomitus.
▶ Place the patient in semi-Fowler's position to help him deep-breathe with less pain and thus prevent pulmonary complications and to help localize purulent exudate in his lower abdomen or pelvis.

After surgery to evacuate the peritoneum:
▶ Maintain parenteral fluid and electrolyte administration, as ordered. Accurately record fluid intake and output, including NG tube and any drain output.
▶ Place the patient in semi-Fowler's position to promote drainage (through drainage tube) by gravity. Move him carefully because the slightest movement will intensify the pain.
▶ Implement other safety measures if fever and pain disorient the patient.
▶ Encourage and assist ambulation as ordered, usually on the first postoperative day.
▶ Watch for signs of dehiscence (the patient may complain that "something gave way") and abscess formation (continued abdominal tenderness and fever).
▶ Frequently assess for peristaltic activity by listening for bowel sounds and checking for gas, bowel movements, and a soft abdomen.

▶ Gradually decrease parenteral fluids and increase oral fluids.

REFERENCES
1. Peralta, R., et al. eMedicine from *WebMD* (2006 August 2). "Peritonitis and Abdominal Sepsis." [Online] Available at *www.emedicine.com/med/topic2737.htm.*
2. McGibbon, A., et al. "An Evidence-Based Manual for Abdominal Paracentesis," *Digestive Diseases and Science* 52(12):3307-15, December 2007.

ULCERATIVE COLITIS

Ulcerative colitis is an inflammatory, usually chronic disease that affects the mucosa of the colon. It invariably begins in the rectum and sigmoid colon and commonly extends upward into the entire colon; it rarely affects the small intestine, except for the terminal ileum. Ulcerative colitis produces edema (leading to mucosal friability) and ulcerations. Severity ranges from a mild, localized disorder to a fulminant disease that may cause a perforated colon, progressing to potentially fatal peritonitis and toxemia.

Causes and incidence
Although the etiology of ulcerative colitis is unknown, it's thought to be related to abnormal immune response in the GI tract, possibly associated with food or bacteria such as *Escherichia coli*. Stress was once thought to be a cause of ulcerative colitis, but studies show that although it isn't a cause, it does increase the severity of the attack.

Although the exact cause of ulcerative colitis is unknown, autoimmune, genetic, and environmental factors are thought to play roles.[1] Researchers believe that an interaction with an environmental agent (maybe a virus) and the body's immune system may trigger the disease or cause damage to the in-

testinal wall which initiates the disease process.[1] Up to 20% of those with the disease may have one or more affected relatives with Crohn's disease or ulcerative colitis, but current research does not show a clear-cut inheritance pattern.[1] People of Jewish ancestry are more likely to get the disease and there is a higher incidence among whites.[2] Ulcerative colitis affects 5 million Americans, with males and females equally affected.[1] It is usually diagnosed around age 30, males are more likely than females to be diagnosed at ages 50 to 60.[1]

Signs and symptoms

The hallmark of ulcerative colitis is recurrent attacks of bloody diarrhea, in many cases containing pus and mucus, interspersed with asymptomatic remissions. The intensity of these attacks varies with the extent of inflammation. It isn't uncommon for a patient with ulcerative colitis to have as many as 15 to 20 liquid, bloody stools daily. Other symptoms include spastic rectum and anus, abdominal pain, irritability, weight loss, weakness, anorexia, nausea, and vomiting.

Ulcerative colitis may lead to complications, such as hemorrhage, stricture, or perforation of the colon. Other complications include joint inflammation, ankylosing spondylitis, eye lesions, mouth ulcers, liver disease, and pyoderma gangrenosum. Scientists think that these complications occur when the immune system triggers inflammation in other parts of the body. These disorders are usually mild and disappear when the colitis is treated.

Patients with ulcerative colitis have an increased risk of developing colorectal cancer; children with ulcerative colitis may experience impaired growth and sexual development.

Complications

▶ Nutritional deficiencies
▶ Perineal sepsis
▶ Anal fistula
▶ Perirectal abscess
▶ Hemorrhage
▶ Toxic megacolon
▶ Arthritis
▶ Coagulation defects
▶ Pyoderma gangrenosum
▶ Uveitis
▶ Pericholangitis
▶ Ankylosing spondylitis
▶ Loss of muscle mass
▶ Peritonitis
▶ Toxemia

Diagnosis

Colonoscopy determines the extent of the disease and evaluates strictured areas and pseudopolyps. Biopsy would then be done during colonoscopy and helps differentiate between Crohn's disease and ulcerative colitis.[3] Sigmoidoscopy can be done when colonoscopy is high risk.[3] Barium enema can assess the extent of the disease and detect complications, such as strictures and carcinoma.

A stool sample should be cultured and analyzed for leukocytes, ova, and parasites. Other supportive laboratory values include decreased serum levels of potassium, magnesium, hemoglobin, and albumin as well as leukocytosis and increased prothrombin time. An elevated erythrocyte sedimentation rate correlates with the severity of the attack.

Treatment

The goals of treatment are to control inflammation, replace nutritional losses and blood volume, and prevent complications. Supportive treatment includes bed rest, I.V. fluid replacement, and a clear-liquid diet. For patients awaiting surgery or showing signs of dehydration and debilitation from excessive diarrhea, total parenteral nutrition (TPN) rests the intestinal tract, decreases stool volume, and restores positive nitrogen balance. Blood transfusions or iron supplements may be needed to correct anemia.

Corticosteroids are used for moderate to severe ulcerative colitis.[4] Since long-term use of corticosteroids is not recommended, aminosalicylates (5-ASA), immunomodulators (azathioprine and 6-MP), and infliximab are used, which help decrease the dose of corticosteroids.[4]

Antispasmodics and antidiarrheals are used only in patients whose ulcerative colitis is under control but who have frequent, loose stools.

HEALTH & SAFETY *Antispasmodics and antidiarrheals may precipitate massive dilation of the colon (toxic megacolon) and are generally contraindicated.*

Surgery is the last resort if the patient has toxic megacolon, fails to respond to drugs and supportive measures, or finds symptoms unbearable. A common surgical technique is proctocolectomy with ileostomy. Another procedure, the ileoanal pull-through, is being performed in more cases. This procedure entails performing a total proctocolectomy and mucosal stripping, creating a pouch from the terminal ileum, and anastomosing the pouch to the anal canal. A temporary ileostomy is created to divert stool and allow the rectal anastomosis to heal. The ileostomy is closed in 2 to 3 months, and the patient can then evacuate stool rectally. This procedure removes all the potentially malignant epithelia of the rectum and colon. Total colectomy and ileorectal anastomosis isn't as common because of its mortality rate (2% to 5%). This procedure removes the entire colon and anastomoses the terminal ileum to the rectum; it requires observation of the remaining rectal stump for any signs of cancer or colitis.

Pouch ileostomy (also known as Kock pouch or continent ileostomy), in which the surgeon creates a pouch from a small loop of the terminal ileum and a nipple valve from the distal ileum, may be an option. The resulting stoma opens just above the pubic hairline and the pouch is emptied periodically through a catheter inserted in the stoma.

In ulcerative colitis, a colectomy may be performed after 10 years of active disease because of the increased incidence of colon cancer in these cases. Performing a partial colectomy to prevent colon cancer is controversial.

Studies done in the United Kingdom and the United States have found that transdermal nicotine may help in the treatment of ulcerative colitis.[5]

Special considerations

Patient care includes close monitoring for changes in status.

▶ Accurately record intake and output, particularly the frequency and volume of stools. Watch for signs of dehydration and electrolyte imbalances, especially signs and symptoms of hypokalemia (muscle weakness and paresthesia) and hypernatremia (tachycardia, flushed skin, fever, and dry tongue). Monitor hemoglobin level and hematocrit, and give blood transfusions as ordered. Provide good mouth care for the patient who's allowed nothing by mouth.

▶ After each of the patient's bowel movements, thoroughly clean the skin around the rectum. Provide an air mattress or sheepskin to help prevent skin breakdown.

▶ Administer medications as ordered. Watch for adverse effects of prolonged corticosteroid therapy (moon face, hirsutism, edema, and gastric irritation). Be aware that corticosteroid therapy may mask infection.

▶ If the patient needs TPN, change dressings as ordered, assess for inflammation at the insertion site, and check capillary blood glucose levels every 4 to 6 hours.

▶ Take precautionary measures if the patient is prone to bleeding. Watch closely for signs of complications, such as a perforated colon and peritonitis (fever, severe abdominal pain, abdominal rigidity and tenderness, and cool, clammy skin) and toxic megacolon (abdominal distention and decreased bowel sounds).

For the patient requiring surgery:

▶ Carefully prepare the patient for surgery, and inform him about ileostomy.

▶ Do a bowel preparation as ordered.

▶ After surgery, provide meticulous supportive care and continue teaching correct stoma care.

▶ Keep the nasogastric tube patent. After removal of the tube, provide a clear-liquid diet and gradually advance to a low-residue diet, as tolerated.

▶ After a proctocolectomy and ileostomy, teach good stoma care. Wash the skin around the stoma with soapy water, and dry it thoroughly. Apply karaya gum around the stoma's base to avoid irritation, and make a watertight seal. Attach the pouch over the karaya ring. Cut an opening in the ring to fit over the stoma, and secure the pouch to the skin. Empty the pouch when it's one-third full.

▶ After a pouch ileostomy, uncork the catheter every hour to allow contents to drain. After 10 to 14 days, gradually increase the length of time the catheter is left corked until it can be opened every 3 hours. Then remove the catheter, and reinsert it every 3 to 4 hours for drainage. Teach the patient how to insert the catheter and how to take care of the stoma.

▶ Encourage the patient to have regular physical examinations.

REFERENCES

1. Crohn's & Colitis Foundation of America. "About Crohn's Disease." [Online]. Available at *www.ccfa.org/info/about/crohns.*

2. National Digestive Diseases Information Clearinghouse (2006 February). "Crohn's Disease," NIH Publication No. 06-3410 [Online]. Available at *http://digestive.niddk.nih. gov/ddiseases/pubs/crohns/index.htm.*

3. Leighton, S.A., et al. "Standards of Practice Committee, American Society for Gastrointestinal Endoscopy. ASGE Guideline: Endoscopy in the Diagnosis and Treatment of Inflammatory Bowel Disease." *Gastrointestinal Endoscopy* 63(4):558-65, April 2006. Available at *www.guideline.gov.*

4. Lichtenstein, G.R., et al. "American Gastroenterological Association Institute Medical Position Statement on Corticosteroids, Immunomodulators, and Infliximab in Inflammatory Bowel Disease," *Gastroenterology* 130(3): 935-39, March 2006. Available at *www.guideline.gov.*

5. Bandolier. "Transdermal Nicotine for Ulcerative Colitis." [Online]. Available at *www.jr2.ox.ac. uk/bandolier/band39/b39-5.html.*

VIRAL HEPATITIS

Viral hepatitis is a fairly common systemic disease, marked by hepatic cell destruction, necrosis, and autolysis, leading to anorexia, jaundice, and hepatomegaly. In most patients, hepatic cells eventually regenerate with little or no residual damage. However, old age and serious underlying disorders make complications more likely. The prognosis is poor if edema and hepatic encephalopathy develop.

Hepatitis occurs in these forms:

▶ Type A (infectious or short-incubation hepatitis) is rising among homosexuals and in people with immunosuppression related to human immunodeficiency virus (HIV) infection.

▶ Type B (serum or long-incubation hepatitis) also is increasing among HIV-positive individuals. Routine screening of donor blood for the hepatitis B surface antigen (HBsAg) has decreased the incidence of posttransfusion cases, but transmission by needles shared by drug abusers remains a major problem.

▶ Type C accounts for about 20% of all viral hepatitis cases and for most posttransfusion cases.

▶ Type D (delta hepatitis) is responsible for about 50% of all cases of fulminant hepatitis, which has a high mortality. Developing in 1% of patients, fulminant hepatitis causes unremitting liver failure with encephalopathy. It progresses to coma and commonly leads to death within 2 weeks. In

the United States, type D is confined to people who are frequently exposed to blood and blood products, such as I.V. drug users and patients with hemophilia.

▶ Type E (formerly grouped with type C under the name non-A, non-B hepatitis) occurs primarily among patients who have recently returned from an endemic area (such as India, Africa, Asia, or Central America); it's more common in young adults and more severe in pregnant women.

▶ Hepatitis G is a recently discovered form of hepatitis. Transmission is by the bloodborne route, and it's more common in those who receive blood transfusions.

Causes and incidence

The major forms of viral hepatitis result from infection with the causative viruses: A, B, C, D, E, or G.

Type A hepatitis is highly contagious and is usually transmitted by the fecal-oral route.[1] However, it may also be transmitted parenterally. Hepatitis A usually results from ingestion of contaminated food, milk, or water. Many outbreaks of this type are traced to ingestion of seafood from polluted water. In 2006, there were more than 3,500 acute cases of hepatitis A infection reported in the United States—the lowest rate ever recorded.[1]

Type B hepatitis, once thought to be transmitted only by the direct exchange of contaminated blood, is now known to be transmitted also by contact with human secretions and feces. As a result, nurses, physicians, laboratory technicians, and dentists are frequently exposed to type B hepatitis, in many cases as a result of wearing defective gloves. Transmission also occurs during intimate sexual contact as well as through perinatal transmission. In 2003, an estimated 73,000 new cases of hepatitis B virus (HBV) and 5,000 deaths from HBV occurred.[2]

Although specific type C hepatitis viruses have been isolated, patients can have false negative and false positive tests. Patients with early infection may not have developed antibodies yet, which account for the false positive test. This type of hepatitis is transmitted through direct contact with human blood. Research suggests that hepatitis C can survive on surfaces at room temperature for at least 16 hours but no longer than 4 days.[3] Hepatitis C accounted for 26,000 new infections in 2004, a decline since the 1980s.[4] Most exposures (60%) occur through the use of illicit I.V. drugs. However, sexual transmission is responsible for 20% of cases. More than 4.1 million Americans have the hepatitis C virus.[4]

Type D hepatitis is found only in patients with an acute or chronic episode of hepatitis B and requires the presence of HBsAg. The type D virus depends on the double-shelled type B virus to replicate. For this reason, type D infection can't outlast a type B infection. About 15 million people are infected with hepatitis D worldwide. It's more common in adults than in children. People with a history of illicit I.V. drug use and people who live in the Mediterranean basin have a higher incidence.

Type E hepatitis is transmitted enterically, much like type A. Because this virus is inconsistently shed in feces, detection is difficult. It is uncommon in the United States.[5] It's typically found in developing countries that lie near the equator. Incidence is highest among people ages 15 to 40.

Type G may be transmitted in a manner similar to that of hepatitis C. It may also be transmitted by sexual contact, and its incidence may be higher than previously suspected. It's associated with acute and chronic liver disease, but studies haven't clearly implicated the hepatitis G virus as an etiologic agent.

Other proposed causative factors, such as non-ABCDE viral hepatitis and type F, are under investigation.

Signs and symptoms

Assessment findings are similar for the different types of hepatitis. Typically, signs and symptoms progress in several stages.

In the prodromal (preicteric) stage, the patient typically complains of easy fatigue and anorexia (possibly with mild weight loss), generalized malaise, depression, headache, weakness, arthralgia, myalgia, photophobia, and nausea with vomiting. He also may describe changes in his senses of taste and smell.

Assessment of the patient's vital signs may reveal a fever of 100° to 102° F (37.8° to 38.9° C). As the prodromal stage ends, usually 1 to 5 days before the onset of the clinical jaundice stage, inspection of urine and stool specimens may reveal dark-colored urine and clay-colored stools.

If the patient has progressed to the clinical jaundice stage, he may report pruritus, abdominal pain or tenderness, and indigestion. Early in this stage, he may complain of anorexia; later, his appetite may return. Inspection of the sclerae, mucous membranes, and skin may reveal jaundice, which can last for 1 to 2 weeks. Jaundice indicates that the damaged liver is unable to remove bilirubin from the blood; however, its presence doesn't indicate the severity of the disease. Occasionally, hepatitis occurs without jaundice.

During the clinical jaundice stage, inspection of the skin may detect rashes, erythematous patches, or urticaria, especially if the patient has hepatitis B or C. Palpation may disclose abdominal tenderness in the right upper quadrant, an enlarged and tender liver and, in some cases, splenomegaly and cervical adenopathy.

During the recovery (posticteric) stage, most of the patient's symptoms decrease or subside. On palpation, a decrease in liver enlargement may be noted. The recovery phase commonly lasts from 2 to 12 weeks, although sometimes this phase lasts longer in the patient with hepatitis B, C, or E. Little is known about hepatitis G.

Complications

▶ Life-threatening fulminant hepatitis causing liver failure and encephalopathy
▶ Pancreatitis
▶ Cirrhosis
▶ Myocarditis
▶ Typical pneumonia
▶ Aplastic anemia
▶ Transverse myelitis
▶ Peripheral neuropathy

Diagnosis

A hepatitis profile, which identifies antibodies specific to the causative virus and establishes the type of hepatitis, is routine in suspected viral hepatitis.
▶ Type A: Detection of an antibody to hepatitis A confirms the diagnosis.
▶ Type B: The presence of HBsAg and hepatitis B antibodies confirm the diagnosis.
▶ Type C: Diagnosis depends on serologic testing for the specific antibody 1 or more months after the onset of acute hepatitis. Until then, the diagnosis is established primarily by obtaining negative test results for hepatitis A, B, and D.
▶ Type D: Detection of intrahepatic delta antigens or immunoglobulin (Ig) antidelta antigens in acute disease (or IgM and IgG in chronic disease) establishes the diagnosis.
▶ Type E: Detection of hepatitis E antigens supports the diagnosis; however, the diagnosis may also be determined by ruling out hepatitis C.
▶ Type G: Detection of hepatitis G antigen supports the diagnosis but doesn't clearly implicate infection; the patient may be otherwise asymptomatic.

Additional findings from liver function studies support the diagnosis:
▶ Serum aspartate aminotransferase and serum alanine aminotransferase levels are increased in the prodromal stage of acute viral hepatitis.

▶ Serum alkaline phosphatase levels are slightly increased.

▶ Serum bilirubin levels are elevated. Levels may continue to be high late in the disease, especially in severe cases.

▶ Prothrombin time is prolonged (more than 3 seconds longer than normal indicates severe liver damage).

▶ White blood cell counts commonly reveal transient neutropenia and lymphopenia followed by lymphocytosis.

▶ Liver biopsy is performed if chronic hepatitis is suspected; however, it's performed for acute hepatitis only if the diagnosis is questionable.

Treatment

No specific drug therapy has been developed for hepatitis, with the exception of hepatitis C, which has been treated somewhat successfully with interferon alpha. Instead, patients are advised to rest in the early stages of the illness and to combat anorexia by eating small, high-calorie, high-protein meals. (Protein intake should be reduced if signs or symptoms of pre-coma—lethargy, confusion, and mental changes—develop.) Large meals are usually better tolerated in the morning because many patients experience nausea late in the day.

In acute viral hepatitis, hospitalization usually is required only for the patient with severe symptoms or complications. Parenteral nutrition may be required if the patient experiences persistent vomiting and is unable to maintain oral intake.

Antiemetics may be given 30 minutes before meals to relieve nausea and prevent vomiting; phenothiazines have a cholestatic effect and should be avoided. For severe pruritus, the resin cholestyramine may be given.

Special considerations

Use enteric precautions when caring for patients with type A or E hepatitis. Practice standard precautions for all patients.

▶ Inform visitors about isolation precautions.

▶ Provide rest periods throughout the day. Schedule treatments and tests so that the patient can rest between bouts of activity.

▶ Because inactivity may make the patient anxious, include diversionary activities as part of his care. Gradually add activities to his schedule as he begins to recover.

▶ Encourage the patient to eat. Don't overload his meal tray or overmedicate him because this will diminish his appetite.

▶ Encourage fluids (at least 4 qt [4 L] per day). Encourage the anorectic patient to drink fruit juice. Also offer chipped ice and effervescent soft drinks to maintain hydration without inducing vomiting.

▶ Administer supplemental vitamins and commercial feedings, as ordered. If symptoms are severe and the patient can't tolerate oral intake, provide I.V. therapy and parenteral nutrition, as ordered by the physician.

▶ Record the patient's weight daily, and keep intake and output records. Observe stools for color, consistency, and amount, and record the frequency of bowel movements.

▶ Watch for signs of fluid shift, such as weight gain and orthostasis.

▶ Watch for signs of hepatic coma, dehydration, pneumonia, vascular problems, and pressure ulcers.

▶ In fulminant hepatitis, maintain electrolyte balance and a patent airway, prevent infections, and control bleeding. Correct hypoglycemia and other complications while awaiting liver regeneration and repair.

▶ Before discharge, emphasize the importance of having regular medical checkups for at least 1 year. The patient will have an increased risk of developing hepatoma. Warn the patient against using alcohol or over-the-counter drugs during this period. Teach him to recognize the signs of a recurrence.

▶ Inform the patient about the availability of support groups for people with all types

of hepatitis, and provide contact information if he's interested.

▶ Inform patients about the Hepatitis A vaccine, which is recommended for all children at age 1 year and for any persons who are at increased risk for the disease.[1]

▶ Inform patients about the Hepatitis B vaccine which is recommended for all babies at birth and all children up to the age of 18 and others who are at increased risk for the disease.[2]

REFERENCES

1. National Center for HIV/AIDS, Viral Hepatitis, STD, and TB Prevention (2007 October 18). "Viral Hepatitis A." [Online]. Available at *www.cdc.gov/ncidod/diseases/hepatitis/a/faqa.htm*.
2. National Center for HIV/AIDS, Viral Hepatitis, STD, and TB Prevention (2007 December 8). "Viral Hepatitis B." [Online]. Available at *www.cdc.gov/ncidod/diseases/hepatitis/b/faqa.htm*.
3. National Center for HIV/AIDS, Viral Hepatitis, STD, and TB Prevention (2007 June 26). "Viral Hepatitis C." [Online]. Available at *www.cdc.gov/ncidod/diseases/hepatitis/c/faqa.htm*.
4. National Center for HIV/AIDS, Viral Hepatitis, STD, and TB Prevention (2007 December 8). "Viral Hepatitis D." [Online]. Available at *www.cdc.gov/ncidod/diseases/hepatitis/d/fact.htm*.
5. National Center for HIV/AIDS, Viral Hepatitis, STD, and TB Prevention (2007 December 8). "Viral Hepatitis E." [Online]. Available at *www.cdc.gov/ncidod/diseases/hepatitis/e/fact.htm*.

Musculoskeletal disorders

CARPAL TUNNEL SYNDROME

Carpal tunnel syndrome, a form of repetitive stress injury, is the most common of the nerve entrapment syndromes. It results from compression of the median nerve within the carpal tunnel at the wrist. This compression neuropathy causes sensory and motor changes in the hand.

Causes and incidence

The carpal tunnel is formed by the carpal bones and the transverse carpal ligament. Inflammation or fibrosis of the tendon sheaths that pass through the carpal tunnel commonly causes edema and compression of the median nerve. The cause of carpal tunnel syndrome may be congenital because the carpal tunnel is smaller in some people.[1] Many conditions have been found to cause the contents or structure of the carpal tunnel to swell and press the median nerve against the transverse carpal ligament. Such conditions include rheumatoid arthritis, flexor tenosynovitis (commonly associated with rheumatic disease), nerve compression, pregnancy, renal failure, menopause, diabetes mellitus, acromegaly, edema following Colles' fracture, hypothyroidism, amyloidosis, myxedema, benign tumors, tuberculosis, and other granulomatous diseases. Another source of damage to the median nerve is dislocation or acute sprain of the wrist.

Carpal tunnel injury is three times more common in women than in men.[1] It usually occurs in women between ages 30 and 60 and poses a serious occupational health problem.

HEALTH & SAFETY *Assembly-line workers, packers, and people who repeatedly use poorly designed tools are most likely to develop this disorder. Any strenuous use of the hands—sustained grasping, twisting, or flexing—aggravates this condition.*

Carpal tunnel syndrome is more common in assembly-line workers than computer users. A Mayo Clinic study found that up to 7 hours of computer use each day didn't increase a person's risk of carpal tunnel syndrome.[1] Another cause may be shearing injuries. Researchers at the Mayo Clinic have found that scar tissue that results from shearing injuries can lead to pressure buildup, which causes the symptoms of carpal tunnel syndrome.[2]

Signs and symptoms

The patient with carpal tunnel syndrome usually complains of weakness, pain, burning, numbness, or tingling in one or both hands. This paresthesia affects the thumb, forefinger, middle finger, and half of the fourth finger. The patient can't clench his

hand into a fist; the nails may be atrophic, the skin dry and shiny. (See *The carpal tunnel.*)

Because of vasodilatation and venous stasis, symptoms are typically worse at night and in the morning. The pain may spread to the forearm and, in severe cases, as far as the shoulder or neck. The patient can usually relieve such pain by shaking or rubbing his hands vigorously or dangling his arms at his side.

Complications

▶ Decreased wrist function
▶ If untreated—permanent nerve damage with loss of movement and sensation

Diagnosis

Physical examination reveals decreased sensation to light touch or pinpricks in the affected fingers. Thenar muscle atrophy occurs in about one-half of all cases of carpal tunnel syndrome, but it's usually a late sign. The patient exhibits a positive Tinel's sign (tingling over the median nerve on light percussion) and responds positively to Phalen's wrist-flexion test (holding the forearms vertically and allowing both hands to drop into complete flexion at the wrists for 1 minute reproduces symptoms of carpal tunnel syndrome). A compression test supports this diagnosis: A blood pressure cuff inflated above systolic pressure and placed on the forearm for 1 to 2 minutes provokes pain and paresthesia along the distribution of the median nerve.

Electromyography and nerve conduction velocity detect a median nerve motor conduction delay of more than 5 milliseconds. Other laboratory tests may identify the underlying disease.

Treatment

Conservative treatment should be tried first, including resting the hands by splinting the wrist in neutral extension for 1 to 2 weeks. Nonsteroidal anti-inflammatory drugs usual-

The carpal tunnel

The carpal tunnel is clearly visible in this palmar view and cross section of a right hand. Note the median nerve, flexor tendons of fingers, and blood vessels passing through the tunnel on their way from the forearm to the hand.

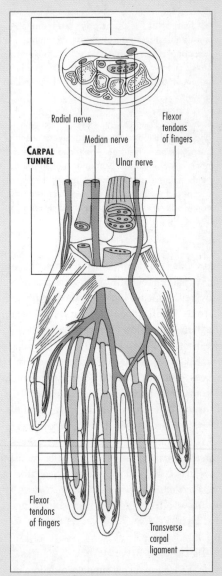

Radial nerve

Median nerve

Flexor tendons of fingers

CARPAL TUNNEL

Ulnar nerve

Flexor tendons of fingers

Transverse carpal ligament

EVIDENCE-BASED PRACTICE

Patient satisfaction with carpal tunnel treatment

Question: *Should adults older than age 70 have nonsurgical therapy for the treatment of carpal tunnel syndrome?*

Research: Carpal tunnel syndrome is common in the general population, and the incidence increases with age. The authors studied 102 patients older than age 70 who have carpal tunnel syndrome. The participants were mailed follow-up questionnaires to assess symptoms, functional status, treatment expectations, and satisfaction with the results of their carpal tunnel treatment at a minimum of 2 years after initial diagnosis.

Conclusion: Patients who were treated with surgery were found to have more severe cases of carpal tunnel syndrome than those treated with nonsurgical methods. Some 93% of surgical patients reported satisfaction with their treatment, compared with only 54% of patients treated conservatively. They also reported better symp-

tom relief and functional status than the nonsurgical patients.

Application: For patients older than age 70, surgery provides greater symptom relief from carpal tunnel syndrome and return to functional status. Nurses should educate their patients about all treatment options for carpal tunnel syndrome, including surgery. Advanced age shouldn't deter the nurse from discussing surgical options for relief of carpal tunnel syndrome.

Source: Ettema, A.M., et al. "Surgery versus Conservative Therapy in Carpal Tunnel Syndrome in People Aged 70 Years and Older," *Plastic and Reconstructive Surgery* 118(4):947-58, September 2006.

---

ly provide symptomatic relief.[3] Injection of the carpal tunnel with hydrocortisone may provide significant but temporary relief.[3] Steroids are effective in high and low doses.[3] If a definite link has been established between the patient's occupation and the development of repetitive stress injury, he may have to seek other work. Effective treatment also may require correction of an underlying disorder. When conservative treatment fails, the only alternative is surgical decompression of the nerve by resecting the entire transverse carpal tunnel ligament or by using endoscopic surgical techniques. (See *Patient satisfaction with carpal tunnel treatment.*) Neurolysis (freeing of the nerve fibers) may also be necessary.

Special considerations

Patient care for carpal tunnel syndrome includes the following:

▶ Administer mild analgesics as needed. Encourage the patient to use his hands as much as possible. If his dominant hand has been impaired, you may have to help with eating and bathing.

▶ Teach the patient how to apply a splint. Tell him not to make it too tight. Show him how to remove the splint to perform gentle range-of-motion exercises, which should be done daily. Make sure the patient knows how to do these exercises before he's discharged.

▶ After surgery, monitor vital signs, and regularly check the color, sensation, and motion of the affected hand.

▶ Advise the patient who's about to be discharged to occasionally exercise his hands in warm water. If the arm is in a sling, tell him to remove the sling several times per day to do exercises for his elbow and shoulder.

▶ Suggest occupational counseling for the patient who has to change jobs because of repetitive stress injury.

REFERENCES

1. National Institute of Neurological Disorders and Stroke (2007 December 11). "Carpal Tunnel Syndrome Fact Sheet," NIH publication No. 03-4898 [Online]. Available at *www.ninds. nih.gov/disorders/carpal_tunnel/detail_carpal_ tunnel.htm.*
2. MayoClinic.com (2006 November 19). "Mayo Clinic Researchers Find Evidence for Traumatic Cause of Carpal Tunnel Syndrome" [Online]. Available at *www.mayoclinic.org/news2006-rst/3763.html.*
3. Piazzini, D.B., et al. "A Systematic Review of Conservative Treatment of Carpal Tunnel Syndrome," *Clinical Rehabilitation* 21(4):299-314, April 2007.

GOUT

Gout, also called *gouty arthritis,* is a metabolic disease marked by urate deposits, which cause painfully arthritic joints. It can strike any joint but favors those in the feet and legs. Gout follows an intermittent course and typically leaves patients totally free from symptoms for years between attacks. It can cause chronic disability or incapacitation and, rarely, severe hypertension and progressive renal disease. The prognosis is good with treatment.

Causes and incidence

Elevated blood levels of uric acid (hyperuricemia), due to overproduction of uric acid or retention of uric acid, cause gout. The overproduction of uric acid is responsible for 10% of primary gout and underexcretion is responsible for 90% of the cases.[1]

Overproduction may be due to a genetic disorder, myeloproliferative and lymphoproliferative disorders, psoriasis, chemotherapy, hemolytic anemias, or obesity.

In secondary gout, which develops during the course of another disease (such as obesity, diabetes mellitus, hypertension, sickle cell anemia, and renal disease), hyperuricemia results from the breakdown of nucleic acids. Renal insufficiency, lead nephropathy, starvation or dehydration, hypothyroidism, hyperparathyroidism, and ethanol abuse are common causes. Secondary gout can also follow drug therapy that interferes with uric acid excretion. Increased concentration of uric acid leads to urate deposits (*tophi*) in joints or tissues and consequent local necrosis or fibrosis. The risk is greater in men, postmenopausal women, and those who use alcohol. Primary gout usually occurs in men and in postmenopausal women; secondary gout occurs in elderly people.

In 2005, 3 million Americans reported having gout.[3]

Signs and symptoms

Gout develops in four stages: asymptomatic, acute, intercritical, and chronic. In asymptomatic gout, serum urate levels rise but produce no symptoms. As the disease progresses, it may cause hypertension or nephrolithiasis, with severe back pain. The first acute attack strikes suddenly and peaks quickly. Although it generally involves only one or a few joints, this initial attack is extremely painful. Affected joints are hot, tender, inflamed, and appear dusky-red or cyanotic. The metatarsophalangeal joint of the great toe usually becomes inflamed first (*podagra*), followed by the instep, ankle, heel, knee, or wrist joints. Sometimes a low-grade fever is present. Mild acute attacks usually subside quickly but tend to recur at irregular intervals. Severe attacks may persist for days or weeks.

Intercritical periods are the symptom-free intervals between gout attacks. Most patients have a second attack within 6 months to 2 years, but in some, the second attack doesn't occur for 5 to 10 years. Delayed attacks are more common in untreated pa-

Gouty deposits

The final stage of gout is marked by painful polyarthritis, with large, subcutaneous, tophaceous deposits in cartilage, synovial membranes, tendons, and soft tissue. The skin over the tophus is shiny, thin, and taut.

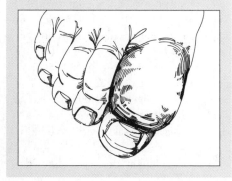

tients and tend to be longer and more severe than initial attacks. Such attacks are also polyarticular, invariably affecting joints in the feet and legs, and are sometimes accompanied by fever. A migratory attack sequentially strikes various joints and the Achilles tendon and is associated with either subdeltoid or olecranon bursitis.

Eventually, chronic polyarticular gout sets in. This final, unremitting stage of the disease is marked by persistent painful polyarthritis, with large, subcutaneous tophi in cartilage, synovial membranes, tendons, and soft tissue. Tophi form in fingers, hands, knees, feet, ulnar sides of the forearms, helix of the ear, Achilles tendons and, rarely, internal organs, such as the kidneys and myocardium. The skin over the tophus may ulcerate and release a chalky, white exudate or pus. Chronic inflammation and tophaceous deposits precipitate secondary joint degeneration, with eventual erosions, deformity, and disability. (See *Gouty deposits*.)

Complications
▶ Chronic renal dysfunction and renal calculi

▶ Urolithiasis
▶ Cardiovascular lesions
▶ Stroke
▶ Coronary thrombosis
▶ Hypertension
▶ Infection occurs with tophi rupture and nerve entrapment

Diagnosis
The presence of monosodium urate monohydrate crystals in synovial fluid taken from an inflamed joint or tophus establishes the diagnosis.

Aspiration of synovial fluid (arthrocentesis) or of tophaceous material reveals needle-like intracellular crystals of sodium urate. Although hyperuricemia isn't specifically diagnostic of gout, serum uric acid is above normal. Urinary uric acid is usually higher in secondary gout than in primary gout. In acute attacks, erythrocyte sedimentation rate and white blood cell (WBC) count may be elevated, and WBC count shifts to the left.

Initially, X-rays are normal. However, in chronic gout, X-rays show "punched out" erosions, sometimes with periosteal overgrowth. Outward displacement of the overhanging margin from the bone contour characterizes gout. X-rays rarely show tophi. (See *Understanding pseudogout*. Also see *Diagnosing gout*, page 210.)

Treatment
Correct management seeks to terminate an acute attack, reduce hyperuricemia, and prevent recurrence, complications, and the formation of renal calculi. Colchicine is effective in reducing pain, swelling, and inflammation; pain typically subsides within 12 hours of treatment and is completely relieved in 48 hours. Treatment for the patient with acute gout consists of bed rest; immobilization and protection of the inflamed, painful joints; and local application of heat or cold, whichever works for the patient. Maximal doses of nonsteroidal anti-inflammatory drugs (NSAIDs) usually provide excellent re-

lief for patients who can tolerate them; doses should be gradually reduced after several days.

Resistant inflammation or the inability to tolerate NSAIDS or colchicine may require oral corticosteroids or intra-articular corticosteroid injection to relieve pain. Treatment for chronic gout aims to decrease serum uric acid level. Continuing maintenance dosage of allopurinol may be given to suppress uric acid formation or control uric acid levels, preventing further attacks. However, this powerful drug should be used cautiously in patients with renal failure. Uricosuric agents promote uric acid excretion and inhibit accumulation of uric acid, but their value is limited in patients with renal impairment. These medications shouldn't be given to patients with renal calculi.

Newer medications are being evaluated for the treatment of gout as well. They include pegylated formulations of uricase and a new potent xanthine oxidase inhibitor, febuxostat. Some cardiovascular drugs have been used as treatment also.[2]

Adjunctive therapy emphasizes a few dietary restrictions, primarily the avoidance of alcohol and purine-rich foods (organ meats, beer, wine, and certain types of fish). Obese patients should try to lose weight because obesity puts additional stress on painful joints.

In some cases, surgery may be necessary to improve joint function or correct deformities. Tophi must be excised and drained if they become infected or ulcerated. They can also be excised to prevent ulceration, improve the patient's appearance, or make it easier for him to wear shoes or gloves.

Special considerations

Patient care for gout includes these interventions:
▶ Encourage bed rest but use a bed cradle to keep bedcovers off extremely sensitive, inflamed joints.

Understanding pseudogout

Also known as *calcium pyrophosphate disease*, pseudogout results when calcium pyrophosphate crystals collect in periarticular joint structures.

SIGNS AND SYMPTOMS

Like true gout, pseudogout causes sudden joint pain and swelling, most commonly of the knee, wrist, and ankle or other peripheral joints.

Pseudogout attacks are self-limiting and triggered by stress, trauma, surgery, severe dieting, thiazide therapy, or alcohol abuse. Associated symptoms resemble those of rheumatoid arthritis.

ESTABLISHING A DIAGNOSIS

Diagnosis of pseudogout hinges on joint aspiration and synovial biopsy to detect calcium pyrophosphate crystals. X-rays show calcium deposits in the fibrocartilage and linear markings along the bone ends. Blood tests may detect an underlying endocrine or metabolic disorder.

RELIEF FOR PRESSURE AND INFLAMMATION

Management of pseudogout may include aspirating the joint to relieve pressure; instilling corticosteroids and administering analgesics, salicylates, phenylbutazone, or other nonsteroidal anti-inflammatory drugs to treat inflammation and, if appropriate, treating the underlying disorder. Without treatment, pseudogout leads to permanent joint damage in about one-half of those it affects, most of whom are older adults.

▶ Give pain medication, as needed, especially during acute attacks. Apply hot or cold packs to inflamed joints according to what the patient finds effective. Administer anti-inflammatory medication and other drugs, as ordered. Watch for adverse effects. Be alert for GI disturbances with colchicine.

Diagnosing gout

Question: *What other tests can be performed to diagnose gout when standard test results are inconclusive?*

Research: Physicians typically use physical examination, medical history, uric acid levels in the blood, and synovial fluid sampling to diagnose gout. At times, test results are inconclusive using these methods. Researchers conducted this study to compare the use of conventional X-ray with high-resolution ultrasound to determine which test was more accurate in helping to arrive at a definitive diagnosis in such patients. The study included 105 patients whose clinical presentation indicated gout. They performed both tests on each participant and analyzed the findings to arrive at their conclusions.

Conclusion: In 19 of the study participants, researchers were unable to reach a definite diagnosis; however, they determined that 55 of the participants had a definite diagnosis of gout, and 31 had a different disease. X-ray results were more specific than ultrasound for diagnos-ing gout, whereas the ultrasound was more sensitive and often provided additional diagnostic information when laboratory findings and X-ray results were negative or inconclusive.

Application: The nurse caring for a patient with suspected gout should be aware that high-resolution ultrasound can be used to confirm or refute the diagnosis when standard testing is inconclusive. This is especially important to ensure appropriate treatment for the patient who's ultimately found to have a different disease. When a patient's diagnosis is made by clinical presentation alone, be sure to confirm by additional testing—whenever possible.

Source: Rettenbacher, T., et al. "Diagnostic Imaging of Gout: Comparison of High-Resolution US versus Conventional X-ray," *European Radiology* 18(3):621-30, March 2008.

▶ Watch for acute gout attacks 24 to 96 hours after surgery. Even minor surgery can precipitate an attack. Before and after surgery, administer colchicine as ordered to help prevent gout attacks.

▶ Tell the patient to avoid high-purine foods, such as anchovies, liver, sardines, kidneys, sweetbreads, lentils, and alcoholic beverages—especially beer and wine—which raise the urate level. Explain the principles of a gradual weight-reduction diet to obese patients.

▶ Advise the patient to report any adverse effects of allopurinol, such as drowsiness, dizziness, nausea, vomiting, urinary frequency, or dermatitis.

REFERENCES

1. Gout.com. Information about Gout and Hypouricemia for You and Your Patients (2008 January 6). [Online]. Available at *www.gout.com/professional/index.aspx*.
2. Schmacher, H.R. Jr., and Chen, L.X. "Newer Therapeutic Approaches: Gout," *Rheumatic Disease Clinics of North America* 32(1):235-44, February 2006.
3. Helmick, C., et al. "Estimates of the Prevalence of Arthritis and Other Rheumatic Conditions in the United States, Part I and Part II," *Arthritis and Rheumatism* 58(1):115-25, January 2008. Available at *www.sciencedaily.com/releases/2008/01/080102142942.htm*.

HERNIATED DISK

Herniated disk, also called *ruptured* or *slipped disk* and *herniated nucleus pulposus,* occurs when all or part of the nucleus pulposus—the soft, gelatinous, central portion of an intervertebral disk—is forced through the disk's weakened or torn outer ring (anulus fibrosus). When this happens, the extruded disk may impinge on spinal nerve roots as they exit from the spinal canal or on the spinal cord itself, resulting in back pain and other signs of nerve root irritation.

Causes and incidence

Herniated disks may result from severe trauma or strain or may be related to intervertebral joint degeneration. Men between the ages of 30 and 50 are most prone to this condition,[1] but elderly people also are at risk because minor trauma may cause herniation in disks that have begun to deteriorate due to age. Other conditions that weaken the disk, besides aging, are improper lifting, smoking, excessive body weight, sudden pressure, and repetitive strenuous activities.[2] Ninety percent of herniation occurs in the lumbar and lumbosacral regions of the spine, 8% in the cervical region, and 1% to 2% in the thoracic region. Patients with a congenitally small lumbar spinal canal or with osteophyte formation on the vertebrae may be more susceptible to nerve root compression by a herniated disk and more likely to have neurologic symptoms.[1]

Signs and symptoms

The overriding symptom of lumbar herniated disk is severe low back pain that radiates to the buttocks, legs, and feet, usually unilaterally. When herniation follows trauma, the pain may begin suddenly, subside in a few days, and then recur at shorter intervals and with progressive intensity. Sciatic pain follows, beginning as a dull pain in the buttocks. Valsalva's maneuver, coughing, sneez- ing, or bending intensify the pain, which is commonly accompanied by muscle spasms.

Complications

▶ Paresthesia or hyperthesia
▶ Sensory and motor loss in the area innervated by the compressed spinal nerve root
▶ Weakness and atrophy of leg muscles

Diagnosis

Obtaining a careful patient history is vital because the events that intensify disk pain are diagnostically significant. The straight-leg–raising test and its variants are perhaps the best tests for herniated disk, but the results may still be negative.

To do this test, have the patient lie in a supine position on the examination table. Place one hand on the patient's ilium, to stabilize the pelvis, and the other hand under the ankle, then slowly raise the patient's leg. The test is positive only if the patient complains of posterior leg (sciatic) pain, not back pain. In the Lasègue test, the patient lies flat while the thigh and knee are flexed to a 90-degree angle. Resistance and pain as well as loss of ankle or knee-jerk reflex indicate spinal root compression.

X-rays of the spine are essential to rule out other abnormalities, but they may not diagnose herniated disk because marked disk prolapse can be present despite a normal X-ray. A thorough check of the patient's peripheral vascular status—including posterior tibial and dorsalis pedis pulses and skin temperature of extremities—helps rule out ischemic disease, another cause of leg pain or numbness. After physical examination and X-rays, myelography, computed tomography scans, and magnetic resonance imaging (MRI) provide the most specific diagnostic information, showing spinal canal compression by herniated disk material. MRI is the method of choice to confirm the diagnosis and determine the exact level of herniation. A myelogram can define the size and location of disk herniation. An electromyogram

can determine the exact nerve root involved. A nerve conduction velocity test may also be performed.

Treatment

Nonsurgical treatment is effective in treating 90% of patients.[2] Unless neurologic impairment progresses rapidly, treatment is initially conservative and consists of several weeks of bed rest (possibly with pelvic traction), administration of heat applications, nonsteroidal anti-inflammatory drugs, and an exercise program. Epidural corticosteroids, short-term oral corticosteroids, nerve root blocks, or physical therapy may be used to decrease pain.[5] Muscle relaxants, such as diazepam, methocarbamol, or cyclobenzaprine, may relieve associated muscle spasms.

A herniated disk that fails to respond to conservative treatment may require surgery. One option: a laminectomy, which excises a portion of the lamina and removes or reshapes the protruding disk. If a laminectomy doesn't alleviate pain and disability, a spinal fusion, which eliminates motion between two or more vertebral segments may be necessary to overcome segmental instability. Laminectomy and spinal fusion are sometimes performed concurrently to stabilize the spine. Lumbar diskectomy is the most common surgical procedure, however, and is used to remove fragments of nucleus pulposus. A study done between 2000 and 2004 compared patients who had a diskectomy with those who were treated nonsurgically over a 2-year period. No statistical difference was found in the outcomes of the two groups, and both improved over the 2-year period.[3]

One nonsurgical intervention involves injecting the enzyme chymopapain into the herniated disk, which produces a loss of water and proteoglycans from the disk, thereby reducing both the disk's size and the pressure in the nerve root. This procedure is as effective as surgery and easier on the patient.[4]

Special considerations

Herniated disk requires supportive care, careful patient teaching, and strong emotional support to help the patient cope with the discomfort and frustration of chronic lower back pain.

▶ If the patient requires myelography, question him carefully about allergies to iodides, iodine-containing substances, or seafood because such allergies may indicate sensitivity to the test's radiopaque dye. Reinforce previous explanations of the need for this test, and tell the patient to expect some pain. Assure him that he'll receive a sedative before the test, if needed, to keep him as calm and comfortable as possible. After the test, urge the patient to remain in bed with his head elevated (especially if metrizamide was used) and to drink plenty of fluids. Monitor intake and output. Watch for seizures and allergic reaction.

▶ During conservative treatment, watch for any deterioration in neurologic status (especially during the first 24 hours after admission), which may indicate an urgent need for surgery. Use antiembolism stockings as prescribed, and encourage the patient to move his legs, as allowed. Provide high-topped sneakers to prevent footdrop. Work closely with the physical therapy department to ensure a consistent regimen of leg- and back-strengthening exercises. Give plenty of fluids to prevent renal stasis, and remind the patient to cough, deep breathe, and use blow bottles or an incentive spirometer to preclude pulmonary complications. Provide good skin care. Assess for bowel and bladder functions. Use a fracture bedpan for the patient on complete bed rest.

▶ After laminectomy, microdiskectomy, or spinal fusion, enforce bed rest, as ordered. If a blood drainage system (Hemovac or Jackson Pratt drain) is in use, check the tubing frequently for kinks and a secure vacuum. Empty the Hemovac at the end of each shift, and record the amount and color of drainage. Report immediately any colorless

moisture on dressings (possible cerebrospinal fluid leakage) or excessive drainage. Observe neurovascular status of the legs (color, motion, temperature, and sensation).

▶ Monitor vital signs, and check for bowel sounds and abdominal distention. Use the logrolling technique to turn the patient. Administer analgesics as ordered, especially 30 minutes before initial attempts at sitting or walking. Give the patient assistance during his first attempt to walk. Provide a straight-backed chair for limited sitting.

▶ Teach the patient who has undergone spinal fusion how to wear a brace. Assist with straight-leg–raising and toe-pointing exercises, as ordered. Before discharge, teach proper body mechanics—bending at the knees and hips (never at the waist), standing straight, and carrying objects close to the body. Advise the patient to lie down when tired and to sleep on his side (never on his abdomen) on an extra-firm mattress or a bed board. Urge maintenance of proper weight to prevent lordosis caused by obesity.

▶ Tell the patient who must receive a muscle relaxant about the possible adverse effects, especially drowsiness. Warn him to avoid activities that require alertness until he has built up a tolerance to the drug's sedative effects.

▶ Provide emotional support. Try to cheer the patient up when he seems frustrated or and depressed. Assure him of his progress, and offer encouragement.

REFERENCES

1. MayoClinic.com (2005 September 8). "Herniated Disk" [Online]. Available at *www.mayoclinic.com/health/herniated-disk/DS00893.*
2. American Academy of Orthopaedic Surgeons (2007 July). "Herniated Disk" [Online]. Available at *http://orthoinfo.aaos.org/topic.cfm?topic=A00334.*
3. Weinstien, J.N., et al. "Surgical vs. Nonoperative Treatment for Lumbar Disk Herniation, the Pine Patient Outcomes Research Trial (SPORT): A Randomized Trial," *JAMA* 296(20):2441-450, November 2006.
4. Yeung, A.T., and Yeung, C.A. "Minimally Invasive Techniques for the Management of Lumbar Disc Herniation," *Orthopedic Clinics of North America* 38(3):363-72, July 2007.
5. Ackerman, W.E. 3rd, and Ahmad, M. "The Efficacy of Lumbar Epidural Steroid Injections in Patients with Lumbar Disc Herniations," *Anesthesia and Analgesia* 104(5):1217-222, May 2007.

OSTEOARTHRITIS

Osteoarthritis, the most common form of arthritis, is a chronic disease that causes deterioration of the joint cartilage and formation of reactive new bone at the margins and subchondral areas of the joints. This degeneration results from a breakdown of chondrocytes, most commonly in the distal interphalangeal and proximal interphalangeal joints, but also in the hip and knee joints.

Disability depends on the site and severity of involvement and can range from minor limitation of the dexterity of the fingers to severe disability in persons with hip or knee involvement. The rate of progression varies, and joints may remain stable for years in an early stage of deterioration.

Causes and incidence

Studies indicate that osteoarthritis is acquired and probably results from a combination of metabolic, genetic, chemical, and mechanical factors. Risk factors include heredity, obesity, joint injury, repeated overuse of a joint, lack of physical activity, nerve injury, and aging.[2] Secondary osteoarthritis usually follows an identifiable predisposing event—most commonly trauma, congenital deformity, or obesity—and leads to degenerative changes.

Osteoarthritis affects nearly 27 million adults.[1] It occurs equally in both sexes. Its earliest symptoms typically begin after age

What happens in osteoarthritis

The characteristic breakdown of articular cartilage is a gradual response to aging or to predisposing factors, such as joint abnormalities or traumatic injury.

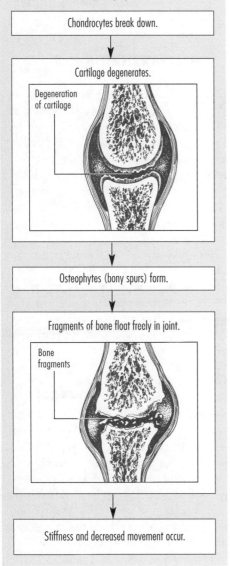

| Chondrocytes break down. |

Cartilage degenerates.

Degeneration of cartilage

Osteophytes (bony spurs) form.

Fragments of bone float freely in joint.

Bone fragments

Stiffness and decreased movement occur.

40 and may progress with advancing age.[2] It's present in almost everyone by age 70.

Before age 45, it's more common in men, but after age 55, the incidence is higher in women.

Signs and symptoms

The most common symptom of osteoarthritis is a deep, aching joint pain, particularly after exercise or a weight-bearing activity, and it's usually relieved by rest. Other symptoms include stiffness in the morning and after exercise (relieved by rest), aching during changes in weather, "grating" of the joint during motion, altered gait contractures, and limited movement. These symptoms increase with poor posture, obesity, and stress on the affected joint.

Osteoarthritis of the interphalangeal joints produces irreversible joint changes and node formation. The nodes eventually become red, swollen, and tender, causing numbness and loss of dexterity. (See *What happens in osteoarthritis.*)

Diagnosis

A thorough physical examination confirms typical symptoms, and absence of systemic symptoms rules out an inflammatory joint disorder. X-rays of the affected joint help confirm diagnosis of osteoarthritis, but may look normal in the early stages. X-rays may require many views and typically show:
▶ narrowing of joint space or margin
▶ cystlike bony deposits in joint space and margins and sclerosis of the subchondral space
▶ joint deformity due to degeneration or articular damage
▶ bony growths at weight-bearing areas
▶ fusion of joints. (See *Digital joint deformities.*)

Treatment

Treatment is aimed at relieving pain, maintaining or improving mobility, and minimizing disability. Medications include nonsteroidal anti-inflammatory drugs (NSAIDS), COX-2 inhibitors (celecoxib) and, in some

cases, intra-articular injections of corticosteroids.

IN THE NEWS *Many patients take glucosamine and chondroitin for joint pain, believing these substances help decrease the pain. New studies have shown that these therapies may not be effective.[3]*

Studies also show that NSAIDS are more effective than acetaminophen in relieving knee and hip pain of osteoarthritis.[4] Injecting artificial joint fluid into the knee can provide relief of pain for up to 6 months.

Effective treatment also reduces stress by weight loss, and by supporting or stabilizing the joint with crutches, braces, cane, walker, cervical collar, or traction. Exercise, such as through physical therapy, is integral to maintaining or improving joint mobility. Other supportive measures include massage, moist heat, paraffin dips for hands, protective techniques to prevent undue stress on the joints, and adequate rest (particularly after activity).

Surgical treatment is reserved for patients who have severe disability or uncontrollable pain. Options include:
▶ Arthroplasty (partial or total): replaces the deteriorated part of a joint with a prosthetic appliance
▶ Arthrodesis: fuses bones surgically, and is used primarily in a spine laminectomy
▶ Osteoplasty: scrapes and lavages the deteriorated bone from the joint
▶ Osteotomy: excises a wedge of bone, or cuts bone, to change the alignment and relieve stress on that bone.

Special considerations
Patient care for osteoarthritis includes the following:
▶ Promote adequate rest, particularly after activity. Plan rest periods during the day, and provide for adequate sleep at night. Moderation is the key—teach the patient to pace daily activities.

Digital joint deformities

Osteoarthritis of the interphalangeal joints produces irreversible changes in the distal joints (Heberden's nodes, below left) and the proximal joints (Bouchard's nodes, below right). Initially painless, these nodes gradually progress or suddenly flare up, resulting in redness, swelling, tenderness, and impaired sensation and dexterity.

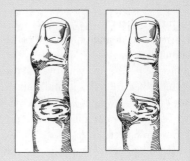

▶ Assist with physical therapy, and encourage the patient to perform gentle, isometric range-of-motion (ROM) exercises.
▶ Provide emotional support and reassurance to help the patient cope with limited mobility. Explain that osteoarthritis *isn't* a systemic disease.

Specific patient care depends on the affected joint:
▶ *Hand:* Apply hot soaks and paraffin dips to relieve pain, as ordered.
▶ *Spine (lumbar and sacral):* Recommend a firm mattress (or bed board) to decrease morning pain.
▶ *Spine (cervical):* Check cervical collar for constriction; watch for redness with prolonged use.
▶ *Hip:* Use moist heat pads to relieve pain, and administer antispasmodic drugs as ordered. Assist with ROM and strengthening exercises, always making sure the patient gets the proper rest afterward. Check crutches, cane, braces, and walker for proper fit,

and teach the patient to use them correctly. For example, the patient with unilateral joint involvement should use an orthopedic appliance such as a walker or a cane. Recommend the use of cushions when sitting as well as the use of an elevated toilet seat.

▶ *Knee:* Twice daily, assist with prescribed ROM exercises, exercises to maintain muscle tone, and progressive resistance exercises to increase muscle strength. Provide elastic supports or braces if needed.

To minimize the long-term effects of osteoarthritis:

▶ Teach the patient to take medication exactly as prescribed, and report adverse effects immediately.

▶ Advise the patient to avoid overexertion. He should take care to stand and walk correctly, to minimize weight-bearing activities, and to be especially careful when stooping or picking up objects.

▶ Instruct the patient to wear proper-fitting, supportive shoes and not to allow the heels to become worn down.

▶ Advise the patient to install safety devices at home such as guard rails in the bathroom.

▶ Instruct the patient to maintain proper body weight to lessen strain on joints.

REFERENCES

1. Helmick C., et al. "Estimates of the Prevalence of Arthritis and Other Rheumatic Conditions in the United States, Part I," *Arthritis and Rheumatism* 58(1):15-25, January 2008.
2. Arthritis Foundation (2005). "Osteoarthritis Fact Sheet" [Online]. Available at *http://ww2.arthritis.org/conditions/Fact_Sheets/OA_Fact_Sheet.asp.*
3. Distler, J., and Anguelouch, A. "Evidence-Based Practice: Review of Clinical Evidence on the Efficacy of Glucosamine and Chondroitin in the Treatment of Osteoarthritis," *Journal of the American Academy of Nurse Practitioners* 18(10):487-93, October 2006.
4. Towheed, T.E., et al. "Acetaminophen for Osteoarthritis," *Cochrane Database of Systematic Reviews* (1):CD004257, January 2006.

OSTEOMYELITIS

Osteomyelitis is a pyogenic bone infection that may be chronic or acute. It commonly results from the combination of an acute infection originating elsewhere in the body and local trauma to the bone, which is usually trivial but results in hematoma formation. Once the bone is infected, osteomyelitis usually remains localized, but it can spread through the bone to the marrow, cortex, and periosteum. Acute osteomyelitis is usually a blood-borne disease, which most commonly affects rapidly growing children. Chronic osteomyelitis, which is rare, is characterized by multiple draining sinus tracts and metastatic lesions. Another hallmark of chronic osteomyelitis is necrotic bone resulting from impaired blood flow related to raised intraosseous pressure.[3]

Causes and incidence

Virtually any pathogenic bacteria can cause osteomyelitis under the right circumstances. Typically, these organisms find a culture site in a hematoma from recent trauma or in a weakened area, such as the site of surgery or local infection (for example, furunculosis), and spread directly to bone. As the organisms grow and form pus within the bone, tension builds within the rigid medullary cavity, forcing pus through the haversian canals. This forms a subperiosteal abscess that deprives the bone of its blood supply and may eventually cause necrosis. In turn, necrosis stimulates the periosteum to create new bone *(involucrum);* the old bone *(sequestrum)* detaches and works its way out through an abscess or the sinuses. By the time sequestrum forms, osteomyelitis is chronic. People at risk for developing osteomyelitis include people with sickle cell anemia, diabetes, decreased immunity, those receiving hemodialysis, I.V. drug abusers, and the elderly.[1]

Osteomyelitis is found in children and adults and is more common in males.[2] Fifty

percent of the cases are preschool-age children.[2] The most common sites in children are the lower end of the femur and the upper end of the tibia, humerus, and radius. In adults, it's usually as a complication of an acute localized infection. The most common sites in adults are the pelvis and vertebrae, generally as a result of contamination associated with surgery or trauma. Other common sites are sternoclavicular, sacroiliac, and symphysis pubis.

Signs and symptoms
Onset of acute osteomyelitis is usually rapid, with sudden pain accompanied by tenderness, heat, swelling, and restricted movement of the affected area. Associated systemic symptoms may include tachycardia, sudden fever, nausea, and malaise. Generally, the clinical features of both chronic and acute osteomyelitis are the same, except that chronic infection can persist intermittently for years, flaring up spontaneously after minor trauma. Chronic osteomyelitis is the relapse of a previously treated or untreated infection.[3] Sometimes, however, the only symptom of chronic infection is the persistent drainage of pus from an old pocket in a sinus tract.

Complications
▶ Chronic infection
▶ Skeletal deformities
▶ Joint deformities
▶ Disturbed bone growth in children
▶ Differing leg lengths
▶ Impaired mobility

Diagnosis
Patient history, physical examination, and blood tests help to confirm osteomyelitis. Aids to diagnosis include the following:
▶ A white blood cell count can show leukocytosis but commonly is normal.
▶ Erythrocyte sedimentation rate or C-reactive protein level diagnostic tests, typically combined, may show an elevated rate or level, but can be nonspecific in acute cases.
▶ Cultures of the lesion indicate the source of the organism. Blood cultures help identify the causative organism.
▶ Magnetic resonance imaging is best for detecting spinal infection.
▶ Computed tomography is best for visualizing islands of dead bone.
▶ Ultrasound may demonstrate abnormalities after 1 to 2 days of symptoms.

X-rays may not show bone involvement until the disease has been active for some time, usually 2 to 3 weeks. Bone scans can detect early infection. Diagnosis must rule out poliomyelitis, rheumatic fever, myositis, and bone fractures. The gold standard for diagnosing osteomyelitis is histopathologic and microscopic examination of bone. (See *Using MRI for diagnosis,* page 218.)

Treatment
Treatment for acute osteomyelitis should begin before definitive diagnosis. Treatment includes administration of antibiotics after blood cultures are taken; early surgical drainage to relieve pressure buildup and sequestrum formation; immobilization of the affected bone by plaster cast, traction, or bed rest; and supportive measures, such as analgesics and I.V. fluids. In chronic cases, the patient may benefit from long-term antibiotics.[4]

If an abscess forms, treatment includes incision and drainage, followed by a culture of the drained fluid. Intracavitary instillation of antibiotics may be done through closed-system continuous irrigation with low intermittent suction; limited irrigation with blood drainage system with suction; or local application of packed, wet, antibiotic-soaked dressings.

In addition to these therapies, chronic osteomyelitis usually requires surgery to remove dead bone (*sequestrectomy*) and to promote drainage (*saucerization*). The area may be filled with bone graft or packing ma-

EVIDENCE-BASED PRACTICE

Using MRI for diagnosis

Question: *Can an MRI be used to accurately diagnose osteomyelitis of the foot and ankle?*

Research: The diagnosis of osteomyelitis of the foot and ankle is typically made using technetium (^{99m}Tc) bone scanning, plain radiography, and white blood cell studies. To determine whether diagnosis by magnetic resonance imaging (MRI) is as accurate as these studies, researchers extracted data from 16 research studies performed between 1966 and June 2006 that included MRI evaluation. Analysis of the data was performed using the calculation of the diagnostic odds ratio.

Conclusion: When a direct comparison could be made between the MRI and each of the other types of tests, the diagnostic odds ratio of the MRI showed markedly superior accuracy in confirming the presence or absence of osteomyelitis.

Application: When the nurse is caring for a patient with suspected osteomyelitis, it's beneficial to know that one noninvasive test, the MRI, can be used to confirm or rule out the diagnosis. This enables appropriate treatment to begin earlier in the course of the disease because multiple test results aren't needed for confirmation. It also places less strain on the patient, who can now be spared multiple testing procedures.

Source: Kapoor, A., et al. "Magnetic Resonance Imaging for Diagnosing Foot Osteomyelitis: A Meta-Analysis," *Archives of Internal Medicine* 167(2):125-32, January 22, 2007.

---

terial to promote new bone tissue. An infected prosthesis is removed and a new one is implanted the same day or after resolution of the infection.

Some centers use hyperbaric oxygen to increase the activity of naturally occurring leukocytes. Free-tissue transfers and local muscle flaps also are used to fill in dead space and increase blood supply.

Special considerations

Focus on controlling infection, protecting the bone from injury, and offering meticulous supportive care.
▶ Use strict sterile technique when changing dressings and irrigating wounds. If the patient is in skeletal traction for compound fractures, cover insertion points of pin tracks with small, dry dressings, and tell him not to touch the skin around the pins and wires (and why).

▶ Administer I.V. fluids to maintain adequate hydration as necessary. Provide a diet high in protein and vitamin C.
▶ Assess—daily—vital signs, wound appearance, and new pain, which may indicate secondary infection.
▶ Carefully monitor suctioning equipment, and the amount of solution it instills and suctions.
▶ Support the affected limb with firm pillows. Keep the limb level with the body; *don't* let it sag. Turn the patient gently every 2 hours, and watch for signs of developing pressure ulcers. Report any signs of pressure ulcer formation immediately.
▶ Support the cast with firm pillows, and smooth rough cast edges by petaling with pieces of adhesive tape or moleskin. Check circulation and drainage; if a wet spot appears on the cast, circle it with a marking pen, and note the time of appearance (on the cast). Be aware of how much drainage is expected. Check the circled spot at least

every 4 hours. Report any enlargement immediately.

▶ Protect the patient from mishaps, such as jerky movements and falls, which may threaten bone integrity. Report sudden pain, crepitus, or deformity immediately. Watch for any sudden malposition of the limb, which may indicate fracture.

▶ Provide emotional support and appropriate diversions. Before discharge, teach the patient how to protect and clean the wound and, most important, how to recognize signs of recurring infection (increased temperature, redness, localized heat, and swelling). Stress the need for follow-up examinations. Instruct the patient to seek prompt treatment for possible sources of recurrence—blisters, boils, styes, and impetigo.

REFERENCES

1. Cleveland Clinic Center for Consumer Health Information (2004 February 6). "Osteomyelitis" [Online]. Available at *www.clevelandclinic.org/health/health-info/docs/2700/2702.asp?index=9495.*
2. Kalyoussef, S., and Tolan, R.W. (2006 May 26). "Osteomyelitis" [Online]. Available at *www.emedicine.com/ped/topic1677.htm.*
3. Johnston, B.L., and Conly, J.M. "Osteomyelitis Management: More Art than Science?" *The Canadian Journal of Infectious Diseases and Medical Microbiology* 18(2):115-18, March-April 2007.
4. Beals, R.K., and Bryant, R.E. "The Treatment of Chronic Open Osteomyelitis of the Tibia in Adults," *Clinics of Orthopaedics and Related Research* (433):212-17, April 2005.

OSTEOPOROSIS

Osteoporosis is a metabolic bone disorder in which the rate of bone resorption accelerates while the rate of bone formation slows down, causing a loss of bone mass. Bones affected by this disease lose calcium and phosphate salts and thus become porous, brittle, and abnormally vulnerable to fractures. Osteoporosis may be primary or secondary to an underlying disease. Primary osteoporosis is commonly called *postmenopausal osteoporosis* because it typically develops in postmenopausal women.

Causes and incidence

Many factors are known to contribute to primary osteoporosis. Poor nutrition, including mild but prolonged negative calcium balance resulting from an inadequate dietary intake of calcium, may be an important contributing factor—as well as low body weight, smoking, excessive alcohol use, and a sedentary lifestyle.[1] Other factors include aging and inherited traits, such as a family history of fractures, a slender body build, fair skin, or Caucasian or Asian ethnicity.[1] Causes of secondary osteoporosis are many: prolonged therapy with steroids or heparin, total immobilization or disuse of a bone (as with hemiplegia, for example), alcoholism, malnutrition, malabsorption, scurvy, lactose intolerance, osteogenesis imperfecta, Sudeck's atrophy (localized to hands and feet, with recurring attacks), and endocrine disorders (hypopituitarism, acromegaly, thyrotoxicosis, long-standing diabetes mellitus, hyperthyroidism). Many diseases and medications used to treat these conditions are risk factors that can increase the risk of osteoporosis and broken bones.[5]

The incidence of osteoporosis is high, with an estimated 10 million U.S. residents suffering from osteoporosis. Incidence is higher in women than in men, with women accounting for 80% of osteoporosis cases.[2] An additional 34 million U.S. residents are thought to have low bone mass, or osteopenia.[2] An estimated 30% of women have osteopenia, which can deteriorate into osteoporosis.

Signs and symptoms

Osteoporosis is usually discovered incidentally on X-rays; the patient may have been

asymptomatic for years. Vertebral collapse, causing a backache with pain that radiates around the trunk, is the most common presenting feature. Any movement or jarring aggravates the backache.

In another common pattern, osteoporosis can develop insidiously, with increasing deformity, kyphosis, and loss of height. Sometimes a dowager hump is present. As bones weaken, there's a greater likelihood for spontaneous wedge fractures, pathologic fractures of the neck or femur, Colles' fractures after a minor fall, and hip fractures.

Complications
▶ Bone fractures

Diagnosis
Differential diagnosis must exclude other causes of rarefying bone disease, especially those affecting the spine, such as metastatic cancer and advanced multiple myeloma. The differential diagnosis should also exclude osteomalacia, osteogenesis imperfecta tarda, skeletal hyperparathyroidism, and hyperthyroidism. Initial evaluation should attempt to identify the specific cause of osteoporosis through the patient history.

HEALTH & SAFETY *Research has shown that early identification of osteoporosis significantly improves patient outcomes.*[6]

▶ Bone mineral density testing is performed in dual-energy X-ray absorptiometry (DEXA) and measures the mineralization of bones. It's the gold standard for evaluating osteoporosis.
▶ A spine computed tomography scan shows demineralization. Quantitative computed tomography can evaluate bone density but is less available and more expensive than DEXA.
▶ X-rays show fracture or vertebral collapse in severe cases.
▶ Urine calcium can provide evidence of bone turnover but is limited in value.

Treatment
Treatment aims to slow down or prevent bone loss, prevent additional fractures, and control pain. A physical therapy program that emphasizes gentle exercise and activity is an important part of the treatment. Medications may include bisphosphonates, such as alendronate, risedronate, and zoledronic acid to prevent bone loss and reduce the risk of fractures.[2] The physician may also recommend adequate calcium and vitamin D intake. Raloxifene and calcitonin may also have been prescribed. Weakened vertebrae should be supported, usually with a back brace. Surgery can correct pathologic fractures of the femur by open reduction and internal fixation. Colles' fracture requires reduction with plaster immobilization for 4 to 10 weeks.

The incidence of primary osteoporosis may be reduced through adequate intake of dietary calcium and regular exercise. Exercise therapy increases bone density at the lumbar spine and hip in postmenopausal women.[3] Hormone therapy (HT) with estrogen and progesterone may retard bone loss and prevent the occurrence of fractures; however, this therapy remains controversial due to adverse effects.[2] HT decreases bone reabsorption and increases bone mass. Secondary osteoporosis can be prevented through effective treatment of the underlying disease as well as corticosteroid therapy, early mobilization after surgery or trauma, careful observation for signs of malabsorption, and prompt treatment of hyperthyroidism. Decreased alcohol consumption and caffeine use as well as smoking cessation are also helpful preventive measures. Although fluoride treatments have been used to increase bone mass density, research shows that fluoride doesn't result in a decrease in vertebral fractures and causes GI adverse effects.[4]

Special considerations

Your care plan should focus on the patient's fragility. Stress careful positioning, ambulation, and prescribed exercises.

▶ Check the patient's skin daily for redness, warmth, and new sites of pain, which may indicate new fractures. Encourage activity; help the patient walk several times daily. As appropriate, perform passive range-of-motion exercises, or encourage the patient to perform active exercises. Make sure the patient regularly attends scheduled physical therapy sessions.

▶ Impose safety precautions. Keep the side rails of the patient's bed in the raised position. Move the patient gently and carefully at all times. Explain to the patient's family and ancillary health care personnel how easily osteoporotic bones can shatter.

▶ Provide a balanced diet high in nutrients that support skeletal metabolism: vitamin D, calcium, and protein. Administer analgesics and heat to relieve pain.

▶ Make sure the patient and her family clearly understand the prescribed drug regimen. Tell them how to recognize significant adverse effects and to report them immediately. The patient should also report any new pain sites immediately, especially after trauma, no matter how slight. Advise the patient to sleep on a firm mattress and avoid excessive bed rest. Make sure she knows how to wear her back brace.

▶ Thoroughly explain osteoporosis to the patient and her family. If the patient and her family don't understand the nature of this disease, the patient may be more susceptible to fractures that could have been prevented if they had been better educated and therefore, more careful.

▶ Teach the patient to use good body mechanics—to stoop before lifting anything and to avoid twisting movements and prolonged bending.

REFERENCES

1. American Academy of Orthopaedic Surgeons (2007 July). "Osteoporosis" [Online]. Available at http://orthoinfo.aaos.org/topic.cfm?topic=A00232.
2. National Osteoporosis Foundation (2007). "Fast Facts" [Online]. Available at www.nof.org/osteoporosis/diseasefacts.htm.
3. Bonaiuti, D., et al. "Exercise for Preventing and Treating Osteoporosis in Postmenopausal Women," Cochrane Database of Systematic Reviews (3):CD000333, 2002.
4. Haguenauer, D., et al. "Fluoride for Treating Postmenopausal Osteoporosis," Cochrane Database of Systematic Reviews (4):CD002825, 2000.
5. NIH Osteoporosis and Related Bone Diseases Resource Center (2007 December). "Osteoporosis" [Online]. Available at www.niams.nih.gov/Health%5FInfo/Bone/Osteoporosis/default.asp.
6. Levine, J.P. "Effective Strategies to Identify Postmenopausal Women at Risk for Osteoporosis," Geriatrics 62(11):22-30, November 2007.

PAGET'S DISEASE

Paget's disease, also called *osteitis deformans*, is a slowly progressive metabolic bone disease characterized by an initial phase of excessive bone resorption (osteoclastic phase), followed by a reactive phase of excessive abnormal bone formation (osteoblastic phase). The new bone structure, which is chaotic, fragile, and weak, causes painful deformities of both external contour and internal structure. Paget's disease usually localizes in one or more areas of the skeleton (most commonly the lower torso), but occasionally skeletal deformity is widely distributed. It can be fatal, particularly when it's associated with heart failure (widespread disease creates a continuous need for high cardiac output), bone sarcoma, or giant-cell tumors. Although bone sarcoma (osteosarcoma) is a rare complication of

Paget's disease with a very low incidence rate, nearly all osteosarcomas that occur in adults older than age 60, do so in patients with Paget's disease.[3]

Causes and incidence

The disease occurs worldwide, but is more common in areas with people of Anglo-Saxon descent such as Western Europe, England, the United States, Australia, and New Zealand.[1] The disease occurs in males and females and affects 1.5% to 8% of people older than age 50.[2] Although the exact cause is unknown, one theory holds that early viral infection causes a dormant skeletal infection that erupts many years later as Paget's disease. There's evidence of measles virus in the bone lesions of Paget's disease.[2] Research continues to explore this cause. Genetic factors are also suspected since Paget's disease can be found in 25% to 40% of relatives with the disease.[1]

Signs and symptoms

Clinical effects of Paget's disease vary. Early stages may not produce symptoms, but when pain does develop, it's usually severe and persistent and may coexist with impaired movement resulting from impingement of abnormal bone on the spinal cord or sensory nerve root. Such pain intensifies with weight bearing.

The patient with skull involvement shows characteristic cranial enlargement over frontal and occipital areas (hat size may increase) and may complain of headaches. Other deformities include kyphosis (spinal curvature due to compression fractures of pagetic vertebrae), accompanied by a barrel-shaped chest and asymmetrical bowing of the tibia and femur, which commonly reduces height. Pagetic sites are warm and tender and are susceptible to pathologic fractures after minor trauma. Pagetic fractures heal slowly and usually incompletely. Hip replacement surgery is increased for patients

who have an associated diagnosis of osteoporosis.[3]

Bony impingement on the cranial nerves may cause blindness and hearing loss with tinnitus and vertigo. Other complications include hypertension, renal calculi, hypercalcemia, gout, heart failure, and a waddling gait (from softening of pelvic bones).

Complications

▶ Slow healing fractures of involved sites after minor trauma
▶ Paraplegia from vertebral collapse or vascular changes that affect the spinal cord
▶ Blindness and hearing loss with tinnitus and vertigo resulting from bony impingement on cranial nerves
▶ Osteoarthritis
▶ Sarcoma
▶ Hypertension
▶ Renal calculi
▶ Hypercalcemia
▶ Gout
▶ Heart failure
▶ Waddling gait from softened pelvic bones

Diagnosis

X-rays taken before overt symptoms develop show increased bone expansion and density. A bone scan, which is more sensitive than X-rays, clearly shows early pagetic lesions (radioisotope collects around areas of active disease).[2] Computed tomography scan or magnetic resonance imaging shows extra bony extension if sarcomatous degeneration occurs. Bone biopsy reveals characteristic mosaic pattern.

Other laboratory findings include:
▶ elevated serum alkaline phosphatase levels (an index of osteoblastic activity and bone formation)
▶ elevated serum calcium.

Increasing use of routine chemistry screens (including serum alkaline phosphatase) is making early diagnosis more common. Serum osteocalcin and N-telopeptide are usually increased.

Treatment

Primary treatment consists of drug therapy and includes one of the following:

▶ Bisphosphonates, such as zoledronic acid, etidronate, alendronate, pamidronate, tiludronate, and risedronate, produce rapid reduction in bone turnover and relieve pain. They also reduce serum alkaline phosphate and urinary hydroxyproline secretion. Therapy produces noticeable improvement after 1 to 3 months. Oral calcium and vitamin D supplements are recommended to decrease hypocalcemia in patients using bisphosphonates.[2]

▶ Calcitonin (subcutaneously) is used to retard bone resorption (which relieves bone lesions and pain) and reduce levels of serum alkaline phosphate and urinary hydroxyproline secretion. Calcitonin is used for patients who can't tolerate bisphosphates.[2]

▶ Analgesics such as acetaminophen, nonsteroidal anti-inflammatory drugs (NSAIDs) or COX-2 inhibitors are used to manage pain.[2]

Orthopedic surgery is used to correct specific deformities in severe cases, reduce or prevent pathologic fractures, correct secondary deformities, or relieve neurologic impairment. For patients who have an associated diagnosis of osteoporosis, the need for hip replacement surgery increases more than threefold.[3] In these instances, joint replacement presents challenges, however. Bonding material (methyl methacrylate) doesn't set properly on pagetic bone.

Other treatment varies according to symptoms. Analgesics or NSAIDs may be given to control pain.

IN THE NEWS *Future goals to manage Paget's disease include preventive treatment measures. Because it's now possible to identify people who are genetically predisposed to developing Paget's disease, early treatment intervention is being investigated. Clinical studies will need to determine how effective it is to treat minimally symptomatic patients with more potent medications in an effort to prevent disease progression.[3]*

Special considerations

Patients with Paget's disease require the following special considerations:

▶ To evaluate the effectiveness of analgesics, and assess the level of pain daily. Watch for new areas of pain or restricted movements, which may indicate new fracture sites, and sensory or motor disturbances, such as difficulty in hearing, seeing, or walking.

▶ Monitor serum calcium and alkaline phosphatase levels.

▶ If the patient is confined to prolonged bed rest, prevent pressure ulcers by providing good skin care. Reposition the patient frequently, and use a flotation mattress. Provide high-topped sneakers to prevent footdrop.

▶ Monitor intake and output. Encourage adequate fluid intake to minimize renal calculi formation.

▶ Demonstrate how to inject calcitonin properly and rotate injection sites or how to perform nasal inhalation if that's the form prescribed. Warn the patient that adverse effects may occur (nausea, vomiting, local inflammatory reaction at injection site, facial flushing, itching of hands, and fever). Give reassurance that these adverse effects are usually mild and infrequent.

▶ To help the patient adjust to the changes in lifestyle imposed by this disease, teach him how to pace activities and, if necessary, how to use assistive devices. Encourage him to follow a recommended exercise program, avoiding both immobilization and excessive activity. Suggest a firm mattress or a bed board to minimize spinal deformities. Warn against imprudent use of analgesics because diminished sensitivity to pain resulting from analgesic use may make the patient unaware of new fractures. To prevent falls at home, advise removal of throw rugs and other obstacles.

▶ Help the patient and his family make use of community support resources, such as a visiting nurse or home health agency. For more information, refer them to the Paget's Foundation. (The Web site for the New York, NY organization is *www.paget.org/.*)

REFERENCES

1. American Academy of Orthopaedic Surgeons (2007 October). "Paget's Disease of Bone" [Online]. Available at: *http://orthoinfo.aaos.org/topic.cfm?topic=A00076.*
2. The Paget Foundation (2007). "A Nurse's Guide to the Management of Paget's Disease of Bone" [Online]. Available at *www.paget.org/pdf/nurse-guide2007.pdf.*
3. Langston, L., and Ralston, S.H. "Management of Paget's Disease of Bone," *British Society for Rheumatology Oxford Journals.* 43(8):955-59, 2004.

RHABDOMYOLYSIS

Rhabdomyolysis is the breakdown of muscle fibers that results in the release of muscle fiber content into the circulation. It results from the toxicity of destroyed muscle cells, causing kidney damage or failure. Predisposing factors include trauma, ischemia, polymyositis, and drug overdose. Toxins and environmental, infectious, and metabolic factors may induce it. Rhabdomyolysis accounts for 8% to 15% of cases of acute renal failure; about 5% of cases result in death.[1]

Causes and incidence

Rhabdomyolysis follows direct injury to the skeletal muscle fibers, specifically the sarcolemma, which then release myoglobin into the bloodstream. Myoglobin is an oxygen-binding protein pigment found in skeletal muscle. When this muscle is damaged, myoglobin is released into the bloodstream. It's then filtered by the kidneys.

Myoglobin may occlude the structures of the kidney, causing damage such as acute tubular necrosis or kidney failure. Myoglobin can also cause kidney failure because it breaks down into potentially toxic compounds. Necrotic skeletal muscle may cause massive fluid shifts from the bloodstream into the muscle, reducing the relative fluid volume of the body and leading to shock and reduced blood flow to the kidneys.

The disorder may be caused by any condition that results in damage to skeletal muscle. Rhabdomyolysis may result from blunt trauma; extensive burn injury; viral, bacterial, or fungal infection (such as legionnaires' disease or, especially, influenza type A or B); prolonged immobilization; near electrocution or near drowning; metabolic or genetic factors; drug therapy; or toxins. Children who engage in heavy exercise may also experience rhabdomyolysis. Other causes include shaken baby syndrome and exposure to extreme cold, heatstroke, or snakebite. Patients taking illicit drugs or multiple prescription drugs are at risk for rhabdomyolysis.[4]

In the United States, rhabdomyolysis affects about 1 in 10,000 people, with a slightly higher incidence in men than in women. It can occur in infants, toddlers, and adolescents who inherited enzyme deficiencies of carbohydrate and lipid metabolism, or in those with inherited myopathies, such as Duchenne's muscular dystrophy, and malignant hyperthermia.[2] Patients with hyperthyroidism have been found to be at an increased risk for developing rhabdomyolysis due to their increased energy consumption and depletion of energy stores.[5]

Signs and symptoms

Signs and symptoms of rhabdomyolysis include myalgia or muscle pain (especially in the thighs, calves, or lower back); weakness, tenderness, malaise, fever, dark urine, nausea, and vomiting. The patient may also experience weight gain, seizures, joint pain, and fatigue. Symptoms may be subtle initial-

ly. Acute renal failure (ARF) and a need for hemodialysis are common complications of rhabdomyolysis. Measurement of the initial serum creatinine level is a predictor of ARF and the need for hemodialysis. The initial blood urea nitrogen test is a predictor of the need for hemodialysis.[3]

Complications
▶ Kidney failure

Diagnosis
Elevations in the following laboratory data—serum CK, serum creatinine, urine myoglobin, hemoglobin, and red blood cells (RBCs)—are indicators of rhabdomyolysis.[4] A serum or urine myoglobin test is positive. Creatine kinase results that are 100 times above normal or higher suggest rhabdomyolysis. A urinalysis may reveal casts and may be positive for hemoglobin without evidence of RBCs on microscopic examination. Serum potassium may be very high (potassium is released from cells into the bloodstream when cell breakdown occurs).

Treatment
Early, aggressive hydration may prevent complications from rhabdomyolysis by rapidly eliminating the myoglobin from the kidneys. Diuretics and I.V. hydration promote diuresis. Diuretic medications, such as mannitol or furosemide, may aid in flushing the pigment out of the kidneys. If urine output is sufficient, bicarbonate may be given to maintain an alkaline urine state, thereby helping to prevent the dissociation of myoglobin into toxic compounds. Hyperkalemia should be treated if present. Kidney failure should be treated as appropriate. Dialysis may be necessary and, in severe cases, kidney transplantation.

Special considerations
▶ Monitor the patient's intake and output, vital signs, electrolyte levels, daily weight, and laboratory results.

▶ Watch for signs of renal failure (such as decreasing urine output and increasing urine specific gravity), fluid overload (such as dyspnea and tachycardia), pulmonary edema, and electrolyte imbalances (such as serum potassium).

▶ Provide reassurance and emotional support for the patient and his family.

▶ To help prevent rhabdomyolysis from occurring, ensure adequate hydration, monitor the patient for adverse reactions to any of his prescribed drugs, and monitor blood transfusion administration carefully.

REFERENCES
1. Rhabdomyolysis Kidney Failure and Damage (2007). Available at *www.rhabdomyolysis.org.*
2. Craid, S. (2006 November 3). "Rhabdomyolysis" [Online]. Available at *www.emedicine.com/emerg/topic508.htm.*
3. Fernandez, W.G., et al. "Factors Predictive of Acute Renal Failure and Need for Hemodialysis among ED Patients with Rhabdomyolysis," *American Journal of Emergency Medicine* 23(1):1-7, January 2005.
4. Melli, G., et al. "Rhabdomyolysis: An Evaluation of 475 Hospitalized Patients." *Medicine* 84(6):377-85, November 2005.
5. Lichtstein, D.M., and Arteaga, R.B. "Rhabdomyolysis Associated with Hyperthyroidism," *American Journal of the Medical Sciences* 332(2):103-105, August 2006.

TENDINITIS AND BURSITIS

*T*endinitis is a painful inflammation of tendons and of tendon-muscle attachments to bone, usually in the shoulder rotator cuff, hip, Achilles tendon, or hamstring. Some common names for various tendinitis problems are tennis elbow, golfer's elbow, pitcher's shoulder, swimmer's shoulder, and jumper's knee.[1] *Bursitis* is a painful inflammation of one or more of the bursae—closed sacs lubricated with small amounts of synovial fluid that facilitate the motion of muscles and tendons over bony promi-

nences. There are more than 150 bursae in the body.[2] Bursitis usually occurs in the subdeltoid, olecranon, trochanteric, calcaneal, or prepatellar bursae.

Causes and incidence

Tendinitis commonly results from overuse or injury (such as strain during sports activity), another musculoskeletal disorder (such as rheumatic diseases or congenital defects). It's more common in middle-age adults.

Bursitis can occur at any age but usually occurs in older individuals due to an inflammatory joint disease (such as rheumatoid arthritis or gout) or recurring trauma that stresses or pressures a joint. Chronic bursitis follows attacks of acute bursitis or repeated trauma and infection. Septic bursitis may result from infection from traumatic injury, septic arthritis, or bacteremia.

Signs and symptoms

The patient with tendinitis of the shoulder complains of restricted shoulder movement, especially abduction, and localized pain, which is most severe at night and usually interferes with sleep. The pain extends from the acromion (the shoulder's highest point) to the deltoid muscle insertion, predominantly in the so-called painful arc—that is, when the patient abducts his arm between 50 and 130 degrees. Fluid accumulation causes swelling. In calcific tendinitis, calcium deposits in the tendon cause proximal weakness and, if calcium erodes into adjacent bursae, acute calcific bursitis.

In bursitis, fluid accumulation in the bursae causes irritation, inflammation, sudden or gradual pain, and limited movement. Other symptoms vary according to the affected site. Subdeltoid bursitis impairs arm abduction, and prepatellar bursitis (housemaid's knee) produces pain when the patient climbs stairs. Hip bursitis causes pain at the hip that can extend to the outside of the thigh area. The pain may get worse with prolonged walking, stair climbing, or squatting.[3]

Complications

▸ Untreated tendinitis can cause scar tissue and subsequent disability.
▸ Untreated bursitis can cause extreme pain and restricted joint movement.

Diagnosis

In tendinitis, X-rays may be normal at first but later show bony fragments, osteophyte sclerosis, or calcium deposits. Arthrography is usually normal, with occasional small irregularities on the undersurface of the tendon. Computed tomography scan and magnetic resonance imaging (MRI) have replaced X-ray and even arthrography of the shoulder as diagnostic tools. An MRI will usually identify tears, partial tears, inflammation, or tumor but can't reveal irregularities of the tendon sheath itself. Diagnosis of tendinitis must rule out other causes of shoulder pain, such as myocardial infarction, cervical spondylosis, degenerative changes, and tendon tear or rupture. Significantly, in tendinitis, heat aggravates shoulder pain; in other painful joint disorders, heat usually provides relief.

Localized pain and inflammation and a history of unusual strain or injury 2 to 3 days before onset of pain are the bases for diagnosing bursitis. During early stages, X-rays are usually normal, except in calcific bursitis, where X-rays may show calcium deposits.

In bursitis, X-rays can't definitively diagnose the problem, yet they're helpful to rule out other causes of pain. Screening for bursitis requires combing through the patient history for related events of overuse and pressure on the affected joint, and physical assessment of the painful joint and surrounding area. Sometimes blood tests and analysis of fluid from the inflamed bursae are examined as a way to rule out other causes.[2]

Treatment

Most cases of tendinitis don't require a physician's care. Treatment for bursitis is similar to that for tendinitis and can usually be done at home.

Treatment to relieve pain includes resting the joint.[4] Other treatments include immobilization with a sling, splint, or cast; nonsteroidal anti-inflammatory drugs (NSAIDs) such as ibuprofen, naproxen, indomethacin, or oxaprozin; analgesics; application of cold or heat, ultrasound, or local injection of an anesthetic and corticosteroids to reduce inflammation. (Mixing a corticosteroid and an anesthetic such as lidocaine generally provides immediate pain relief.) Extended-release injections of a corticosteroid, such as triamcinolone or prednisolone, offer longer-term pain relief. Until the patient is free from pain and able to perform range-of-motion (ROM) exercises easily, treatment also includes oral NSAIDs (as mentioned above). Short-term analgesics include propoxyphene, codeine, acetaminophen with codeine and, occasionally, oxycodone.

Supplementary treatment for tendinitis includes fluid removal by aspiration and heat therapy. For calcific tendinitis, recommended treatment includes ice packs, physical therapy, ultrasonography, or hydrotherapy to help the patient maintain or recover ROM. It may be necessary to delay treatment until the acute attack is over to ensure maximum patient compliance. Rarely does calcific tendinitis require surgical removal of calcium deposits. Similarly, in bursitis, surgical removal of the affected bursae is seldom necessary.[2] Long-term control of chronic bursitis and tendinitis may require changes in lifestyle to prevent recurring joint irritation.

The Mayo Clinic offers these preventive measures for bursitis: stretch and strengthen muscles, take frequent breaks from repetitive tasks, cushion joints, don't sit for long periods, and practice good posture. Preventive measures for tendinitis include avoiding exercises that place excessive stress on tendons, adding variety to exercises, using proper technique, stretching, warming up before a workout, and using proper ergonomics at work.[1]

Special considerations

When treating patients with tendinitis or bursitis, remember to consider the following:
▶ Assess the severity of pain and the ROM to determine effectiveness of the treatment.
▶ Before injecting corticosteroids or local anesthetics, ask the patient about his drug allergies.
▶ Assist with intra-articular injection. Scrub the patient's skin thoroughly with povidone-iodine or a comparable solution. After the injection, massage the area to ensure penetration through the tissue and joint space. Apply ice intermittently for about 4 hours to minimize pain. Avoid applying heat to the area for 2 days.
▶ Tell the patient to take anti-inflammatory agents with milk to minimize GI distress and to report any signs of distress immediately.
▶ Advise the patient to perform strengthening exercises and avoid activities that aggravate the joint.
▶ Remind the patient to wear a splint or sling during the first few days of an attack of subdeltoid bursitis or tendinitis to support the arm and protect the shoulder, particularly at night. Demonstrate how to wear the sling so it won't put too much weight on the shoulder.
▶ Advise the patient to maintain joint mobility and prevent muscle atrophy by performing exercises or physical therapy when he's free from pain.

REFERENCES

1. MayoClinic.com (2007 November 3). "Tendinitis" [Online]. Available at *www.mayo clinic.com/health/tendinitis/DS00153.*
2. MayoClinic.com (2007 September 27). "Bursitis" [Online]. Available at *www.mayo clinic.com/health/bursitis/DS00032.*

3. American Academy of Orthopaedic Surgeons (2007 August). "Hip Bursitis" [Online]. Available at *http://orthoinfo.aaos.org/topic. cfm?topic=A00409.*

4. American College of Rheumatology (2005 May). "Tendinitis/Bursitis" [Online]. Available at *www.rheumatology.org/public/factsheets/ tendonitis_new.asp.*

6

Renal and urologic disorders

ACUTE POSTSTREPTOCOCCAL GLOMERULONEPHRITIS

Acute poststreptococcal glomerulonephritis (APSGN), also known as *acute glomerulonephritis,* is a relatively common bilateral inflammation of the glomeruli. The condition usually follows a streptococcal infection of the respiratory tract or, less commonly, a skin infection such as impetigo.[1]

Causes and incidence

APSGN results from the entrapment and collection of antigen-antibodies (produced as an immune response to streptococcus) in the glomerular capillary membranes. This induces inflammatory damage and impedes glomerular function. Sometimes, the immune complement further damages the glomerular membrane. The damaged and inflamed glomerulus loses the ability to be selectively permeable, and allows red blood cells (RBCs) and proteins to filter through as the glomerular filtration rate (GFR) falls. Uremic poisoning may result.

APSGN is most common in children ages 4 to 12, but it can occur at any age and it's more prevalent in males. Incidence of APSGN is decreasing.[1] Up to 95% of children and up to 70% of adults with APSGN recover fully; the rest may progress to chron-

ic renal failure within months. A relatively high proportion of patients can present with hypertension-reduced renal function and increased microalbuminuria 5 years after streptococcal infection.[2]

Signs and symptoms

APSGN can begin within 1 to 3 weeks after untreated pharyngitis. Symptoms include mild to moderate edema, oliguria (less than 400 ml/24 hours), proteinuria, azotemia, hematuria, and fatigue. Mild to severe hypertension may result from either sodium or water retention (due to decreased GFR) or inappropriate renin release. Heart failure from hypervolemia leads to pulmonary edema.

Complications

- Glomerulosclerosis and hypertension
- Acute kidney failure
- Chronic kidney failure
- High blood pressure
- Nephrotic syndrome

Diagnosis

Diagnosis requires a detailed patient history and assessment of clinical symptoms and laboratory tests.

Urinalysis typically reveals proteinuria and hematuria. RBCs, white blood cells, and mixed cell casts are common in urinary sediment. Elevated serum creatinine levels and

low creatinine clearance accompany impaired glomerular filtration. Elevated antistreptolysin-O titers (in 80% of patients), elevated streptozyme and antideoxyribonuclease-B titers, and low serum complement levels verify recent streptococcal infection. A throat culture may also show group A betahemolytic streptococcus. Renal ultrasound may show a normal or slightly enlarged kidney. A renal biopsy may confirm the diagnosis or assess renal tissue status.

HEALTH & SAFETY *Although there's no prevention for APSGN, early treatment of a strep infection causing a sore throat and maintaining normal blood pressure and blood glucose levels may help reduce kidney damage and the likeliness of APSGN.*[3]

Treatment

The goals of treatment are relief of symptoms and prevention of complications. Vigorous supportive care includes bed rest, fluid and dietary sodium restrictions, and correction of electrolyte imbalances (possibly with dialysis, although this is rarely necessary). Therapy may include diuretics to reduce extracellular fluid overload and an antihypertensive. The use of antibiotics is recommended for 7 to 10 days if staphylococcal infection is documented. Otherwise, antibiotic use is controversial.

Special considerations

APSGN usually resolves within 2 weeks, so patient care is primarily supportive.
▶ Check vital signs and electrolyte values. Monitor intake and output and daily weight. Assess renal function daily through serum creatinine, blood urea nitrogen, and urine creatinine clearance levels. Watch for and immediately report signs of acute renal failure (oliguria, azotemia, and acidosis).
▶ Consult a dietitian to provide a diet high in calories and low in protein, sodium, potassium, and fluids.

▶ Protect the debilitated patient against secondary infection by providing good nutrition, using good hygienic technique, and preventing contact with infected persons.
▶ Bed rest is necessary during the acute phase. Allow the patient to *gradually* resume normal activities as symptoms subside.
▶ Provide emotional support for the patient and his family. If the patient is on dialysis, explain the procedure fully.
▶ Advise the patient with a history of chronic upper respiratory tract infections to immediately report signs of infection, such as fever or a sore throat.
▶ Tell the patient that follow-up examinations are necessary to detect chronic renal failure. Stress the need for regular blood pressure, urinary protein, and renal function assessments during the convalescent months to detect recurrence. After APSGN, gross hematuria may recur during nonspecific viral infections; abnormal urinary findings may persist for years.
▶ Encourage pregnant females with a history of APSGN to have frequent medical evaluations because pregnancy further stresses the kidneys and increases the risk of chronic renal failure.

REFERENCES

1. Hahn, R.G., et al. "Evaluation of Poststreptococcal Illness," *American Family Physician* 71(10):1949-954, May 2005.
2. Sesso, R., and Pinto, D.W. "Five-Year Follow-Up of Patients with Epidemic Glomerulonephritis Due to Streptococcus Zooepidemicus" *Nephrology Dialysis Transplantation* 20(9):1808-812, September 2005.
3. Mayo Clinic Staff (2007 April 5). "Glomerulonephritis" [Online]. Available at *www.MayoClinic.com*.

ACUTE PYELONEPHRITIS

Acute pyelonephritis (also known as *acute infective tubulointerstitial nephritis*) is a sudden inflammation caused by bacteria that primarily affects the interstitial area and the renal pelvis or, less commonly, the renal tubules. It's one of the most common renal diseases. There are approximately 250,000 newly diagnosed cases of acute pyelonephritis each year in the United States, resulting in more than 100,000 hospitalizations. With treatment and continued follow-up care, the prognosis is good, and extensive permanent damage is rare.

Causes and incidence

Acute pyelonephritis results from bacterial infection of the kidneys. Infecting bacteria usually are normal intestinal and fecal flora that grow readily in urine. The most common causative organism is *Escherichia coli,* but *Staphylococcus saprophyticus, Klebsiella pneumoniae, Proteus, Pseudomonas, Staphylococcus aureus,* and *Enterococcus faecalis* may also cause this infection.[1]

Typically, the infection spreads from the bladder to the ureters, then to the kidneys, as in vesicoureteral reflux due to congenital weakness at the junction of the ureter and the bladder. Bacteria refluxed to intrarenal tissues may create colonies of infection within 24 to 48 hours. Infection may also result from instrumentation (such as catheterization, cystoscopy, or urologic surgery), from a hematogenic infection (as in septicemia or endocarditis), or possibly from lymphatic infection.

Pyelonephritis may also result from an inability to empty the bladder (for example, in patients with neurogenic bladder), urinary stasis, or urinary obstruction due to tumors, strictures, or benign prostatic hyperplasia.

Pyelonephritis is more common in females,[1] probably because of a shorter urethra and the proximity of the urinary meatus to the vagina and the rectum—both conditions allow bacteria to reach the bladder more easily—and a lack of the antibacterial prostatic secretions produced in the male. Few women younger than age 50 are hospitalized with pyelonephritis.

Incidence increases with age and is higher in the following groups:

▶ *Sexually active females:* Intercourse increases the risk of bacterial contamination.
▶ *Pregnant females:* About 5% develop asymptomatic bacteriuria; if untreated, about 40% develop pyelonephritis.
▶ *Diabetic people:* Neurogenic bladder causes incomplete emptying and urinary stasis; glycosuria may support bacterial growth in the urine.
▶ *People with other renal diseases:* Compromised renal function aggravates susceptibility.

Signs and symptoms

Typical clinical features include urgency, frequency, burning during urination, dysuria, nocturia, and hematuria (usually microscopic but may be gross). Urine may appear cloudy and have an ammonia-like or fishy odor. Other common symptoms include a temperature of 102° F (38.9° C) or higher, shaking chills, flank pain, anorexia, and general fatigue.

These symptoms characteristically develop rapidly over a few hours or a few days. Although these symptoms may disappear within days, even without treatment, residual bacterial infection is likely and may cause symptoms to recur later.

Complications

▶ Secondary arteriosclerosis
▶ Calculus formation
▶ Renal damage
▶ Renal abscesses with possible metastasis to other organs
▶ Septic shock
▶ Chronic pyelonephritis

Chronic pyelonephritis

Chronic pyelonephritis is a persistent kidney inflammation that can scar the kidneys and may lead to chronic renal failure. Its etiology may be bacterial, metastatic, or urogenous. This disease is most common in patients who are predisposed to recurrent acute pyelonephritis, such as those with urinary obstructions or vesicoureteral reflux.

Patients with chronic pyelonephritis may have a childhood history of unexplained fevers or bedwetting. Clinical effects may include flank pain, anemia, low urine specific gravity, proteinuria, leukocytes in urine and, especially in late stages, hypertension. Uremia rarely develops from chronic pyelonephritis unless structural abnormalities exist in the excretory system. Bacteriuria may be intermittent. When no bacteria are found in the urine, diagnosis depends on excretory urography (the renal pelvis may appear small and flattened) and renal biopsy.

Effective treatment of chronic pyelonephritis requires control of hypertension, elimination of the existing obstruction (when possible), and long-term antimicrobial therapy.

Diagnosis

Diagnosis is confirmed by urinalysis and culture. Typical findings include:

▶ Pyuria (pus in urine): Urine sediment reveals the presence of leukocytes singly, in clumps, and in casts; and, possibly, a few red blood cells.

▶ Significant bacteriuria: Urine culture reveals more than 10,000 colony forming organisms/mm².

▶ Low specific gravity and osmolality: These findings result from a temporarily decreased ability to concentrate urine.

▶ Slightly alkaline urine pH.

▶ Proteinuria, glycosuria, and ketonuria: These conditions are less common.

Excretory urography or computed tomography scan of the kidneys, ureters, and bladder also help in the evaluation of acute pyelonephritis by revealing calculi, tumors, or cysts in the kidneys and the urinary tract. In addition, excretory urography may show asymmetrical kidneys.

Treatment

The ultimate goal of treatment is to decrease the incidence of infection in order to protect the kidneys.[2] Treatment centers on antibiotic therapy appropriate to the specific infecting organism after identification by urine culture and sensitivity studies. When the infecting organism can't be identified, therapy usually consists of a broad-spectrum antibiotic. Levofloxacin and gatifloxacin are gaining popularity for use against urinary tract infections (UTIs).[3] Urinary analgesics are also appropriate. If the patient is pregnant, antibiotics must be prescribed cautiously.

Symptoms may disappear after several days of antibiotic therapy. Although urine usually becomes sterile within 48 to 72 hours, the course of such therapy is 10 to 14 days. Follow-up treatment may include reculturing urine 1 week after drug therapy stops, then periodically for the next year to detect residual or recurring infection. Most patients with uncomplicated infections respond well to therapy and don't suffer reinfection.

In infection from obstruction or vesicoureteral reflux, antibiotics may be less effective; surgery may be necessary to relieve the obstruction or correct the anomaly. Patients at high risk for recurring UTIs and kidney infections, such as those with prolonged use of an indwelling catheter or maintenance antibiotic therapy, require long-term follow-up. Recurrent episodes of acute pyelonephritis can eventually result in chronic pyelonephritis. (See *Chronic pyelonephritis*.)

Special considerations

Patient care is supportive during antibiotic treatment of the underlying infection.

▶ Administer antipyretics for fever.

▶ Encourage fluids to achieve urine output of more than 2,000 ml/day. This helps to empty the bladder of contaminated urine. Don't encourage intake of more than 2 to 3 qt (2 to 3 L) because this may decrease the effectiveness of the antibiotics.

▶ Teach the patient the proper technique for collecting a clean-catch urine specimen. Be sure to refrigerate or culture a urine specimen within 30 minutes of collection to prevent overgrowth of bacteria.

▶ Make sure the patient knows how important it is to complete the prescribed antibiotic therapy, even after symptoms subside. Encourage long-term follow-up care for high-risk patients.

To prevent acute pyelonephritis:

▶ Observe strict sterile technique during catheter insertion and care.

▶ Instruct females to prevent bacterial contamination by wiping the perineum from front to back after defecation.

▶ Advise routine checkups for patients with a history of UTIs. Teach them to recognize signs of infection, such as cloudy urine, burning on urination, urgency, and frequency, especially when accompanied by a low-grade fever.

▶ Carefully monitor pregnant patients for the development of a UTI. UTIs should be treated promptly in this population to prevent the development of pyelonephritis.[4]

REFERENCES

1. Ramakrishnan, K., and Scheid, D.C. "Diagnosis and Management of Acute Pyelonephritis in Adults," *American Family Physician* 71(5):933-42, March 2005.
2. Dulczak, S., and Kirk, J. "Overview of the Evaluation, Diagnosis, and Management of Urinary Tract Infections in Infants and Children," *Urologic Nursing* 25(3):185-91, June 2005.
3. Liu, H., and Mulholland, S.G. "Appropriate Antibiotic Treatment of Genitourinary Infections in Hospitalized Patients," *American Journal of Medicine* 118(Suppl 7A):14S-20S, July 2005.
4. Morgan, K.L. "Management of UTIs during Pregnancy," *American Journal of Maternal and Child Nursing* 29(4):254-58, July-August 2004.

ACUTE RENAL FAILURE

Acute renal failure (also called *acute kidney injury*) is the sudden interruption of kidney function due to obstruction, reduced circulation, or renal parenchymal disease. It's usually reversible with medical treatment; otherwise, it may progress to end-stage renal disease, uremic syndrome, and death.

Causes and incidence

The causes of acute renal failure are classified as prerenal, intrinsic (or parenchymal), and postrenal. Prerenal failure is associated with diminished blood flow to the kidneys, possibly resulting from hypovolemia, shock, severe anaphylaxis, embolism, blood loss, sepsis, pooling of fluid in ascites or burns; or from cardiovascular disorders, such as heart failure, arrhythmias, and tamponade.

Intrinsic renal failure results from damage to the kidneys themselves, usually due to acute tubular necrosis, but possibly due to acute poststreptococcal glomerulonephritis, systemic lupus erythematosus, periarteritis nodosa, vasculitis, sickle-cell disease, bilateral renal vein thrombosis, nephrotoxins, chronic misuse of nonsteroidal anti-inflammatory drugs, radiopaque contrast agents, ischemia, renal myeloma, acute pyelonephritis, and exposure to heavy metals, such as lead or mercury.

Postrenal failure results from bilateral obstruction of urinary outflow. Its multiple causes include renal calculi, blood clots, papillae from papillary necrosis, tumors, benign prostatic hyperplasia, strictures, and urethral edema from catheterization.

In the United States, the annual incidence of acute renal failure is 100 cases for every million people. It's diagnosed in 1% of hos-

Renal failure: preoperative risk factors

Question: *Is there a way to determine which patients are at a higher risk for acute renal failure after surgery?*

Research: Surgical procedures are a known risk factor for acute renal failure. In an effort to determine which patients may be most at risk, the authors completed an observational, prospective study of 15,102 patients—all of whom had major, noncardiac surgery, and a preoperative creatinine clearance of greater than 80 ml/minute. The authors identified seven additional preoperative risk factors for acute renal failure: age, emergency surgery, liver disease, body mass index, high-risk surgery, peripheral vascular occlusive disease, and chronic obstructive pulmonary disease that requires chronic bronchodilator therapy.

Conclusion: Patients who had several risk factors for acute renal failure were more likely to develop acute renal failure after surgery than patients with fewer risk factors. A total of 121 patients developed acute renal failure, with 14 requiring renal replacement therapy.

Application: Nurses should be aware of their preoperative patient's risk factors for acute renal failure. When a patient with several risk factors returns to the unit after surgery, the nurse should pay special attention to the urine output, creatinine clearance, and renal function laboratory tests for that patient. This may help prevent high-risk patients from developing acute renal failure postoperatively.

Source: Kheterpal, S., et al. "Predictors of Post-Operative Acute Renal Failure after Noncardiac Surgery in Patients with Previously Normal Renal Function," *Anesthesiology* 107(6):892-902, December 2007.

---

pital admissions. Hospital-acquired acute renal failure occurs in 4% of all admitted patients and 20% of patients who are admitted to intensive care units. (See *Renal failure: preoperative risk factors.*)

Signs and symptoms

Acute renal failure is a critical illness. Its early signs are oliguria, azotemia and, rarely, anuria. Electrolyte imbalance, metabolic acidosis, and other severe effects follow, as the patient becomes increasingly uremic and renal dysfunction disrupts other body systems:

▶ *GI:* anorexia, nausea, vomiting, diarrhea or constipation, stomatitis, bleeding, hematemesis, dry mucous membranes, uremic breath
▶ *Central nervous system (CNS):* headache, drowsiness, irritability, confusion, peripheral neuropathy, seizures, coma

▶ *Cutaneous:* dryness, pruritus, pallor, purpura and, rarely, uremic frost
▶ *Cardiovascular:* early in the disease, hypotension; later, hypertension, arrhythmias, fluid overload, heart failure, systemic edema, anemia, altered clotting mechanisms
▶ *Respiratory:* pulmonary edema, Kussmaul's respirations.

Complications
▶ Renal shutdown
▶ Electrolyte imbalance
▶ Metabolic acidosis
▶ Acute pulmonary edema
▶ Hypertensive crisis
▶ Hyperkalemia
▶ Infection
▶ Death

Diagnosis

The patient's history may include a disorder that can cause renal failure. Blood test results indicating acute renal failure include elevated blood urea nitrogen, serum creatinine, and potassium levels and low blood pH, bicarbonate, hematocrit (HCT), and hemoglobin (Hb) level. Urine specimens show casts, cellular debris, decreased specific gravity and, in glomerular diseases, proteinuria and urine osmolality close to serum osmolality. Urine sodium level is less than 20 mEq/L if oliguria is due to decreased perfusion; more than 40 mEq/L if due to an intrinsic problem. Ultrasound is used for patients with previously undiagnosed renal failure to differentiate between acute renal failure and chronic renal failure.[1] Other studies include kidney-ureter-bladder X-rays, cautious use of excretory urography, renal scan, and nephrotomography.

Treatment

The goal of treatment is to correct or eliminate any reversible causes of kidney failure, such as obstructive uropathy, volume depletion, or the use of kidney-toxic medications. Supportive measures include supplemental vitamins, restricted fluids, and a diet high in calories but low in protein, sodium, and potassium. Meticulous electrolyte monitoring is essential to detect hyperkalemia. If hyperkalemia occurs, acute therapy may include dialysis, I.V. administration of hypertonic glucose, insulin infusion, sodium bicarbonate, and administration of a potassium exchange resin (orally or by enema) to remove potassium from the body.

If measures fail to control uremic symptoms, hemodialysis or peritoneal dialysis may be necessary. Continuous arteriovenous hemodiafiltration and continuous venovenous hemodiafiltration are alternative hemodialysis techniques for the treatment of acute renal failure. They're generally reserved for when intermittent dialysis fails to control hypervolemia or uremia, or for patients for whom peritoneal dialysis isn't possible.

Special considerations

Patient care includes careful monitoring and dietary education.

▶ Measure and record intake and output, including all body fluids, such as wound drainage, nasogastric output, and diarrhea. Weigh the patient daily.

▶ Assess Hb levels and HCT, and replace blood components, as ordered.

▶ Monitor vital signs. Watch for and report any signs of pericarditis (pleuritic chest pain, tachycardia, pericardial friction rub), inadequate renal perfusion (hypotension), and acidosis.

▶ Maintain proper electrolyte balance. Strictly monitor potassium levels. Watch for symptoms of hyperkalemia (malaise, anorexia, paresthesia, or muscle weakness) and electrocardiogram changes (tall, peaked T waves, widening QRS segment, and disappearing P waves), and report them immediately. Don't administer medications containing potassium.

▶ If a patient with impaired renal function is scheduled for a procedure with contrast medium, administer N-acetylcysteine before the procedure to help protect the kidneys.[3]

▶ Assess the patient frequently, especially during emergency treatment to lower potassium levels. If the patient receives hypertonic glucose and insulin infusions, monitor potassium levels. If you give sodium polystyrene sulfonate rectally, prevent bowel perforation by making sure the patient doesn't retain it and become constipated.

▶ Consult a dietitian and maintain nutritional status. Provide a high-calorie, low-protein, low-sodium, and low-potassium diet, with vitamin supplements. Give the anorectic patient small, frequent meals. If enteral nutrition is required, use renal formulas that avoid excessive amounts of vitamins C and A, and make sure protein needs are met.[2]

▶ Use sterile technique, because the patient with acute renal failure is highly susceptible to infection. Personnel with upper respiratory tract infections shouldn't provide care for the patient.

▶ Prevent complications of immobility by encouraging frequent coughing and deep breathing, and by performing passive range-of-motion exercises. Help the patient walk as soon as possible.

▶ Provide good mouth care frequently because mucous membranes are dry. If stomatitis occurs, an antibiotic solution may be ordered. Have the patient swish the solution around in his mouth before swallowing.

▶ Monitor for GI bleeding by guaiac testing all stools for blood. Administer medications carefully, especially antacids and stool softeners. Use aluminum-hydroxide–based antacids; magnesium-based antacids can cause serum magnesium levels to rise to critical levels.

▶ Use appropriate safety measures, such as side rails and restraints because the patient with CNS involvement may be dizzy or confused.

▶ Provide emotional support to the patient and his family. Give reassurance by clearly explaining all procedures.

▶ If the patient requires hemodialysis, check the blood access site (arteriovenous fistula, subclavian or femoral catheter) as per facility protocol or every 2 hours for patency and signs of clotting. Don't use the arm with the shunt or fistula for taking blood pressures or drawing blood. Weigh the patient before beginning dialysis. During dialysis, monitor vital signs, clotting times, blood flow, the function of the vascular access site, and arterial and venous pressures. Watch for complications, such as septicemia, embolism, hepatitis, and rapid fluid and electrolyte loss. After dialysis, monitor vital signs and the vascular access site; weigh the patient;

watch for signs of fluid and electrolyte imbalances.[4]

▶ During peritoneal dialysis, position the patient carefully. Elevate the head of the bed to reduce pressure on the diaphragm and aid respiration. Be alert for signs of infection (cloudy drainage, elevated temperature) and, rarely, bleeding. If pain occurs, reduce the amount of dialysate. Monitor the diabetic patient's blood glucose periodically, and administer insulin as ordered. Watch for complications, such as peritonitis, atelectasis, hypokalemia, pneumonia, and shock.

▶ Use standard precautions when handling all blood and body fluids.

REFERENCES

1. Bush, W.H., et al. (2008 April 7). "Renal Failure" [Online]. Available at *www.guideline. gov/summary/summary.aspx?doc_id=8283& nbr=004615&string=renal+AND+failure.*
2. Cotton, A.B. "Medical Nutrition Therapy in Acute Kidney Injury," *Nephrology Nursing Journal* 34(4):444-46, July-August 2007.
3. Marthaler, M.T., and Keresztes, P.A. "Evidence-based Practice for the Use of N-acetylcysteine," *Dimensions in Critical Care Nursing* 23(6):270-73, November-December 2004.
4. National Kidney Foundation NKF/KDOQI Guidelines. "Clinical Practice Guidelines and Clinical Practice Recommendations for Hemodialysis Adequacy, 2006 Update" [Online]. Available at *www.kidney.org/ professionals/kdoqi/guideline_upHD_PD_VA/ index.htm.*

ACUTE TUBULAR NECROSIS

Acute tubular necrosis (ATN), also known as *acute tubulointerstitial nephritis,* accounts for about 75% of all cases of acute renal failure and is the most common cause of acute renal failure in critically ill patients. Over 95% of cases re-

sult from infection or an allergic drug reaction. ATN injures the tubular segment of the nephron, causing renal failure and uremic syndrome. Mortality ranges from 40% to 70%, depending on complications from underlying diseases. Nonoliguric forms of ATN have a better prognosis.

Causes and incidence

ATN results from ischemic or nephrotoxic injury, most commonly in debilitated patients, such as the critically ill or those who have undergone extensive surgery. In ischemic injury, disruption of blood flow to the kidneys may result from circulatory collapse, severe hypotension, trauma, hemorrhage, dehydration, cardiogenic or septic shock, surgery, anesthetics, or reactions to transfusions. Nephrotoxic injury may follow ingestion of certain chemical agents or result from a hypersensitive reaction of the kidneys.[3] (See *Rise in nephrotoxic injury*.) Because nephrotoxic ATN doesn't damage the basement membrane of the nephron, it's potentially reversible. However, ischemic ATN can damage the epithelial and basement membranes and can cause lesions in the renal interstitium. ATN may result from:
▶ a diseased tubular epithelium that allows leakage of glomerular filtrate across the membranes and reabsorption of filtrate into the blood
▶ obstruction of urine flow by the collection of damaged cells, casts, red blood cells (RBCs), and other cellular debris within the tubular walls
▶ ischemic injury to glomerular epithelial cells, resulting in cellular collapse and decreased glomerular capillary permeability
▶ ischemic injury to vascular endothelium, eventually resulting in cellular swelling and obstruction.

Signs and symptoms

Nephrotoxic injury causes multiple symptoms similar to those of renal failure, particularly azotemia, anemia, acidosis, overhy-

Rise in nephrotoxic injury

The incidence of acute tubular necrosis (ATN) due to ingestion or inhalation of toxic substances is rising. Hospitalized patients may present with ATN following exposure to toxic agents, such as antibiotics, chemotherapeutic agents, or contrast material. Other nephrotoxic agents include pesticides, fungicides, heavy metals (for example, mercury, arsenic, lead, bismuth, uranium), and organic solvents containing carbon tetrachloride or ethylene glycol, such as cleaning fluids or industrial solvents. Ingestion of these substances may be accidental or intentional.

dration, and hypertension. Some patients may also experience fever, rash, and eosinophilia. However, ATN is usually difficult to recognize in its early stages because the effects of the critically ill patient's primary disease may mask the symptoms of ATN. The first recognizable effect may be decreased urine output. Generally, hyperkalemia and the characteristic uremic syndrome soon follow, with oliguria (or, rarely, anuria) and confusion, which may progress to uremic coma.

Complications
▶ Heart failure
▶ Uremic pericarditis
▶ Pulmonary edema
▶ Uremic lung
▶ Anemia
▶ Anorexia
▶ Intractable vomiting
▶ Poor wound healing due to debilitation
▶ Fever and chills (This may signal the onset of infection, which is associated with the leading cause of death in ATN.)

Diagnosis

Diagnosis is usually delayed until the condition has progressed to an advanced stage.

The most significant laboratory clues are urinary sediment containing RBCs and casts, and dilute urine of a low specific gravity (1.010), low osmolality (less than 400 mOsm/kg, and high sodium level (40 to 60 mEq/L). Blood studies reveal elevated blood urea nitrogen and serum creatinine levels, anemia, defects in platelet adherence, metabolic acidosis, and hyperkalemia. An electrocardiogram may show arrhythmias (due to electrolyte imbalances) and, with hyperkalemia, widening QRS segment, disappearing P waves, and tall, peaked T waves. Renal ultrasound, computed tomography scan, or magnetic resonance imaging measures renal size and thickness and looks for obstructive uropathy.[2]

Treatment

Treatment consists of identifying the nephrotoxic substance, eliminating its use, and removing it from the body, possibly by hemodialysis or hemoperfusion in extreme cases. Initial treatment may include administration of diuretics and infusion of a large volume of fluids to flush out tubules of cellular casts and debris, and to replace fluid loss. However, this treatment carries a risk of fluid overload. Long-term fluid management requires daily replacement of projected and calculated losses (including insensible loss). Diet may be high in carbohydrates and low in protein, sodium, and potassium to minimize the buildup of these nutrients in the body. During the course of acute renal failure, treatment is supportive.

Other appropriate measures to control complications include transfusion of packed RBCs for anemia and administration of antibiotics for infection. Epogen may be given to stimulate RBC production as an alternative to blood transfusion. Hyperkalemia may require emergency I.V. administration of 50% glucose, regular insulin, and sodium bicarbonate. Sodium polystyrene sulfonate with sorbitol may be given by mouth or by enema to reduce extracellular potassium lev-

els. Peritoneal dialysis or hemodialysis may be needed if the patient is catabolic.

Acute tubular necrosis can be prevented. Studies show that giving aminoglycosides in once-a-day doses can decrease the incidence of nephrotoxicity. Monitor blood levels of cyclosporin and tacrolimus to maintain therapeutic levels. Give isotonic sodium chloride solution (0.9%) before giving radiocontrast dye. Studies show that giving calcium channel blockers during kidney transplant surgery reduces the chance of acute tubular necrosis after the operation.[1]

Special considerations

Patient care is largely supportive.

▶ Maintain fluid balance. Watch for fluid overload, a common complication of therapy. Accurately record intake and output, including wound drainage, nasogastric output, and hemodialysis and peritoneal dialysis balances. Weigh the patient daily.

▶ Monitor hemoglobin (Hb) levels and hematocrit, and administer blood products as needed.

▶ Maintain electrolyte balance. Monitor laboratory results, and report imbalances. Enforce dietary restriction of foods containing sodium and potassium, such as bananas, orange juice, and baked potatoes. Check for potassium content in prescribed medications (for example, potassium penicillin). Provide adequate calories and essential amino acids, while restricting protein intake to maintain an anabolic state. Total parenteral nutrition may be indicated in the severely debilitated or catabolic patient.

▶ Use sterile technique, particularly when handling catheters because the debilitated patient is vulnerable to infection. Immediately report fever, chills, delayed wound healing, or flank pain if the patient has an indwelling catheter in place.

▶ Watch for complications. If anemia worsens (pallor, weakness, lethargy with decreased Hb level), administer RBCs as ordered. For acidosis, give sodium bicarbonate,

or assist with dialysis in severe cases as ordered. Watch for signs of diminishing renal perfusion (hypotension and decreased urine output). Encourage coughing and deep breathing to prevent pulmonary complications.

▶ Perform passive range-of-motion exercises. Provide good skin care; apply lotion or bath oil for dry skin. Help the patient walk as soon as possible, but guard against exhaustion.

▶ Provide reassurance and emotional support. Encourage the patient and his family to express their fears. Fully explain each procedure; repeat the explanation each time the procedure is done. Help the patient and his family set realistic goals according to individual prognosis.

▶ To prevent ATN, make sure patients are well hydrated before surgery or after X-rays that use a contrast medium. Administer mannitol, as ordered, to high-risk patients before and during these procedures. Carefully monitor patients receiving blood transfusions to detect early signs of transfusion reaction (fever, rash, chills), and discontinue such transfusion immediately.

REFERENCES
1. Shilliday, I.R., and Sherif, M. "Calcium Channel Blockers for Preventing Acute Tubular Necrosis in Kidney Transplant Recipients," *Cochrane Database of Systematic Reviews* (1):CD003421, 2004.
2. Merck Manual, Professional (2005 November). "Tubulointerstitial Nephritis" [Online]. Available at *www.merck.com/mmpe/sec17/ch236/ch236c.html.*
3. Tumlin, J., et al. "Pathophysiology of Contrast-induced Nephropathy," *American Journal of Cardiology* 98(6A):14K-20K, September 2006.

BENIGN PROSTATIC HYPERPLASIA

Although most males older than age 50 have some prostatic enlargement, in benign prostatic hyperplasia (BPH), also known as *benign prostatic hypertrophy,* the prostate gland enlarges sufficiently to compress the urethra and cause some overt urinary obstruction. Depending on the size of the enlarged prostate, the age and health of the patient, and the extent of obstruction, BPH is treated symptomatically or surgically.

Causes and incidence

Evidence suggests a link between BPH and hormonal activity. As males age, production of androgenic hormones decreases, causing an imbalance in androgen and estrogen levels, and high levels of dihydrotestosterone, the main prostatic intracellular androgen. Other causes include neoplasm, arteriosclerosis, diabetes, inflammation, and metabolic or nutritional disturbances. (See *Do vegetables help fight BPH?* page 240.)

Whatever the cause, BPH begins with changes in periurethral glandular tissue. As the prostate enlarges, it may extend into the bladder and obstruct urinary outflow by compressing or distorting the prostatic urethra. BPH may also cause a pouch to form in the bladder that retains urine when the rest of the bladder empties. This retained urine may lead to calculus formation or cystitis.

The likelihood of developing an enlarged prostate increases with age. More than 50% of men have symptoms by age 60 and as many as 90% have symptoms by ages 70 and 80.[1] It's estimated that 115 million men age 50 and older will develop BPH. The incidence rate is highest in Blacks (224.3 cases per 10,000 people), who tend to be diagnosed later, with more advanced disease, and thus, have a poorer prognosis. In Whites, however, the incidence rate is 150.3 per

100,000, while in Asians, it's 82.2 cases per 100,000.

Signs and symptoms

Clinical features of BPH depend on the extent of prostatic enlargement and the lobes affected. Characteristically, the condition starts with a group of symptoms known as *prostatism*: reduced urinary stream caliber and force, urinary hesitancy, and difficulty starting micturition (resulting in straining, feeling of incomplete voiding, and an interrupted stream). As the obstruction increases, it causes frequent urination with nocturia, dribbling, urine retention, incontinence, and possibly hematuria. Physical examination indicates a visible midline mass above the symphysis pubis that represents an incompletely emptied bladder; rectal palpation discloses an enlarged prostate. Examination may detect secondary anemia and, possibly, renal insufficiency secondary to obstruction. As BPH worsens, complete urinary obstruction may follow infection or use of decongestants, tranquilizers, alcohol, antidepressants, or anticholinergics.

Complications

▶ Infection
▶ Renal insufficiency
▶ Hemorrhage
▶ Shock

Diagnosis

Clinical features and a digital rectal examination are usually sufficient for diagnosis.

A prostate-specific antigen (PSA) blood test is used in conjunction with the rectal exam for men over the age of 50. The PSA test tests for a protein produced by prostate cells that's usually elevated in men who have prostate cancer. The PSA test is done to rule out cancer.[2] Other findings help to confirm it:

▶ Excretory urography may indicate urinary tract obstruction, hydronephrosis, calculi or tumors, and filling and emptying defects in the bladder.

▶ Elevated blood urea nitrogen and serum creatinine levels suggest renal dysfunction.

▶ Urinalysis and urine culture show hematuria, pyuria and, when the bacterial count exceeds 100,000/µl, urinary tract infection (UTI).

When symptoms are severe, a cystourethroscopy is definitive, but this test is performed only immediately before surgery to help determine the best procedure. It can show prostate enlargement, bladder wall changes, and a raised bladder.

HEALTH & SAFETY *Use of nonsteroidal anti-inflammatory drugs may prevent or delay the development of BPH.[4]*

Treatment

Conservative therapy includes prostate massages, sitz baths, fluid restriction for bladder distention, and antimicrobials for infection. If symptoms are mild, self-care may include avoidance of alcohol and caffeine, especially after dinner; urinating when the urge is initially felt; avoiding over-the-counter cold and sinus medications that contain decongestants or antihistamines because they can increase BPH symptoms; keeping warm and exercising regularly because cold weather and lack of physical activity may worsen symptoms; performing pelvic strengthening exercises (Kegel exercises); and reducing

stress, because nervousness and tension can lead to more frequent urination. Regular ejaculation may help relieve prostatic congestion. If patients ask about saw palmetto berries, an herb used as an alternative treatment, caution them that researchers have recently found that saw palmetto berries are no more effective than a placebo.[3]

Drug therapy includes finasteride and dutasteride, which lower levels of hormones produced by the prostate, reduce the size of the prostate gland, increase urine flow rate, and decrease symptoms of BPH. Advise patients who are candidates for these drugs that they may not see any significant improvement in symptoms for 3 to 6 months. Also explain that potential adverse effects related to finasteride include decreased sex drive and impotence.

Terazosin, doxazosin, tamsulosin, and alfuzosin all relax smooth muscle of the bladder neck and the prostate and therefore improve urine flow and reduce bladder outlet obstruction.[1]

Surgery is the only effective therapy to relieve acute urine retention, hydronephrosis, severe hematuria, recurrent UTIs, and other intolerable symptoms. A transurethral resection may be performed if the prostate weighs less than 2 oz (56.7 g). In this procedure, a resectoscope removes tissue with a wire loop and electric current. In high-risk patients, continuous drainage with an indwelling urinary catheter alleviates urine retention. Transurethral needle ablation may be used to heat and destroy prostate tissue by radiofrequency; this helps spare surrounding tissue.

The following procedures involve open surgical removal:

▶ *suprapubic (transvesical) resection:* most common and useful when prostatic enlargement remains within the bladder
▶ *retropubic (extravesical) resection:* allows direct visualization; potency and continence are usually maintained.

Balloon dilatation of the prostate is still being investigated. Balloon dilatation or balloon urethroplasty involves passing a flexible balloon catheter through the urethra at the level of the prostate while being guided by fluoroscope. The balloon is inflated for a short time to distend the prostatic urethra.

Special considerations

Prepare the patient for diagnostic tests and surgery, as appropriate.

▶ Monitor and record the patient's vital signs, intake and output, and daily weight. Watch closely for signs of postobstructive diuresis (such as increased urine output and hypotension), which may lead to serious dehydration, lowered blood volume, shock, electrolyte loss, and anuria.

▶ Administer antibiotics, as ordered, for UTI, urethral instrumentation, and cystoscopy.

▶ If urine retention is present, insert an indwelling urinary catheter (although this is usually difficult in a patient with BPH). If the catheter can't be passed transurethrally, assist with suprapubic cystostomy (under local anesthetic). Watch for rapid bladder decompression.

After prostatic surgery:

▶ Maintain patient comfort, and watch for and prevent postoperative complications. Observe for immediate dangers of prostatic bleeding (shock and hemorrhage). Check the catheter often (every 15 minutes for the first 2 to 3 hours) for patency and urine color; check dressings for bleeding.

▶ Postoperatively, many urologists insert a three-way catheter and establish continuous bladder irrigation. Keep the catheter open at a rate sufficient to maintain returns that are clear and light pink. Watch for fluid overload from absorption of the irrigating fluid into systemic circulation. If a regular catheter is used, observe it closely. If drainage stops because of clots, irrigate the catheter, as ordered, usually with 80 to 100 ml of

normal saline solution, while maintaining *strict* sterile technique.

▶ Watch for septic shock, the most serious complication of prostatic surgery. Immediately report severe chills, sudden fever, tachycardia, hypotension, or other signs of shock. Start rapid infusion of antibiotics I.V. as ordered.

▶ Watch for pulmonary embolus, heart failure, and renal shutdown. Monitor vital signs, central venous pressure, and arterial pressure continuously. The patient may need intensive supportive care in the intensive care unit.

▶ Administer anticholinergics, as ordered, to relieve painful bladder spasms that commonly occur after transurethral resection.

▶ Offer comfort measures to the patient after an open procedure: provide suppositories (except after perineal prostatectomy), analgesic medication to control incisional pain, and frequent dressing changes.

▶ Continue infusing I.V. fluids until the patient can drink sufficient fluids (2 to 3 qt [2 to 3 L]/day) to maintain adequate hydration.

▶ Administer stool softeners and laxatives, as ordered, to prevent straining. *Don't* check for fecal impaction because a rectal examination may precipitate bleeding.

▶ After the catheter is removed, the patient may experience frequency, dribbling, and occasional hematuria. Reassure him that he'll gradually regain urinary control.

▶ Reinforce prescribed limits on activity. Warn the patient against lifting, strenuous exercise, and long automobile rides because these increase bleeding tendency. Also caution the patient to restrict sexual activity for at least several weeks after discharge from the hospital.

▶ Instruct the patient to follow the prescribed oral antibiotic drug regimen, and tell him the indications for using gentle laxatives. Urge him to seek medical care immediately if he can't void, if he passes bloody urine, or if he develops a fever.

REFERENCES

1. National Kidney and Urologic Diseases Information Clearinghouse (2006 June). "Prostate Enlargement: Benign Prostatic Hyperplasia," NIH Publication No. 07-3012 [Online]. Available at *http://kidney.niddk.nih.gov/kudiseases/pubs/prostateenlargement/*.
2. National Cancer Institute (2007 August 21). "The Prostate-Specific Antigen (PSA) Test: Questions and Answers" [Online]. Available at *www.cancer.gov/cancertopics/factsheet/Detection/PSA*.
3. Bent S., et al. "Saw Palmetto for Benign Prostatic Hyperplasia," *New England Journal of Medicine* 354(6):557-66, February 2006.
4. St. Sauver, J.L., et al. "Protective Association between Nonsteroidal Antiinflammatory Drug Use and Measures of Benign Prostatic Hyperplasia," *American Journal of Epidemiology* 164(8):760-68, October 2006.
5. Rohrmann, S., et al. "Fruit and Vegetable Consumption, Intake of Micronutrients, and Benign Prostatic Hyperplasia in US Men," *American Journal of Clinical Nutrition* 85(2):523-29, February 2007.

CHRONIC RENAL FAILURE

Chronic renal failure (chronic kidney disease) is usually the end result of a gradually progressive loss of renal function; occasionally, it's the result of a rapidly progressive disease of sudden onset. Few symptoms develop until after more than 75% of glomerular filtration is lost; then the remaining normal parenchyma deteriorates progressively, and symptoms worsen as renal function decreases. The Kidney Disease Outcomes Quality Initiative of the National Kidney Foundation defines chronic kidney disease as kidney damage for greater than or equal to 3 months or a decreased glomerular filtration rate (GFR) of less than 60 ml/min/1.73m^2 for 3 or more months.[1] If this condition continues unchecked, uremic toxins accumulate and produce potentially fatal phys-

iologic changes in all major organ systems. If the patient can tolerate it, maintenance dialysis or kidney transplantation can sustain life.

Causes and incidence

Diabetes and hypertension are the primary causes of chronic renal failure, accounting for two-thirds of cases. Other causes of chronic renal failure include:

▶ chronic glomerular disease such as glomerulonephritis
▶ chronic infections, such as chronic pyelonephritis or tuberculosis
▶ congenital anomalies such as polycystic kidneys
▶ vascular diseases such as renal nephrosclerosis
▶ obstructive processes such as calculi
▶ collagen diseases such as systemic lupus erythematosus
▶ nephrotoxic agents such as long-term aminoglycoside therapy.

These conditions gradually destroy the nephrons and eventually cause irreversible renal failure. Similarly, acute renal failure that fails to respond to treatment becomes chronic renal failure.

According to the National Kidney Foundation chronic kidney diseases progress through the following stages:

Stage 1: kidney damage with normal or increased GFR (GFR ≥ 90 ml/min/1.73m²)

Stage 2: kidney damage with mildly decreased GFR (GFR 60 to 89 ml/min/1.73m²)

Stage 3: moderate reduction of GFR (GFR 30 to 59 ml/min/1.73m²)

Stage 4: severe reduction of GFR (GFR 15 to 29 ml/min/1.73m²)

Stage 5: kidney failure (GFR < 15 ml/min/1.73m² or dialysis) [1]

It's estimated that about 11% of people (about 19.2 million) in the United States have chronic kidney disease.[6] Even though chronic kidney disease affects all ages and races, the incidence is higher in people older than age 65, and is four times higher in Blacks than in Whites.

HEALTH & SAFETY *Obesity may be a significant risk factor for chronic renal failure. Losing weight and maintaining it may be one way to reduce the risk of chronic renal failure.* [2]

Signs and symptoms

Chronic renal failure produces major changes in all body systems:

▶ *Renal and urologic:* Initially, salt-wasting and consequent hyponatremia produce hypotension, dry mouth, loss of skin turgor, listlessness, fatigue, and nausea; later, somnolence and confusion develop. As the number of functioning nephrons decreases, so does the kidneys' capacity to excrete sodium, resulting in salt retention and overload. Accumulation of potassium causes muscle irritability and muscle weakness as the potassium level continues to rise. Fluid overload and metabolic acidosis also occur. Urine output decreases; urine is very dilute and contains casts and crystals.

▶ *Cardiovascular:* Renal failure leads to hypertension, arrhythmias (including life-threatening ventricular tachycardia or fibrillation), cardiomyopathy, uremic pericarditis, pericardial effusion with possible cardiac tamponade, heart failure, and periorbital and peripheral edema.

▶ *Respiratory:* Pulmonary changes include reduced pulmonary macrophage activity with increased susceptibility to infection, pulmonary edema, pleuritic pain, pleural friction rub and effusions, crackles, thick sputum, uremic pleuritis and uremic lung (or uremic pneumonitis), dyspnea due to heart failure, and Kussmaul's respirations as a result of acidosis.

▶ *GI:* Inflammation and ulceration of GI mucosa cause stomatitis, gum ulceration and bleeding and, possibly, parotitis, esophagitis, gastritis, duodenal ulcers, lesions on the small and large bowel, uremic colitis, pancreatitis, and proctitis. Other GI symptoms

include a metallic taste in the mouth, uremic fetor (ammonia smell to breath), anorexia, nausea, and vomiting.

▶ *Cutaneous:* Typically, the skin is pallid, yellowish bronze, dry, and scaly. Other cutaneous symptoms include severe itching; purpura; ecchymoses; petechiae; uremic frost (most common in critically ill or terminal patients); thin, brittle fingernails with characteristic lines; and dry, brittle hair that may change color and fall out easily.

▶ *Neurologic:* Restless leg syndrome, one of the first signs of peripheral neuropathy, causes pain, burning, and itching in the legs and feet, which may be relieved by voluntarily shaking, moving, or rocking them. Eventually, this condition progresses to paresthesia and motor nerve dysfunction (usually bilateral footdrop) unless dialysis is initiated. Other signs and symptoms include muscle cramping and twitching, shortened memory and attention span, apathy, drowsiness, irritability, confusion, coma, and seizures. EEG changes indicate metabolic encephalopathy.

▶ *Endocrine:* Common endocrine abnormalities include stunted growth patterns in children (even with elevated growth hormone levels), infertility and decreased libido in both sexes, amenorrhea and cessation of menses in females, and impotence, decreased sperm production, and testicular atrophy in males. Increased aldosterone secretion (related to increased renin production) and impaired carbohydrate metabolism (increased blood glucose levels similar to diabetes mellitus) may also occur.

▶ *Hematopoietic:* Anemia, decreased red blood cell (RBC) survival time, blood loss from dialysis and GI bleeding, mild thrombocytopenia, and platelet defects occur. Other problems include increased bleeding and clotting disorders, demonstrated by purpura, hemorrhage from body orifices, easy bruising, ecchymoses, and petechiae.

▶ *Skeletal:* Calcium-phosphorus imbalance and consequent parathyroid hormone imbalances cause muscle and bone pain, skeletal demineralization, pathologic fractures, and calcifications in the brain, eyes, gums, joints, myocardium, and blood vessels. Arterial calcification may produce coronary artery disease. In children, renal osteodystrophy (renal rickets) may develop.

Complications
▶ Anemia
▶ Peripheral neuropathy
▶ Cardiopulmonary complications
▶ GI complications
▶ Sexual dysfunction
▶ Skeletal defects

Diagnosis
Diagnosis of chronic renal failure is based on clinical assessment, a history of chronic progressive debilitation, and gradual deterioration of renal function as determined by creatinine clearance tests. The following laboratory findings also aid in diagnosis:

▶ Blood studies show elevated blood urea nitrogen, serum creatinine, and potassium levels; decreased arterial pH and bicarbonate; and low hemoglobin (Hb) level and hematocrit (HCT).

▶ Urine specific gravity becomes fixed at 1.010; urinalysis may show proteinuria, glycosuria, erythrocytes, leukocytes, and casts, depending on the etiology.

▶ X-ray studies include kidney-ureter-bladder films, excretory urography, nephrotomography, renal scan, and renal arteriography.

▶ Renal or abdominal computed tomography scan, magnetic resonance imaging, or ultrasound indicate changes associated with chronic renal failure, including abnormally small size in both kidneys. Ultrasound is used for patients with previously undiagnosed renal failure to differentiate between acute renal failure and chronic renal failure.[3]

▶ Kidney biopsy allows histologic identification of the underlying pathology.

Treatment

Treatment focuses on controlling the symptoms, minimizing complications, and slowing the progression of the disease. Associated diseases such as hypertension that cause or result from chronic renal failure must be controlled. Conservative treatment aims to correct specific symptoms. A low-protein diet reduces the production of end products of protein metabolism that the kidneys can't excrete. (A patient receiving continuous peritoneal dialysis should have a high-protein diet.) A high-calorie diet that prevents ketoacidosis and the negative nitrogen balance that results in catabolism and tissue atrophy, and restricts sodium and potassium.

Maintaining fluid balance requires careful monitoring of vital signs, weight changes, and urine volume (if present). If some renal function remains, administration of loop diuretics such as furosemide, and fluid restriction can reduce fluid retention. Cardiac glycosides may be used to mobilize edema fluids; antihypertensives, to control blood pressure and associated edema. Antiemetics taken before meals may relieve nausea and vomiting; cimetidine or ranitidine may decrease gastric irritation. Methylcellulose or docusate can help prevent constipation.

Treatment may also include regular stool analysis (guaiac test) to detect occult blood and, as needed, cleaning enemas to remove blood from the GI tract. Anemia necessitates iron and folate supplements; severe anemia requires infusion of fresh frozen packed cells or washed packed cells. However, transfusions relieve anemia only temporarily. Epoetin alpha (erythropoietin) increases RBC production.

Drug therapy usually relieves associated symptoms: an antipruritic, such as trimeprazine or diphenhydramine, can be used for itching. Aluminum hydroxide gel can lower serum phosphate levels. The patient may also benefit from supplementary vitamins (particularly B vitamins and vitamin D) and essential amino acids. Careful monitoring of serum potassium levels is necessary to detect hyperkalemia. Emergency treatment for severe hyperkalemia includes dialysis therapy and administration of 50% hypertonic glucose I.V., regular insulin, calcium gluconate I.V., sodium bicarbonate I.V., and caution exchange resins such as sodium polystyrene sulfonate. Cardiac tamponade resulting from pericardial effusion may require emergency pericardial tap or surgery.

Blood gas measurements may indicate acidosis; intensive dialysis and thoracentesis can relieve pulmonary edema and pleural effusions.

Hemodialysis or peritoneal dialysis (particularly continuous ambulatory peritoneal dialysis and continuous cyclic peritoneal dialysis) can help control most manifestations of end-stage renal disease; altering dialyzing bath fluids can correct fluid and electrolyte disturbances. (See *Comparing peritoneal dialysis and hemodialysis,* page 246. Also see *Continuous ambulatory peritoneal dialysis,* page 247.) However, anemia, peripheral neuropathy, cardiopulmonary and GI complications, sexual dysfunction, and skeletal defects may persist. Maintenance dialysis itself may produce complications, such as protein wasting, refractory ascites, and dialysis dementia. Kidney transplants may eventually be the treatment of choice for some patients with end-stage renal disease.

Special considerations

Because chronic renal failure has such widespread clinical effects, it requires meticulous and carefully coordinated supportive care.
▶ Good skin care is important. Bathe the patient daily, using superfatted soaps, oatmeal baths, and skin lotion without alcohol to ease pruritus. Don't use soaps containing glycerin because they dry skin. Give good perineal care, using mild soap and water. Pad the side rails to guard against ecchymoses. Turn the patient often, and use a

Comparing peritoneal dialysis and hemodialysis

Advantages, disadvantages, and complications of peritoneal dialysis and hemodialysis are described below.

TYPE	ADVANTAGES	DISADVANTAGES	POSSIBLE COMPLICATIONS
Peritoneal dialysis	▪ Can be performed immediately ▪ Requires less complex equipment and less specialized personnel than hemodialysis ▪ Requires small amounts of heparin or none at all ▪ No blood loss; minimal cardiovascular stress ▪ Can be performed by patient anywhere (continuous ambulatory peritoneal dialysis), without assistance and with minimal patient teaching ▪ Allows patient independence without long interruptions in daily activities because exchange may be done at night while he sleeps ▪ Lower infection rate ▪ Lower cost	▪ Contraindicated within 72 hours of abdominal surgery ▪ Requires 48 to 72 hours for significant response to treatment ▪ Severe protein loss necessitates high-protein diet (up to 100 g/day) ▪ High risk of peritonitis; repeated bouts may cause scarring, preventing further treatments with peritoneal dialysis ▪ Urea clearance less than with hemodialysis (60%)	▪ Bacterial or chemical peritonitis ▪ Pain (abdominal, lower back, shoulder) ▪ Shortness of breath, or dyspnea ▪ Atelectasis and pneumonia ▪ Severe loss of protein into the dialysis solution in the abdominal cavity (10 to 20 g/day) ▪ Fluid overload ▪ Excessive fluid loss ▪ Constipation ▪ Catheter site inflammation, infection, or leakage ▪ Anorexia ▪ Hypertriglyceridemia ▪ Abdominal hernias
Hemodialysis	▪ Takes only 3 to 5 hours per treatment ▪ Faster results in an acute situation ▪ Total number of hours of maintenance treatment that's only half that of peritoneal dialysis ▪ In an acute situation, can use an I.V. route without a surgical access route	▪ Requires surgical creation of a vascular access between circulation and dialysis machine ▪ Requires complex water treatment, dialysis equipment, and highly trained personnel ▪ Requires administration of larger amounts of heparin ▪ Confines patient to special treatment unit	▪ Septicemia ▪ Air emboli ▪ Rapid fluid and electrolyte imbalance (disequilibrium syndrome) ▪ Hemolytic anemia ▪ Metastatic calcification ▪ Increased risk of hepatitis ▪ Hypotension or hypertension ▪ Itching ▪ Pain (generalized or in chest) ▪ Heparin overdose, possibly causing hemorrhage ▪ Leg cramps ▪ Nausea and vomiting ▪ Headache

convoluted foam mattress to prevent skin breakdown.

▶ Provide good oral hygiene. Brush the patient's teeth often with a soft brush or sponge tip to reduce breath odor. Sugarless

Continuous ambulatory peritoneal dialysis

Continuous ambulatory peritoneal dialysis is a useful alternative to hemodialysis in patients with renal failure. Using the peritoneum as a dialysis membrane, it allows almost uninterrupted exchange of dialysis solution. With this method, four to six exchanges of fresh dialysis solution are infused each day. The approximate dwell time for daytime exchanges is 5 hours; for overnight exchanges, the dwell time is 8 to 10 hours. After each dwell time, the patient removes the dialyzing solution by gravity drainage. An alternative method uses a continuous cycler-assisted peritoneal dialysis machine while the patient sleeps. The machine performs three to five exchanges during the night and can be used in the morning with one dwell time that lasts the entire day.[4] This form of dialysis offers the unique advantages of a simple, easily taught procedure and patient independence from a special treatment center.

In this procedure, a Tenckhoff catheter is surgically implanted in the abdomen, just below the umbilicus. A bag of dialysis solution is attached using sterile technique to the tube, and the fluid is allowed to flow into the peritoneal cavity (this takes about 10 minutes).

The fluid is then drained out of the peritoneal cavity through gravity flow by unrolling the bag and suspending it below the pelvis (drainage takes about 20 minutes). After the fluid drains, the patient uses sterile technique to connect a new bag of dialyzing solution and fills the peritoneal cavity again. He repeats this procedure four to six times per day.

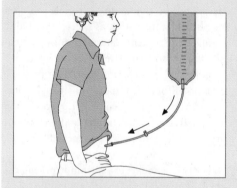

The dialyzing fluid remains in the peritoneal cavity for 4 to 6 hours.[4] During this time, the bag may be rolled up and placed under a shirt or blouse, and the patient can go about normal activities while dialysis takes place.

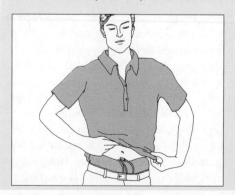

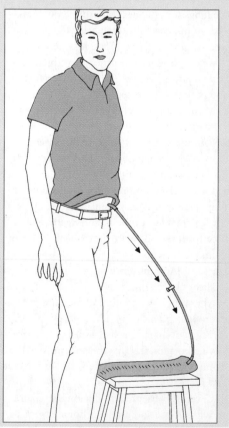

hard candy and mouthwash minimize bad taste in the mouth and alleviate thirst.

▶ Offer small, palatable meals that are also nutritious; try to provide favorite foods within dietary restrictions. Encourage intake of high-calorie foods. Instruct the outpatient to avoid high-sodium and high-potassium foods. Encourage adherence to fluid and protein restrictions. To prevent constipation, stress the need for exercise and sufficient dietary bulk.

▶ Watch for hyperkalemia. Observe for cramping of the legs and abdomen, and diarrhea. As potassium levels rise, watch for muscle irritability and a weak pulse rate. Monitor the electrocardiogram for tall, peaked T waves, widening QRS segment, prolonged PR interval, and disappearance of P waves, indicating hyperkalemia.

▶ Assess hydration status carefully. Check for jugular vein distention, and auscultate the lungs for crackles. Measure daily intake and output carefully, including all drainage, emesis, diarrhea, and blood loss. Record daily weight, presence or absence of thirst, axillary sweat, dryness of tongue, hypertension, and peripheral edema.

▶ Monitor for bone or joint complications. Prevent pathologic fractures by turning the patient carefully and ensuring his safety. Provide passive range-of-motion exercises for the bedridden patient.

▶ Encourage deep breathing and coughing to prevent pulmonary congestion. Listen often for crackles, rhonchi, and decreased breath sounds. Be alert for clinical effects of pulmonary edema (dyspnea, restlessness, crackles). Administer diuretics and other medications, as ordered.

▶ Maintain strict sterile technique. Use a micropore filter during I.V. therapy. Watch for signs of infection (listlessness, high fever, and leukocytosis). Urge the patient to avoid contact with infected persons during the cold and flu season.

▶ Carefully observe and document seizure activity. Infuse sodium bicarbonate for aci-dosis, and sedatives or anticonvulsants for seizures, as ordered. Pad the side rails and keep an oral airway and suction setup at bedside. Assess neurologic status periodically, and check for Chvostek's and Trousseau's signs, indicators of low serum calcium levels.

▶ Observe for signs of bleeding. Watch for prolonged bleeding at puncture sites and at the vascular access site used for hemodialysis. Monitor Hb levels and HCT, and check stools, urine, and vomitus for blood.

▶ Report signs of pericarditis, such as a pericardial friction rub and chest pain.

▶ Watch for the disappearance of friction rub, with a drop of 15 to 20 mm Hg in blood pressure during inspiration (paradoxical pulse)—an early sign of pericardial tamponade.

▶ Schedule medications carefully. Give iron before meals, aluminum hydroxide gels after meals, and antiemetics, as necessary, a half hour before meals. Administer antihypertensives at appropriate intervals. If the patient requires a rectal infusion of sodium polystyrene sulfonate for dangerously high potassium levels, apply an emollient to soothe the perianal area. Make sure the sodium polystyrene sulfonate enema is expelled; otherwise, it will cause constipation and won't lower potassium levels. Recommend antacid cookies as an alternative to aluminum hydroxide gels needed to bind GI phosphate.

If the patient requires dialysis:

▶ Prepare the patient by fully explaining the procedure. Make sure that he understands how to protect and care for the arteriovenous shunt, fistula, or other vascular access. Check the vascular access site per facility protocol or every 2 hours for patency and the extremity for adequate blood supply and intact nervous function (temperature, pulse rate, capillary refill, and sensation). If a fistula is present, feel for a thrill (a buzzing sensation), and listen for a bruit. Use a gentle touch to avoid occluding the fistula. Report signs of possible clotting. Don't use the arm with the vascular access site to take

blood pressure readings, draw blood, or give injections because these procedures may rupture the fistula or occlude blood flow.

▶ Withhold the 6 a.m. (or morning) dose of antihypertensive on the morning of dialysis, and instruct the outpatient to do the same.

▶ Use standard precautions when handling body fluids and needles.

▶ Monitor Hb levels and HCT. Assess the patient's tolerance of his levels. Some individuals are more sensitive to lower levels than others. Instruct the anemic patient to conserve energy and to rest frequently.

▶ After dialysis, check for disequilibrium syndrome, a result of sudden correction of blood chemistry abnormalities. Symptoms range from a headache to seizures. Also, check for excessive bleeding from the dialysis site. Apply pressure dressing or absorbable gelatin sponge, as indicated. Monitor blood pressure carefully after dialysis.[5]

▶ A patient undergoing dialysis is under a great deal of stress, as is his family. Refer them to appropriate counseling agencies for assistance in coping with chronic renal failure.

REFERENCES

1. National Kidney Foundation (2002). "K/DOQI Clinical Practice Guidelines for Chronic Kidney Disease: Evaluation, Classification, and Stratification. Part 4. Definition and Classification of Stages of Chronic Kidney Disease" [Online]. Available at *www.kidney.org/professionals/ KDOQI/guidelines_ckd/p4_class_g1.htm.*

2. Ejerblad, E., et al. "Obesity and Risk for Chronic Renal Failure," *Journal of the American Society of Nephrology* 17(6):1695-702, June 2006.

3. Bush, W.H., et al. (2008 April 7). "Renal Failure" [Online]. Available at *www.guideline. gov/summary/summary.aspx?doc_id=8283& nbr=004615&string=renal+AND+failure.*

4. National Kidney and Urologic Diseases Information Clearinghouse (2006 May). "Treatment Methods for Kidney Failure: Peritoneal Dialysis," NIH Publication No. 06-4688 [Online]. Available at *http://kidney.niddk.nih.gov/ kudiseases/pubs/peritoneal/.*

5. National Kidney Foundation NKF/KDOQI Guidelines. "Clinical Practice Guidelines and Clinical Practice Recommendations for Hemodialysis Adequacy, 2006 Update" [Online]. Available at *www.kidney.org/professionals/ kdoqi/guideline_upHD_PD_VA/index.htm.*

6. Ryan, T.P., et al. "Chronic Kidney Disease Prevalence and Rate of Diagnosis," *American Journal of Medicine* 120(11):981-86, November 2007.

LOWER URINARY TRACT INFECTION

Cystitis and urethritis are the two forms of lower urinary tract infection (UTI), a condition common in females.[1] In males and children, lower UTIs are commonly related to anatomic or physiologic abnormalities and therefore require extremely close evaluation. UTIs usually respond readily to treatment, but recurrence is possible, as is resistant bacterial flare-up during therapy.

UTIs account for 8.3 million visits to physicians each year.[2]

Causes and incidence

Most lower UTIs result from ascending infection by a single, gram-negative, enteric bacterium, such as *Escherichia coli, Klebsiella, Proteus, Enterobacter, Pseudomonas,* or *Serratia.* However, in a patient with neurogenic bladder, an indwelling catheter, or a fistula between the intestine and bladder, a lower UTI may result from simultaneous infection with multiple pathogens. Studies suggest that infection results from a breakdown in local defense mechanisms in the bladder that allows bacteria to invade the bladder mucosa and multiply. These bacteria can't be readily eliminated by normal micturition.

Bacterial flare-up during treatment is generally caused by the pathogenic organism's resistance to the prescribed antimicrobial therapy. The presence of even a small number (less than 10,000/µl) of bacteria in a

midstream urine specimen obtained during treatment casts doubt on the effectiveness of treatment.

Almost 20% of women who have a UTI will have a second UTI, and 30% of those will have one after that. Of those 30%, 80% will suffer another UTI. [2] In 99% of patients, recurrent lower UTI results from reinfection by the same organism or from some new pathogen; in the remaining 1%, recurrence reflects persistent infection, usually from renal calculi, chronic bacterial prostatitis, or a structural anomaly that may become a source of infection.

UTIs are nearly 10 times more common in females than in males and affect approximately 20% of all females at least once. Lower UTI is also a prevalent bacterial disease in children, with females again most commonly affected.

The high incidence of lower UTI among females may result from the shortness of the female urethra ($1\frac{1}{4}''$ to $2''$ [3 to 5 cm]), which predisposes females to infection caused by bacteria from the vagina, perineum, rectum, or a sexual partner. Males are less vulnerable because their urethras are longer ($7''$ [18.4 cm]) and because prostatic fluid serves as an antibacterial shield. However, in men older than age 60, incidence rates match those of women. In both males and females, infection usually ascends from the urethra to the bladder. Incomplete emptying of the bladder and chronic urine retention are risk factors associated with UTIs. Other conditions that put people at risk for UTIs include enlarged prostate, diabetes, or other disease that suppresses the immune system, abnormalities of the urinary tract, and diaphragm use.[2]

Signs and symptoms

Lower UTI usually produces urgency, frequency, dysuria, cramps or spasms of the bladder, itching, a feeling of warmth during urination, nocturia, and possibly urethral discharge in males. Inflammation of the bladder wall also causes hematuria and fever. Other common features include lower back pain, malaise, nausea, vomiting, abdominal pain or tenderness over the bladder area, chills, and flank pain. In elderly patients, the most common initial symptoms of a lower UTI are lethargy and a change in mental status.

Complications

▶ Infection of adjacent organs and structures

Diagnosis

Characteristic clinical features and a microscopic urinalysis showing red blood cells and white blood cells greater than 10 per high-power field suggest lower UTI. A clean-catch midstream urine specimen revealing a bacterial count above 100,000/µl confirms the diagnosis.

Lower counts don't necessarily rule out infection, especially if the patient is voiding frequently because bacteria require 30 to 45 minutes to reproduce in urine. Careful midstream, clean-catch collection is preferred to catheterization, which can reinfect the bladder with urethral bacteria.

Sensitivity testing determines the appropriate therapeutic antimicrobial agent. If patient history and physical examination warrant, a blood test or a stained smear of the discharge rules out venereal disease. Voiding cystoureterography or excretory urography may detect congenital anomalies that predispose the patient to recurrent UTIs.

Treatment

Appropriate antimicrobials are the treatment of choice for most initial lower UTIs. A course of antibiotic therapy lasting from 7 to 10 days is standard. Recent studies suggest that 3 days of antibiotic therapy is similar to an antibiotic regimen of 5 to 10 days in achieving symptomatic cure during uncomplicated UTIs, whereas the longer treatment time is more effective in obtaining bacterio-

logical cure.[3] A urine culture taken 1 to 2 weeks later indicates whether the infection has been eradicated. Research has also shown that nonpregnant women who have had several UTIs are less likely to have another infection if they take antibiotics for 6 to 12 months.[4]

Recurrent infections due to infected renal calculi, chronic prostatitis, or structural abnormality may necessitate surgery; prostatitis also requires long-term antibiotic therapy. In patients without these predisposing conditions, long-term, low-dosage antibiotic therapy is the treatment of choice.

Special considerations

The care plan should include careful patient teaching, supportive measures, and proper specimen collection.

▶ Explain the nature and purpose of antimicrobial therapy. Emphasize the importance of completing the prescribed course of therapy or, with long-term prophylaxis, of adhering strictly to the ordered dosage. Urge the patient to drink plenty of water (at least eight glasses per day). Stress the need to maintain a consistent fluid intake of about 2 qt (2 L)/day. More or less than this amount may alter the effect of the prescribed antimicrobial. Fruit juices, especially cranberry juice, and oral doses of vitamin C may help acidify the urine and enhance the action of the medication.

▶ Watch for GI disturbances from antimicrobial therapy. Nitrofurantoin macrocrystals, taken with milk or a meal, prevent such distress. If therapy includes phenazopyridine, warn the patient that this drug may turn urine red-orange.

▶ Suggest warm sitz baths for relief of perineal discomfort. If baths aren't effective, apply heat sparingly to the perineum but be careful not to burn the patient. Apply topical antiseptics, such as povidone-iodine ointment, on the urethral meatus as necessary.

▶ Collect all urine specimens for culture and sensitivity testing carefully and promptly.

Teach the female patient how to clean the perineum properly and keep the labia separated during voiding. A noncontaminated midstream specimen is essential for accurate diagnosis.

▶ To prevent recurrent lower UTIs, teach the female patient to carefully wipe the perineum from front to back and to clean it thoroughly with soap and water after defecation. Advise an infection-prone woman to void immediately after sexual intercourse. Stress the need to drink plenty of fluids routinely and to avoid postponing urination. Recommend frequent comfort stops during long car trips. Also stress the need to completely empty the bladder. Cranberry juice may decrease the incidence of UTIs in females with recurrent UTIs, but current evidence doesn't support its prophylactic effectiveness for other groups.[5] Further study is needed to define dosage and method of administration.[5] To prevent recurrent infections in males, urge prompt treatment of predisposing conditions such as chronic prostatitis. Have the patient use a commode rather than a bedpan to promote sitting up, which assists in emptying the bladder.

REFERENCES

1. Howes, D.S., and Henry, S. (2008 January 31). "Urinary Tract Infection, Female" [Online]. Available at *www.emedicine.com/EMERG/topic626.htm.*
2. National Kidney and Urologic Diseases Information Clearinghouse (2005 December). "Urinary Tract Infection in Adults," NIH Publication No. 07-2097 [Online]. Available at *http://kidney.niddk.nih.gov/kudiseases/pubs/uti adult/.*
3. Albert, X., et al. "Antibiotics for Preventing Recurrent Urinary Tract Infection in Non-Pregnant Women," *Cochrane Database of Systematic Reviews* (2):CD001209, July 2004.
4. Mil, G., et al. "Duration of Antibacterial Treatment for Uncomplicated Urinary Tract Infection in Women," *Cochrane Database of Systematic Reviews* (2):CD004682, April 2005.

5. Jepson, R.G., and Craid, J.C. "Cranberries for Preventing Urinary Tract Infection," *Cochrane Database of Systematic Reviews* (4): CD001321, January 2008.

NEPHROTIC SYNDROME

Nephrotic syndrome is a condition characterized by marked proteinuria, hypoalbuminemia, hyperlipidemia, and edema.[1] (See *What happens in nephrotic syndrome.*) Although nephrotic syndrome isn't a disease itself, it results from a specific glomerular defect and indicates renal damage. The prognosis is highly variable, depending on the underlying cause. Some forms may progress to end-stage renal failure.

Causes and incidence

About 75% of nephrotic syndrome cases result from primary (idiopathic) glomerulonephritis. Classifications include:

▶ *Minimal change nephritic syndrome,* the main cause of nephrotic syndrome in children, may be difficult to detect initially because the glomerulus looks normal by light microscopy. Some tubules may contain increased lipid deposits.

▶ *Membranous glomerulonephritis,* the most common lesion in adult idiopathic nephrotic syndrome, is characterized by uniform thickening of the glomerular basement membrane containing dense deposits and eventually progresses to renal failure.

▶ *Focal glomerulosclerosis* can develop spontaneously at any age, follow renal transplantation, or result from heroin abuse. Reported incidence of this condition is 10% in children with nephrotic syndrome and up to 20% in adults. Lesions initially affect the deeper glomeruli, causing hyaline sclerosis, with later involvement of the superficial glomeruli. These lesions generally cause slowly progressive deterioration in renal function. Remissions occur occasionally.

▶ In *membranoproliferative glomerulonephritis,* slowly progressive lesions develop in the subendothelial region of the basement membrane. Lesions may follow infection, particularly streptococcal infection. This disease occurs primarily in children and young adults.

Other causes of nephrotic syndrome include metabolic diseases such as diabetes mellitus; collagen-vascular disorders, such as systemic lupus erythematosus and periarteritis nodosa; circulatory diseases, such as heart failure, sickle cell anemia, and renal vein thrombosis; nephrotoxins, such as mercury, gold, and bismuth; allergic reactions; and infections, such as tuberculosis or enteritis. Other possible causes are pregnancy, hereditary nephritis, multiple myeloma, and other neoplastic diseases. These diseases increase glomerular protein permeability, leading to increased urinary excretion of protein, especially albumin, and subsequent hypoalbuminemia.

Nephrotic patients have an increased risk of infection, particularly of peritonitis.

In children, nephrotic syndrome occurs in about two to five cases per 100,000 children.[2] In the general population, the incidence rate is about 15.5 per 100,000.

Signs and symptoms

The dominant clinical feature of nephrotic syndrome is mild to severe dependent edema of the ankles or sacrum, or periorbital edema, especially in children. Edema may lead to ascites, pleural effusion, and swollen external genitalia. Accompanying symptoms may include orthostatic hypotension, lethargy, anorexia, depression, and pallor.

Complications

▶ Malnutrition
▶ Infection
▶ Coagulation disorders
▶ Thromboembolic vascular occlusion, and accelerated atherosclerosis. (See *Deep vein*

What happens in nephrotic syndrome

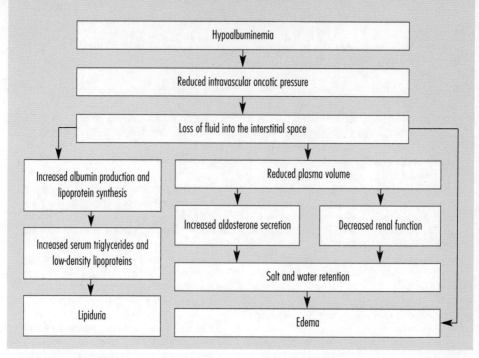

thrombosis and nephrotic syndrome, page 254.)

Diagnosis

Consistent proteinuria in excess of 3.5 g/ 24 hours strongly suggests nephrotic syndrome; examination of urine also reveals an increased number of hyaline, granular, and waxy, fatty casts, and oval fat bodies. Serum values that support the diagnosis are increased cholesterol, phospholipids, and triglycerides and decreased albumin levels. Histologic identification of the lesion requires kidney biopsy. Other tests may be done to rule out metabolic causes.

Treatment

The goals of treatment of nephrotic syndrome are to relieve symptoms, prevent complications, and delay progressive kidney damage. Treatment of the causative dis-

order—possibly lifelong—is necessary to control nephrotic syndrome. Corticosteroid, immunosuppressive, antihypertensive, and diuretic medications may help control symptoms. Antibiotics may be needed to control infections. Angiotensin-converting enzyme inhibitors may significantly reduce the degree of protein loss in urine and are therefore typically prescribed for the treatment of nephrotic syndrome.

Treatment of hypertension and of high cholesterol and triglyceride levels is also recommended to reduce the risk of atherosclerosis and complications. Dietary limitation of cholesterol and saturated fats may be of little benefit because the high levels that accompany this condition seem to result from overproduction by the liver rather than from excessive fat intake. Alteration in protein intake isn't indicated. Sodium may be restricted to help control edema. Vitamin D

Deep vein thrombosis and nephrotic syndrome

Question: *Can deep vein thrombosis or pulmonary embolism be caused by nephrotic syndrome?*

Research: Two audits of patient records were conducted in southwest Scotland after a patient—who was diagnosed as having deep vein thrombosis (DVT)—was treated with anticoagulants, and needed two additional hospitalizations before being diagnosed with nephrotic syndrome caused by membranous nephropathy. The first audit was of diagnostic discharge codes for nephrotic syndrome and venous thromboembolism in southwest Scotland from 1997 to 2006. The second was an audit of 98 patients, diagnosed by Doppler as having DVT from July 2005 to July 2006, to determine whether urine testing for protein had been conducted.

Conclusion: The first audit results showed that 32 patients had been diagnosed with nephrotic syndrome during the time period studied. Four of the 32 patients, or 12.5%, had presented initially with either DVT or pulmonary embolism. The second audit showed that only 1 of

the 98 patients reviewed had received urine testing for protein. The researchers concluded that, although nephrotic syndrome is not a common cause of DVT, health care practitioners should consider testing for it in all patients with DVT or pulmonary embolism.

Application: The nurse caring for a patient with DVT or pulmonary embolism should carefully review the results of laboratory studies, in particular the serum albumin levels, to explore the possibility of a nephrotic syndrome etiology. Low or low-normal serum albumin levels would indicate the need for further testing. In addition, all patients with DVT or pulmonary embolism should have their urine screened for protein.

Source: Ambler, B., et al. "Nephrotic Syndrome Presenting as Deep Vein Thrombosis or Pulmonary Embolism," *Emergency Medicine Journal* 25(4):241-42, April 2008.

---

may need to be replaced if nephrotic syndrome is chronic and unresponsive to therapy. Oral anticoagulants may be required to treat or prevent clot formation because it's well-documented that nephrotic syndrome is associated with an increased risk of thromboembolic complications, such as deep vein thrombosis, renal vein thrombosis, and pulmonary embolism. Each case must be examined separately weighing the benefits of oral anticoagulants against the risk of increased bleeding.[2]

Diuretics are given for edema. Research shows that interventions to prevent infection, such as oral antibiotics, are no longer indicated.[3]

Some patients respond to an 8-week course of corticosteroid therapy (such as prednisone), followed by a maintenance dose. Others respond better to a combination course of prednisone and azathioprine or cyclophosphamide. Research indicates that continuing to take corticosteroid medication for several months after the first episode of nephritic syndrome reduces the risk of relapse.[3]

Special considerations

Patient care includes identification and treatment of the underlying cause accompanied by supportive care during treatment.

▶ Frequently check urine protein. (Urine containing protein appears frothy.)

▶ Measure blood pressure while the patient is supine and also while he's standing; immediately report a drop in blood pressure that exceeds 20 mm Hg.

▶ After kidney biopsy, watch for bleeding and shock.

▶ Monitor intake and output, and check weight at the same time each morning—after the patient voids and before he eats—and while he's wearing the same kind of clothing. Ask the dietitian to plan a low-sodium diet.

▶ Provide good skin care because the patient with nephrotic syndrome usually has edema.

▶ To avoid thrombophlebitis, encourage activity and exercise, and provide antiembolism stockings as ordered.

▶ Watch for and teach the patient and his family how to recognize adverse drug effects, such as bone marrow toxicity from cytotoxic immunosuppressants and cushingoid symptoms (muscle weakness, mental changes, acne, moon face, hirsutism, girdle obesity, purple striae, amenorrhea) from long-term steroid therapy. Other steroid complications include masked infections, increased susceptibility to infections, ulcers, GI bleeding, and steroid-induced diabetes; a steroid crisis may occur if the drug is discontinued abruptly. To prevent GI complications, administer steroids with an antacid or with cimetidine or ranitidine. Explain that steroid adverse effects will subside when therapy stops.

▶ Offer the patient and his family reassurance and support, especially during the acute phase, when edema is severe and the patient's body image changes.

REFERENCES

1. National Kidney and Urologic Diseases Information Clearinghouse (2007 February). "Nephrotic Syndrome in Adults," NIH Publication No. 07-4624 [Online]. Available at *http://kidney.niddk.nih.gov/kudiseases/pubs/nephrotic/*.

2. Glassock, R.J. "Prophylactic Anticoagulation in Nephrotic Syndrome: A Clinical Conundrum," *Journal of the American Society of Nephrology* 18(8):2221-225, August 2007.

3. Wu, H.M., et al. "Interventions for Preventing Infection in Nephrotic Syndrome," *Cochrane Database of Systematic Reviews* (2): CD003964, April 2004.

4. Hodson, E.M., et al. "Corticosteroid Therapy for Nephrotic Syndrome in Children," *Cochrane Database of Systematic Reviews* (4):CD001533, August 2007.

NEUROGENIC BLADDER

Neurogenic bladder (also known as *neuromuscular dysfunction of the lower urinary tract, neurologic bladder dysfunction,* and *neuropathic bladder*) refers to all types of bladder dysfunction caused by an interruption of normal bladder innervation. Subsequent complications include incontinence, residual urine retention, urinary infection, calculus formation, and renal failure. A neurogenic bladder can be spastic (hypertonic, reflex, or automatic) or flaccid (hypotonic, atonic, nonreflex, or autonomous).

Causes and incidence

At one time, neurogenic bladder was thought to result primarily from spinal cord injury; now, it appears to stem from a host of underlying conditions. These include:

▶ cerebral disorders, such as stroke, brain tumor (meningioma and glioma), Parkinson's disease, multiple sclerosis, dementia, and incontinence caused by aging

▶ spinal cord disease or trauma, such as herniated vertebral disks, spina bifida, myelomeningocele, spinal stenosis (causing cord compression) or arachnoiditis (causing adhesions between the membranes covering the cord), cervical spondylosis, myelopathies from hereditary or nutritional deficiencies and, rarely, tabes dorsalis

▶ disorders of peripheral innervation, including autonomic neuropathies resulting from endocrine disturbances such as diabetes mellitus (most common)

▶ metabolic disturbances, such as hypothyroidism, porphyria, or uremia (infrequent)
▶ acute infectious diseases such as transverse myelitis
▶ heavy metal toxicity
▶ chronic alcoholism
▶ collagen diseases such as systemic lupus erythematosus
▶ vascular diseases such as atherosclerosis
▶ distant effects of cancer such as primary oat cell carcinoma of the lung
▶ herpes zoster
▶ sacral agenesis.

An upper motor neuron lesion (above S2 to S4) causes spastic neurogenic bladder, with spontaneous contractions of detrusor muscles, elevated intravesical voiding pressure, bladder wall hypertrophy with trabeculation, and urinary sphincter spasms. A lower motor neuron lesion (below S2 to S4) causes flaccid neurogenic bladder, with decreased intravesical pressure, increased bladder capacity and large residual urine retention, and poor detrusor contraction.

There's some evidence that neurogenic bladder occurs in people with diabetes at earlier ages than in those without diabetes.[1]

Signs and symptoms

Neurogenic bladder produces a wide range of clinical effects, depending on the underlying cause and its effect on the structural integrity of the bladder. Usually, this disorder causes some degree of incontinence, changes in initiation or interruption of micturition, loss of the urge to void when the bladder is full, leakage of urine and the inability to empty the bladder completely. Other effects of neurogenic bladder include vesicoureteral reflux, deterioration or infection in the upper urinary tract, and hydroureteral nephrosis.

Depending on the site and extent of the spinal cord lesion, spastic neurogenic bladder may produce involuntary or frequent scanty urination, without a feeling of bladder fullness, and possibly spontaneous spasms of the arms and legs. Anal sphincter tone may be increased. Tactile stimulation of the abdomen, thighs, or genitalia may precipitate voiding and spontaneous contractions of the arms and legs. With cord lesions in the upper thoracic (cervical) level, bladder distention can trigger hyperactive autonomic reflexes, resulting in severe hypertension, bradycardia, and headaches.

Flaccid neurogenic bladder may be associated with overflow incontinence, diminished anal sphincter tone, and a greatly distended bladder (evident on percussion or palpation), but without the accompanying feeling of bladder fullness due to sensory impairment.

Diagnosis

When neurogenic bladder is suspected, the nervous system, including the brain, and the bladder itself are examined.[2] The patient's history may include a condition or disorder that can cause neurogenic bladder, incontinence, and disruptions of micturition patterns. Voiding cystourethrography evaluates bladder neck function, vesicoureteral reflux, and continence. Urodynamic studies help evaluate how urine is stored in the bladder, how well the bladder empties, and the rate of movement of urine out of the bladder during voiding. These studies consist of four components:
▶ Urine flow study (uroflow) shows diminished or impaired urine flow.
▶ Cystometry evaluates bladder nerve supply, detrusor muscle tone, and intravesical pressures during bladder filling and contraction.
▶ Urethral pressure profile determines urethral function with respect to the length of the urethra and the outlet pressure resistance.
▶ Sphincter electromyelography correlates the neuromuscular function of the external sphincter with bladder muscle function during bladder filling and contraction. This

evaluates how well the bladder and urinary sphincter muscles work together.

▶ Retrograde urethrography reveals the presence of strictures and diverticula. This test may not be performed on a routine basis.

Treatment

The goals of treatment are to maintain the integrity of the upper urinary tract, control infection, and prevent urinary incontinence through evacuation of the bladder, drug therapy, surgery or, less commonly, neural blocks and electrical stimulation.

Techniques of bladder evacuation include Credé's method, Valsalva's maneuver, and intermittent self-catheterization. Credé's method—application of manual pressure over the lower abdomen—promotes complete emptying of the bladder. After appropriate instruction, most patients can perform this maneuver themselves. Even when patients perform this maneuver properly, however, Credé's method isn't always successful and doesn't always eliminate the need for catheterization.

Intermittent self-catheterization—more effective than either Credé's method or Valsalva's maneuver—has proved to be a major advance in the treatment of neurogenic bladder because it allows complete emptying of the bladder without the risks that an indwelling catheter poses. Generally, a male can perform this procedure more easily but a female can learn it with the help of a mirror. Intermittent self-catheterization, in conjunction with a bladder-retraining program, is especially useful for patients with flaccid neurogenic bladder. Although most patients are taught to self-catheterize during the day hours, nighttime catheterizations are also recommended as a way to prevent bladder nighttime overdistention, and to reverse or prevent bladder and upper tract deterioration.[2]

Drug therapy for neurogenic bladder may include bethanechol and phenoxybenzamine to facilitate bladder emptying and propantheline, methantheline, flavoxate, dicyclomine, darifenacin, hyoscyamine, and imipramine to facilitate urine storage and stop urge incontinence. Conjugated estrogen is used to increase the tone of urethral muscles. Antispasmodic drugs also are used to relax smooth muscles and increase bladder capacity including oxybutynin, tolterodine, and trospium.

Other treatments include pelvic floor exercises, biofeedback and electrical stimulation, and bladder training.[3] Diet therapy is also used. This involves removing certain foods from the diet that can worsen symptoms of urinary frequency and urge incontinence. These foods include spicy foods, chocolate, and citrus juices.

When conservative treatment fails, surgery may correct the structural impairment through transurethral resection of the bladder neck, urethral dilatation, external sphincterotomy, or urinary diversion procedures. Implantation of an artificial urinary sphincter may be necessary if permanent incontinence follows surgery for neurogenic bladder. Intravesical electrotherapy is also used to help increase bladder compliance. It has been shown to help increase feelings of bladder fullness.[4]

Special considerations

Care for patients with neurogenic bladder varies according to the underlying cause and method of treatment.

▶ Explain all diagnostic tests clearly so the patient understands the procedure, time involved, and possible results. Assure the patient that the lengthy diagnostic process is necessary to identify the most effective treatment plan. After the treatment plan is chosen, explain it to the patient in detail.

▶ Use strict sterile technique during insertion of an indwelling catheter (a temporary measure to drain the incontinent patient's bladder). Don't interrupt the closed drainage system for any reason. Obtain urine speci-

mens with a syringe and small-bore needle inserted through the aspirating port of the catheter itself (below the junction of the balloon instillation site). Irrigate in the same manner if ordered.

▶ Clean the catheter insertion site with soap and water at least twice per day. Don't allow the catheter to become encrusted. Use a sterile applicator to apply antibiotic ointment around the meatus after catheter care. Keep the drainage bag below the tubing, and don't raise the bag above the level of the bladder. Clamp the tubing, or empty the bag before transferring the patient to a wheelchair or stretcher to prevent accidental urine reflux. If urine output is considerable, empty the bag more frequently than once every 8 hours because bacteria can multiply in standing urine and migrate up the catheter and into the bladder.

▶ Watch for signs of infection (fever, cloudy or foul-smelling urine). Encourage the patient to drink plenty of fluids to prevent calculus formation and infection from urinary stasis. Try to keep the patient as mobile as possible. Perform passive range-of-motion exercises if necessary.

▶ If a urinary diversion procedure is to be performed, arrange for consultation with an enterostomal therapist, and coordinate the care plans.

▶ Before discharge, teach the patient and his family evacuation techniques as necessary (Credé's method, intermittent catheterization). Counsel him regarding sexual activities. Remember, the incontinent patient feels embarrassed and distressed. Provide emotional support.

▶ Teach the motivated patient to do intermittent self-catheterization using clean technique with good hand-washing technique and a sterile catheter or a nonsterile clean catheter. Clean intermittent catheterization results in lower infection rates than use of an indwelling catheter.[3] For an older patient or one with a weak immune system, sterile technique should be taught. Further research is needed to establish whether clean technique or sterile technique is better for this group.

REFERENCES

1. National Diabetes Information Clearinghouse (2004 June). "Sexual and Urologic Problems of Diabetes," NIH Publication No. 04-5135 [Online]. Available at *http://diabetes.niddk.nih .gov/dm/pubs/sup/index.htm*.
2. Canon, S., et al. "Nocturnal Bladder Emptying for Reversing Urinary Tract Deterioration Due to Neurogenic Bladder," *Current Urology Reports* 8(1):60-65, January 2007.
3. Brigham and Women's Hospital (2007 October 26). "Neurogenic Bladder" [Online]. Available at *http://healthlibrary.brighamandwomens.org/ Search/85,P01487*.
4. Hagerty, J.A., et al. "Intravesical Electrotherapy for Neurogenic Bladder Dysfunction: A 22-Year Experience," *Journal of Urology* 178(4 Pt 2):1680-83, October 2007.

POLYCYSTIC KIDNEY DISEASE

Polycystic kidney disease (PKD) is an inherited disorder characterized by multiple, bilateral, grapelike clusters of fluid-filled cysts that grossly enlarge the kidneys, compressing and eventually leading to reduced kidney function and kidney failure. (See *Polycystic kidney.*) The disease appears in two distinct forms: Autosomal recessive PKD (ARPKD), the infantile form, typically causes stillbirth or early neonatal death, although some infants may survive for 2 years, then develop fatal renal, cardiac, or respiratory failure. Autosomal dominant PKD (ADPKD), the adult form, begins insidiously but usually becomes obvious between ages 30 and 40.[1] In the adult form, renal deterioration is more gradual but, as in the infantile form, progresses relentlessly to fatal uremia.

The prognosis in adults is extremely variable. Progression may be slow, even after

symptoms of renal insufficiency appear. However, after uremic symptoms develop, PKD is usually fatal within 4 years, unless the patient receives treatment with dialysis, kidney transplantation, or both. More than 60% develop kidney failure or end-stage renal diseases. PKD accounts for 8% to 10% of patients on dialysis.[1]

Causes and incidence

While both types of PKD are genetically transmitted, the incidence in two distinct age-groups and different inheritance patterns suggest two unrelated disorders. The infantile type appears to be inherited as an autosomal recessive trait, whereas the adult type seems to be an autosomal dominant trait. The gene has been located on chromosome 6, supporting the premise that this is a single genetic disease with variable phenotype presentation.

KD reportedly affects 1 in 500 to 1 in 1,000 Americans or about 600,000 people.[1] Both types of PKD affect males and females equally.

Signs and symptoms

The neonate with infantile polycystic disease commonly has pronounced epicanthal folds, a pointed nose, a small chin, and floppy, low-set ears (Potter facies). At birth, he has huge bilateral masses on the flanks that are symmetrical, tense, and can't be transilluminated. He characteristically shows signs of respiratory distress and heart failure. Eventually, he develops uremia and renal failure. Accompanying hepatic fibrosis may cause portal hypertension and bleeding varices to develop, requiring sclerotherapy or portacaval shunting.[3]

Adult PKD commonly produces no symptoms through the patient's 40s but may induce nonspecific symptoms, such as hypertension, polyuria, and recurrent urinary tract infections (UTIs). Later, the patient develops overt symptoms related to the enlarging kidney mass, such as lumbar pain, widening

Polycystic kidney

In polycystic kidney disease, cysts are seen in grapelike clusters, as shown below.

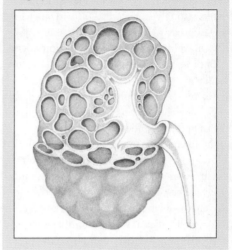

girth, and swollen or tender abdomen. Abdominal pain is usually worsened by exertion and relieved by lying down. In advanced stages, this disease may cause recurrent hematuria, life-threatening retroperitoneal bleeding resulting from cyst rupture, proteinuria, and colicky abdominal pain from the ureteral passage of clots or calculi. Generally, about 10 years after symptoms appear, progressive compression of kidney structures by the enlarging mass produces renal failure and uremia. Hypertension is found in about 20% to 30% of children and up to 75% of adults due to intrarenal ischemia, which activates the renin-angiotensin system.

Complications

▶ Hematura
▶ Retroperitoneal bleeding from ruptured cysts
▶ Proteinuria
▶ Colicky abdominal pain
▶ Renal failure

Diagnosis

New therapeutic approaches are being evaluated to measure disease progression earlier and to initiate treatment of ADPKD. A family history and a physical examination revealing large bilateral, irregular masses in the flanks strongly suggest PKD. In advanced stages, grossly enlarged and palpable kidneys make the diagnosis obvious. In patients with these findings, the following laboratory results are typical:

▶ Excretory urography reveals enlarged kidneys, with elongation of pelvis, flattening of the calyces, and indentations caused by cysts. Excretory urography of the neonate shows poor excretion of contrast medium.

▶ Ultrasound, computed tomography, and magnetic resonance imaging scan show kidney enlargement and the presence of cysts; tomography demonstrates multiple areas of cystic damage. Ultrasonography is the preferred imaging technique because it's less expensive, doesn't require contrast or radiation exposure, and is easily and safely performed on children and pregnant females.[2]

▶ Urinalysis and creatinine clearance tests are nonspecific tests that evaluate renal function and reveal urine protein or blood in the urine.

Diagnosis must rule out the presence of renal tumors.

There are new therapeutic approaches being evaluated to measure disease progression earlier and to initiate treatment of ADPKD.

Treatment

PKD can't be cured. The primary goal of treatment is preserving renal parenchyma and preventing infectious complications. Management of secondary hypertension will also help prevent rapid deterioration in function. Progressive renal failure requires treatment similar to that for other types of renal disease, including dialysis or, rarely, kidney transplantation.

When adult PKD is discovered in the asymptomatic stage, careful monitoring is required, including urine cultures and creatinine clearance tests every 6 months. Prompt and vigorous antibiotic treatment is needed when a urine culture reveals infection—even when the patient is asymptomatic. As renal impairment progresses, selected patients may undergo dialysis, transplantation, or both. Cystic abscess or retroperitoneal bleeding may require surgical drainage; intractable pain (a rare symptom) also may require surgery. However, because this disease affects both kidneys, nephrectomy usually isn't recommended because it increases the risk of infection in the remaining kidney.

Special considerations

Because PKD is usually relentlessly progressive, comprehensive patient teaching and emotional support are essential.

▶ Refer the young adult patient or the parents of infants with PKD for genetic counseling. Parents will probably have many questions about the risk to other offspring.[3]

▶ Provide supportive care to minimize any associated symptoms. Carefully assess the patient's lifestyle and his physical and mental status; determine how rapidly the disease is progressing. Use this information to plan individualized patient care.

▶ Acquaint yourself with all aspects of end-stage renal disease, including dialysis and transplantation, so you can provide appropriate care and patient teaching as the disease progresses.

▶ Explain all diagnostic procedures to the patient or to his family if the patient is an infant. Before beginning excretory urography or other procedures that use an iodine-based contrast medium, determine whether the patient has ever had an allergic reaction to iodine or shellfish. Even if the patient has no history of allergy, watch for an allergic reaction after performing the procedures.

▶ Administer antibiotics as ordered for UTI. Stress to the patient the need to take the medication exactly as prescribed, even if symptoms are minimal or absent.

REFERENCES

1. PKD Foundation "ARPKD: Autosomal Recessive Polycystic Kidney Disease" [Online]. Available at *www.pkdcure.org/site/PageServer*.
2. National Kidney and Urologic Disease Information Clearinghouse (2007 November). "Polycystic Kidney Disease," NIH Publication No. 08-4008 [Online]. Available at *http://kidney.niddk.nih.gov/kudiseases/pubs/polycystic/*.
3. Chapman, A.B. "Autosomal Dominant Polycystic Kidney Disease: Time for a Change?" *Journal of the American Society of Nephrology* 18(5):1399-407, May 2007.

PROSTATITIS

Prostatitis, inflammation of the prostate gland, may present as acute bacterial prostatitis, chronic bacterial prostatitis, chronic prostatitis/chronic pelvic pain syndrome (CPPS) or asymptomatic inflammatory prostatitis.

Acute prostatitis most commonly results from gram-negative bacteria and is easy to recognize and treat. However, chronic prostatitis, the most common cause of recurrent urinary tract infections (UTIs) in males, is less easy to recognize. CPPS is the most common form of prostatitis, accounting for 90% of the cases.

Prostatitis (acute, chronic, or noninfectious) is treated based on type; treatment can include antimicrobials, muscle relaxants, and lifestyle changes

Causes and incidence

The most common cause of bacterial prostatitis is infection by *Escherichia coli;* the rest are due to infection by *Klebsiella, Enterobacter, Proteus, Pseudomonas, Streptococcus,* or *Staphylococcus*.[2] These organisms probably spread to the prostate by the bloodstream or from ascending urethral infection, invasion of rectal bacteria via lymphatics, reflux of infected bladder urine into the prostate ducts or, less commonly, sexual intercourse or such procedures as cystoscopy or catheterization. Chronic bacterial prostatitis usually results from recurrent UTIs but is associated with an underlying defect in the prostate which becomes the focal point for bacteria in the urinary tract.[3] Chronic prostatitis/CPPS is the least understood type. It can be inflammatory or noninflammatory, and symptoms are present without evidence of an infecting organism. About 5% to 8% of males eventually have bacteria in their urine or prostatic fluid.[4]

It's estimated that 25% of males who seek outpatient care do so because of prostatitis.[3]

In patients younger than 35 years, acute bacterial prostate is the most common. About 10% of males ages 20 to 74 years have prostatitis symptoms.

Signs and symptoms

Acute prostatitis begins with fever, chills, lower back pain, myalgia, perineal fullness, and arthralgia. Urination is frequent and urgent. Dysuria, nocturia, and urinary obstruction also may occur. The urine may appear cloudy. When palpated rectally, the prostate is tender, indurated, swollen, firm, and warm.

Chronic bacterial prostatitis sometimes produces no symptoms but usually elicits the same urinary symptoms as the acute form but to a lesser degree. Other possible signs and symptoms include painful ejaculation, hemospermia, persistent urethral discharge, vague suprapubic discomfort, and sexual dysfunction. Dysuria and suprapubic discomfort can be the only symptoms of prostatitis but aren't specific to prostatitis. One study showed that although dysuria associated with prostatitis resolved after treatment with antibiotics, it was later diagnosed as a symptom associated with prostatic adenoma.[1]

Chronic prostatitis/CPPS is characterized by urinary and genital pain for at least 3 months out of 6.

EVIDENCE-BASED PRACTICE

Acupuncture and pelvic pain

Question: *Can acupuncture relieve the pain associated with chronic prostatitis/chronic pelvic pain syndrome?*

Research: Chronic prostatitis/chronic pelvic pain syndrome (CP/CPPS), also called *chronic nonbacterial prostatitis* or *prostatodynia*, is a disabling condition of unknown origin affecting men of all ages and ethnic groups. This study, comparing the efficacy of acupuncture to sham acupuncture for the relief of CP/CPPS was conducted because conventional therapies offer little or no proven relief of symptoms. The researchers used the National Institutes of Health (NIH) consensus criteria for CP/CPPS and the NIH Chronic Prostatitis Symptom Index for the selection of participants, with participants having symptoms for at least 3 of the preceding 6 months. The study consisted of 89 participants who were divided into two groups: 44 participants placed in the acupuncture group and 45 in the sham acupuncture group. They received twice-weekly, 30-minute sessions for 10 weeks without needle stimulation, herbs, or adjuvants.

Conclusion: Of the 44 participants in the acupuncture group, 32 (73%) responded favorably, with long-term responses (24 weeks after completing therapy) in 14 (32%) patients. In the sham acupuncture group of 45 participants, 21 (47%) responded favorably, with long-term responses in 6 (13%) patients. Participants receiving acupuncture were almost twice as likely as sham treatment participants to experience improvement in CP/CPPS symptoms.

Application: CP/CPPS is the most prevalent form of prostatitis and also the most challenging to treat because there's currently no effective relief for the disabling symptoms it produces. When caring for a patient with CP/CPPS, the nurse should provide information about recommended treatment modalities; non-prostate-centered treatment strategies, such as physical therapy and relaxation techniques; and alternative therapies such as acupuncture.

Source: Lee, S.W., et al. "Acupuncture versus Sham Acupuncture for Chronic Prostatitis/Chronic Pelvic Pain," *American Journal of Medicine* 121(1):79, January 2008.

Complications

▶ UTI is the most common
▶ Prostatic abscess
▶ Acute urine retention
▶ Pyelonephritis
▶ Epididymitis

Diagnosis

Characteristic rectal examination findings suggest prostatitis. In many cases, a urine culture can identify the causative infectious organism. A firm diagnosis depends on urine cultures of specimens obtained by the Meares and Stamey technique. This test requires four specimens: one collected when the patient starts voiding (voided bladder one); another midstream; another after the patient stops voiding and the physician massages the prostate to produce secretions (expressed prostate secretions); and a final voided specimen. A significant increase in colony count in the prostatic specimen confirms prostatitis.

Treatment

Systemic antibiotic therapy chosen according to the infecting organism is the treatment of choice for acute prostatitis. If sepsis is likely, I.V. antibiotics may be given until sensitivity test results are known. If test results and clinical response are favorable, parenteral therapy continues for 48 hours to 1 week, after which an oral agent is substituted for 30 days. Supportive therapy includes bed

rest, adequate hydration, and administration of analgesics, antipyretics, sitz baths, and stool softeners as necessary. Diet therapy includes avoiding substances that irritate the bladder, such as alcohol, caffeinated food and beverages, citrus juices, and hot or spicy foods. Increasing the intake of fluids encourages frequent urination that will help flush the bacteria from the bladder. In symptomatic chronic prostatitis, regular massage of the prostate is most effective. Regular ejaculation may help promote drainage of prostatic secretions. Anticholinergics and analgesics may help relieve nonbacterial prostatitis symptoms. (See *Acupuncture and pelvic pain*).

If drug therapy is unsuccessful, treatment may include transurethral resection of the prostate, which requires removal of all infected tissue. However, this procedure usually isn't performed on young adults because it may cause retrograde ejaculation and sterility. Total prostatectomy is curative but may cause impotence and incontinence.

Special considerations

Patient care is primarily supportive.

▶ Ensure bed rest and adequate hydration. Provide stool softeners and administer sitz baths, as ordered.

▶ As necessary, prepare to assist with suprapubic needle aspiration of the bladder or a suprapubic cystostomy.

▶ Emphasize the need for strict adherence to the prescribed drug regimen. Instruct the patient to drink at least eight glasses of water per day. Have him report adverse drug reactions (rash, nausea, vomiting, fever, chills, and GI irritation).

REFERENCES

1. Canavese, C., et al. "An Asymptomatic Patient with Multiple Solid Renal Masses: Errors in Diagnosis," *Nephrology, Dialysis, Transplantation* 20(10):2274-278, October 2005.
2. Stevermer, J., and Easley, S. K. "Treatment of Prostatitis," *American Family Physician* 61(10):3015-3026, May 2000.
3. National Kidney and Urologic Disease Information Clearinghouse (2003 December). "Prostatitis: Disorders of the Prostate," NIH Publication No. 04-4553 [Online]. Available at *http://kidney.niddk.nih.gov/kudiseases/pubs/prostatitis/*.
4. Clemens, J.Q., et al. "Prevalence of and Risk Factors for Prostatitis: Population Based Assessment Using Physician Assigned Diagnoses," *Journal of Urology* 178(4 Pt 1):1333-337, October 2007.

RENAL CALCULI

Renal calculi or nephrolithiasis (commonly called *kidney stones*) may form anywhere in the urinary tract but usually develop in the renal pelvis or the calyces of the kidneys. Calculi formation follows precipitation of substances normally dissolved in the urine, such as calcium oxalate, calcium phosphate, magnesium ammonium phosphate or, occasionally, urate or cystine. (See *How urine pH affects calculi formation*, page 264.) Renal calculi vary in size and may be solitary or multiple. They may remain in the renal pelvis or enter the ureter and may damage renal parenchyma; large calculi cause pressure necrosis. In certain locations, calculi cause obstruction, with resultant hydronephrosis, and tend to recur.

Causes and incidence

Although the exact cause of renal calculi is unknown, predisposing factors include:

▶ *Dehydration:* Decreased urine production concentrates calculus-forming substances.

▶ *Infection:* Infected, damaged tissue serves as a site for calculus development; pH changes provide a favorable medium for calculus formation (especially for magnesium ammonium phosphate or calcium phosphate calculi); or infected calculi (usually magnesium ammonium phosphate or staghorn calculi) may develop if bacteria serve as the nu-

How urine pH affects calculi formation

The pH of the urine influences the types of calculi that may form.

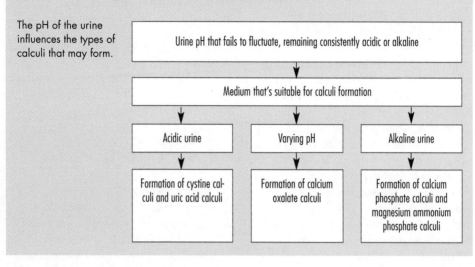

| Urine pH that fails to fluctuate, remaining consistently acidic or alkaline |

↓

| Medium that's suitable for calculi formation |

| Acidic urine | Varying pH | Alkaline urine |

| Formation of cystine calculi and uric acid calculi | Formation of calcium oxalate calculi | Formation of calcium phosphate calculi and magnesium ammonium phosphate calculi |

cleus in calculus formation. Infections may promote destruction of renal parenchyma.

▶ *Obstruction:* Urinary stasis (as in immobility from spinal cord injury) allows calculus constituents to collect and adhere, forming calculi. Obstruction also promotes infection, which, in turn, compounds the obstruction.

▶ *Metabolic factors:* These factors may predispose to renal calculi: hyperparathyroidism, renal tubular acidosis, elevated uric acid (usually with gout), defective metabolism of oxalate, genetic defect in metabolism of cystine, and excessive intake of vitamin D or dietary calcium. Hypercalciuria may be the cause of calculi in more than 50% of people. In this condition, calcium is lost into the urine and causes crystals of calcium oxalate or calcium phosphate to form.[1]

Among Americans, renal calculi develop in 2% to 10% of the population, with people living in southeastern states having an increased risk. They're more common in men, who have a 12% lifetime prevalence. Women have a 7% lifetime prevalence.[2] They're rare in children. They're three to

four times more common in white males than black males.[2]

Some types of calculi tend to be familial; some are associated with other conditions, such as bowel disease, ileal bypass for obesity, or renal tubule defects. Calcium calculi are most common, accounting for more than 75% of all calculi. They're two to three times more common in males, usually appearing between ages 20 and 30. The calcium may combine with other substances, such as oxalate (the most common substance), phosphate, or carbonate, to form the calculus. Oxalate is present in certain foods. Diseases of the small intestine increase the tendency to form calcium oxalate calculi. Recurrence is likely.

Uric acid calculi also are more common in males and make up about 6% of all calculi. These calculi are associated with gout and chemotherapy. Cystine calculi, which make up about 2% of all calculi, may form in people with cystinuria, a hereditary disorder affecting both males and females. Struvite calculi, accounting for about 15% of all calculi, are mainly found in females as a result of a urinary tract infection (UTI). They can grow

Types of renal calculi

Multiple small calculi may vary in size; they may remain in the renal pelvis or pass down the ureter.

A staghorn calculus (a cast of the calyceal and pelvic collecting system) may form from a calculus that stays in the kidney.

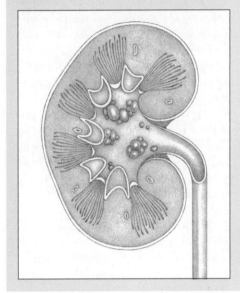

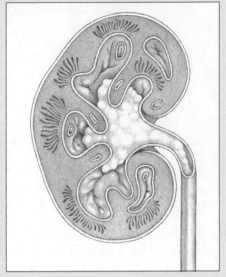

very large and may obstruct the kidney, ureter, or bladder.

Indinavir calculi appear in patients with human immunodeficiency virus who are treated with the protease inhibitor indinavir.

Signs and symptoms

Sometimes there are no symptoms when a person has renal calculi. Many times, renal calculi are diagnosed during a nonrelated medical treatment. Classic symptoms are usually increased pain, hematuria, and recurrent UTIs.[2]

Clinical effects vary with calculi size, location, and etiology. Pain, the key symptom, usually results from obstruction; large, rough calculi occlude the opening to the ureter and increase the frequency and force of peristaltic contractions. The pain of classic renal colic travels from the costovertebral angle to the flank, to the suprapubic region

and external genitalia. The intensity of this pain fluctuates and may be excruciating at its peak. If calculi are in the renal pelvis and calyces, pain may be more constant and dull. Back pain (from calculi that produce an obstruction within a kidney) and severe abdominal pain (from calculi traveling down a ureter) may also occur. (See *Types of renal calculi.*) Nausea and vomiting usually accompany severe pain.

Other associated signs include fever, chills, hematuria (when calculi abrade a ureter), abdominal distention, pyuria and, rarely, anuria (from bilateral obstruction, or unilateral obstruction in the patient with one kidney).

Complications

▶ Calculi that remain in the renal pelvis cause damage to renal parenchyma

▶ Large calculi in the kidneys cause pressure necrosis
▶ Hydronephrosis
▶ Intractable pain
▶ Bleeding

Diagnosis

Diagnosis is based on the clinical picture and the following tests:
▶ Computed tomography scan or magnetic resonance imaging are highly sensitive for identifying hydronephrosis and detecting small renal and urethral calculi.
▶ Excretory urography may be used for diagnosis of obstruction by urinary calculus.
▶ Kidney-ureter-bladder X-rays reveal most renal calculi.
▶ Calculus analysis shows mineral content.
▶ Excretory urography confirms the diagnosis and determines size and location of calculi.
▶ Kidney ultrasonography is an easily performed, noninvasive, nontoxic test to detect obstructive changes such as hydronephrosis.
▶ Urine culture of midstream specimen may indicate UTI.
▶ Urinalysis may be normal, or may show increased specific gravity and acid or alkaline pH suitable for different types of calculus formation. Other urinalysis findings include hematuria (gross or microscopic), crystals (urate, calcium, or cystine), casts, and pyuria with or without bacteria and white blood cells.
▶ A 24-hour urine collection is evaluated for calcium oxalate, phosphorus, and uric acid excretion levels.
▶ Serial blood calcium and phosphorus levels detect hyperparathyroidism and show increased calcium level in proportion to normal serum protein.

Increased blood uric acid levels may indicate gout as the cause. Diagnosis must rule out appendicitis, cholecystitis, peptic ulcer, and pancreatitis as potential sources of pain.

Treatment

Because 90% of renal calculi are smaller than 5 mm in diameter, treatment usually consists of measures to promote their natural passage. Along with vigorous hydration, such treatment includes antimicrobial therapy (varying with the cultured organism) for infection, analgesics such as stadol for pain, and diuretics to prevent urinary stasis and further calculus formation (thiazides decrease calcium excretion into the urine). Nonsteroidal anti-inflammatory drugs are also used for pain; studies have shown them to be as effective as opioid analgesics.[2] Prophylaxis to prevent calculus formation includes a low-calcium diet for absorptive hypercalciuria, parathyroidectomy for hyperparathyroidism, allopurinol for uric acid calculi, and daily administration of ascorbic acid by mouth to acidify the urine.[4]

Calculi too large for natural passage may require surgical removal. When a calculus is in the ureter, a cystoscope may be inserted through the urethra and the calculus manipulated with catheters or retrieval instruments. Extraction of calculi from other areas (kidney calyx, renal pelvis) may necessitate a flank or lower abdominal approach. Percutaneous ultrasonic lithotripsy and extracorporeal shock wave lithotripsy shatter the calculus into fragments for removal by suction or natural passage. Studies comparing ureteroscopic removal of calculi with extracorporeal shock wave lithotripsy show that ureteroscopic removal achieves a higher calculus-free state but with higher complications and a longer hospital stay.[3] (See *Surgery options and outcomes*.)

Special considerations

Patient care includes confirming the diagnosis, facilitating passage of the calculus, and prevention of future occurrences.
▶ To aid diagnosis, maintain a 24- to 48-hour record of urine pH, with nitrazine pH paper; strain all urine through gauze or a

EVIDENCE-BASED PRACTICE

Surgery options and outcomes

Question: *Is percutaneous nephrolithotomy in the supine position safe and effective?*

Research: Percutaneous nephrolithotomy for renal calculi can be performed in the supine or prone positions. Researchers studied 322 consecutive percutaneous nephrolithotomies performed by one surgeon on patients in the supine position between 1999 and 2006 to determine the safety, effectiveness, and suitability of supine positioning for this procedure.

Conclusion: Of the 322 procedures studied, only 1 resulted in failed access with the patient's kidney being punctured. There were no complications reported in the remaining patients, including those with bilateral stones and staghorn calculi. The procedures resulted in a 91% calculi clearance rate. Benefits of supine positioning were determined to be a reduction in the overall operative time and a decreased length of hospitalization compared with the traditional prone position.

Application: The nurse caring for a patient about to undergo a percutaneous nephrolithotomy for renal calculi should be aware that the patient can be placed in either a prone or supine position. Although it isn't the traditional position for this procedure, the supine position is safe and provides for effective calculi clearance. In addition, the nurse can anticipate a faster recovery and discharge of the patient who was positioned supine.

Source: Steele, D., and Marshall, V. "Percutaneous Nephrolithotomy in the Supine Position: A Neglected Approach?" *Journal of Endourology* 21(12):1433-37, December 2007.

---

tea strainer, and save all solid material recovered for analysis.

▶ To facilitate spontaneous passage, encourage the patient to walk if possible. Also promote sufficient intake of fluids to maintain a urine output of 3 to 4 L/day (urine should be very dilute and colorless). To help acidify urine, offer fruit juices, particularly cranberry juice. If the patient can't drink the required amount of fluid, supplemental I.V. fluids may be given. Record intake and output and daily weight to assess fluid status and renal function.

▶ Stress the importance of proper diet and compliance with drug therapy. For example, if the patient's calculus is caused by a hyperuricemic condition, advise him (or whoever prepares his meals) to avoid foods high in purine. Restrict protein to 60 g/day to decrease calcium and uric acid, and limit sodium to 3 to 4 g/day. Oxalate foods are restricted.

▶ If surgery is necessary, give reassurance by supplementing and reinforcing what the surgeon has told the patient about the procedure. The patient is apt to be fearful, especially if surgery includes removal of a kidney, so emphasize the fact that the body can adapt well to one kidney. If he's to have an abdominal or flank incision, teach deep-breathing and coughing exercises.

▶ After surgery, the patient will probably have an indwelling catheter or a nephrostomy tube. Unless one of his kidneys was removed, expect bloody drainage from the catheter. Never irrigate the catheter without a physician's order. Check dressings regularly for bloody drainage, and know how much drainage to expect. Immediately report suspected hemorrhage (excessive drainage, rising pulse rate). Use sterile technique when changing dressings or providing catheter care.

▶ Watch for signs of infection (rising fever, chills), and give antibiotics as ordered. To prevent pneumonia, encourage frequent position changes, and ambulate the patient as soon as possible. Have him hold a small pillow over the operative site to splint the incision and thereby facilitate deep-breathing and coughing exercises.

▶ Before discharge, teach the patient and his family the importance of following the prescribed dietary and medication regimens to prevent recurrence of calculi. Encourage increased fluid intake. If appropriate, show the patient how to check his urine pH, and instruct him to keep a daily record. Tell him to immediately report symptoms of acute obstruction (pain, inability to void).

REFERENCES

1. National Kidney and Urologic Disease Information Clearinghouse (2007 October). "Kidney Stones in Adults," NIH Publication No. 08-2495 [Online]. Available at *http://kidney.niddk.nih.gov/Kudiseases/pubs/stonesadults/#cause.*

2. MayoClinic.com (2008 April 8). "Kidney Stones" [Online]. Available at *www.mayoclinic.com/health/kidney-stones/DS00282.*

3. Nabi, G., et al. "Extra-Corporeal Shock Wave Lithotripsy (ESWL) versus Ureteroscopic Management for Ureteric Calculi," *Cochrane Database of Systematic Reviews* (1):CD006029, January 2007.

4. Park, S., and Pearle, M.S. "Pathophysiology and Management of Calcium Stones," *Urology Clinics of North America* 34(3):323-34, August 2007.

RENOVASCULAR HYPERTENSION

Renovascular hypertension is a rise in systemic blood pressure resulting from stenosis of the major renal arteries or their branches or from intrarenal atherosclerosis. This narrowing or sclerosis may be partial or complete, and the resulting blood pressure elevation, benign or malignant. About 10% of patients with high blood pressure have secondary hypertension which results from an underlying cause.[1] Renal artery stenosis is the most common cause of secondary hypertension.

Causes and incidence

Stenosis or occlusion of the renal artery stimulates the affected kidney to release the enzyme renin, which converts angiotensinogen—a plasma protein—to angiotensin I. As angiotensin I circulates through the lungs and liver, it converts to angiotensin II, which causes peripheral vasoconstriction, increased arterial pressure and aldosterone secretion and, eventually, hypertension.

Atherosclerosis (especially in older males) accounts for about two-thirds of cases of renovascular hypertension. Fibromuscular diseases of the renal artery wall layers—such as medial fibroplasia and, less commonly, intimal and subadventitial fibroplasias, is the cause of about one-third of renovascular hypertension cases.[2] Together, they're the primary causes in 95% of all patients with renovascular hypertension. Fibromuscular dysplasia is more common among younger patients and in women.[2] Other causes include arteritis, anomalies of the renal arteries, embolism, trauma, tumor, and dissecting aneurysm. Less than 5% of patients with high blood pressure display renovascular hypertension; it's most common in persons younger than age 30 or older than age 50.

Signs and symptoms

In addition to elevated systemic blood pressure, renovascular hypertension usually produces symptoms common to hypertensive states, such as headache, palpitations, tachycardia, anxiety, light-headedness, decreased tolerance of temperature extremes, retinopathy, and mental sluggishness.

Complications

▶ Heart failure
▶ Myocardial infarction

▶ Stroke
▶ Renal failure

Diagnosis

The definitive diagnostic procedure is done by arterial digital subtraction angiography with assays of venous rennin. When stenosis is significant, transluminal angioplasty can be done during the same procedure.

Diagnosis is confirmed by the following tests:

▶ Gadolinium enhanced magnetic resonance angiography can identify turbulent blood flow indicative of renal stenosis.
▶ Duplex Doppler ultrasonography scans the renal artery and will reveal stenosis, but results vary.
▶ Oral captopril renography is the simplest noninvasive test for detection of renovascular hypertension but has a relatively high false-positive rate.

Treatment

Surgery, the treatment of choice, is performed to restore adequate circulation and to control severe hypertension or severely impaired renal function by renal artery bypass, endarterectomy, arterioplasty or, as a last resort, nephrectomy. Balloon catheter renal artery dilation is used in selected cases to correct renal artery stenosis without the risks and morbidity of surgery. Symptomatic measures include antihypertensives, diuretics, and a sodium-restricted diet.

Medications that may be used in an attempt to control blood pressure include diuretics, beta-adrenergic blockers, calcium channel blockers, angiotensin-converting enzyme inhibitors, angiotensin-receptor blockers, and alpha-adrenergic blockers. Diazoxide or nitroprusside may be given in the hospital if symptoms are acute. Response to medications is highly individual, and the dosage or specific drug used may need frequent adjustment.

Lifestyle changes may be recommended, including weight reduction, exercise, dietary modifications, smoking cessation, and avoidance of alcohol. These habits add to the effects of hypertension in causing complications.

Special considerations

The care plan must emphasize helping the patient and his family understand renovascular hypertension and the importance of following the prescribed treatment.

▶ Accurately monitor intake and output and daily weight. Check blood pressure in both arms regularly, with the patient lying down and standing. A drop of 20 mm Hg or more on arising may necessitate an adjustment in antihypertensive medications. Assess renal function daily.
▶ Maintain fluid and sodium restrictions. Explain the purpose of a low-sodium diet.
▶ Explain the diagnostic tests, and prepare the patient appropriately; for example, adequately hydrate the patient before tests that use contrast media. Make sure the patient isn't allergic to the dye used in diagnostic tests. After excretory urography or arteriography, watch for complications.
▶ If a nephrectomy is necessary, reassure the patient that the remaining kidney is adequate for renal function.
▶ Postoperatively, watch for bleeding and hypotension. If the sutures around the renal vessels slip, the patient can quickly go into shock because kidneys receive 25% of cardiac output.
▶ Provide a quiet, stress-free environment if possible. Urge the patient and his family members to have regular blood pressure screenings.

REFERENCES

1. Vascular Disease Foundation (2007 December 5). "Renovascular Hypertension: What Is It?" [Online]. Available at *www.vdf.org/diseaseinfo/ras/*.
2. Merck Manuals Online Medical Library (2007 July). "Renovascular Hypertension" [Online]. Available at *www.merck.com/mmpe/sec07/ch071/ch071b.html*.

Immune disorders

ACQUIRED IMMUNODEFICIENCY SYNDROME

Acquired immunodeficiency syndrome (AIDS) is a serious secondary immunodeficiency disorder caused by the human immunodeficiency virus (HIV). Both diseases are characterized by the progressive destruction of cell-mediated (T-cell) immunity with subsequent effects on humoral (B-cell) immunity because of the pivotal role of the CD4+ helper T cells in immune reactions. The resultant immunodeficiency makes the patient susceptible to opportunistic infections, unusual cancers, and other abnormalities. (See *Common infections and neoplasms in HIV and AIDS.*)

The Centers for Disease Control and Prevention (CDC) first described AIDS in 1981. Since then, the CDC has declared a case surveillance definition for AIDS and modified it several times, most recently in January 2006.

Causes and incidence

AIDS results from infection with HIV, which has two forms: HIV-1 and HIV-2. Both forms of HIV have the same modes of transmission and similar opportunistic infections associated with AIDS, but studies indicate that HIV-2 develops more slowly and presents with milder symptoms than HIV-1.

Transmission occurs through contact with infected blood or body fluids and is associated with identifiable high-risk behaviors. It's disproportionately represented in:

▶ homosexual and bisexual men
▶ persons who use illicit I.V. drugs
▶ neonates of infected females
▶ recipients of contaminated blood or blood products (the incidence has dramatically decreased since mid-1985)
▶ heterosexual partners of persons in the former groups.

The CDC's case surveillance data collection system as of July 2006 has been established in 45 states and 5 U.S. territories.[1] As a national comprehensive data collection system is implemented, prevalence data will become more accurate. However, HIV screening still remains voluntary except for prenatal care settings.[4] The CDC recently submitted its recommendations (to health care providers) to incorporate routine HIV testing as a part of their assessment to improve the number of patients who volunteer to be tested.

IN THE NEWS *The CDC estimates there are a quarter million Americans who are unaware of their HIV positive status.*[2]

Data from 2003 estimates the prevalence of HIV in the United States to be 1.04 to 1.185 million, which includes those who are unaware of their HIV positive status.

Of the people living with HIV, 24% to 27% were undiagnosed.[1] Of new cases diagnosed between 2001 and 2004 (with 33 states reporting), 29% were women and 66% were people of color. Non–Hispanic blacks accounted for 51% of cases. Male-to male sexual contact remains the major transmission carrier, accounting for 44% of new cases; while 34% are due to high-risk heterosexual contact.[1]

Signs and symptoms

A person with acute HIV presents with symptoms such as a rash, acute viral infection, myalgia, fever, malaise, fatigue, headache, and lymphadenopathy. A person with HIV may then remain asymptomatic for months or years. Initially, laboratory evidence or seroconversion to HIV antibodies may be the only clinical evidence of infection. However, as the disease progresses, the patient may develop generalized adenopathy and nonspecific signs and symptoms, such as weight loss, fatigue, night sweats, and fevers. As the patient's T-cell count lowers further, neurologic symptoms, opportunistic infections, and certain normally rare cancers may develop. HIV also destroys lymph nodes and immunologic organs, leading to major dysfunctions of the immunologic system. Eventually, HIV advances to AIDS. (Some individuals, termed *nonprogressors,* develop AIDS very slowly or not at all. They seem to have genetic differences that prevent the virus from attaching to certain immune receptors.) The clinical course varies slightly in children, who have a shorter incubation time (typically, a mean of 17 months).

Complications

▶ Opportunistic infections
▶ Unusual cancers
▶ Lymphoid interstitial pneumonia
▶ Arthritis
▶ Hypergammaglobulinemia
▶ Production of autoimmune antibodies
▶ AIDS dementia complex

Common infections and neoplasms in HIV and AIDS

The disorders listed below are commonly seen in patients with human immunodeficiency virus (HIV) and acquired immunodeficiency syndrome (AIDS). AIDS is diagnosed when a patient who has tested positive for HIV shows a CD4+ T-cell count of less than 200 cells/µl. The first group of infections are common in patients with HIV; the next three are associated with the progressively lower CD4+ T-cell counts found in AIDS patients.

■ Common infections in a patient with a CD4+ count less than 350 cells/µl include:
– herpes simplex virus
– herpes zoster
– *Mycobacterium tuberculosis*
– non–Hodgkin's lymphoma
– oral or vaginal thrush.
■ Common infections in a patient with a CD4+ count less than 200 cells/µl include:
– *Candida* esophagitis
– *Pneumocystis carinii* pneumonia.
■ Common infections in a patient with a CD4+ count less than 100 cells/µl include:
– AIDS dementia
– Cryptococcal meningitis
– progressive multifocal leukoencephalopathy
– toxoplasmosis encephalitis
– wasting syndrome.
■ Common infections in a patient with a CD4+ count less than 50 cells/µl include:
– *Cytomegalovirus* infection
– *Mycobacterium avium.*
■ Common neoplasms in patients with HIV and AIDS include:
– Hodgkin's disease
– Kaposi's sarcoma
– malignant lymphoma.

▶ HIV encephalopathy
▶ Peripheral neuropathies

HEALTH & SAFETY *Early diagnosis of HIV positive status, medical treatment, and a healthy lifestyle may delay*

the onset of AIDS—a chronic and life-threatening condition caused by HIV. [5]

Diagnosis

Signs and symptoms may occur at any time after infection with HIV, but AIDS isn't officially diagnosed until the patient's CD4+ T-cell count falls below 200 cells/µl.[1] If acute HIV is suspected, the p24 antigen test and HIV ribonucleic acid (RNA) test should be ordered. Almost all persons with acute HIV have HIV RNA copies greater than 50,000 copies/ml.

The most commonly performed tests, antibody tests, indicate HIV infection indirectly by revealing HIV antibodies. However, antibody testing isn't reliable. Because people produce detectable levels of antibodies at different rates—a "window" varying from a few weeks to as long as 35 months in one documented case—an HIV–infected person can test negative for HIV antibodies. Antibody tests are also unreliable in neonates because transferred maternal antibodies persist for 6 to 10 months.

The recommended protocol requires initial screening of individuals and blood products with an enzyme-linked immunosorbent assay (ELISA). A positive ELISA should be repeated and then confirmed by an alternate method, usually the Western blot or an immunofluorescence assay. The radioimmunoprecipitation assay is considered more sensitive and specific than the Western blot, but because it requires radioactive materials, it's a poor choice for routine screening. To overcome such problems, direct tests are used, including antigen tests (p24 antigen), HIV cultures, nucleic acid probes of peripheral blood lymphocytes, and the polymerase chain reaction. (See *Laboratory tests for diagnosing and tracking HIV and assessing immune status.*)

Additional tests to support the diagnosis and help evaluate the severity of immunosuppression include CD4+ and CD8+ T-lymphocyte subset counts, erythrocyte sedimentation rate, complete blood cell count, serum beta$_2$-microglobulin, p24 antigen, neopterin levels, and anergy testing. Because many opportunistic infections in AIDS patients are reactivations of previous infections, patients also are tested for associated neoplasms, infections, and sexually transmitted diseases.

Treatment

There's no cure for either HIV or AIDS. However, significant advances have been made to help patients control signs and symptoms and impair disease progression.

Early diagnosis is critical in order for people with HIV to receive life-extending therapy.[4] Because HIV can become resistant to any drug, health care professionals use combination treatments and multiple drug regimens to suppress the virus. Patients on medication remain infectious.

Highly active antiretroviral therapy (HAART) is an effective method of treatment; however, these drugs are known to cause elevated liver enzyme levels and liver injury. This adverse effect is referred to as antiretroviral drug-related liver injury (ARLI). ARLI is a common cause of morbidity, mortality, and discontinuation of treatment in HIV infected patients.[3] HAART aims to reduce the number of HIV particles in the blood as measured by viral load, thus increasing T-cell counts and improving the immunologic system's functioning. A regular and vigilant medication regimen is critical, or resistance will develop because HIV strains mutate and can become resistant to HAART relatively easily. The *nucleoside analogues* (sometimes called reverse transcriptase inhibitors) have been the mainstay of AIDS therapy in recent years. These drugs interfere with viral reverse transcriptase, which impairs HIV's ability to turn its RNA into deoxyribonucleic acid for insertion into the host cell.

According to guidelines by the International AIDS Society-USA, antiretroviral

Laboratory tests for diagnosing and tracking HIV and assessing immune status

The chart below lists several laboratory tests that are used to diagnose HIV infection and their findings.

TEST	FINDINGS IN HIV INFECTION
Human immunodeficiency virus (HIV) antibody tests	
■ Enzyme-linked immunosorbent assay (ELISA)	■ Positive test results must be confirmed by Western blot
■ Western blot	■ Positive
■ Indirect immunofluorescence assay	■ Positive test results must be confirmed by Western blot
■ Radioimmunoprecipitation assay	■ Positive, more sensitive and specific than Western blot
■ Home sample collection (dried blood spot, oral mucosa fluid, urine)	■ Findings confirmed with ELISA or Western blot
HIV tracking	
■ p24 antigen	■ Positive for free viral protein
■ Polymerase chain reaction	■ Detection of HIV ribonucleic acid (RNA) or DNA
■ Branch deoxyribonucleic acid (bDNA)	■ Detection of HIV RNA
■ Nucleic acid sequence-based amplification	■ Detection of HIV RNA
■ Peripheral blood mononuclear cell culture for HIV-1	■ Positive when two consecutive assays detect reverse transcriptase or p24 antigen in increasing magnitude
■ Quantitative cell culture	■ Measures viral load within cells
■ Quantitative plasma culture	■ Measures viral load by free infectious virus in the plasma
■ β_2 microglobulin	■ Protein is increased with disease progression
■ Serum neopterin	■ Increased levels seen with disease progression
Immune status	
■ Number of CD4+ cells	■ Decreased
■ Percentage of CD4+ cells	■ Decreased
■ CD4+:CD8+ ratio	■ Decreased
■ White blood cell count	■ Normal to decreased
■ Immunoglobulin levels	■ Increased
■ CD4+ cell function tests	■ CD4+ T cells have decreased ability to respond to antigen
■ Skin test sensitivity reaction	■ Decreased to absent

therapy should begin in all symptomatic patients or when the patient's CD4+ T-cell count drops to less than 350/µl.[2] Most clinicians recommend starting the patient on a combination of these drugs in an attempt to gain the maximum benefit and to inhibit the production of resistant mutant strains of HIV. The drug combinations and dosages are then altered, depending on the patient's response.

Increasingly, physicians are basing changes in therapy on the patient's viral load rather than on his CD4+ T-cell count. Because the CD4+ count is influenced by the total white blood cell count, changes in the CD4+ count may have nothing to do with

EVIDENCE-BASED PRACTICE

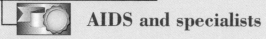

AIDS and specialists

Question: *Are patients with AIDS commonly referred to specialists for treatment?*

Research: The complexity and rapid development of new drugs for treating human immunodeficiency virus (HIV) and acquired immunodeficiency syndrome (AIDS) has made it difficult for physicians in family practice to stay current with treatment protocols.

Researchers conducted a follow-up study to a 1994 cohort study that examined how family physicians in Massachusetts cared for patients infected with HIV because they wanted to determine how care and referral patterns had changed during the previous 11 years. Data was obtained from a cross-sectional survey mailed to the active membership of the Massachusetts Academy of Family Physicians.

Conclusion: Data analysis showed that 85.3% of the physicians who responded to the survey said that they were more likely to refer patients with HIV or AIDS to specialists immediately, compared with their own practice patterns a decade ago. Although the number of HIV positive patients in individual practices had remained about the same in both studies, the current study showed that the number of practices

that had no patients with AIDS was significantly higher. In the current study, 61.7% of physicians indicated that they referred patients with AIDS immediately, 36.8% co-managed these patients, and 1.5% managed them alone, compared with the 1994 study, in which 18.3% had made immediate referrals, 74.3% had co-managed HIV patients, and 7.4% had managed them alone. The care and referrals for patients who were HIV positive showed similar changes.

Application: It's important for all nurses, but especially those working in family-practice settings, to be aware of ongoing changes in the care and treatment of patients who are HIV positive and those with AIDS. The nurse can help the patient understand why referral to a specialist is necessary, especially with patients who are reluctant to see new, unfamiliar providers.

Source: Fournier, P.O., et al. "A Shift in Referral Patterns for HIV/AIDS Patients," *Journal of Family Practice* 57(2):E1-9, February 2008.

changes in the patient's HIV status. Many physicians suggest that patients on antiretroviral therapy have their viral load checked every 3 months.

The increasing use of protease inhibitors (PIs) has greatly increased the life expectancy of patients with AIDS. These drugs block the enzyme protease, which HIV needs to produce virions, the viral particles that spread the virus to other cells. The use of PIs dramatically reduces viral load—sometimes to undetectable levels—while producing a corresponding increase in the CD4+ T-cell count. Because they act at a different site than nucleoside analogues, the PIs don't produce additional adverse effects when added to a patient's regimen.

Antiviral therapy includes the use of multiple combined drug therapies that suppress the replication of the HIV virus in the body. After antiviral therapy is initiated, treatment should be aggressive. Initially, highly active antiviral therapy, consisting of a triple drug therapy regimen—a PI and two nonnucleoside reverse transcriptase inhibitors—is recommended. In addition to these primary treatments, anti-infectives are used to combat opportunistic infections (some are used prophylactically to help patients resist opportunistic infections), and antineoplastic drugs are used to fight associated neoplasms. Supportive treatments help maintain nutritional status and relieve pain and other dis-

tressing physical and psychological symptoms. (See *AIDS and specialists.*)

Special considerations

▶ Advise health care workers and the public to use precautions in all situations where there's a risk of exposure to blood, body fluids, and secretions. Diligently practicing standard precautions can prevent the inadvertent transmission of AIDS and other infectious diseases that are transmitted by similar routes.

▶ Recognize that a diagnosis of AIDS is profoundly distressing because of the disease's social impact and discouraging prognosis. The patient may lose his job and financial security as well as the support of family and friends. Do your best to help him cope with an altered body image, the emotional burden of serious illness, and the threat of death, and encourage and assist the patient in learning about AIDS societies and support programs.

REFERENCES

1. Glynn, M.K., et al. "The Status of National HIV Case Surveillance, United States 2006," *Public Health Reports* 122(Suppl 1): 63-71, 2007.
2. CDC National Center for HIV, STD, and TB Prevention (September 21, 2006 press release), "CDC Recommends Routine, Voluntary HIV Screening in Health Care Settings."
3. Soriano, V., et al. Medscape Nurses. "Anti-Retroviral Drugs and Liver Injury," January 9, 2008 [Online]. Available at *www.medscape.com/viewarticle/568415_7.*
4. Cotton, D.J. "Time to Make HIV Screening Routine in the U.S.?" *AIDS Clinical Care* 3(3):1, March, 2005.
5. MayoClinic.com (2007 December 1). "HIV Testing: What Tests and When to Get Tested" [Online]. Available at *www.mayoclinic.com/health/hiv-testing/ID00050.*

ALLERGIC RHINITIS

Allergic rhinitis is a reaction to airborne (inhaled) allergens. Depending on the allergen, the resulting rhinitis and conjunctivitis may occur seasonally (hay fever) or year-round (perennial allergic rhinitis).

Causes and incidence

Hay fever reflects an immunoglobulin (Ig) E-mediated type I hypersensitivity response to an environmental antigen (allergen) in a genetically susceptible individual. In most cases, it's induced by windborne pollens: in the spring by tree pollens (oak, elm, maple, alder, birch, and cottonwood), in the summer by grass pollens (sheep sorrel and English plantain), and in the fall by weed pollens (ragweed). Occasionally, hay fever is induced by allergy to fungal spores. In addition to individual sensitivity and geographical differences in plant population, the amount of pollen in the air can be a factor in determining whether symptoms develop. Hot, dry, windy days have more pollen than cool, damp, rainy days.

In perennial allergic rhinitis, inhaled allergens provoke antigen responses that produce recurring symptoms year-round. The allergens trigger antibody production and histamine release, producing itching, swelling, and mucus. The major perennial allergens and irritants include dust mites, feather pillows, mold, cigarette smoke, upholstery, and animal dander. Seasonal pollen allergy may exacerbate signs and symptoms of perennial rhinitis.

Allergic rhinitis is the most common atopic allergic reaction, affecting more than 40 million Americans.[1] The estimated costs for physician visits and medications, lost work and school total $2 billion annually in the United States.[2] It's most prevalent in young children and adolescents—80% of cases are diagnosed by the time an individual reaches age 20—but it can occur in all age-

groups. In childhood, it's more common in boys, but in adulthood, prevalence is equal among men and women.[1] Allergic rhinitis may be a precursor to asthma development in children.[3]

Signs and symptoms

In seasonal allergic rhinitis, the key signs and symptoms are paroxysmal sneezing, profuse watery rhinorrhea, nasal obstruction or congestion, and pruritus of the nose and eyes. It's usually accompanied by pale, cyanotic, edematous nasal mucosa; red and edematous eyelids and conjunctivae; excessive lacrimation; and headache or sinus pain. Some patients also complain of itching in the throat and malaise.

In perennial allergic rhinitis, conjunctivitis and other extranasal effects are rare, but chronic nasal obstruction is common. In many cases, this obstruction extends to eustachian tube obstruction, particularly in children.

In both types of allergic rhinitis, dark circles may appear under the patient's eyes ("allergic shiners") because of venous congestion in the maxillary sinuses. The severity of signs and symptoms may vary from season to season and from year to year.

Complications

▶ Sinus and middle ear infection
▶ Nasal polyps

Diagnosis

Microscopic examination of sputum and nasal secretions reveals large numbers of eosinophils. Blood chemistry shows normal or elevated IgE. A definitive diagnosis is based on the patient's personal and family history of allergies as well as physical findings during a symptomatic phase. Skin testing paired with tested responses to environmental stimuli can pinpoint the responsible allergens given the patient's history. In patients who can't tolerate skin testing, the radioallergosorbent test may be helpful in determining specific allergen sensitivity.

To distinguish between allergic rhinitis and other nasal mucosa disorders, remember these differences:

▶ In chronic vasomotor rhinitis, rhinorrhea is mucoid, and both eye symptoms and seasonal variation are absent.
▶ In infectious rhinitis (the common cold), the nasal mucosa is beet red; nasal secretions contain polymorphonuclear, not eosinophilic, exudate; and signs and symptoms include fever and sore throat. This condition isn't a recurrent seasonal phenomenon.
▶ Chronic rhinitis is associated with the development of sinusitis. Sinusitis is commonly preceded by rhinitis and usually occurs with rhinitis.[4]
▶ In rhinitis medicamentosa, which results from excessive use of nasal sprays or drops, nasal drainage and mucosal redness and swelling disappear when such medication is withheld.
▶ In children, differential diagnosis should rule out a nasal foreign body, such as a bean or a button.

Treatment

Treatment aims to control symptoms by eliminating the environmental antigen, if possible, and providing drug therapy and immunotherapy.

Antihistamines block histamine effects but commonly produce anticholinergic adverse effects (sedation, dry mouth, nausea, dizziness, blurred vision, and nervousness). Antihistamines, such as cetirizine, loratadine, and fexofenadine, produce fewer adverse effects and are less likely to cause sedation.

Inhaled intranasal steroids produce local anti-inflammatory effects with minimal systemic adverse effects. The most commonly used intranasal steroids are fluticasone, mometasone, and triamcinolone. These drugs are effective when symptoms aren't relieved by antihistamines alone.

Advise the patient to use intranasal steroids regularly as prescribed for optimal effectiveness. Cromolyn may be helpful in treating hay fever, but this drug may take up to 4 weeks to produce a satisfactory effect and must be taken regularly during allergy season. Eyedrop versions of cromolyn and antihistamines are available for itchy, blood-shot eyes.

Long-term management includes im-munotherapy, or desensitization with injec-tions of extracted allergens, administered be-fore or during allergy season, or perennially. Seasonal allergies require particularly close dosage regulation.

Special considerations
▶ Before desensitization injections, assess the patient's symptom status. Afterward, watch for adverse reactions, including ana-phylaxis and severe localized erythema.
▶ Keep epinephrine and emergency resusci-tation equipment available, and observe the patient for 30 minutes after the injection. In-struct the patient to call the physician if a delayed reaction occurs.

The following protocol is recommended for allergic rhinitis:
▶ Monitor the patient's compliance with prescribed drug treatment regimens. Also carefully note any changes in the control of his symptoms or any signs of drug misuse.
▶ To reduce environmental exposure to air-borne allergens, suggest that the patient sleep with the windows closed, avoid the countryside during pollination seasons, use air conditioning to filter allergens and mini-mize moisture and dust, and eliminate dust-collecting items, such as wool blankets, deep-pile carpets, and heavy drapes, from the home.
▶ In severe and resistant cases, suggest that the patient consider drastic changes in lifestyle such as relocation to a pollen-free area either seasonally or year-round.

▶ Be aware that some patients may develop chronic complications, including sinusitis and nasal polyps.

REFERENCES
1. Sheikh, J. (2007 November 8). "Rhinitis, Aller-gic" [Online]. Available at *www.emedicine.com/MED/topic104.htm*.
2. Weber, R.W. "Allergic Rhinitis," *Primary Care: Clinics in Office Practice* 35(1) 1-10, March 2008.
3. Masuda, S., et al. "High Prevalence and Young Onset of Allergic Rhinitis in Children with Bronchial Asthma," *Pediatric Allergy and Im-munology,* January 2008.
4. American Academy of Otolaryngology-Head and Neck Surgery. "Fact Sheet: Allergic Rhini-tis, Sinusitis, and Rhinosinusitis" [Online]. Available at *www.entnet.org/HealthInforma-tion/rhinitis.cfm*.

ANAPHYLAXIS

Anaphylaxis is a dramatic, acute atopic reaction marked by the sud-den onset of rapidly progressive ur-ticaria and respiratory distress. A severe re-action may precipitate vascular collapse, leading to systemic shock and, sometimes, death. Anaphylaxis reaction is the result of an antigen body response; an anaphylactoid response results from a nonantibody trigger. There's no difference in clinical presentation and treatment.[2]

Causes and incidence
The source of anaphylactic reactions is in-gestion of, or other systemic exposure to, sensitizing drugs or other substances. Such substances may include:
▶ allergen extracts
▶ diagnostic chemicals (sulfobromo-phthalein, sodium dehydrocholate, and radi-ographic contrast media)
▶ enzymes (L-asparaginase)

Penicillin guidelines

The following recommendations can prevent an allergic response when administering penicillin or its derivatives, such as ampicillin.

■ Have an emergency kit available to treat allergic reactions.

■ Take a detailed patient history, including penicillin allergy and other allergies. In an infant who's younger than three months old, check for penicillin allergy in the mother.

■ Never give penicillin to a patient who has had an allergic reaction to it.

■ Before giving penicillin to a patient with suspected penicillin allergy, refer the patient for skin and immunologic tests to confirm it.

■ Always tell a patient he's going to receive penicillin before he takes the first dose.

■ Observe the patient carefully for adverse effects for at least a half hour after penicillin administration.

■ Be aware that penicillin derivatives also elicit an allergic reaction.

▶ foods, especially legumes, nuts, berries, seafood, and egg albumin; and sulfite-containing food additives
▶ hormones
▶ insect venom (honeybees, wasps, hornets, yellow jackets, fire ants, mosquitoes, and certain spiders)
▶ local anesthetics
▶ penicillin and other antibiotics
▶ polysaccharides
▶ ruptured hydatid cyst (in rare instances)
▶ salicylates
▶ serums (usually horse serum)
▶ sulfonamides
▶ vaccines

HEALTH & SAFETY *Anaphylaxis reactions related to food allergies are estimated at 30,000 annually in the United States. And approximately 200 deaths per year occur from anaphylaxis reactions related to food allergies.* [3]

A common cause of anaphylaxis is penicillin, which induces anaphylaxis in 1% to 10% of patients treated with it. Penicillin is most likely to induce anaphylaxis after parenteral administration or prolonged therapy, and in atopic patients with an allergy to other drugs or foods. (See *Penicillin guidelines.*) An anaphylactic reaction requires previous sensitization or exposure to the specific antigen, resulting in the production of specific immunoglobulin (Ig) E antibodies by plasma cells. This antibody production takes place in the lymph nodes and is enhanced by helper T cells. IgE antibodies then bind to membrane receptors on mast cells (found throughout connective tissue) and basophils.

On reexposure, the antigen binds to adjacent IgE antibodies or cross-linked IgE receptors, activating a series of cellular reactions that trigger degranulation—the release of powerful chemical mediators (such as histamine, eosinophil chemotactic factor of anaphylaxis, and platelet-activating factor) from mast cell stores. IgG or IgM enters into the reaction and activates the release of complement fractions.

At the same time, two other chemical mediators, bradykinin and leukotrienes, induce vascular collapse by stimulating contraction of certain groups of smooth muscles and by increasing vascular permeability. In turn, increased vascular permeability leads to decreased peripheral resistance and plasma leakage from the circulation to extravascular tissues (which lowers blood volume, causing hypotension, hypovolemic shock, and cardiac dysfunction).

Signs and symptoms

An anaphylactic reaction produces sudden physical distress within seconds or minutes (although a delayed or persistent reaction may occur for up to 24 hours) after exposure to an allergen. The reaction's severity is inversely related to the interval between exposure to the allergen and the onset of symptoms. Usually, the first signs and symptoms

include a feeling of impending doom or fright, weakness, sweating, sneezing, shortness of breath, nasal pruritus, urticaria, and angioedema, followed rapidly by signs and symptoms in one or more target organs.

Cardiovascular symptoms include hypotension, shock and, sometimes, cardiac arrhythmias. If untreated, arrhythmia may precipitate circulatory collapse. Respiratory symptoms can occur at any level in the respiratory tract and commonly include nasal mucosal edema, profuse watery rhinorrhea, itching, nasal congestion, and sudden sneezing attacks. Edema of the upper respiratory tract results in hypopharyngeal and laryngeal obstruction (hoarseness, stridor, and dyspnea). This is an early sign of acute respiratory failure, which can be fatal. GI and genitourinary symptoms include severe stomach cramps, nausea, diarrhea, and urinary urgency and incontinence.

Complications
▶ Respiratory obstruction
▶ Systemic vascular collapse
▶ Death

Diagnosis
Anaphylaxis can be diagnosed by the rapid onset of severe respiratory or cardiovascular signs and symptoms after ingestion or injection of a drug, vaccine, diagnostic agent, food, or food additive or after an insect sting. If these symptoms occur without a known allergic stimulus, rule out other possible causes of shock (acute myocardial infarction, status asthmaticus, or heart failure). Skin tests or in vitro tests determine the presence of specific IgE antibodies and can identify the cause of anaphylaxis, whether the trigger is specific foods, medications, or stinging insects.[2]

Treatment
Anaphylaxis is always an emergency. It requires an *immediate* injection of epinephrine

1:1,000 aqueous solution, 0.2 to 0.5 ml, repeated every 5 minutes as needed.[1]

In the early stages of anaphylaxis, when the patient hasn't lost consciousness and is normotensive, give epinephrine I.M. or subcutaneously and help it move into circulation faster by massaging the injection site. In severe reactions, when the patient has lost consciousness and is hypotensive, give epinephrine I.V.

Maintain airway patency. Observe for early signs of laryngeal edema (hoarseness, stridor, and dyspnea), which will probably require endotracheal tube insertion or a tracheotomy and oxygen therapy.

In case of cardiac arrest, begin cardiopulmonary resuscitation, including closed-chest heart massage, assisted ventilation, and other therapies as indicated by clinical response.

Watch for hypotension and shock, and maintain circulatory volume with volume expanders (plasma, plasma expanders, saline, and albumin) as needed. Stabilize blood pressure with the I.V. vasopressors norepinephrine and dopamine. Monitor blood pressure, central venous pressure, and urine output as a response index.

After the initial emergency, administer other medications as ordered: subcutaneous epinephrine, longer-acting epinephrine, corticosteroids, and I.V. diphenhydramine for long-term management and I.V. aminophylline over 10 to 20 minutes for bronchospasm. Rapid infusion of aminophylline may cause or aggravate severe hypotension.

Special considerations
▶ To prevent anaphylaxis, teach the patient to avoid exposure to known allergens. A person allergic to certain foods or drugs must learn to avoid the offending food or drug in all its forms. A person allergic to insect stings should avoid open fields and wooded areas during the insect season. An epinephrine kit (epinephrine, diphenhydramine) should also be carried whenever the patient with known severe allergic reac-

tions goes outdoors. In addition, every patient prone to anaphylaxis should wear a medical identification bracelet identifying his allergies.

▶ If a patient must receive a drug to which he's allergic, prevent a severe reaction by making sure he receives careful desensitization with gradually increasing doses of the antigen or advance administration of steroids. Of course, a person with a known allergic history should receive a drug with a high anaphylactic potential only after cautious pretesting for sensitivity. Closely monitor the patient during testing, and make sure you have resuscitation equipment and epinephrine ready. When any patient needs a drug with a high anaphylactic potential (particularly parenteral drugs), make sure he receives each dose under close medical observation.

▶ Closely monitor a patient undergoing diagnostic tests that use radiographic contrast media, such as excretory urography, cardiac catheterization, and angiography.

REFERENCES

1. Joint Task Force on Practice Parameters, et al. "The Diagnosis and Management of Anaphylaxis: An Updated Practice Parameter," *Journal of Allergy and Clinical Immunology* 115(3 Suppl 2):S483-523, March 2005.
2. Scarlet, C. "Anaphylaxis," *Journal of Infusion Nurses* 29(1):39-44, January-February 2000.
3. Burks, A. Wesley, M.D. "Factoring PAF in Anaphylaxis," *New England Journal of Medicine* 358(1):79-81, January 2008.

● ASTHMA

Asthma is a reversible lung disease characterized by obstruction or narrowing of the airways, which are typically inflamed and hyperresponsive to various stimuli. It may resolve spontaneously or with treatment. Its symptoms range from mild wheezing and dyspnea to life-threatening respiratory failure. (See *Determining asthma's severity.*) Symptoms of bronchial airway obstruction may persist between acute episodes. If untreated, the airways become remodeled, which results in permanent lung damage and a decrease in lung function.[1]

Causes and incidence

Asthma that results from sensitivity to specific external allergens is known as *extrinsic*. In cases in which the allergen isn't obvious, asthma is referred to as *intrinsic*. Allergens that cause extrinsic asthma include pollen, animal dander, house dust or mold, cockroach allergen, kapok or feather pillows, food additives containing sulfites, and any other sensitizing substance. Extrinsic (atopic) asthma usually begins in childhood and is accompanied by other manifestations of atopy (type I, immunoglobulin [Ig] E-mediated allergy), such as eczema and allergic rhinitis. In intrinsic (nonatopic) asthma, no extrinsic allergen can be identified. Most cases are preceded by a severe respiratory infection. Tobacco smoke, emotional stress, dust mites, air pollution, temperature, and humidity may aggravate intrinsic asthma attacks.[2] There's also a genetic component to asthma; more than 20 genes have been identified.[3] In many asthmatics, intrinsic and extrinsic asthmas coexist.

Several drugs and chemicals may provoke an asthma attack without using the IgE pathway. Apparently, they trigger release of mast-cell mediators by way of prostaglandin inhibition. Examples of these substances include aspirin, various nonsteroidal anti-inflammatory drugs (such as indomethacin and mefenamic acid), and tartrazine, a yellow food dye. Exercise may also provoke an asthma attack. In exercise-induced asthma, bronchospasm may follow heat and moisture loss in the upper airways.

The allergic response has two phases. When the patient inhales an allergenic substance, sensitized IgE antibodies trigger mast-cell degranulation in the lung intersti-

Determining asthma's severity

Asthma is classified by severity. The following factors are used to determine whether a patient's asthma is considered mild intermittent, mild persistent, moderate persistent, or severe persistent:
• frequency, severity, and duration of symptoms
• degree of airflow obstruction (spirometry measure) or peak expiratory flow (PEF)
• frequency of nighttime symptoms and the degree that the asthma interferes with daily activities.

Severity can change over time, and even milder cases can become severe in an uncontrolled attack. Long-term therapy depends on the level of severity. For all patients, quick relief can be obtained by using a short-acting bronchodilator (2 to 4 puffs of short-acting inhaled beta$_2$-adrenergic agonists as needed for symptoms). However, if a patient who has intermittent asthma begins to use a short-acting bronchodilator more than twice per week, or a patient with persistent asthma finds himself using the bronchodilator daily or with increasing frequency, that may indicate the need to initiate or increase long-term control therapy.

MILD INTERMITTENT ASTHMA
The signs and symptoms of mild intermittent asthma include:
• daytime symptoms no more than twice per week
• nighttime symptoms no more than twice per month
• lung function testing (either PEF or forced expiratory volume in 1 second) is 80% of predicted value or higher
• PEF varies no more than 20%.

Severe exacerbations, separated by long, symptomless periods of normal lung function, indicate mild intermittent asthma. A course of systemic corticosteroids is recommended for these exacerbations; otherwise, daily medication isn't required.

MILD PERSISTENT ASTHMA
The signs and symptoms of mild persistent asthma include:
• daytime symptoms 3 to 6 days per week
• nighttime symptoms 3 to 4 times per month

• lung function testing is 80% of predicted value or higher
• PEF varies between 20% and 30%.

The preferred treatment for mild persistent asthma is low-dose inhaled corticosteroids, but alternative treatments include cromolyn, leukotriene modifier, nedocromil, or sustained-release theophylline.

MODERATE PERSISTENT ASTHMA
The signs and symptoms of moderate persistent asthma include:
• daily daytime symptoms
• at least weekly nighttime symptoms
• lung function testing is 60% to 80% of predicted value
• PEF varies more than 30%.

The preferred treatment for moderate persistent asthma is low- or medium-dose inhaled corticosteroids combined with a long-acting inhaled beta$_2$-adrenergic agonist. Alternative treatments include increasing inhaled corticosteroids within the medium-dose range or low- or medium-dose inhaled corticosteroids with either a leukotriene modifier or theophylline.

For recurring exacerbations, the preferred treatment is to increase inhaled corticosteroids within the medium-dose range and add a long-acting inhaled beta$_2$-adrenergic agonist. The alternative treatment is to increase inhaled corticosteroids within the medium-dose range and add either a leukotriene modifier or theophylline.

SEVERE PERSISTENT ASTHMA
The signs and symptoms of severe persistent asthma include:
• continual daytime symptoms
• frequent nighttime symptoms
• lung function testing is 60% of predicted value or lower
• PEF varies more than 30%.

The preferred treatment for severe persistent asthma includes high-dose inhaled corticosteroids combined with long-acting inhaled beta$_2$-adrenergic agonists. Long-term administration of corticosteroid tablets or syrup (2 mg/kg/day, not to exceed 60 mg/day) may be used to reduce the need for systemic corticosteroid therapy.

tium, releasing histamine, cytokines, prosta-glandins, thromboxanes, leukotrienes, and eosinophil chemotaxic factors. Histamine then attaches to receptor sites in the larger bronchi, causing irritation, inflammation, and edema. In the late phase, inflammatory cells flow in. The influx of eosinophils provides additional inflammatory mediators and contributes to local injury.

About 20 million people in the United States have asthma; 9 million of them are children.[4] Although this common condition can strike at any age, one-half of all cases first occur in children younger than age 10. Nearly 1 in 13 children have asthma, and the rates are increasing worldwide. In childhood, asthma is more prevalent in boys than girls. By age 40, however, women and men are equally represented. Blacks are also more susceptible than whites; they're more likely to be hospitalized for asthma attacks and to die from them.[4] Emergency department visits, hospitalizations, and mortality from asthma have been increasing for more than 20 years, especially among children and blacks.

Signs and symptoms

An asthma attack may begin dramatically, with simultaneous onset of many severe symptoms, or insidiously, with gradually increasing respiratory distress. It typically includes progressively worsening shortness of breath, coughing, wheezing, and chest tightness or some combination of these signs or symptoms.

During an acute attack, the cough sounds tight and dry. As the attack subsides, tenacious mucoid sputum is produced (except in young children, who don't expectorate). Characteristic wheezing may be accompanied by coarse rhonchi, but fine crackles aren't heard unless associated with a related complication. Between acute attacks, breath sounds may be normal.

The intensity of breath sounds in symptomatic asthma is typically reduced. A pro-longed phase of forced expiration is typical of airflow obstruction. Evidence of lung hyperinflation (use of accessory muscles, for example) is particularly common in children. Acute attacks may be accompanied by tachycardia, tachypnea, and diaphoresis. In severe attacks, the patient may be unable to speak more than a few words without pausing for breath. Cyanosis, confusion, and lethargy indicate the onset of respiratory failure.

Complications
▶ Status asthmaticus
▶ Respiratory failure

Diagnosis

Laboratory studies in patients with asthma commonly show these abnormalities:
▶ Pulmonary function studies reveal signs of airway obstruction (decreased peak expiratory flow rates and forced expiratory volume in 1 second), low-normal or decreased vital capacity, and increased total lung and residual capacity. However, pulmonary function studies may be normal between attacks.
▶ Pulse oximetry may reveal decreased arterial oxygen saturation (SaO_2).
▶ Arterial blood gas (ABG) analysis provides the best indications of an attack's severity. In acutely severe asthma, the partial pressure of arterial oxygen is less than 60 mm Hg, the partial pressure of arterial carbon dioxide ($PaCO_2$) is 40 mm Hg or more, and pH is usually decreased.
▶ Complete blood count with differential reveals increased eosinophil count.
▶ Chest X-rays may show hyperinflation with areas of focal atelectasis.

Before initiating tests for asthma, rule out other causes of airway obstruction and wheezing. In children, such causes include cystic fibrosis, tumors of the bronchi or mediastinum, and acute viral bronchitis; in adults, other causes include obstructive pulmonary disease, heart failure, and epiglottiditis.

Treatment

Treatment of acute asthma aims to decrease bronchoconstriction, reduce bronchial airway edema, and increase pulmonary ventilation. After an acute episode, treatment focuses on avoiding or removing precipitating factors, such as environmental allergens or irritants.

If asthma is known to be caused by a particular antigen, it may be treated by desensitizing the patient through a series of injections of limited amounts of the antigen. The aim is to curb the patient's immune response to the antigen.

If asthma results from an infection, antibiotics are prescribed. Drug therapy is most effective when begun soon after the onset of signs and symptoms. For relief of symptoms in adults and children older than age 5, short-acting inhaled beta$_2$-adrenergic agonists for bronchodilation may be used, and a course of systemic corticosteroids may be needed. The goal of therapy is asthma control with minimal or no adverse effects from medication.

Acute attacks that don't respond to self-treatment may require hospital care, beta$_2$-adrenergic agonists by inhalation or subcutaneous (subQ) injection (in three doses over 60 to 90 minutes), and—possibly—oxygen for hypoxemia. If the patient responds poorly, systemic corticosteroids and, possibly, subQ epinephrine may help. Beta$_2$-adrenergic agonist inhalation continues hourly. I.V. aminophylline may be added to the regimen, and I.V. fluid therapy is started. Patients who don't respond to this treatment, whose airways remain obstructed, and who have increasing respiratory difficulty are at risk for status asthmaticus and may require mechanical ventilation.

Treatment of status asthmaticus consists of aggressive drug therapy with a beta$_2$-adrenergic agonist by nebulizer every 30 to 60 minutes, possibly supplemented with subQ epinephrine, I.V. corticosteroids, I.V. aminophylline, oxygen administration, I.V.

fluid therapy, and intubation and mechanical ventilation for hypercapnic respiratory failure ($Paco_2$ of 40 mm Hg or more). (See *How status asthmaticus progresses,* pages 284 and 285.)

Special considerations

During an acute attack, proceed as follows:
▶ First, assess the severity of asthma.
▶ Administer the prescribed treatments, and assess the patient's response.
▶ Place the patient in high Fowler's position. Encourage pursed-lip and diaphragmatic breathing. Help him to relax.
▶ Monitor the patient's vital signs. Keep in mind that developing or increasing tachypnea may indicate worsening asthma or drug toxicity. Blood pressure readings may reveal pulsus paradoxus (a decrease in systolic blood pressure of more than 10 mm Hg with inspiration) indicating severe asthma. Hypertension may indicate asthma-related hypoxemia.
▶ Administer prescribed humidified oxygen by nasal cannula at 2 L/minute to ease breathing and to increase Sao_2. Later, adjust oxygen according to the patient's vital signs and ABG levels.
▶ Anticipate intubation and mechanical ventilation if the patient fails to maintain adequate oxygenation.
▶ Observe the frequency and severity of your patient's cough, and note whether it's productive. Then auscultate his lungs, noting adventitious or absent breath sounds. If his cough isn't productive and rhonchi are present, teach him effective coughing techniques. If the patient can tolerate postural drainage and chest percussion, perform these procedures to clear secretions. Suction an intubated patient as needed.
▶ Treat dehydration with I.V. fluids until the patient can tolerate oral fluids, which will help loosen secretions.
▶ If conservative treatment fails to improve the airway obstruction, anticipate bron-

How status asthmaticus progresses

A potentially fatal complication, status asthmaticus arises when impaired gas exchange and heightened airway resistance increase the work of breathing. This flow chart shows the stages of status asthmaticus.

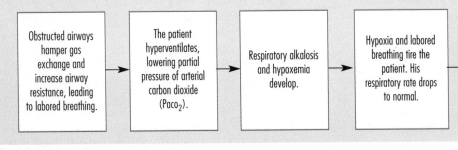

Obstructed airways hamper gas exchange and increase airway resistance, leading to labored breathing. → The patient hyperventilates, lowering partial pressure of arterial carbon dioxide ($Paco_2$). → Respiratory alkalosis and hypoxemia develop. → Hypoxia and labored breathing tire the patient. His respiratory rate drops to normal.

choscopy or bronchial lavage when a lobe or larger area collapses.

During long-term care, proceed as follows:

▶ Monitor the patient's respiratory status to detect baseline changes, to assess response to treatment, and to prevent or detect complications.

▶ Auscultate the lungs frequently, noting the degree of wheezing and quality of air movement.

▶ Review ABG levels, pulmonary function test results, and Sao_2 readings.

▶ If the patient is taking systemic corticosteroids, observe for complications, such as elevated blood glucose levels, friable skin, and bruising.

▶ Cushingoid effects resulting from the long-term use of oral corticosteroids may be minimized by alternate-day dosage or use of prescribed inhaled corticosteroids.

▶ If the patient is taking corticosteroids by inhaler, watch for signs of candidal infection in the mouth and pharynx. Using an extender device and rinsing the mouth afterward may prevent this.

▶ Observe the patient's anxiety level. Keep in mind that measures that reduce hypoxemia and breathlessness should help relieve anxiety.

▶ Keep the room temperature comfortable, and use an air conditioner or a fan in hot, humid weather.

▶ Control exercise-induced asthma by instructing the patient to use a bronchodilator or cromolyn 30 minutes before exercise. Also instruct him to use pursed-lip breathing while exercising.

Make sure the patient and his family know how to:

▶ avoid known allergens and irritants

▶ recognize symptoms of viral infections, and why it's important to contact the health provider as soon as an infection sets in

▶ use a metered-dose inhaler (If he has difficulty using an inhaler, he may need an extender device to optimize drug delivery and lower the risk of candidal infection with orally inhaled corticosteroids.)

▶ use a peak flow meter to measure the degree of airway obstruction (useful for patients with moderate to severe asthma) Tell the patient to keep a record of peak flow readings and bring it to medical appointments. Explain the importance of calling the physician at once if the peak flow drops suddenly (since this may signal severe respiratory problems).

▶ do diaphragmatic and pursed-lip breathing, and effective coughing techniques.

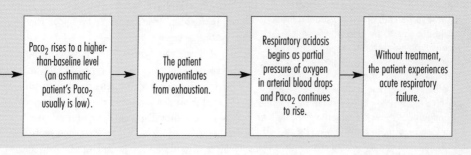

Paco$_2$ rises to a higher-than-baseline level (an asthmatic patient's Paco$_2$ usually is low). → The patient hypoventilates from exhaustion. → Respiratory acidosis begins as partial pressure of oxygen in arterial blood drops and Paco$_2$ continues to rise. → Without treatment, the patient experiences acute respiratory failure.

Caution the patient or his family to notify the physician if the patient develops a fever above 100.4° F (37.8° C), chest pain, shortness of breath without coughing or exercising, or uncontrollable coughing. An uncontrollable asthma attack requires immediate attention.

Also, make sure the patient and his family know:
▶ names, dosages, actions, adverse effects and any special instructions for using prescribed drugs
▶ importance of inhaled steroids in preventing remodeling of lung tissue
▶ importance of drinking plenty of fluids daily to help loosen secretions and maintain hydration.

REFERENCES
1. Ten Hacken, N.H., et al. "Airway Remodeling and Long-Term Decline in Lung Function in Asthma," *Current Opinion in Pulmonary Medicine* 9(1):9-14, January 2003.
2. Department of Health and Human Services, Centers for Disease Control and Prevention. "Asthma," Available at *www.cdc.gov/asthma/faqs.htm.*
3. McCance, K.L., and Heuther, S.E., eds. *Pathophysiology: The Biologic Basis for Disease in Adults and Children,* 5th ed. St. Louis: Elsevier Mosby, 2006.
4. National Heart Lung and Blood Institute (2006 May). "Who is at Risk for Asthma" [Online]. Available at *www.nhlbi.nih.gov/health/dci/Diseases/Asthma/Asthma_WhoIsAtRisk.html.*

BLOOD TRANSFUSION REACTION

Mediated by immune or nonimmune factors, a transfusion reaction accompanies or follows I.V. administration of blood components. Its severity varies from mild (fever and chills) to severe (acute renal failure or complete vascular collapse and death), depending on the amount of blood transfused, the type of reaction, and the patient's general health. The practice came under systematic scrutiny in the 1980s, largely because of concerns about transfusion-related infection. Thanks to advances in medical technology, other issues—including transfusion-related acute lung injury, the age of transfused blood, and effects of transfused blood on the immune system[3]—have moved to the fore. Concern about these issues has led to methodical examinations. It also drives the current debate over transfusion practice.

Understanding the Rh system

The rhesus (Rh) blood group system contains more than 30 antibodies and antigens. Eighty-five percent of people around the world are said to be Rh-positive, which means that their red blood cells carry the D or Rh antigen. The remaining 15% are Rh-negative; they *don't* carry this antigen.

When Rh-negative people first receive Rh-positive blood, they become sensitized to the D antigen but show no immediate reaction to it. If they receive Rh-positive blood a second time, they then develop a massive hemolytic reaction. For example, an Rh-negative mother who delivers a baby who is Rh-positive is sensitized by the baby's Rh-positive blood. If she has a second Rh-positive pregnancy, her sensitized blood would cause a hemolytic reaction in fetal circulation. Thus, the Rh-negative mother should receive Rh(D) immune globulin (human) I.M. within 72 hours after delivering her first Rh-positive baby to prevent formation of antibodies against Rh-positive blood.

Causes and incidence

Hemolytic reactions follow transfusion of mismatched blood. Transfusion of serologically incompatible blood triggers the most serious reaction, marked by intravascular agglutination of red blood cells (RBCs).

HEALTH & SAFETY *There are no universal blood donors. At one time, blood donors with the blood type O/Rh were considered "universal donors," meaning that this blood type could be received by anyone without the risk of a reaction. That's no longer considered true.*[2]

The recipient's antibodies (immunoglobulin [Ig] G or IgM) attach to the donated RBCs, leading to widespread clumping and destruction of the recipient's RBCs and, possibly, the development of disseminated intravascular coagulation (DIC) and other serious effects.

Transfusion of Rh-incompatible blood triggers a less serious reaction within several days to 2 weeks. Rh reactions are most common in females sensitized to RBC antigens by prior pregnancy or by unknown factors (such as bacterial or viral infection) and in people who have received more than five transfusions. (See *Understanding the Rh system.*)

Allergic reactions are the most common type of reaction.[1] In this type of reaction, transfused soluble antigens react with surface IgE molecules on mast cells and basophils, causing degranulation and release of allergic mediators. Antibodies against IgA in an IgA-deficient recipient can also trigger a severe allergic reaction (anaphylaxis).

Febrile nonhemolytic reactions apparently develop when cytotoxic or agglutinating antibodies in the recipient's plasma attack antigens on transfused lymphocytes, granulocytes, or plasma cells.

Although fairly uncommon, *bacterial contamination* of donor blood can occur during donor phlebotomy. Offending organisms are usually gram-negative, especially *Pseudomonas* species, *Citrobacter freundii,* and *Escherichia coli.*

All blood is tested for hepatitis, cytomegalovirus, and human immunodeficiency virus.

Most acute transfusion reactions occur in people over 60 years because the most transfusions are administered in that population.[2] Allergic reactions occur in 1 case per 333 population, and febrile nonhemolytic reactions occurs in 1 case per 200 population.[2] Anaphylactic reactions occur in 1 case per 20,000 to 50,000 population.[2]

Signs and symptoms

Immediate effects of a hemolytic transfusion reaction develop within a few minutes or hours after the start of the transfusion and may include chills, fever, urticaria, tachycardia, dyspnea, nausea, vomiting, tightness in the chest, chest and back pain, hypotension, bronchospasm, angioedema, and signs and

symptoms of anaphylaxis, shock, pulmonary edema, heart failure, and renal failure. In a surgical patient under anesthesia, these symptoms are masked, but blood oozes from mucous membranes or the incision site.

Delayed hemolytic reactions can occur up to several weeks after a transfusion, causing fever, an unexpected fall in serum hemoglobin (Hb) level, and jaundice.

Allergic reactions are typically afebrile and characterized by urticaria and angioedema, possibly progressing to cough, respiratory distress, nausea, vomiting, diarrhea, abdominal cramps, vascular instability, shock, and coma.

The hallmark of febrile nonhemolytic reactions is mild to severe fever that may begin at the start of transfusion or within 2 hours after its completion.

Bacterial contamination produces a high fever, nausea, vomiting, diarrhea, abdominal cramps and, possibly, shock. Symptoms of viral contamination may not appear for several weeks after transfusion.

Complications
▶ Bronchospasm
▶ Tubular necrosis
▶ Acute renal failure
▶ Anaphylactic shock
▶ Vascular collapse
▶ DIC

Diagnosis
Confirming a hemolytic transfusion reaction requires proof of blood incompatibility and evidence of hemolysis, such as hemoglobinuria, anti-A or anti-B antibodies.

If you suspect such a reaction, have the patient's blood retyped and crossmatched with the donor's blood. After a hemolytic transfusion reaction, laboratory tests will show increased indirect bilirubin levels, decreased haptoglobin levels, increased serum Hb levels, and Hb in the urine. As the reaction progresses, tests may show signs of DIC (thrombocytopenia, increased prothrombin time, and decreased fibrinogen level) and acute tubular necrosis (increased blood urea nitrogen and serum creatinine levels).

A blood culture to isolate the causative organism should be done when bacterial contamination is suspected.

Treatment
At the first sign of a hemolytic reaction, *stop the transfusion immediately.* Depending on the nature of the patient's reaction, prepare to:
▶ monitor vital signs every 15 to 30 minutes, watching for signs of shock
▶ maintain a patent I.V. line with normal saline solution; insert an indwelling catheter, and monitor intake and output
▶ cover the patient with blankets to ease chills, and explain what's happening
▶ deliver supplemental oxygen at low flow rates through a nasal cannula or bag-valve-mask (handheld resuscitation bag)
▶ give drugs as ordered: an I.V. antihypotensive drug and normal saline solution to combat shock, epinephrine to treat dyspnea and wheezing, diphenhydramine to combat cellular histamine released from mast cells, corticosteroids to reduce inflammation, and mannitol or furosemide to maintain urinary function. Administer parenteral antihistamines and corticosteroids for allergic reactions. (Severe reactions such as anaphylaxis may require epinephrine.) Administer antipyretics for nonhemolytic febrile reactions and appropriate I.V. antibiotics for bacterial contamination.

Special considerations
▶ Remember to fully document the transfusion reaction on the patient's chart, noting the transfusion's duration, the amount of blood absorbed, and a complete description of the reaction and of any interventions.
▶ To prevent a hemolytic transfusion reaction, make sure you know your hospital's policy about giving blood before you give a blood transfusion. Then make sure you have

the right blood and the right patient. Check and double-check the patient's name, hospital number, ABO blood group, and Rh status. If you find even a small discrepancy, don't give the blood. Notify the blood bank immediately, and return the unopened unit.
▶ In the case of a reaction, return all equipment and blood to the lab for testing.

REFERENCES

1. American Cancer Society (2006 November 28). "Possible Risks of Blood Product Transfusions" [Online]. Available at *www.cancer.org/docroot/ ETO/content/ETO_1_4x_Possible_Risks_of_ Blood_Product_Transfusions.asp*.
2. MayoClinic.com (2006 December 28). "Universal Blood Donor Type: Is There Such a Thing?" [Online]. Available at *www.mayo clinic.com/health/universal-blood-donor-type/ HQ00949*.
3. Corwin, H.L., and Carson, J.L. "Blood Transfusion—When Is More Really Less?" *New England Journal of Medicine* 356(16):1667-69, April 19, 2007.

CHRONIC FATIGUE SYNDROME

Sometimes called *chronic Epstein-Barr virus,* or *myalgic encephalomyelitis,* chronic fatigue and immune dysfunction syndrome is typically marked by debilitating fatigue, neurologic abnormalities, and persistent symptoms that suggest chronic mononucleosis.

Causes and incidence

The cause of chronic fatigue syndrome (CFS) is unknown. Some researchers suggest that *Chlamydia pneumoniae* is the infectious agent responsible for the disease. The Centers for Disease Control and Prevention (CDC) has found that CFS isn't caused by a single recognized agent and found no association with Epstein-Barr virus, human retroviruses, human herpes virus 6, enteroviruses, rubella, *Candida albicans,* bornaviruses, and

Mycoplasma.[2] Recent studies have shown that inflammation of nervous system pathways, acting as an immune or autoimmune response, may play a role as well. CFS may also be associated with a reaction to viral illness that's complicated by dysfunctional immune response and by other factors that may include gender, age, genetic disposition, prior illness, stress, and environment.

It commonly occurs in young to middle-age adults and is found primarily in females.

Signs and symptoms

CFS has specific symptoms and signs, based on the exclusion of other possible causes. Its characteristic symptom is prolonged, often overwhelming fatigue that's commonly associated with a varying complex of other symptoms that are similar to those of many infections, including myalgia and cephalgia. It may develop within a few hours and can last for 6 months or more. Fatigue isn't relieved by rest and is severe enough to restrict activities of daily living by at least 50%.

Decreased motor function is an undisputable symptom associated with CFS. Low effort capacity and reduced effort tolerance are two areas of CFS being evaluated to determine if one has a greater effect on CFS. Reduced effort tolerance might be the primary disturbance in CFS.[1]

To aid in disease identification, the CDC uses a "working case definition" to group symptoms and severity.

Diagnosis

Because the cause and nature of CFS are still unknown, no single test unequivocally confirms its presence. Therefore, physicians base this diagnosis on the patient's history and the CDC's criteria. (See *CDC criteria for diagnosing chronic fatigue syndrome.*) Because the CDC criteria is admittedly a work in progress, which may not include all forms of this disease, and is based on symptoms that can result from other diseases, diagnosis is

difficult and uncertain. Including a review of medications and a physical examination, a mental status screen test and other lab tests—along with the patient history—can help with diagnosis.[3] There are also several questionnaires that can assist with identification of CFS.[3]

Treatment

No treatment is known to cure CFS. Symptomatic treatment may involve the use of medications to treat depression, anxiety, pain, discomfort, and fever. Hidden yeast infections may be present and should be treated. Antiviral drugs such as acyclovir, and selected immunomodulating agents, such as I.V. gamma globulin, ampligen, and transfer factor, may be of assistance.

Special considerations

▶ Some patients may benefit from avoiding environmental irritants and certain foods.
▶ Because patients with CFS may benefit from supportive contact with others who share this disease, refer the patient to the CFS Association of America (*www. cfids.org/*)for information and to local support groups. Patients also may benefit from psychological counseling.

REFERENCES

1. Van Houdenhove, B. "Rehabilitation of Decreased Motor Performance in Patients with Chronic Fatigue Syndrome: Should We Treat Low Effort Capacity or Reduced Effort Tolerance?" *Clinical Rehabilitation* (12):1121-142, December 2007.
2. Centers for Disease Control and Prevention (2006 July 11). "Chronic Fatigue Syndrome, Possible Causes" [Online]. Available at *www.cdc.gov/cfs/cfscauses.htm.*
3. Centers for Disease Control and Prevention (2006 July 11). "CFS Toolkit for Health Care Professionals: Diagnosing CFS" [Online]. Available at *www.cdc.gov/cfs/pdf/Diagnosing_CFS.pdf.*

CDC criteria for diagnosing chronic fatigue syndrome

To meet the Centers for Disease Control and Prevention (CDC) definition of chronic fatigue syndrome, a patient must meet two criteria:

Unexplained, persistent fatigue that is not due to ongoing exertion, isn't relieved by rest, is of new onset, (not lifelong) and results in significant reduction in previous levels of activity. [3]

Four or more of the following symptoms are present for 6 months or more:
• Impaired memory or concentration
• Postexertional malaise
• Unrefreshing sleep
• Muscle pain
• Multijoint pain without swelling or redness
• Headaches of a new type or severity
• Sore throat that's frequent or recurring
• Tender cervical or axillary lymph nodes [3]

LATEX ALLERGY

L atex is a substance found in an increasing number of products both on the job and in the home environment. Also on the rise is the number of latex allergies. Latex allergy is a hypersensitivity reaction to products that contain natural latex, which is derived from the sap of a rubber tree, not synthetic latex. These hypersensitivity reactions range from local dermatitis to a life-threatening anaphylactic reaction.

Causes and incidence

Approximately 1% of the general population has a latex allergy.[1] Anyone who's in frequent contact with latex-containing products is at risk for developing a latex allergy. (See *Products that contain latex*, page 290.) The more frequent the exposure, the higher the risk. The populations at highest risk are medical and dental professionals, workers in

Products that contain latex

Many medical and everyday items contain latex, which can be a threat to the patient with latex allergy. Common items that contain latex include:

MEDICAL PRODUCTS
- Adhesive bandages
- Airways, nasogastric tubes
- Blood pressure cuff, tubing, and bladder
- Catheter leg straps
- Catheters
- Dental dams
- Elastic bandages
- Electrode pads
- Fluid-circulating hypothermia blankets
- Handheld resuscitation bag
- Hemodialysis equipment
- I.V. catheters
- Latex or rubber gloves
- Medication vials
- Pads for crutches
- Protective sheets
- Reservoir breathing bags
- Rubber airway and endotracheal tubes
- Tape
- Tourniquets

NONMEDICAL PRODUCTS
- Adhesive tape
- Balloons (excluding Mylar)
- Cervical diaphragms
- Condoms
- Disposable diapers
- Elastic stockings
- Glue
- Latex paint
- Nipples and pacifiers
- Rubber bands
- Tires

latex companies, chefs/restaurant workers, and patients with spina bifida. Eight percent to 17% of health care workers and up to 68% of children with spina bifida have latex allergies.[1]

Other individuals at risk include:
▶ patients with a history of asthma or other allergies, especially to bananas, avocados, kiwi, papaya, chestnuts, peaches, or nectarines[2]
▶ patients with a history of multiple intra-abdominal or genitourinary surgeries
▶ patients who require frequent intermittent urinary catheterization.

Signs and symptoms
Early signs that a life-threatening hypersensitivity reaction may be occurring include hypotension, tachycardia, and oxygen desaturation. Other clinical findings include urticaria, flushing, bronchospasm, difficulty breathing, pruritus, palpitations, abdominal pain, and syncope. Mild signs and symptoms may include itchy skin, swollen lips, nausea, diarrhea, and red, swollen, teary eyes. (See *Spina bifida and latex allergies*.)

Complications
▶ Respiratory obstruction
▶ Systemic vascular collapse
▶ Death

Diagnosis
A patient who describes even the mildest symptoms during a history and physical assessment should be suspected of having a latex allergy. The patient may describe dermatitis or mild respiratory distress when using latex gloves, inflating a balloon, or coming in contact with other latex products. A skin test should be performed only by specialized allergy centers. The skin is pricked and exposed to small amounts of latex on the forearm or back to determine latex sensitivity.[3] A blood test for latex sensitivity can confirm the diagnosis. This test, which measures specific immunoglobulin E antibodies against latex, should be used only when latex allergy is suspected; it isn't recommended as a screening tool.

Spina bifida and latex allergies

Question: *How can the nurse predict which children with spina bifida are most likely to have an allergic reaction to latex?*

Research: Children with spina bifida are among those who exhibit a higher incidence of latex allergies. Researchers conducted this study to evaluate the prevalence of latex allergy in a group of children with spina bifida and to assess the relationship of early and frequent exposure to latex products and other risk factors to the development of allergic reactions. The 80 children who participated in the study had each undergone multiple surgical procedures, implants of latex-containing materials, and catheterization. The data collected was obtained from a questionnaire, skin-prick test to latex, and a blood test to determine the presence of the specific serum immunoglobulin (Ig) E to latex.

Conclusion: A latex sensitization with specific IgE was identified in 32 of the 80 participants (40%), with only 12 of those demonstrating clinical latex allergic reactions. Repeated or continuous exposure to latex early in life and the disease-associated propensity for latex sensitization were strongly linked to those children who demonstrated clinical latex allergic reactions. The number of surgical procedures performed on the child also had a direct relationship to the child's development of a clinical reaction after exposure.

Application: The nurse caring for a child with spina bifida should be aware of the increased disease-related risk of latex allergy in children with spina bifida The use of latex-free equipment and supplies should be required for all procedures performed on the child, regardless of the child's other risk factors, to prevent a potentially life-threatening allergic reaction. Latex-free precautions should be instituted from birth because the potential for sensitization increases with early and repeated latex exposure.

Source: Ausili, E., et al. "Prevalence of Latex Allergy in Spina Bifida: Genetic and Environmental Risk Factors," *European Review of Medical and Pharmacological Sciences* 11(3):149-53, May-June 2007.

Treatment

The best treatment of latex allergy is prevention; the more a latex-sensitive person is exposed to latex, the worse his symptoms will become. To avoid exposure, advise the patient to substitute products made of silicone and vinyl for those made of latex, and avoid foods that can trigger latex reactions. If the patient has a severe allergy, he may need to carry injectable epinephrine with him at all times.[3]

When a latex allergy is suspected or known, the patient may receive medications before and after surgery or other invasive procedures. Premedications may include prednisone, diphenhydramine, and cimetidine. Postmedications may include hydrocortisone, diphenhydramine, nonsedating antihistamines such as fexofenadine, and famotidine. There's no known treatment for an allergic reaction to latex. Care is supportive in nature. The patient's airway, breathing, and circulation must be monitored. An artificial airway, oxygen therapy, cardiopulmonary resuscitation, and fluid management may be necessary. During an acute reaction, epinephrine, diphenhydramine, and hydrocortisone are commonly administered by I.V. infusion.

Special considerations

▶ Make sure that items that aren't available in a latex-free form, such as stethoscopes and blood pressure cuffs, are wrapped in

cloth before they come in contact with a hypersensitive patient's skin.

▶ Place the patient in a private room or with another patient who requires a latex-free environment.

▶ When adding medication to an I.V. bag, inject the drug through the spike port, not the rubber latex port.

▶ Urge the patient to wear an identification tag mentioning his latex allergy.

▶ Teach the patient and family members how to use an epinephrine autoinjector.

▶ Teach the patient to be aware of all latex-containing products and to use vinyl or silicone products instead. Advise him that Mylar balloons don't contain latex.

REFERENCES

1. American Latex Allergy Association, "Latex Allergy Statistics" [Online]. Available at *www.latexallergyresources.org/topics/LatexAllergyStatistics.cfm.*
2. Behrman, A.J. (2007 November 28). "Latex Allergy" [Online]. Available: *www.emedicine.com/emerg/topic814.htm.*
3. MayoClinic.com (2007 December 1). "Latex Allergy" [Online]. Available at *www.mayoclinic.com/health/latex-allergy/DS00621.*

LUPUS ERYTHEMATOSUS

A chronic inflammatory disorder of the connective tissues, lupus erythematosus appears in two forms. *Discoid lupus erythematosus* affects only the skin. (See *Discoid lupus erythematosus.*) *Systemic lupus erythematosus* (SLE) affects multiple organ systems as well as the skin and can be fatal. Like rheumatoid arthritis, SLE is characterized by recurring remissions and exacerbations, especially common during the spring and summer. The prognosis improves with early detection and treatment, but remains poor for patients who develop cardiovascular, renal, or neurologic complications or severe bacterial infections.

Causes and incidence

The exact cause of SLE remains a mystery, but evidence points to interrelated immunologic, environmental, hormonal, and genetic factors. Autoimmunity is thought to be the prime causative mechanism. In autoimmunity, the body produces antibodies against its own cells such as the antinuclear antibody. Auto-antibodies are produced against red blood cells, neutrophils, platelets, lymphocytes, or almost any organ or tissue in the body. The formed antigen-antibody complexes can suppress the body's normal immunity and damage tissues.

Certain predisposing factors may make a person susceptible to SLE. Physical or mental stress, streptococcal or viral infections, exposure to sunlight or ultraviolet light, immunization, pregnancy, and abnormal estrogen metabolism may all affect this disease's development.

SLE also may be triggered or aggravated by treatment with certain drugs, most commonly, procainamide, hydralazine, and quinidine.[1] Others include anticonvulsants, penicillins, sulfa drugs, and hormonal contraceptives.

The Lupus Foundation of America estimates that 1.5 to 2 million Americans have lupus, and 90% of them are women. Lupus affects people all over the world, but is most prevalent among Asians, Blacks, Native Americans, and Latinos.[1] SLE affects 1 out of 250 Blacks and 1 out of 1,000 Whites. Most cases—80%—occur in women of childbearing age. [2]

Signs and symptoms

The onset of SLE may be acute or insidious and produces no characteristic clinical pattern. However, its symptoms commonly include fever, weight loss, malaise, and fatigue as well as rashes and polyarthralgia. SLE may involve every organ system. In 90% of patients, joint involvement is similar to that in rheumatoid arthritis. Skin lesions are most commonly erythematous rashes in areas ex-

posed to light. The classic butterfly rash over the nose and cheeks occurs in fewer than 50% of the patients. (See *Butterfly rash*, page 294.) Ultraviolet rays commonly provoke or aggravate skin eruptions. Vasculitis can develop (especially in the digits), possibly leading to infarctive lesions, necrotic leg ulcers, or digital gangrene. Raynaud's phenomenon appears in about 20% of patients. Patchy alopecia and painless ulcers of the mucous membranes are common.

Constitutional symptoms of SLE include aching, malaise, fatigue, low-grade or spiking fever, chills, anorexia, and weight loss. Lymph node enlargement (diffuse or local, and nontender), abdominal pain, nausea, vomiting, diarrhea, and constipation may occur. Females may experience irregular menstrual periods or amenorrhea during the active phase of SLE.

About 50% of SLE patients develop signs of cardiopulmonary abnormalities, such as pleuritis, pericarditis, and dyspnea. Myocarditis, endocarditis, tachycardia, parenchymal infiltrates, and pneumonitis may occur. Renal effects may include hematuria, proteinuria, urine sediment, and cellular casts, which may progress to total kidney failure.

Urinary tract infections may result from heightened susceptibility to infection. Seizure disorders and mental dysfunction may indicate neurologic damage. Central nervous system (CNS) involvement may produce emotional instability, psychosis, and organic mental syndrome. Headaches, irritability, and depression are common. (See *Signs of systemic lupus erythematosus*, page 294.)

Complications
▶ Pleurisy
▶ Pleural effusions
▶ Pneumonitis
▶ Pulmonary hypertension
▶ Pulmonary infection
▶ Pericarditis
▶ Myocarditis
▶ Endocarditis
▶ Coronary atherosclerosis
▶ Renal failure
▶ Seizures
▶ Mental dysfunction

Discoid lupus erythematosus

Discoid lupus erythematosus (DLE) is a form of lupus erythematosus marked by chronic skin eruptions that, left untreated, can lead to scarring and permanent disfigurement. About 1 of 20 patients with DLE later develops systemic lupus erythematosus (SLE). The exact cause of DLE is unknown, but some evidence suggests an autoimmune defect. An estimated 60% of patients with DLE are women in their late 20s or older. This disease is rare in children.

DLE lesions are raised, red, scaling plaques, with follicular plugging and central atrophy. The raised edges and sunken centers give them a coinlike appearance. Although these lesions can appear anywhere on the body, they usually erupt on the face, scalp, ears, neck, and arms or on any part of the body that's exposed to sunlight. Such lesions can resolve completely or may cause hypopigmentation or hyperpigmentation, atrophy, and scarring. Facial plaques sometimes assume the butterfly pattern characteristic of SLE. Hair tends to become brittle or may fall out in patches.

As a rule, patient history and the appearance of the rash itself are diagnostic. Lupus erythematosus cell test is positive in fewer than 10% of patients. Skin biopsy of lesions reveals immunoglobulins or complement components. SLE must be ruled out.

Patients with DLE should avoid prolonged exposure to the sun, fluorescent lighting, or reflected sunlight. They should wear protective clothing, use sunscreening agents, avoid engaging in outdoor activities during periods of most intense sunlight (10 a.m. to 2 p.m.), and report any changes in the lesions. Drug treatment consists of topical, intralesional, or systemic medication, as in SLE.

Butterfly rash

In the classic butterfly rash, lesions appear on the cheeks and the bridge of the nose, creating a characteristic butterfly pattern. The rash may vary in severity from malar erythema to discoid lesions (plaque).

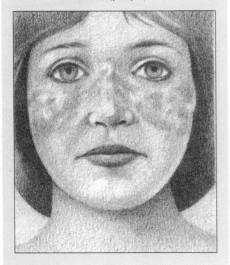

Diagnosis

Diagnostic tests for patients with SLE include a complete blood count with differential (for signs of anemia and decreased white blood cell [WBC] count); platelet count (may be decreased); erythrocyte sedimentation rate (commonly elevated); and serum electrophoresis (may show hypergammaglobulinemia).

Specific tests for SLE include:
▶ antinuclear antibody panel, including anti-deoxyribonucleic acid (DNA) and anti-Smith antibodies—generally positive for lupus alone. (Because the anti-DNA test is rarely positive in other conditions, it's the most specific test for SLE. However, if the patient is in remission, anti-DNA may be reduced or absent [correlates with disease activity, especially renal involvement, and helps monitor response to therapy].[2] Other

tests may be performed as needed to rule out other disorders.)
▶ urine studies—may show red blood cell counts and WBCs, urine casts and sediment, and significant protein loss (more than 0.5 g/24 hours)
▶ blood studies—decreased serum complement (C3 and C4) levels indicate active disease
▶ chest X-ray—may show pleurisy or lupus pneumonitis
▶ electrocardiogram—may show conduction defect with cardiac involvement or pericarditis
▶ kidney biopsy—determines disease stage and extent of renal involvement.

Some patients show a positive lupus anticoagulant test and a positive anticardiolipin test. Such patients are prone to antiphospholipid syndrome (thrombosis and thrombocytopenia).

Signs of systemic lupus erythematosus

Diagnosing systemic lupus erythematosus (SLE) is difficult because SLE commonly mimics other diseases; symptoms may be vague and vary greatly from patient to patient.

Under revised criteria for SLE, the patient must have four or more of the following signs:
• abnormal titer of antinuclear antibody
• hemolytic disorder
• malar rash
• discoid rash
• arthritis
• oral ulcerations
• photosensitivity
• serositis
• renal disorder
• neurologic disorder
• immunologic disorder.

Treatment

Patients with mild disease require little or no medication. Nonsteroidal anti-inflammatory drugs, such as ibuprofen, naproxen, and aspirin control arthritis symptoms in many patients. Anti-malarial drugs such as hydroxychloroquine (also considered a disease modifying antirheumatic drug) can improve symptoms in 1 to 3 months.[3] Skin lesions need topical treatment. Corticosteroid creams are recommended for acute lesions.

Refractory skin lesions are treated with intralesional corticosteroids or antimalarials such as hydroxychloroquine. Because hydroxychloroquine can cause retinal damage, such treatment requires ophthalmologic examination every 6 months.

Corticosteroids are used for serious disease related to vital organ systems, such as pleuritis, pericarditis, lupus nephritis, vasculitis, and CNS involvement. Initial doses equivalent to 60 mg or more of prednisone usually bring noticeable improvement within 48 hours. As soon as symptoms are under control, steroid dosage is tapered slowly. (Rising serum complement levels and decreasing anti-DNA titers indicate patient response.) Diffuse proliferative glomerulonephritis, a major complication of SLE, requires treatment with large doses of steroids. If renal failure occurs, dialysis or kidney transplant may be necessary. In some patients, cytotoxic drugs may delay or prevent deteriorating renal status. Antihypertensive drugs and dietary changes also may be warranted in renal disease. SLE may have related symptoms as some systemic manifestations of infectious diseases such as leptospirosis infection. Incorrect diagnosis could increase the risk morbidity and mortality of SLE.[4]

The photosensitive patient should wear protective clothing (hat, sunglasses, long sleeves, and slacks) and use a screening agent, with a sun protection factor of at least 15, when outdoors. Because SLE usually strikes females of childbearing age, questions about pregnancy commonly arise. Available evidence indicates that a woman with SLE can have a safe, successful pregnancy if she has no serious renal or neurologic impairment.

Special considerations

Careful assessment, supportive measures, emotional support, and patient education are all important parts of the care plan for patients with SLE.

▶ Watch for constitutional symptoms: joint pain or stiffness, weakness, fever, fatigue, and chills. Observe for dyspnea, chest pain, and any edema of the extremities. Note the size, type, and location of skin lesions. Check urine for hematuria, scalp for hair loss, and skin and mucous membranes for petechiae, bleeding, ulceration, pallor, and bruising.

▶ Provide a balanced diet. Renal involvement may mandate a low-sodium, low-protein diet.

▶ Urge the patient to get plenty of rest. Schedule diagnostic tests and procedures to allow adequate rest. Explain all tests and procedures. Tell the patient that several blood samples are needed initially, then periodically, to monitor progress.

▶ Apply heat packs to relieve joint pain and stiffness. Encourage regular exercise to maintain full range of motion (ROM) and prevent contractures. Teach ROM exercises as well as body alignment and postural techniques. Arrange for physical therapy and occupational counseling as appropriate.

▶ Explain the expected benefit of prescribed medications. Watch for adverse effects, especially when the patient is taking high doses of corticosteroids.

▶ Advise the patient receiving cyclophosphamide to maintain adequate hydration. If prescribed, give mesna to prevent hemorrhagic cystitis and ondansetron to prevent nausea and vomiting.

▶ Monitor vital signs, intake and output, weight, and laboratory reports. Check pulse

rates, and observe for orthopnea. Check stools and GI secretions for blood.

▶ Observe for hypertension, weight gain, and other signs of renal involvement.

▶ Assess for signs of neurologic damage: personality change, paranoid or psychotic behavior, ptosis, or diplopia. Take seizure precautions. If Raynaud's phenomenon is present, warm and protect the patient's hands and feet.

▶ If the patient is a female and uses makeup, offer cosmetic tips such as suggesting the use of hypoallergenic makeup. If you know of a hairdresser who specializes in scalp disorders, provide the patient with a referral.

▶ Advise the patient to purchase medications in quantity, if possible. Warn against "miracle" drugs for relief of arthritis symptoms.

▶ Refer the patient to the Lupus Foundation of America and the Arthritis Foundation, if that would be helpful.

REFERENCES

1. Lupus Foundation of America. "About Lupus" [Online]. Available at *www.lupus.org*.
2. Lamont, D.W., et al. (2006 January 17). "Systemic Lupus Erythematosus" [Online]. Available at *www.emedicine.com/emerg/topic564.htm*.
3. American College of Rheumatology (2006 October). "Hydroxychloroquine" [Online]. Available at *www.rheumatology.org/public/factsheets/hydroxychloroquine.asp*.
4. Barnabe, C., and Fahlman, N. "Overlapping Clinical Features of Lupus and Leptospirosis" *Clinical Rheumatology,* January 10, 2008.

RHEUMATOID ARTHRITIS

A chronic, systemic, inflammatory disease, rheumatoid arthritis (RA) primarily attacks peripheral joints and surrounding muscles, tendons, ligaments, and blood vessels. Spontaneous remissions and unpredictable exacerbations mark the course of this potentially crippling disease.

RA usually requires lifelong treatment and, sometimes, surgery. In most patients, the disease follows an intermittent course and allows normal activity, although 10% suffer total disability from severe articular deformity, associated extra-articular symptoms, or both. The prognosis worsens with the development of nodules, vasculitis, and high titers of rheumatoid factor (RF).

Causes and incidence

What causes the chronic inflammation characteristic of RA isn't known, but various theories point to infectious, genetic, and endocrine factors (hormonal influence in women may be a factor). Currently, it's believed that a genetically susceptible individual develops abnormal or altered immunoglobulin (Ig) G antibodies when exposed to an antigen. This altered IgG antibody isn't recognized as "self," and the individual forms an antibody against it—an antibody known as RF. By aggregating into complexes, RF generates inflammation. Eventually, cartilage damage by inflammation triggers additional immune responses, including activation of complement. This in turn attracts polymorphonuclear leukocytes and stimulates release of inflammatory mediators, which enhance joint destruction. Some scientists believe that RA is triggered by an infectious agent, but more research is needed.[1]

Much more is known about the pathogenesis of RA than about its causes. If unarrested, the inflammatory process within the joints occurs in four stages. First, synovitis develops from congestion and edema of the synovial membrane and joint capsule. Formation of pannus—thickened layers of granulation tissue—marks the second stage's onset. Pannus covers and invades cartilage and eventually destroys the joint capsule and bone. Progression to the third stage is characterized by fibrous ankylosis—fibrous invasion of the pannus and scar formation that occludes the joint space. Bone atrophy and malalignment cause visible deformities and

disrupt the articulation of opposing bones, causing muscle atrophy and imbalance and, possibly, partial dislocations or subluxations. In the fourth stage, fibrous tissue calcifies, resulting in bony ankylosis and total immobility.

RA occurs worldwide, striking three times more females than males. Although it can occur at any age, it usually begins between ages 25 and 50. This disease affects more than 2 million people in the United States alone. [1]

Studies show that RA improves in 75% to 95% of pregnant females.

Signs and symptoms

RA usually develops insidiously. At first, it produces nonspecific signs and symptoms, such as fatigue, malaise, anorexia, persistent low-grade fever, weight loss, lymphadenopathy, and vague articular symptoms. Later, more specific localized articular symptoms develop, commonly in the fingers at the proximal interphalangeal, metacarpophalangeal, and metatarsophalangeal joints. RA usually affects the smaller joints first, including hands, wrists, feet, and ankles, progressing to larger joints such as knees, hips, and shoulders. The disease is also marked by exacerbations where symptoms become active, followed by periods of remission where symptoms are relaxed.[3]

These symptoms usually occur bilaterally and symmetrically. The affected joints stiffen after inactivity, especially upon rising in the morning. The fingers may assume a spindle shape from marked edema and joint congestion. The joints become tender and painful, at first only when the patient moves them, but eventually even at rest. They commonly feel hot to the touch. Ultimately, joint function is diminished.

Deformities are common if active disease continues. (See *Joint deformities*.) Proximal interphalangeal joints may develop flexion deformities or become hyperextended. Metacarpophalangeal joints may swell dor-

Joint deformities

In advanced rheumatoid arthritis, marked edema and congestion cause spindle-shaped interphalangeal joints and severe flexion deformities.

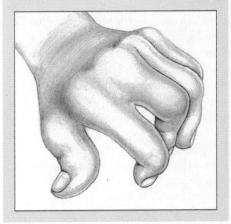

sally, and volar subluxation and stretching of tendons may pull the fingers to the ulnar side (ulnar drift). The fingers may become fixed in a characteristic "swan's neck" appearance, or "boutonnière" deformity. The hands appear foreshortened, the wrists boggy; carpal tunnel syndrome from synovial pressure on the median nerve causes tingling paresthesia in the fingers.

The most common extra-articular finding is the gradual appearance of rheumatoid nodules—subcutaneous, round or oval, nontender masses—usually on pressure areas such as the elbows.

Complications

▶ Vasculitis can lead to skin lesions, leg ulcers, and multiple systemic complications.
▶ Peripheral neuropathy may produce numbness or tingling in the feet or weakness and loss of sensation in the fingers. Stiff, weak, or painful muscles are common.
▶ Other common extra-articular effects include pericarditis, pulmonary nodules or fibrosis, pleuritis, scleritis, and episcleritis.

▶ Another complication is destruction of the odontoid process, part of the second cervical vertebra.

▶ Rarely, cord compression may occur, particularly in patients with long-standing deforming disease. Upper motor neuron signs and symptoms, such as a positive Babinski's sign and muscle weakness, may also develop.

▶ RA can also cause temporomandibular joint disease, which impairs chewing and causes earaches.

▶ Other extra-articular findings may include infection, osteoporosis, myositis, cardiopulmonary lesions, lymphadenopathy, and peripheral neuritis.

Diagnosis

Typical clinical features suggest this disorder, but a definitive diagnosis is based on laboratory and other test results:

▶ X-rays: In early stages, they show bone demineralization and soft-tissue swelling; later, loss of cartilage and narrowing of joint spaces; and finally, cartilage and bone destruction and erosion, subluxations, and deformities.

▶ rheumatoid factor test: Results are positive in 75% to 80% of patients as indicated by a titer of 1:160 or higher. Some people who don't have RA will test positive.[1]

▶ synovial fluid analysis: This reveals increased volume and turbidity but decreased viscosity and complement (C3 and C4) levels; white blood cell count usually exceeds 10,000/μl.

▶ erythrocyte sedimentation rate: This is elevated in 85% to 90% of patients. (It may be useful to monitor response to therapy because elevation commonly parallels disease activity.)

▶ complete blood count: This usually reveals moderate anemia and slight leukocytosis.

A C-reactive protein test can help monitor response to therapy.

IN THE NEWS *Magnetic resonance imaging scans are useful to view actual changes to the bones in RA process. They're also a way to measure disease progression and response to therapy.*[2]

Treatment

Nonsteroidal anti-inflammatory drugs (NSAIDS), such as aspirin, naproxen, and ibuprofen, are the mainstay of RA therapy because they decrease inflammation and relieve joint pain. Corticosteroids also decrease inflammation and joint pain and are more potent than NSAIDS; therefore, they're used for shorter periods during flare-ups or when NSAIDS aren't helpful.[3]

Disease-modifying antirheumatic drugs (DMARDs) are used in conjunction with NSAIDs. DMARDs prevent joint destruction and deformity and can promote remission. DMARDs include hydroxychloroquine, sulfasalazine, methotrexate, gold salts, and penicillamine. Immunosuppressants, such as cyclophosphamide, methotrexate, and azathioprine, are also therapeutic and more commonly used in early disease. (See *Drug therapy for arthritis.*)

Supportive measures include 8 to 10 hours of sleep every night, frequent rest periods between daily activities, and splinting to rest inflamed joints. A physical therapy program that includes range-of-motion exercises and carefully individualized therapeutic exercises forestalls joint function loss; application of heat relaxes muscles and relieves pain. Moist heat usually works best for patients with chronic disease. Ice packs are effective during acute episodes.

Advanced disease may require synovectomy, joint reconstruction, or total joint arthroplasty.

Useful surgical procedures in RA include metatarsal head and distal ulnar resectional arthroplasty, insertion of a Silastic prosthesis between the metacarpophalangeal and proximal interphalangeal joints, and arthrodesis

Drug therapy for arthritis

This chart lists relevant information about drugs commonly used in RA therapy. Other drugs—not listed here—that may be used in resistant cases include prednisone, chloroquine, azathioprine, and cyclophosphamide.

DRUG AND ADVERSE EFFECTS

CLINICAL CONSIDERATIONS

Aspirin

Prolonged bleeding time; GI disturbances, including nausea, dyspepsia, anorexia, ulcers, and hemorrhage; hypersensitivity reactions ranging from urticaria to anaphylaxis; salicylism (mild toxicity: tinnitus, dizziness; moderate toxicity: restlessness, hyperpnea, delirium, marked lethargy; and severe toxicity: coma, seizures, severe hyperpnea)

- Don't use in patients with GI ulcers, bleeding, or hypersensitivity or in neonates.
- Tell the patient to take the drug with food, milk, antacid, or a large glass of water to reduce GI adverse effects.
- Monitor the patient's salicylate level. Remember that toxicity can develop rapidly in febrile, dehydrated children.
- Teach the patient to reduce the dose, one tablet at a time, if tinnitus occurs.
- Teach the patient to watch for signs of bleeding, such as bruising, melena, and petechiae.

Fenoprofen, ibuprofen, naproxen, piroxicam, sulindac, and tolmetin

Prolonged bleeding time; central nervous system abnormalities (headache, drowsiness, restlessness, dizziness, and tremor); GI disturbances, including hemorrhage and peptic ulcer; increased blood urea nitrogen and liver enzyme levels

- Don't use in patients with renal disease, in patients with asthma who have nasal polyps, or in children.
- Use cautiously in patients with GI and cardiac disease or if a patient is allergic to other nonsteroidal anti-inflammatory drugs (NSAIDs).
- Tell the patient to take the drug with milk or meals to reduce GI adverse effects.
- Tell the patient that the drug effect may be delayed for 2 to 3 weeks.
- Monitor the patient's kidney, liver, and auditory functions in long-term therapy. Stop the drug if abnormalities develop.
- Use cautiously in elderly patients; they may experience severe GI bleeding without warning.

Hydroxychloroquine and sulfasalazine

Blood dyscrasias, GI irritation, corneal opacities, and keratopathy or retinopathy

- Don't use in patients with retinal or visual field changes.
- Use cautiously in patients with hepatic disease, alcoholism, glucose-6-phosphate dehydrogenase deficiency, or psoriasis.
- Perform complete blood count (CBC) and liver function tests before therapy and during chronic therapy. The patient should also have regular ophthalmologic examinations.
- Tell the patient to take the drug with food or milk to minimize GI adverse effects.
- Warn the patient that dizziness may occur.

(continued)

Drug therapy for arthritis *(continued)*

DRUG AND ADVERSE EFFECTS	CLINICAL CONSIDERATIONS
Gold (oral and parenteral)	
Dermatitis, pruritus, rash, stomatitis, nephrotoxicity, blood dyscrasias and, with oral form, GI distress and diarrhea	■ Watch for and report adverse effects. Observe for nitritoid reaction (flushing, fainting, and sweating). ■ Check the patient's urine for blood and albumin before giving each dose. If positive, hold the drug and notify the physician. Stress to the patient the need for regular follow-up, including blood and urine testing. ■ To avoid local nerve irritation, mix the drug well, and give it via a deep I.M. injection in the buttock. ■ Advise the patient not to expect improvement for 3 to 6 months. ■ Tell the patient to report rash, bruising, bleeding, hematuria, or oral ulcers.
Methotrexate	
Tubular necrosis, bone marrow depression, leukopenia, thrombocytopenia, pulmonary interstitial infiltrates, hyperuricemia, stomatitis, rash, pruritus, dermatitis, alopecia, diarrhea, dizziness, cirrhosis, and hepatic fibrosis	■ Don't give to women who are pregnant or breast-feeding or to patients who are alcoholic. ■ Monitor the patient's uric acid levels, CBC, and intake and output. ■ Warn the patient to report promptly any unusual bleeding (especially GI) or bruising. ■ Warn the patient to avoid alcohol, aspirin, and NSAIDs. ■ Advise the patient to follow the prescribed regimen.

(joint fusion). Arthrodesis sacrifices joint mobility for stability and pain relief. Synovectomy (removal of destructive, proliferating synovium, usually in the wrists, knees, and fingers) may halt or delay the course of this disease. Osteotomy (the cutting of bone or excision of a wedge of bone) can realign joint surfaces and redistribute stresses. Tendons may rupture spontaneously, requiring surgical repair. Tendon transfers may prevent deformities or relieve contractures. (See *When arthritis requires surgery.*)

Special considerations

▶ Assess all joints carefully. Look for deformities, contractures, immobility, and inability to perform everyday activities.

▶ Monitor the patient's vital signs, and note weight changes, sensory disturbances, and level of pain. Administer analgesics as ordered, and watch for adverse effects.

▶ Provide meticulous skin care. Check for rheumatoid nodules as well as pressure ulcers and breakdowns due to immobility, vascular impairment, corticosteroid treatment, or improper splinting. Use lotion or cleaning oil, not soap, for dry skin.

▶ Explain all diagnostic tests and procedures. Tell the patient to expect multiple blood samples to allow firm diagnosis and accurate monitoring of therapy.

▶ Monitor the duration, not the intensity, of morning stiffness because duration more accurately reflects the disease's severity. En-

When arthritis requires surgery

Arthritis severe enough to necessitate total knee or total hip arthroplasty calls for comprehensive preoperative teaching and postoperative care.

BEFORE SURGERY

• Explain preoperative and surgical procedures. Show the patient the prosthesis, if available.

• Teach the patient postoperative exercises such as isometrics, and supervise his practice. Also, teach deep-breathing and coughing exercises that will be necessary after surgery.

• Explain that total hip or knee arthroplasty requires frequent range-of-motion exercises of the leg after surgery; total knee arthroplasty requires frequent leg-lift exercises.

• Show the patient how to use a trapeze to move himself about in bed after surgery, and make sure he has a fracture bedpan handy.

• Tell the patient what kind of dressings to expect after surgery. After total knee arthroplasty, the patient's knee may be placed in a constant-passive-motion device to increase postoperative mobility and prevent emboli. After total hip arthroplasty, he'll have an abduction pillow between the legs to help keep the hip prosthesis in place.

AFTER SURGERY

• Closely monitor and record vital signs. Watch for complications, such as steroid crisis and shock in patients receiving steroids. Monitor distal leg pulses often, marking them with a waterproof marker to make them easier to find.

• As soon as the patient awakens, have him do active dorsiflexion; if he can't, report this imme-

diately. Supervise isometric exercises every 2 hours. After total hip arthroplasty, check traction for pressure areas, and keep the bed's head raised between 30 and 45 degrees.

• Change or reinforce dressings, as needed, using sterile technique. Check wounds for hematoma, excessive drainage, color changes, or foul odor—all possible signs of hemorrhage or infection. (Wounds on rheumatoid arthritis patients may heal slowly.) Avoid contaminating dressings while helping the patient use the urinal or bedpan.

• Administer blood replacement products, antibiotics, and pain medication, as ordered. Monitor serum electrolyte and hemoglobin levels and hematocrit.

• Have the patient turn, cough, and deep-breathe every 2 hours; then percuss his chest.

• After total knee arthroplasty, keep the patient's leg extended and slightly elevated.

• After total hip arthroplasty, keep the patient's hip in abduction to prevent dislocation by using such measures as a wedge pillow. Prevent external rotation, and avoid hip flexion greater than 90 degrees. Watch for and immediately report any inability to rotate the hip or bear weight on it, increased pain, or a leg that appears shorter—all may indicate dislocation.

• Once the physician gives the okay, help the patient get out of bed and sit in a chair, keeping his weight on the unaffected side. When the patient is ready to walk, consult with the physical therapist who can provide walking instruction and aids.

---

courage the patient to take hot showers or baths at bedtime or in the morning to reduce the need for pain medication.

▶ Apply splints carefully and correctly. Observe for pressure ulcers if the patient is in traction or wearing splints.

▶ Explain the nature of the disease. Make sure the patient and his family understand that RA is a chronic disease that requires

major changes in lifestyle. Emphasize that there are no miracle cures, despite claims to the contrary.

▶ Encourage a balanced diet, but make sure the patient understands that special diets won't cure RA. Stress the need for weight control because obesity adds further stress to joints.

▶ Urge the patient to perform activities of daily living (ADLs), such as practicing good hygiene and dressing and feeding himself. Suggest ADL aids, such as a long-handled shoehorn; elastic shoelaces; zipper-pulls; button hooks; easy-to-handle cups, plates, and silverware; elevated toilet seats; and battery-operated toothbrushes. Household cleaning devices such as long-handled dustpans are also available. Patients who have trouble maneuvering fingers into gloves should wear mittens.

▶ ADLs that can be done in a sitting position should be encouraged. Allow the patient enough time to calmly perform these tasks.

▶ Provide emotional support. Remember that the patient with chronic illness easily becomes depressed, discouraged, and irritable. Encourage the patient to discuss his fears concerning dependency, sexuality, body image, and self-esteem. Refer him to an appropriate social service agency as needed.

▶ Discuss sexual aids: alternative positions, pain medication, and moist heat to increase mobility.

▶ Before discharge, make sure the patient knows how and when to take prescribed medication and how to recognize possible adverse effects.

▶ Teach the patient how to stand, walk, and sit correctly: upright and erect. Tell him to sit in chairs with high seats and armrests; he'll find it easier to get up from a chair if his knees are lower than his hips. If he doesn't own a chair with a high seat, recommend putting blocks of wood under a favorite chair's legs. Suggest an elevated toilet seat.

▶ Mobility aids are very helpful. Many medical and commercial stores offer assistive and supportive devices that promote self-care, including an overhead grasping trapeze to get out of bed, easy-to-open drawers, handheld shower nozzles, handrails, and grab bars.

▶ Instruct the patient to pace daily activities, resting for 5 to 10 minutes out of each hour and alternating sitting and standing tasks. Adequate sleep and correct sleeping posture are important. He should sleep on his back on a firm mattress and should avoid placing a pillow under his knees, which encourages flexion deformity.

▶ Teach the patient to avoid putting undue stress on joints and to use the largest joint available for a given task, to support weak or painful joints as much as possible, to avoid positions of flexion and promote positions of extension, to hold objects parallel to the knuckles as briefly as possible, to always use his hands toward the center of his body, and to slide—not lift—objects whenever possible. Enlist the aid of the occupational therapist to teach how to simplify activities and protect arthritic joints. Stress the importance of shoes with proper support.

Refer the patient to the Arthritis Foundation for more information on coping with the disease.

REFERENCES

1. Arthritis Foundation. "Disease Center, Rheumatoid Arthritis" [Online]. Available at *www.arthritis.org/disease-center.php? disease_id=31.*
2. Hodgson, R.J. "MRI of Rheumatoid Arthritis—Image Quantitation for the Assessment of Disease Activity, Progression and Response to Therapy," *Rheumatology* 47(1):13-21, January 2008.
3. MayoClinic.com (2007 November 2). "Rheumatoid Arthritis" [Online]. *www.mayoclinic.com/ health/rheumatoid-arthritis/DS00020.*

SCLERODERMA

Scleroderma, a systemic sclerosis that's also known as *progressive systemic sclerosis,* is a diffuse connective tissue disease characterized by fibrotic, degenerative, and occasionally inflammatory changes in skin, blood vessels, synovial membranes, skeletal muscles, and internal organs (especially the esophagus, intestinal tract, thyroid, heart, lungs, and kidneys). Additional study

Health problems and scleroderma

Question: *What are the main health problems of patients with scleroderma, based on sub-type and disease duration?*

Research: Scleroderma is a chronic, often disabling autoimmune disease of the connective tissues. The most common sub-type of scleroderma is the systemic form of the disease, which can be subdivided into diffuse cutaneous systemic sclerosis and limited cutaneous systemic sclerosis. The subtypes differ in their course, complications, and prognosis. Researchers interested in determining the main health problems of patients with systemic sclerosis (based on the disease subtype), and the effects of disease duration on symptom intensification, studied 63 patients. All had been diagnosed with systemic sclerosis according to the criteria of the American Rheumatism Association. The participants were divided into two groups: 47 with limited systemic sclerosis and 16 with diffuse systemic sclerosis; 29 participants (46%) had been ill for 5 to 14 years and 17 (27%) for more than 15 years. Data was compiled from a survey questionnaire completed by the participants.

Conclusion: Analysis of the data showed that participants with diffuse systemic sclerosis were more likely to experience quick fatigability and a feeling of tiredness, joint and muscle pain, reduction in range of motion, renal crisis, increased blood pressure, and a significant incidence of lung, kidney, GI, and myocardial involvement. Participants with limited systemic sclerosis were more likely to experience pain connected with easily inflicted skin injuries and ulcers that are difficult to heal; an inability to cope with the disease; problems involving the GI system, including difficulties with opening the mouth, swallowing, heartburn and belching, diarrhea or constipation; and a significant incidence of pulmonary hypertension, skin calcifications, telangiectasia, and lung fibrosis. Raynaud's phenomenon was present in almost all participants (93.7%) in both groups, regardless of disease duration. Self-care difficulties intensified with disease duration, especially with limited systemic sclerosis. The disease had a profound effect on the mental attitudes of participants in both groups, an influence that increased with disease duration, limiting their social and professional activities.

Application: It's important for the nurse caring for a patient with scleroderma to recognize the individual care problems of the patient. The primary nursing care goals should include pain reduction, infection prevention, rapid identification of life-threatening conditions, and patient education that enables the patient to perform self-care, and enhances the patient's ability to cope with the disease in daily life.

Source: Sierakowska, M., et al. "Nursing Problems of Patients with Systemic Sclerosis," *Advances in Medical Sciences* 52 Suppl 1:147-52, 2007.

is needed to understand more about how systemic sclerosis progresses. Presently, additional research is being done to improve methods to measure disease activity in systemic sclerosis. The goal is to create a global standard to measure disease activity as a way to improve treatment.[3] (See *Health problems and scleroderma*.)

This disease occurs in distinctive forms:

▶ *CREST syndrome*—a benign form characterized by calcinosis, Raynaud's phenomenon, esophageal dysfunction, sclerodactyly, and telangiectasia
▶ *diffuse systemic sclerosis*—characterized by generalized skin thickening and invasion of internal organ systems
▶ *localized scleroderma*—characterized by patchy skin changes with a droplike appearance known as morphea. Although localized

scleroderma presents on the skin, it's characterized as an organ-specific autoimmune disorder that differs from systemic sclerosis.[4]

▶ *linear scleroderma*—characterized by a band of thickened skin on the face or extremities that severely damages underlying tissues, causing atrophy and deformity (most common in childhood.)

Other forms include chemically induced localized scleroderma, eosinophilia myalgia syndrome (recently associated with ingestion of L-tryptophan), toxic oil syndrome (associated with contaminated oil), and graft-versus-host disease.

Causes and incidence

The cause of scleroderma is unknown. Inheritance may play a role as well as the environment.[1] Known risk factors include exposure to silica dust and polyvinyl chloride.

It's estimated that 300,000 people in the United States have scleroderma.[2] Scleroderma affects more females than men, and onset is between ages 25 and 55.[2] Approximately 30% of patients with scleroderma die within 5 years of onset.

Signs and symptoms

Scleroderma typically begins with Raynaud's phenomenon—blanching, cyanosis, and erythema of the fingers and toes in response to stress or exposure to cold. Progressive phalangeal resorption may shorten the fingers.

Compromised circulation, which results from abnormal thickening of the arterial intima, may cause slowly healing ulcerations on the tips of the fingers or toes that may lead to gangrene. Raynaud's phenomenon may precede scleroderma by months or years.

Later symptoms include pain, stiffness, and finger and joint swelling. Skin thickening produces taut, shiny skin over the entire hand and forearm. Facial skin also becomes tight and inelastic, causing a masklike appearance and "pinching" of the mouth. As

tightening progresses, contractures may develop.

GI dysfunction causes frequent reflux, heartburn, dysphagia, and bloating after meals. These symptoms may cause the patient to decrease food intake and lose weight. Other GI effects include abdominal distention, diarrhea, constipation, and malodorous floating stools.

Complications

▶ Cardiac and pulmonary fibrosis producing arrhythmias and dyspnea
▶ Pulmonary artery hypertension
▶ Renal involvement, usually accompanied by malignant hypertension, the main cause of death

Diagnosis

Typical cutaneous changes provide the first clue to diagnosis. Results of diagnostic tests include:

▶ blood studies—slightly elevated erythrocyte sedimentation rate, positive rheumatoid factor in 25% to 35% of patients, and positive antinuclear antibody test
▶ anticentromere antibody is found in the CREST form of scleroderma; anti-scl 70 antibody is found in the diffuse form of scleroderma[1]
▶ chest X-rays—bilateral basilar pulmonary fibrosis
▶ electrocardiogram—possible nonspecific abnormalities related to myocardial fibrosis
▶ GI X-rays—distal esophageal hypomotility and stricture, duodenal loop dilation, small-bowel malabsorption pattern, and large diverticula
▶ hand X-rays—terminal phalangeal tuft resorption, subcutaneous calcification, and joint space narrowing and erosion
▶ pulmonary function studies—decreased diffusion and vital capacity and restrictive lung disease
▶ skin biopsy—may show changes consistent with the disease's progress, such as

marked thickening of the dermis and occlusive vessel changes
- urinalysis—proteinuria, microscopic hematuria, and casts (with renal involvement).

Treatment

Currently, no cure exists for scleroderma. Treatment aims to preserve normal body functions and minimize complications. Use of an immunosuppressant such as chlorambucil is a common palliative measure. Corticosteroids and colchicine seem to stabilize symptoms; D-penicillamine may be helpful. Blood platelet levels need to be monitored throughout drug therapy.

Other treatments vary according to symptoms:
- for chronic digital ulcerations—a digital plaster cast to immobilize the area, minimize trauma, and maintain cleanliness; possibly surgical debridement
- for esophagitis with stricture—antacids, cimetidine, periodic esophageal dilatation, and a soft, bland diet
- for hand debilitation—physical therapy to maintain function and promote muscle strength, heat therapy to relieve joint stiffness, and patient teaching to make performance of daily activities easier
- for Raynaud's phenomenon—various vasodilators and antihypertensive agents (such as methyldopa or calcium channel blockers), intermittent cervical sympathetic blockade or, rarely, thoracic sympathectomy
- for scleroderma kidney (with malignant hypertension and impending renal failure)—dialysis, antihypertensives, and calcium channel blockers
- for small-bowel involvement (diarrhea, pain, malabsorption, and weight loss)—broad-spectrum antibiotics, such as erythromycin or tetracycline, to counteract bacterial overgrowth in the duodenum and jejunum related to hypomotility.

Special considerations

- Assess the patient's motion restrictions, pain, vital signs, intake and output, respiratory function, and daily weight.
- Because of compromised circulation, warn against fingerstick blood tests.
- Remember that air conditioning may aggravate Raynaud's phenomenon.
- Help the patient and his family adjust to the patient's new body image and to the limitations and dependence that these changes cause.
- Teach the patient to avoid fatigue by pacing activities and organizing schedules to include necessary rest.
- Stress to the patient and his family the need to accept the fact that this condition is incurable. Encourage them to express their feelings and help them cope with their fears and frustrations by offering information about the disease, its treatment, and relevant diagnostic tests.
- Whenever possible, let the patient participate in treatment by measuring his own intake and output, planning his own diet, assisting in dialysis, giving himself heat therapy, and doing prescribed exercises.
- Direct the patient to seek out support groups, which can be found in every state. Instruct the patient to call 1-800-722-HOPE, or go to *www.scleroderma.org* (if possible) to determine the closest location.

REFERENCES

1. Shiel, W.C. (2007 March 7). "Scleroderma" [Online]. Available at *www.medicinenet.com/scleroderma/article.htm.*
2. Scleroderma Foundation. "Overview of Scleroderma" [Online]. Available at *www.scleroderma.org/medical/overview.shtm.*
3. Hudson, M., et al. "Update on Indices of Disease Activity in Systemic Sclerosis," *Seminars in Arthritis and Rheumatism* 37(2): 93-98, October 2007.
4. Takehara, K., and Sato, S. "Localized Scleroderma Is an Autoimmune Disorder," *Rheumatology* 44(3):274-279, March 2005.

VASCULITIS

Vasculitis includes a broad spectrum of disorders characterized by inflammation and necrosis of blood vessels. Its clinical effects, which reflect tissue ischemia caused by blood flow obstruction, and confirming laboratory procedures, depend on the vessels involved. The prognosis is variable. For example, hypersensitivity vasculitis is usually a benign disorder limited to the skin, but more extensive polyarteritis nodosa can be rapidly fatal. Vasculitis can occur at any age, except for mucocutaneous lymph node syndrome, which occurs only during childhood. Vasculitis may be a primary disorder or occur secondary to other disorders, such as rheumatoid arthritis or systemic lupus erythematosus.

Causes

How vascular damage develops in vasculitis isn't well understood. It has been associated with a history of serious infectious disease, such as hepatitis B, exposure to chemicals, medications, cancers such as lymphoma or multiple myeloma, and rheumatic diseases.[1] Current theory holds that it's initiated by excessive circulating antigen, which triggers the formation of soluble antigen-antibody complexes. These complexes can't be effectively cleared by the reticuloendothelial system, so they're deposited in blood vessel walls (type III hypersensitivity). Increased vascular permeability associated with release of vasoactive amines by platelets and basophils enhances such deposition. The deposited complexes activate the complement cascade, resulting in chemotaxis of neutrophils, which release lysosomal enzymes. In turn, these enzymes cause vessel damage and necrosis, which may precipitate thrombosis, occlusion, hemorrhage, and ischemia.

Another mechanism that may contribute to vascular damage is the cell-mediated (T-cell) immune response. In this response, circulating antigen triggers the release of sol-uble mediators by sensitized lymphocytes, which attracts macrophages. The macrophages release intracellular enzymes, which cause vascular damage. They can also transform into the epithelioid and multinucleated giant cells that typify the granulomatous vasculitides. Phagocytosis of immune complexes by macrophages enhances granuloma formation.

Incidence is different depending on the type of scleroderma. Henoch-Schönlein purpura occurs in 13.5 cases per 100,000 children. Kawasaki syndrome occurs in 1 to 3 per 10,000 children. Polyarteritis nodosa occurs in 0.7 per 100,000 people, and Wegener's granulomatosis occurs in 1 to 3 cases per 100,000 adults.[2]

Signs and symptoms

The clinical effects of vasculitis vary according to the blood vessels involved. (See *Types of vasculitis.*)

Complications

- ▶ Renal failure
- ▶ Renal hypertension
- ▶ Glomerulitis
- ▶ Fibrous scarring of lung tissue
- ▶ Stroke
- ▶ GI bleeding
- ▶ Necrotizing vasculitis
- ▶ Spontaneous hemorrhage
- ▶ Intestinal obstruction
- ▶ Myocardial infarction
- ▶ Pericarditis
- ▶ Rupture of mesenteric aneurysms

Diagnosis

Because the signs and symptoms of vasculitis may resemble many other conditions, diagnosis is done through medical history, physical exam, and ruling out other causes. The following tests may be helpful: blood tests such as erythrocyte sedimentation rate, C-reactive protein, red blood cell count, white blood cell count, platelets, rheumatoid factor, antineutrophil cytoplasmic antibod-

Types of vasculitis

Vasculitis occurs in various forms; diagnosis depends on the presenting signs and symptoms.

TYPE	VESSELS INVOLVED	SIGNS AND SYMPTOMS	DIAGNOSIS
Polyarteritis nodosa	Small to medium arteries throughout the body (Lesions tend to be segmental, occur at bifurcations and branchings of arteries, and spread distally to arterioles. In severe cases, lesions circumferentially involve adjacent veins.)	Hypertension, abdominal pain, myalgia, headache, joint pain, and weakness	History of symptoms; elevated erythrocyte sedimentation rate (ESR); leukocytosis; anemia; thrombocytosis; depressed C3 complement; rheumatoid factor more than 1:60; circulating immune complexes; tissue biopsy showing necrotizing vasculitis
Allergic angiitis and granulomatosis (Churg-Strauss syndrome)	Small to medium arteries (including arterioles, capillaries, and venules), mainly of the lungs but also other organs	Resembles polyarteritis nodosa with hallmark of severe pulmonary involvement	History of asthma; eosinophilia; tissue biopsy showing granulomatous inflammation with eosinophilic infiltration
Polyangiitis overlap syndrome	Small to medium arteries (including arterioles, capillaries, and venules) of the lungs and other organs	Combines symptoms of polyarteritis nodosa, allergic angiitis, and granulomatosis	Possible history of allergy; eosinophilia; tissue biopsy showing granulomatous inflammation with eosinophilic infiltration
Wegener's granulomatosis	Small to medium vessels of the respiratory tract and kidney	Fever, pulmonary congestion, cough, malaise, anorexia, weight loss, and mild to severe hematuria	Tissue biopsy showing necrotizing vasculitis with granulomatous inflammation; leukocytosis; elevated ESR and immunoglobulin (Ig) A and IgG levels; low titer rheumatoid factor; circulating immune complexes; antineutrophil cytoplasmic antibody in more than 90% of patients
Temporal arteritis	Medium to large arteries, most commonly branches of the carotid artery	Fever, myalgia, jaw claudication, visual changes, and headache (associated with polymyalgia rheumatica syndrome)	Decreased hemoglobin (Hb) level; elevated ESR; tissue biopsy showing panarteritis with infiltration of mononuclear cells, giant cells within vessel wall, fragmentation of internal elastic lamina, and proliferation of intima

(continued)

Types of vasculitis *(continued)*

TYPE	VESSELS INVOLVED	SIGNS AND SYMPTOMS	DIAGNOSIS
Takayasu's arteritis (aortic arch syndrome)	Medium to large arteries, particularly the aortic arch, its branches and, possibly, the pulmonary artery	Malaise, pallor, nausea, night sweats, arthralgia, anorexia, weight loss, pain or paresthesia distal to affected area, bruits, loss of distal pulses, syncope and, if a carotid artery is involved, diplopia and transient blindness; may progress to heart failure or stroke	Decreased Hb level; leukocytosis; positive lupus erythematosus cell preparation and elevated ESR; arteriography showing calcification and obstruction of affected vessels; tissue biopsy showing inflammation of adventitia and intima of vessels, and thickening of vessel walls
Hypersensitivity vasculitis	Small vessels, especially of the skin	Palpable purpura, papules, nodules, vesicles, bullae, ulcers, or chronic or recurrent urticaria	History of exposure to antigen, such as a microorganism or drug; tissue biopsy showing leukocytoclastic angiitis, usually in postcapillary venules, with infiltration of polymorphonuclear leukocytes, fibrinoid necrosis, and extravasation of erythrocytes
Mucocutaneous lymph node syndrome (Kawasaki disease)	Small to medium vessels, primarily of the lymph nodes; may progress to involve coronary arteries	Fever; nonsuppurative cervical adenitis; edema; congested conjunctivae; erythema of oral cavity, lips, and palms; and desquamation of fingertips; may progress to arthritis, myocarditis, pericarditis, myocardial infarction, and cardiomegaly	History of symptoms; elevated ESR; tissue biopsy showing intimal proliferation and infiltration of vessel walls with mononuclear cells; echocardiography necessary
Behçet's disease	Small vessels, primarily of the mouth and genitalia, but also of the eyes, skin, joints, GI tract, and central nervous system	Recurrent oral ulcers, eye lesions, genital lesions, and cutaneous lesions	History of symptoms
Necrotizing vasculitis	Any blood vessel	Red to purple papule skin lesions, pain, infarction, joint pain, numbness, weakness, fever, fatigue, dysmenorrhea, pyrosis, dysphonia, and dysphagia	History of symptoms, muscle biopsy, chest X-ray, and sedimentation rate

ies; magnetic resonance imaging, computed tomography, blood vessel biopsy, and urine test.[3] Laboratory tests performed to confirm a diagnosis of vasculitis depend on the blood vessels involved. (See *Types of vasculitis*.)

Treatment

Treatment of vasculitis aims to minimize irreversible tissue damage associated with ischemia. In primary vasculitis, treatment may involve removal of an offending antigen or use of anti-inflammatory or immunosuppressant drugs. For example, antigenic drugs, food, and other environmental substances should be identified and eliminated, if possible.

Drug therapy in primary vasculitis commonly involves low-dose cyclophosphamide (2 mg/kg orally daily) with daily corticosteroids. In rapidly fulminant vasculitis, cyclophosphamide dosage may be increased to 4 mg/kg daily for the first 2 to 3 days, followed by the regular dose. Prednisone should be given in a dose of 1 mg/kg/day in divided doses for 7 to 10 days, with consolidation to a single morning dose by 2 to 3 weeks. When the vasculitis appears to be in remission or when prescribed cytotoxic drugs take full effect, corticosteroids are tapered down to a single daily dose. Finally, an alternate-day schedule of steroids may continue for 3 to 6 months before slow discontinuation of steroids.

In secondary vasculitis, treatment focuses on the underlying disorder.

Special considerations

▶ Assess patients with Wegener's granulomatosis for dry nasal mucosa. Instill nose drops to lubricate the mucosa and help diminish crusting, or irrigate the nasal passages with warm normal saline solution.
▶ Monitor vital signs. Use a Doppler ultrasonic flowmeter, if available, to auscultate blood pressure in patients with Takayasu's arteritis, because peripheral pulses are generally difficult to palpate in those patients.
▶ Monitor intake and output. Check daily for edema. Keep the patient well hydrated (3 L daily) to reduce the risk of hemorrhagic cystitis associated with cyclophosphamide therapy.

▶ Provide emotional support to help the patient and his family cope with an altered body image—the result of the disorder or its therapy. (For example, Wegener's granulomatosis may be associated with saddle nose, steroids may cause weight gain, and cyclophosphamide may cause alopecia.)
▶ Teach the patient how to recognize drug adverse effects. Monitor the patient's white blood cell count during cyclophosphamide therapy to prevent severe leukopenia.

REFERENCES

1. Shiel, W.C. (2006 September 25). "Vasculitis" [Online]. Available *www.medicinenet.com/vasculitis/article.htm.*
2. Home, C. (2006 March 30). "Vasculitis and Thrombophlebitis" [Online]. Available at *www.emedicine.com/ped/topic2390.htm.*
3. MayoClinic.com (2007 October 10). "Vasculitis" [Online]. Available at *ww.mayoclinic.com/health/vasculitis/DS00513.*

Hematologic disorders

APLASTIC ANEMIAS

Aplastic, or hypoplastic, anemias result from injury to or destruction of stem cells in bone marrow or the bone marrow matrix, causing pancytopenia (anemia, granulocytopenia, and thrombocytopenia) and bone marrow hypoplasia. Although commonly used interchangeably with other terms for bone marrow failure, aplastic anemias properly refer to pancytopenia resulting from the decreased functional capacity of a hypoplastic, fatty bone marrow. These disorders generally produce fatal bleeding or infection, particularly when they're idiopathic or stem from chloramphenicol or from infectious hepatitis. Mortality for aplastic anemias with severe pancytopenia is 80% to 90%.

Causes and incidence

Aplastic anemias usually develop when damaged or destroyed stem cells inhibit red blood cell (RBC) production. Less commonly, they develop when damaged bone marrow microvasculature creates an unfavorable environment for cell growth and maturation. About one-half of such anemias result from drugs (antibiotics and anticonvulsants), toxic agents (such as benzene and chloramphenicol), or radiation. The rest may result from immunologic factors (unconfirmed), severe disease (especially hepatitis), or preleukemic and neoplastic infiltration of bone marrow.[3]

Idiopathic anemias may be congenital. Two such forms of aplastic anemia have been identified: Congenital hypoplastic anemia (Blackfan-Diamond anemia) develops between ages 2 and 3 months; Fanconi's syndrome, between birth and age 10. In Fanconi's syndrome, chromosomal abnormalities are usually associated with multiple congenital anomalies, such as dwarfism, and hypoplasia of the kidneys and spleen. In the absence of a consistent familial or genetic history of aplastic anemia, researchers suspect that these congenital abnormalities result from an induced change in the fetus' development.

Incidence is 0.6 to 6.1 cases per 1 million people. There's no racial predilection in the United States but prevalence is increased in the Far East. Incidence peaks in childhood, in people ages 20 to 25, and in adults older than age 60.

Signs and symptoms

Clinical features of aplastic anemias vary with the severity of pancytopenia but develop insidiously in many cases. Anemic symptoms include progressive weakness and fatigue, shortness of breath, headache, pallor and, ultimately, tachycardia and heart failure. Thrombocytopenia leads to ecchymosis, petechiae, and hemorrhage, especially from

the mucous membranes (nose, gums, rectum, and vagina) or into the retina or central nervous system. Neutropenia may lead to infection (fever, oral and rectal ulcers, and sore throat) but without characteristic inflammation.

Complications

▶ Life threatening hemorrhage from mucous membranes
▶ Opportunistic infections

Diagnosis

Confirmation of aplastic anemia requires a series of laboratory tests:
▶ RBCs are usually normochromic and normocytic with a total count of 1 million/µl or less. However, macrocytosis (larger-than-normal erythrocytes) and anisocytosis (excessive variation in erythrocyte size) may exist. Absolute reticulocyte count is very low.
▶ Serum iron level is elevated (unless bleeding occurs), but total iron-binding capacity is normal or slightly reduced. Hemosiderin (a derivative of hemoglobin [Hb]) is present, and tissue iron storage is visible microscopically.
▶ Platelet, neutrophil, and white blood cell counts fall.
▶ Coagulation tests (bleeding time), reflecting decreased platelet count, are abnormal.
▶ Bone marrow aspiration from several sites may yield a "dry tap," and biopsy will show severely hypocellular or aplastic marrow, with varied amounts of fat, fibrous tissue, or gelatinous replacement; absence of tagged iron (because iron is deposited in the liver rather than bone marrow) and megakaryocytes (platelet precursors); and depression of erythroid elements.

Differential diagnosis must rule out paroxysmal nocturnal hemoglobinuria and other diseases in which pancytopenia is common.

Treatment

Effective treatment must eliminate any identifiable cause and provide vigorous supportive measures, such as packed RBC, platelet, and experimental histocompatibility locus antigen-matched leukocyte transfusions. Even after elimination of the cause, recovery can take months. Bone marrow transplantation is the treatment of choice for anemia due to severe aplasia and for patients who need constant RBC transfusions.[3] (See *Bone marrow transplantation*, page 312.)

Patients with low leukocyte counts need special measures to prevent infection. The infection itself may require specific antibiotics; however, these aren't given prophylactically because they tend to encourage resistant strains of organisms. Patients with low Hb levels may need respiratory support with oxygen in addition to blood transfusions.

For patients older than age 60 or for those who don't have a matched bone marrow donor, antithymocyte globulin (ATG) along with cyclosporine is used.[1] ATG is a horse serum that contains antibodies against human T cells. It may be used in an attempt to suppress the body's immune system, allowing the bone marrow to resume its blood cell-generating function. Other immunosuppressant agents, such as cyclosporine, may also be used.

Other treatments may include corticosteroids such as methylprednisolone, which are commonly given with other immunosuppressants.[2] Bone marrow-stimulating agents such as such as epoetin alfa may help stimulate the bone marrow to make new cells.[2] Colony stimulation factors can be given to encourage growth of specific cellular components.

Special considerations

▶ If the platelet count is low (less than 20,000/µl), prevent bleeding by avoiding I.M. injections, suggest the use of an electric razor and a soft toothbrush, humidify oxygen to prevent drying of mucous mem-

Bone marrow transplantation

In bone marrow transplantation, usually 500 to 700 ml of marrow is aspirated from the pelvic bones of a human leukocyte antigen (HLA)-compatible donor (allogeneic) or of the recipient himself during complete remission (autologous). The aspirated marrow is filtered and then infused into the recipient in an attempt to repopulate the patient's marrow with normal cells. This procedure has contributed to long-term, healthy survival in about 50% of patients with severe aplastic anemia. Bone marrow transplantation may also be effective in patients with acute leukemia, certain immunodeficiency diseases, and solid tumor neoplasms.

Because bone marrow transplantation carries serious risks, it requires strict adherence to infection control and strict sterile techniques and a primary nurse to provide consistent care and continuous monitoring of the patient's status.

BEFORE TRANSPLANTATION

• Explain that the success rate depends on the stage of the disease and an HLA-identical match.
• After bone marrow aspiration is completed under local anesthetic, apply pressure dressings to the donor's aspiration sites. Observe the sites for bleeding. Relieve pain with analgesics and ice packs, as needed.
• Assess the patient's understanding of bone marrow transplantation. If necessary, correct any misconceptions about this procedure and provide additional information, as appropriate. Prepare the patient to expect an extended hospital stay. Explain that chemotherapy and possible radiation treatments are necessary to destroy cells that may cause the body to reject the transplant.
• Various treatment protocols are used. For example, I.V. cyclophosphamide may be used with additional chemotherapeutic agents or total body irradiation and requires aggressive hydration to prevent hemorrhagic cystitis. Control nausea and vomiting as needed with an antiemetic, such as ondansetron, prochlorperazine, metoclopramide, or lorazepam. Give allopurinol, as prescribed, to prevent hyperuricemia resulting from tumor breakdown prod-

ucts. Because alopecia is a common adverse effect of high-dose cyclophosphamide therapy, encourage the patient to choose a wig or scarf before treatment begins.
• Total body irradiation (in one dose or several daily doses) follows chemotherapy, inducing total marrow aplasia. Warn the patient that cataracts, GI disturbances, and sterility are possible adverse effects.

DURING MARROW INFUSION

• Monitor vital signs every 15 minutes.
• Watch for complications of marrow infusion, such as pulmonary embolus and volume overload.
• Reassure the patient throughout the procedure.

AFTER THE INFUSION

• Continue to monitor the patient's vital signs every 15 minutes for 2 hours after infusion, then every 4 hours. Watch for fever and chills, which may be the only signs of infection. Give prophylactic antibiotics as prescribed. To reduce the possibility of bleeding, don't administer medications rectally or I.M.
• Administer methotrexate or cyclosporine, as prescribed, to prevent graft-versus-host (GVH) reaction, a potentially fatal complication of allogeneic transplantation. Watch for signs or symptoms of GVH reaction, such as maculopapular rash, pancytopenia, jaundice, joint pain, and generalized edema.
• Administer vitamins, steroids, and iron and folic acid supplements, as appropriate. Administration of blood products, such as platelets and packed red blood cells, may also be indicated, depending on the results of daily blood studies.
• Provide good mouth care every 2 hours. Use hydrogen peroxide and nystatin mouthwash or oral fluconazole, for example, to prevent candidiasis and other mouth infections. Also provide meticulous skin care, paying special attention to pressure points and open sites, such as aspiration and I.V. openings.

branes, avoid enemas and rectal temperatures, and promote regular bowel movements through the use of a stool softener and a proper diet to prevent constipation. Be sure to apply pressure to venipuncture sites until bleeding stops. Detect bleeding early by checking for blood in urine and stool, and assessing the skin for petechiae.

▶ Take safety precautions to prevent falls that could lead to prolonged bleeding or hemorrhage.

▶ Help prevent infection by washing your hands thoroughly before entering the patient's room, by making sure he's receiving a nutritious diet (high in vitamins and proteins) to improve his resistance, and by encouraging meticulous mouth and perianal care.

▶ Watch for life-threatening hemorrhage, infection, adverse effects of drug therapy, or blood transfusion reaction. Make sure routine throat, urine, nose, rectal, and blood cultures are done regularly and correctly to check for infection. Teach the patient to recognize signs of infection, and tell him to report them immediately.

▶ If the patient has a low Hb level, which causes fatigue, schedule frequent rest periods. Administer oxygen therapy as needed. If blood transfusions are necessary, assess for a transfusion reaction by checking the patient's temperature and watching for the development of other signs and symptoms, such as rash, hives, itching, back pain, restlessness, and shaking chills.

▶ Reassure and support the patient and his family by explaining the disease and its treatment, particularly if he has recurring acute episodes. Explain the purpose of all prescribed drugs and discuss possible adverse effects, including which ones he should report promptly. Encourage the patient who doesn't require hospitalization to continue his normal lifestyle, with appropriate restrictions (such as regular rest periods), until remission occurs.

HEALTH & SAFETY *To prevent aplastic anemia, monitor blood studies carefully in the patient receiving anemia-inducing drugs.*

▶ Support efforts to educate the public about the hazards of toxic agents. Tell parents to keep toxic agents out of the reach of children. Encourage people who work with radiation to wear protective clothing and a radiation-detecting badge and to observe plant safety precautions. Those who work with benzene (solvent) should know that 10 parts per million is the highest safe environmental level and that a delayed reaction to benzene may develop.

REFERENCES

1. Aplastic Anemia & MDS International Foundation, Inc. (2006, November 10). "Aplastic Anemia" [Online]. Available at *www.aplastic.org/aplastic/disease_information/about_the_diseases/aplastic_anemia.php*.
2. MayoClinic.com (2007, March 8). "Aplastic Anemia-Treatment" [Online]. Available at *www.mayoclinic.com/health/aplastic-anemia/DS00322/DSECTION=6*.
3. Young, N.S., et al. "Current Concepts in the Pathophysiology and Treatment of Aplastic Anemia," *Blood* 108(8):2509-19, October 2006.

DISSEMINATED INTRAVASCULAR COAGULATION

Disseminated intravascular coagulation (DIC) occurs as a life-threatening complication of diseases and conditions that accelerate clotting, causing small blood vessel occlusion, organ necrosis, depletion of circulating clotting factors and platelets, and activation of the fibrinolytic system.[2] This, in turn, can provoke severe hemorrhage. (See *Three mechanisms of DIC,* page 314.) Clotting in the microcirculation usually affects the kidneys and extremities but may occur in the brain, lungs, pituitary and adrenal glands, and GI mucosa. Other

Three mechanisms of DIC

No matter how disseminated intravascular coagulation (DIC) begins, accelerated clotting (characteristic of DIC) usually results in excess thrombin. This, in turn, causes fibrinolysis with excess fibrin formation and fibrin degradation products (FDP), activation of fibrin-stabilizing factor (factor XIII), consumption of platelet and clotting factors and, eventually, hemorrhage.

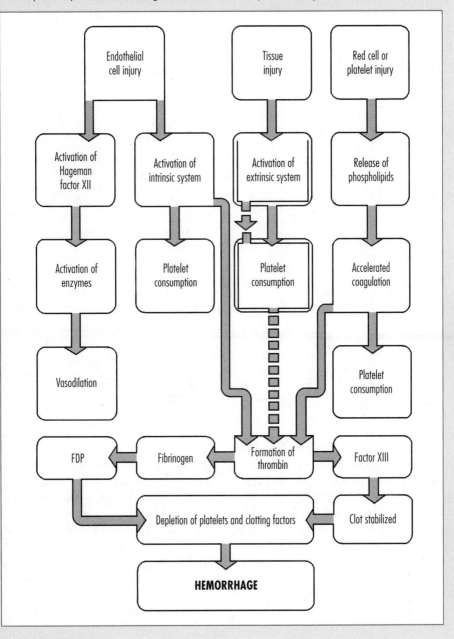

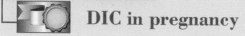

DIC in pregnancy

Question: *What's the most common cause of disseminated intravascular coagulation in obstetric patients?*

Research: Disseminated intravascular coagulation (DIC) can result from obstetric complications, such as abruptio placentae, gestational hypertension, and amniotic fluid embolism. Researchers reviewed the records of 25 obstetric patients with a diagnosis of overt DIC to determine the frequency of its occurrence, causes, and response to treatment. All of the individuals studied were patients in a specific hospital between January 1993 and December 2005.

Conclusion: The study findings indicated that overt DIC occurred once in every 1,355 deliveries. The number of patients with each of the main complications that led to DIC during the study was: abruptio placentae, 6; gestational hypertension, 5; amniotic fluid embolism, 4; acute fatty liver of pregnancy, 4; and HELLP syndrome, 3. Treatment consisted of blood component replacement in all of the patients, cesarean birth in 10 patients, and hysterectomy in 9 patients. Treatment wasn't effective in pre-venting maternal mortality in 6 cases (3 from amniotic fluid embolism) or fetal mortality in 13 cases (all 6 with abruptio placentae, 4 out of 5 with gestational hypertension, and 2 out of 4 with amniotic fluid embolism). Researchers concluded that early diagnosis with prompt treatment, including rapid surgical intervention and eradication of predisposing conditions would minimize maternal morbidity and mortality.

Application: Various pregnancy-related complications can predispose a patient to DIC development. The nurse should be aware of the risk of DIC in such patients and closely monitor for signs and symptoms of DIC, including abnormal laboratory test results.

Source: Kor-anantakul, O., and Lekhakula, A. "Overt Disseminated Intravascular Coagulation in Obstetric Patients," *Journal of the Medical Association of Thailand* 90(5):857-64, May 2007.

conditions, such as vitamin K deficiency, hepatic disease, and anticoagulant therapy, may cause a similar hemorrhage. DIC, also called *consumption coagulopathy* or *defibrination syndrome,* is generally an acute condition but may be chronic in cancer patients. The prognosis depends on early detection and treatment, the hemorrhage's severity, and treatment of the underlying disease or condition.[2]

Causes and incidence

DIC may result from:

▶ infection—gram-negative or gram-positive septicemia; viral, fungal, or rickettsial infection; protozoal infection[4]

▶ obstetric complications—abruptio placentae, amniotic fluid embolism, retained dead fetus, septic abortion, and eclampsia (see *DIC in pregnancy*)

▶ neoplastic disease—acute leukemia, metastatic carcinoma, and aplastic anemia

▶ disorders that produce necrosis—extensive burns and trauma, brain tissue destruction, transplant rejection, and hepatic necrosis

▶ other factors—heatstroke, shock, poisonous snakebite, cirrhosis, fat embolism, incompatible blood transfusion, cardiac arrest, surgery necessitating cardiopulmonary bypass, giant hemangioma, severe venous thrombosis, and purpura fulminans.

It isn't clear why such disorders lead to DIC, nor is it certain that they lead to it through a common mechanism. In many patients, the triggering mechanisms may be the

entrance of foreign protein into the circulation and vascular endothelial injury. Regardless of how DIC begins, the typical accelerated clotting results in generalized activation of prothrombin and a consequent excess of thrombin. Excess thrombin converts fibrinogen to fibrin, producing fibrin clots in the microcirculation. This process consumes exorbitant amounts of coagulation factors (especially fibrinogen, prothrombin, platelets, and factor V and factor VIII), causing hypofibrinogenemia, hypoprothrombinemia, thrombocytopenia, and deficiencies in factor V and factor VIII. Circulating thrombin activates the fibrinolytic system, which lyses fibrin clots into fibrin degradation products. The hemorrhage that occurs may be due largely to the anticoagulant activity of fibrin degradation products as well as depletion of plasma coagulation factors.

It's estimated that 30% to 50% of patients with sepsis get DIC; it occurs equally in males and females and in people of all ages.

Signs and symptoms

The most significant feature of DIC is abnormal bleeding, *without* a history of a serious hemorrhagic disorder. Principal signs of such bleeding include cutaneous oozing, petechiae, ecchymoses, and hematomas caused by bleeding into the skin. Bleeding from surgical or I.V. sites and from the GI tract are equally significant signs, as are acrocyanosis (cyanosis of the extremities) and signs of acute tubular necrosis. Related signs, symptoms, and other effects include nausea, vomiting, dyspnea, oliguria, seizures, coma, shock, major organ failure, confusion, epistaxis, hemoptysis, and severe muscle, back, abdominal, and chest pain.

Complications

▶ Renal failure
▶ Hepatic damage
▶ Stroke
▶ Ischemic bowel

▶ Respiratory distress
▶ Hypoxia
▶ Anorexia
▶ Shock
▶ Coma
▶ Small vessel occlusion
▶ Fibrinolysis and fatal hemorrhage of vital organs

Diagnosis

Abnormal bleeding in the absence of a known hematologic disorder suggests DIC but may be late in the pathophysiologic process. Initial laboratory findings reflect coagulation factor deficiencies:
▶ decreased platelet count—less than 100,000/µl
▶ decreased fibrinogen level—less than 150 mg/dl.

As the excessive clot breaks down, hemorrhagic diathesis occurs, and test results reflect coagulation abnormalities:
▶ prolonged prothrombin time—more than 15 seconds; 50% to 75% of patients have prolonged values
▶ prolonged activated partial thromboplastin time—only 50% to 60% of patients have prolonged times
▶ increased fibrin degradation products—commonly more than 100 mcg/ml.

Other supportive data include positive fibrin monomers, diminished levels of factors V and VIII, fragmentation of red blood cells (RBCs), and decreased hemoglobin (Hb) level (less than 10 g/dl). Assessment of renal status demonstrates reduction in urine output (less than 30 ml/ hour) and elevated blood urea nitrogen (more than 25 mg/dl) and serum creatinine (more than 1.3 mg/dl) levels.

A positive D-dimer test (results greater than 500 and decreased levels of factors II, V, and VIII) is the most specific and reliable test for DIC. Confirming the diagnosis may be difficult because many of these test results also occur in other disorders (primary fibrinolysis, for example).

DIC may also be diagnosed using the Acute Physiology and Chronic Health Evaluation (APACHE) II and Logistic Organ Dysfunction scoring systems. An increased score on these tests indicates an increased likelihood of DIC and mortality.[3]

Treatment

Successful management of DIC necessitates prompt recognition and adequate treatment of the underlying disorder. Treatment may be supportive when the underlying disorder is self-limiting or highly specific. If the patient isn't bleeding, supportive care alone may reverse DIC. However, bleeding may require administration of blood, fresh frozen plasma, platelets, or packed RBCs to support hemostasis.[2] Cryoprecipitates may also be used if fibrinogen is significantly decreased. Heparin is used in the early stages to prevent micro-clotting and is sometimes used in combination with replacement therapy. Heparin doesn't break up clots but it can block new clots from forming.[1] Heparin can't be used if the patient has had recent surgery or GI or central nervous system bleeding.[1] Recombinant human activated protein C has an antithrombotic effect and restores the normal physiologic anticoagulant pathway.[1]

Special considerations

Patient care must focus on early recognition of abnormal bleeding, prompt treatment of the underlying disorders, and prevention of further bleeding.

▶ To avoid dislodging clots and causing fresh bleeding, don't scrub bleeding areas. Use pressure, cold compresses, and topical hemostatic agents to control bleeding.

▶ To prevent injury, enforce complete bed rest during bleeding episodes. If the patient is agitated, pad the side rails.

▶ Check all I.V. and venipuncture sites frequently for bleeding. Apply pressure to injection sites for at least 20 minutes. Alert other personnel to the patient's tendency to hemorrhage.

▶ Monitor intake and output hourly in acute DIC, especially when administering blood products. Watch for transfusion reactions and signs of fluid overload. To measure the amount of blood lost, weigh dressings and linen, and record drainage. Weigh the patient daily, particularly if there's renal involvement.

▶ Watch for bleeding from the GI and genitourinary tracts. If you suspect intra-abdominal bleeding, measure the patient's abdominal girth at least every 4 hours and monitor closely for signs of shock.

▶ Monitor the results of serial blood studies (particularly hematocrit, Hb levels, and coagulation times).

▶ Explain all diagnostic tests and procedures. Allow time for questions.

▶ Inform the patient's family of his progress. Prepare them for his appearance (I.V. lines, nasogastric tubes, bruises, and dried blood). Provide emotional support for the patient and his family. As needed, enlist the aid of a social worker, chaplain, and other members of the health care team in providing such support.

REFERENCES

1. Dressler, D.K. "DIC: Coping with a Coagulation Crisis," *Nursing* 34(5):58-62, May 2004.
2. Levi, M. "Disseminated Intravascular Coagulation," *Critical Care Medicine* 35(9):2191-95, September 2007.
3. Angstwurm, M.W., et al. "New Disseminated Intravascular Coagulation Score: A Useful Tool to Predict Mortality in Comparison with Acute Physiology and Chronic Health Evaluation II and Logistic Organ Dysfunction Scores," *Critical Care Medicine* 34(2):314-20, February 2006.
4. Kinasewitz, G.T., et al. "Prognostic Value of a Simple Evolving Disseminated Intravascular Coagulation Score in Patients with Severe Sepsis," *Critical Care Medicine* 33(10):2214-21, October 2005.

HEMOPHILIA

Hemophilia is a hereditary bleeding disorder that results from a deficiency of specific clotting factors. After a person with hemophilia forms a platelet plug at a bleeding site, the clotting factor deficiency impairs the blood's capacity to form a stable fibrin clot. Bleeding occurs primarily into large joints, especially after trauma or surgery. Spontaneous intracranial bleeding can occur and may be fatal.

Advances in treatment have greatly improved the prognosis for patients with hemophilia, many of whom live normal life spans. Surgical procedures can be done safely at special treatment centers under the guidance of a hematologist.

Causes and incidence

Both hemophilia A and B are inherited as X-linked recessive traits. This means that female carriers have a 50% chance of transmitting the gene to each daughter, who would then be a carrier, and a 50% chance of transmitting the gene to each son, who would be born with hemophilia. Hemophilia A (classic hemophilia), which affects more than 80% of patients with hemophilia, results from a deficiency of factor VIII-C; hemophilia B (Christmas disease), which affects approximately 15% of patients with hemophilia, results from a deficiency of factor IX-C.

The factor VIII gene is located within the Xq28 region, and the factor IX gene is located within Xq27. Females with one defective factor VIII gene are carriers of hemophilia. A large number of disease-causing mutations have been identified in both genes. A specific inversion mutation in the noncoding region of the factor VIII gene is present in approximately 45% of families with severe hemophilia A. Hemophilia A is the most common X-linked genetic disease, occurring in approximately 1 in 5,000 live male births.[1]

Hemophilia B occurs in 1 in 10,000 live male births.[1]

Signs and symptoms

Hemophilia produces abnormal bleeding, which may be mild, moderate, or severe, depending on the degree of factor deficiency.

Mild hemophilia commonly goes undiagnosed until adulthood because the patient doesn't bleed spontaneously or after minor trauma but has prolonged bleeding if challenged by major trauma or surgery. Postoperative bleeding continues as a slow ooze or ceases and starts again, up to 8 days after surgery.

Severe hemophilia causes spontaneous bleeding. In many cases, the first sign of severe hemophilia is excessive bleeding after circumcision. Later, spontaneous bleeding or severe bleeding after minor trauma may produce large subcutaneous and deep intramuscular hematomas. Bleeding into joints (hemarthrosis) and muscles causes pain, swelling, extreme tenderness and, possibly, permanent deformity.

Moderate hemophilia causes symptoms similar to severe hemophilia but produces only occasional spontaneous bleeding episodes.

Bleeding near peripheral nerves may cause peripheral neuropathy, pain, paresthesia, and muscle atrophy.

Complications

▶ If bleeding impairs blood flow through a major vessel, it can cause ischemia and gangrene.

▶ Pharyngeal, lingual, intracardial, intracerebral, and intracranial bleeding may all lead to shock and death.

Diagnosis

Development of a large cephalohematoma or intracranial hemorrhage after prolonged labor or delivery by forceps or vacuum extraction may be the first indication of a bleeding problem. After the neonatal period, a history

Factor replacement products

CRYOPRECIPITATE
- Contains factor VIII (70 to 100 units/bag); doesn't contain factor IX
- Can be stored frozen up to 12 months but must be used within 6 hours after it thaws
- Given through a blood filter; compatible with normal saline solution only
- No longer treatment of choice because of the risk of human immunodeficiency virus and hepatitis infection; can still contain viruses despite greatly improved screening and purification procedures for viral inactivation in blood products

LYOPHILIZED FACTOR VIII OR IX
- Freeze-dried
- Can be stored up to 2 years at about 36° to 46° F (2° to 8° C), up to 6 months at room temperature not exceeding 88° F (31.1° C)
- Labeled with exact units of factor VIII or IX contained in vial
- 200 to 1,500 units of factor VIII or IX per vial; 20 to 40 ml after reconstitution with diluent
- No blood filter needed; usually given by slow I.V. push through a butterfly infusion set

FRESH FROZEN PLASMA
- Contains approximately 0.75 unit/ml of factor VII and approximately 1 unit/ml of factor IX; not practical for most people with hemophilia because a large volume is needed to raise factors to hemostatic levels
- Can be stored frozen up to 12 months but must be used within 2 hours after it thaws
- Given through a blood filter; compatible with normal saline solution only

of prolonged bleeding after surgery (including dental extractions) or trauma or of episodes of spontaneous bleeding into muscles or joints usually indicates some defect in the hemostatic mechanism. Hemophilia A and B may be clinically indistinguishable, but specific coagulation factor assays can diagnose the type and severity of the disease. A positive family history, prenatal diagnosis, and carrier testing can also help diagnose hemophilia, but nearly one-third of all patients have no family history.

Characteristic findings in hemophilia A include:
▶ factor VIII-C assay, 0% to 30% of normal
▶ prolonged partial thromboplastin time (PTT)
▶ normal platelet count and function, bleeding time, and prothrombin time.

Characteristics of hemophilia B include:
▶ deficient factor IX-C
▶ baseline coagulation results similar to hemophilia A, with normal factor VIII.

In both types of hemophilia, the degree of factor deficiency determines severity:
▶ mild hemophilia—factor levels 5% to 40% of normal
▶ moderate hemophilia—factor levels 1% to 5% of normal
▶ severe hemophilia—factor levels less than 1% of normal.

Treatment
Hemophilia isn't curable, but treatment can prevent crippling deformities and prolong life expectancy. Correct treatment quickly stops bleeding by increasing plasma levels of deficient clotting factors to help prevent disabling deformities that result from repeated bleeding into muscles and joints. (See *Factor replacement products*.)

Desmopressin (DDAVP) administered I.V. or intranasally is usually sufficient to manage bleeding episodes in children and adolescents with mild hemophilia A.

Persons with moderate to severe hemophilia A require commercially prepared factor VIII concentrates to treat bleeding episodes. Concentrates derived from human plasma are virally attenuated by one or more available methods, significantly minimizing the risk for human immunodeficiency virus (HIV)-1, HIV-2, hepatitis B, and hepatitis C contamination. However, no currently available method has been successful in eradicating parvovirus B19 from blood products.[2] Factor VIII concentrate derived from recombinant technology (rFVIII) has been shown in multiple clinical trials to be as effective as virally attenuated plasma-derived concentrate. Risk for viral contamination is essentially nonexistent in preparations of rFVIII that avoid human serum albumin as a stabilizer.

In hemophilia B, administration of factor IX concentrate during bleeding episodes increases factor IX levels.

The United States National Hemophilia Foundation first recommended prophylaxis with factor concentrates in 1994 after investigators in Sweden demonstrated repeated success with this approach. The ultimate goal is to prevent irreversible destructive arthritis that results from repeated hemarthrosis and synovial hypertrophy. Prophylaxis for persons with hemophilia A or B may begin as early as age 1 or 2. Recommendations were updated in 2007 and suggest that prophylaxis start prior to the onset of frequent bleeding.[3]

A person with hemophilia who undergoes surgery needs careful management by a hematologist with expertise in hemophilia care. The patient will require replacement of the deficient factor before and after surgery, possibly even for minor surgery such as a dental extraction. (DDAVP may be given before dental extractions and surgery to prevent bleeding.) In addition, epsilon-aminocaproic acid is commonly used for oral bleeding to inhibit the active fibrinolytic system present in the oral mucosa.

Development of factor VIII or factor XI inhibitors occurs in up to 3.5% of children with severe hemophilia A and up to 3% of those with hemophilia B. Studies indicate that certain gene mutations predispose the patient to an increased risk of inhibitor development. Patients with hemophilia who can't achieve hemostasis after use of previously effective factor concentrate doses should be evaluated for factor inhibitors.

Preventive measures include teaching the patient how to avoid trauma, manage minor bleeding, and recognize bleeding that requires immediate medical intervention.

IN THE NEWS *Patients are now being taught how to infuse factor VIII themselves on a regular basis to help prevent acute bleeding episodes. This has shown promise in decreasing joint bleeds and hospitalizations.[4]*

Genetic counseling helps carriers understand how this disease is transmitted. (See *Managing hemophilia.*)

Special considerations

During bleeding episodes:
▶ Give clotting agents as ordered. The body uses up factor VIII in 48 to 72 hours, so repeat infusions, as ordered, until bleeding stops.
▶ Apply cold compresses or ice bags and raise the injured part.
▶ To prevent recurrence of bleeding, restrict activity for 48 hours after bleeding is under control.
▶ Control pain with an analgesic, such as acetaminophen, propoxyphene, codeine, or meperidine, as ordered. Avoid I.M. injections because of possible hematoma formation at the injection site. Aspirin and aspirin-containing medications are contraindicated because they decrease platelet adherence and may increase the bleeding. Caution should be used when trying other nonsteroidal anti-inflammatory drugs, for example, ibuprofen or ketoprofen.

Managing hemophilia

The following guidelines can help parents care for their child with hemophilia.

• Instruct parents to notify the physician immediately after even a minor injury, but especially after an injury to the head, neck, or abdomen. Such injuries may require special blood factor replacement. Also, tell parents to check with the physician before allowing dental extractions or any other surgery.

• Educate the patient and his parents on the early signs and symptoms of hemarthrosis: stiffness, tingling, or ache in joint, followed by decreased range of motion. If signs and symptoms are recognized early, treatment can begin earlier, potentially decreasing the possibility of long-term disability.

• Stress the importance of regular, careful toothbrushing with a soft-bristled toothbrush to prevent the need for dental surgery.

• Teach parents to be alert for signs of severe internal bleeding, such as severe pain or swelling in a joint or muscle, stiffness, decreased joint movement, severe abdominal pain, blood in urine, black tarry stools, and severe headache.

• Advise parents that the child is at risk for hepatitis from blood components. Early signs—headache, fever, decreased appetite, nausea, vomiting, abdominal tenderness, and pain over the liver—may appear 3 weeks to 6 months after treatment with blood components. Tell them to discuss with their physician the possibility of hepatitis vaccination.

• Discuss the increased risk of human immunodeficiency virus (HIV) infection if the child received a blood product before routine screening of blood products for HIV began. Tell parents to ask the physician about periodic testing for HIV.

• Urge parents to make sure their child wears a medical identification bracelet at all times.

• Teach parents never to give their child aspirin, which can aggravate the tendency to bleed. Advise them to give acetaminophen instead.

• Instruct parents to protect their child from injury, but to avoid unnecessary restrictions that impair his normal development. For example, they can sew padded patches into the knees and elbows of a toddler's clothing to protect these joints during falls. They should forbid an older child to participate in contact sports such as football but can encourage him to swim or to play golf.

• Teach parents to elevate and apply cold compresses or ice bags to an injured area and to apply light pressure to a bleeding site. To prevent recurrence of bleeding, advise parents to restrict the child's activity for 48 hours after bleeding is under control.

• If parents have been trained to administer blood factor components at home to avoid frequent hospitalization, make sure they know proper venipuncture and infusion techniques and don't delay treatment during bleeding episodes.

• Instruct parents to keep blood factor concentrate and infusion equipment on hand at all times, even on vacation.

• Emphasize the importance of having the child keep routine medical appointments at the local hemophilia center.

• Daughters of individuals with hemophilia should undergo genetic screening to determine if they're hemophilia carriers. Affected males should undergo counseling as well. If they produce offspring with a non-carrier, all of their daughters will be carriers; if they produce offspring with a carrier, each child has a 25% chance of being affected.

• For more information, refer parents to the National Hemophilia Foundation. The Web site can be found at www.hemophilia.org/NHFWeb/MainPgs/MainNHF.aspx?menuid=0&contentid=1.

If the patient has bled into a joint:
▶ Immediately elevate the joint.

▶ To restore joint mobility, begin range-of-motion exercises, if ordered, at least 48 hours after the bleeding is controlled. Tell

the patient to avoid weight bearing until bleeding stops and swelling subsides.

After bleeding episodes and surgery:
▶ Watch closely for signs of further bleeding, such as increased pain and swelling, fever, or symptoms of shock.
▶ Closely monitor PTT.
▶ Teach parents special precautions to prevent bleeding episodes.
▶ Refer a newly diagnosed patient to a hemophilia treatment center for evaluation. The center will devise a treatment plan for the patient's primary physician and is a resource for other medical and school personnel, dentists, and others involved in the patient's care.
▶ Persons who have been exposed to HIV through contaminated blood products need special support.
▶ Refer patients and carriers for genetic counseling.

REFERENCES
1. The National Hemophilia Foundation. "About Bleeding Disorders" [Online]. Available at *www.hemophilia.org/NHFWeb/MainPgs/Main NHF.aspx?menuid=259&contentid=476.*
2. Cunningham, D., and Rennels, M.B. (2006, November 9) "Parvovirus B19 Infection" [Online]. Available at *www.emedicine.com/ PED/topic192.htm.*
3. National Hemophilia Foundation. "Recommendation #179. MASAC Recommendation Concerning Prophylaxis (Regular Administration of Clotting Factor Concentrate to Prevent Bleeding)" [Online]. Available at *www.hemophilia.org/NHFWeb/MainPgs/ MainNHF.aspx?menuid=57&contentid=1007.* Copyright 2007, National Hemophilia Foundation.
4. Khair, K., and Geraghty, S.J. "Haemophilia A: Meeting the Needs of Individual Patients," *British Journal of Nursing* 16(16):987-93, September 2007.

HYPERSPLENISM

Hypersplenism is a syndrome marked by exaggerated splenic activity and, possibly, splenomegaly. This disorder results in peripheral blood cell deficiency as the spleen traps and destroys peripheral blood cells.

Causes

Hypersplenism may be idiopathic (primary) or secondary to an extrasplenic disorder, such as chronic malaria, polycythemia vera, or rheumatoid arthritis. (See *Causes of splenomegaly.*) In hypersplenism, the spleen's normal filtering and phagocytic functions accelerate indiscriminately, automatically removing antibody-coated, aging, and abnormal cells, even though some cells may be functionally normal. The spleen may also temporarily sequester normal platelets and red blood cells (RBCs), withholding them from circulation. In this manner, the enlarged spleen may trap as much as 90% of the body's platelets and up to 45% of its RBC mass.

Signs and symptoms

Most patients with hypersplenism develop anemia, leukopenia, or thrombocytopenia, in many cases with splenomegaly. They may contract bacterial infections frequently, bruise easily, hemorrhage spontaneously from the mucous membranes and GI or genitourinary tract, and suffer ulcerations of the mouth, legs, and feet. They commonly develop fever, weakness, and palpitations. Patients with secondary hypersplenism may have other clinical abnormalities, depending on the underlying disease.[1]

Complications

▶ Bleeding
▶ Postsplenectomy infection and thromboembolic disease

Diagnosis

Diagnosis requires evidence of abnormal splenic destruction or sequestration of RBCs or platelets and splenomegaly.

The most definitive test measures erythrocytes in the spleen and liver after I.V. infusion of chromium-labeled RBCs or platelets. A high spleen-liver ratio of radioactivity indicates splenic destruction or sequestration.

Complete blood count shows decreased hemoglobin level (as low as 4 g/dl), white blood cell count (less than 4,000/µl), and platelet count (less than 125,000/µl) and an elevated reticulocyte count (more than 75,000/µl). Splenic biopsy, scan, and angiography may be useful; biopsy is hazardous and should be avoided if possible. In sequestration, the spleen is palpable. Use abdominal palpation cautiously because it may create injury, bleeding, or rupture. If confirmation of splenomegaly is necessary, ultrasound is the best choice for examination.[2]

Treatment

Splenectomy is indicated only in transfusion-dependent patients who are refractory to medical therapy. Splenectomy seldom cures the patient, but it does correct the effects of cytopenia. Postoperative complications may include infection and thromboembolic disease. Occasionally, splenectomy may result in accelerated blood cell destruction in the bone marrow and liver. Secondary hypersplenism necessitates treatment of the underlying disease.

Special considerations

▶ If splenectomy is scheduled, administer preoperative transfusions of blood or blood products (fresh frozen plasma and platelets) to replace deficient blood elements. Also treat symptoms or complications of any underlying disorder.

▶ Postoperatively, monitor vital signs. Check for any excessive drainage or apparent bleeding. Watch for infection, thrombo-

Causes of splenomegaly

INFECTIOUS
- Acute (abscesses, subacute infective endocarditis), chronic (tuberculosis, malaria, Felty's syndrome)

CONGESTIVE
- Cirrhosis, thrombosis

HYPERPLASTIC
- Hemolytic anemia, polycythemia vera

INFILTRATIVE
- Gaucher's disease, Niemann-Pick disease

CYSTIC OR NEOPLASTIC
- Cysts, leukemia, lymphoma, myelofibrosis

embolism, and abdominal distention. Keep the nasogastric tube patent; listen for bowel sounds. Instruct the patient to perform deep-breathing exercises, and encourage early ambulation to prevent respiratory complications and venous stasis.

REFERENCES

1. Liangpunsakul, S., et al. "Predictors and Implications of Severe Hypersplenism in Patients with Cirrhosis," *American Journal of the Medical Sciences* 326(3):111-16, September 2003.
2. The Merck Manuals Online Medical Library (2005, November). "Splenomegaly" [Online]. Available at *www.merck.com/mmpe/sec11/ch138/ch138b.html#sec11-ch138-ch138b-594*.

IDIOPATHIC THROMBOCYTOPENIC PURPURA

Idiopathic thrombocytopenic purpura (ITP), also known as *primary immune thrombocytopenic purpura* and *autoim-*

mune thrombocytopenic purpura, is thrombocytopenia that results from immunologic platelet destruction. ITP can be acute (postviral thrombocytopenia) or chronic (Werlhof's disease, purpura hemorrhagica, essential thrombocytopenia, and autoimmune thrombocytopenia). The prognosis for acute ITP is excellent; nearly four out of five patients recover without treatment. The prognosis for chronic ITP is good; remissions lasting weeks or years are common, especially among women.

Causes and incidence

ITP may be an autoimmune disorder, because antibodies that reduce the lifespan of platelets have been found in nearly all patients. The spleen probably helps to remove platelets modified by the antibodies. Acute ITP usually follows a viral infection, such as rubella or chickenpox, and can follow immunization with a live virus vaccine. Chronic ITP seldom follows infection and is commonly linked to immunologic disorders such as systemic lupus erythematosus and drug reactions. ITP frequently occurs in patients who have abused alcohol, heroin, or morphine, and in patients with acquired immunodeficiency syndrome who are exposed to the rubella virus.

The incidence of ITP in adults is about 66 per 1 million cases per year; in children it's about 50 per 1 million.[1] Acute ITP usually affects children between ages 2 and 4; chronic ITP mainly affects adults ages 20 to 50, with a higher incidence in women than in men (female to male ratio 2.6:1).[1] About 40% of patients are younger than age 10.[1]

Signs and symptoms

Clinical features of ITP common to all forms of thrombocytopenia include petechiae (superficial bleeding into the skin, usually on the lower legs),[2] ecchymoses, and mucosal bleeding from the mouth, nose, or GI tract. Generally, hemorrhage is a rare physical finding. Purpuric lesions may occur in vital organs, such as the lungs, kidneys, or brain, and may prove fatal. The onset of acute ITP is usually sudden, causing easy bruising, epistaxis, and bleeding gums, whereas the onset of chronic ITP is insidious.

Complications

▶ Hemorrhage
▶ Cerebral hemorrhage
▶ Fatal purpuric lesions in vital organs

Diagnosis

A platelet count less than 20,000/μl suggests ITP. Platelet size and morphologic appearance may be abnormal and anemia may be present if bleeding has occurred. As in thrombocytopenia, bone marrow studies show an abundance of megakaryocytes and a shortened circulating platelet survival time (hours or days). Occasionally, platelet antibodies may be found in vitro, but this diagnosis is usually inferred from platelet survival data and the absence of an underlying disease.

Treatment

Acute ITP may be allowed to run its course without intervention or may be treated with glucocorticoids or immune globulin. For chronic ITP, corticosteroids, such as methylprednisolone or prednisone, are the initial treatment of choice.[2] I.V. immunoglobulin (IVIG) is used for patients who need a rapid, temporary rise in platelet count.[1] I.V. anti-(Rh)D has been shown, in recent studies, to increase platelet count faster than using steroids.[1] (See *Treatment of ITP.*)

Patients who fail to respond within 4 months or who need high steroid dosage are candidates for splenectomy, which may be successful in 50% of cases.

Before splenectomy, the patient may require blood, blood components, and vitamin K to correct anemia and coagulation defects. After splenectomy, he may need blood and component replacement and platelet concen-

EVIDENCE-BASED PRACTICE

Treatment of ITP

Question: *What treatments are most effective for patients with immune thrombocytopenic purpura (ITP)?*

Research: Researchers reviewed clinical trials and other studies to determine whether British guidelines for the diagnosis and treatment of immune thrombocytopenic purpura should be updated because they were based mainly on expert opinion rather than outcomes derived from clinical trials.

Conclusion: The data obtained and analyzed during the study indicated that most adults tolerate immune thrombocytopenic purpura well. Adults with a chronic form of the disease were best treated with splenectomy, although such treatments as anti-D, rituximab, or dexamethasone may delay or prevent splenectomy if hemostatic platelet count is attained. The patient's platelet count determines whether he should receive any treatment or just be closely moni-

tored. However, age, lifestyle, and other medical conditions that may contribute to the risk of serious bleeding should be considered in all treatment decisions.

Application: When caring for an adult with immune thrombocytopenic purpura, the nurse should be aware that disease management can range from no treatment to splenectomy. Closely monitor all patients with the disease and focus attention on the signs and symptoms of a low platelet count, especially in those receiving no treatment.

Source: Godeau, B. et al. "Immune Thrombocytopenic Purpura in Adults," *Current Opinion in Hematology* 14(5):535-56, September 2007.

trate. Normally, platelets increase spontaneously after splenectomy.

Special considerations
Patient care for ITP is essentially the same as for other types of thrombocytopenia, with emphasis on teaching the patient to observe for petechiae, ecchymoses, and other signs of recurrence. Monitor patients receiving immunosuppressants for signs of bone marrow depression, infection, mucositis, GI ulcers, and severe diarrhea or vomiting. Tell the patient to avoid aspirin, ibuprofen, and warfarin, as these drugs interfere with platelet function and blood clotting.

REFERENCES
1. Silverman, M.A. (2007, January 18). "Idiopathic Thrombocytopenic Purpura" [Online]. Available at *www.emedicine.com/EMERG/ topic282.htm.*

2. MayoClinic.com (2006, October 30). "Idiopathic Thrombocytopenic Purpura" [Online]. Available at *www.mayoclinic.com/health/ idiopathic-thrombocytopenicpurpura/ DS00844/DSECTION=7.*

IRON DEFICIENCY ANEMIA

Iron deficiency anemia is caused by an inadequate supply of iron for optimal formation of red blood cells (RBCs), resulting in smaller (microcytic) cells with less color on staining. Body stores of iron (including plasma iron) decrease, as do levels of transferrin, which binds with and transports iron. Insufficient body stores of iron lead to a depleted RBC mass and, in turn, to a decreased hemoglobin (Hb) concentration (hypochromia) and decreased oxygen-carrying capacity

Absorption and storage of iron

Iron, which is essential to erythropoiesis, is abundant throughout the body. Two-thirds of total body iron is found in hemoglobin (Hb); the other third, mostly in the reticuloendothelial system (liver, spleen, bone marrow), with small amounts in muscle, blood serum, and body cells.

Adequate dietary ingestion of iron and recirculation of iron released from disintegrating red cells maintain iron supplies. The duodenum and upper part of the small intestine absorb dietary iron. Such absorption depends on gastric acid content, the amount of reducing substances (ascorbic acid, for example) present in the alimentary canal, and dietary iron intake. If iron intake is deficient, the body gradually depletes its iron stores, causing decreased Hb levels and, eventually, symptoms of iron deficiency anemia.

of the blood. (See *Absorption and storage of iron.*)

Causes and incidence

Iron deficiency anemia can result from:

▶ inadequate dietary intake of iron (less than 1 to 2 mg/day), such as in prolonged unsupplemented breast-feeding or bottle-feeding of infants, or during periods of stress such as rapid growth in children and adolescents

▶ iron malabsorption, such as in chronic diarrhea, partial or total gastrectomy, chronic diverticulosis, and malabsorption syndromes, such as celiac disease and pernicious anemia

▶ blood loss secondary to drug-induced GI bleeding (from anticoagulants, aspirin, and steroids) or due to heavy menses, hemorrhage from trauma, GI ulcers, esophageal varices, or cancer

▶ pregnancy, which diverts maternal iron to the fetus for erythropoiesis

▶ intravascular hemolysis-induced hemoglobinuria or paroxysmal nocturnal hemoglobinuria

▶ mechanical erythrocyte trauma caused by a prosthetic heart valve or vena cava filters.

A common disease worldwide, iron deficiency anemia affects 4% to 8% of premenopausal women in North America and Europe. It's rare in men and postmenopausal women unless bleeding is present. Persons who are at increased risk for iron deficiency include those of low socioeconomic status who don't get a well-balanced diet that includes iron-rich foods.

Signs and symptoms

Because of the gradual progression of iron deficiency anemia, many patients are initially asymptomatic except for symptoms of any underlying condition. They tend not to seek medical treatment until anemia is severe. At advanced stages, decreased Hb levels and the consequent decrease in the blood's oxygen-carrying capacity cause the patient to develop dyspnea on exertion, fatigue, listlessness, pallor, inability to concentrate, irritability, headache, and a susceptibility to infection. Decreased oxygen perfusion causes the heart to compensate with increased cardiac output and tachycardia.

In chronic iron deficiency anemia, nails become spoon-shaped and brittle, the mouth's corners crack, and the tongue turns smooth. The patient usually complains of dysphagia and may develop pica. Associated neuromuscular effects include vasomotor disturbances, numbness and tingling of the extremities, and neuralgic pain.

Complications

▶ Infection and pneumonia
▶ Pica
▶ Bleeding
▶ Hemochromatosis from over-replacement of iron
▶ Iron poisoning (in children)

Diagnosis

Blood studies (serum iron levels, total iron-binding capacity, and ferritin levels) and stores in bone marrow may confirm iron deficiency anemia. However, the results of these tests can be misleading because of complicating factors, such as infection, pneumonia, blood transfusion, or iron supplements. Characteristic blood test results include:

▶ low Hb levels (in males, less than 12 g/dl; in females, less than 10 g/dl)

▶ low hematocrit (in males, less than 39%; in females, less than 35%)

▶ low serum iron levels, with high binding capacity

▶ low serum ferritin levels

▶ low RBC count, with microcytic and hypochromic cells (in early stages, RBC count may be normal, except in infants and children)

▶ decreased mean corpuscular Hb in severe anemia.

Other blood tests that are gaining popularity in use for diagnosing anemia include reticulocyte hemoglobin content, percentage of hypochromic red RBCs, and soluble transferrin receptor.

Bone marrow studies reveal depleted or absent iron stores (done by staining) and normoblastic hyperplasia.

Diagnosis must rule out other forms of anemia, such as those that result from thalassemia minor, cancer, and chronic inflammatory, hepatic, and renal disease.

Treatment

The first priority of treatment is to determine the underlying cause of anemia. After this is determined, iron replacement therapy can begin. Treatment of choice is an oral preparation of iron or a combination of iron and ascorbic acid (which enhances iron absorption). However, in some cases, iron may have to be administered parenterally—for example, when the patient is noncompliant with taking the oral preparation, he needs more iron than he can take orally, malabsorption prevents adequate iron absorption, or a maximum rate of Hb regeneration is desired.

Because total dose I.V. infusion of supplemental iron is painless and requires fewer injections, it's usually preferred to I.M. administration.[2] Pregnant patients and geriatric patients with severe anemia, for example, should receive a total dose infusion of iron dextran in normal saline solution over 8 hours. To minimize the risk of an allergic reaction to iron, an I.V. test dose of 0.5 ml should be given first. (For more patient care information, see *Supportive management of patients with anemia,* page 328.)

Special considerations

▶ Monitor the patient's compliance with the prescribed iron supplement therapy. Advise the patient not to stop therapy, even if he feels better, because replacement of iron stores takes time.

▶ Tell the patient he may take iron supplements with a meal to decrease gastric irritation. Advise him to avoid milk, milk products, and antacids because they interfere with iron absorption; however, vitamin C can increase absorption.

▶ Warn the patient that iron supplements may result in dark green or black stools and can cause constipation.

▶ Instruct the patient to drink liquid supplemental iron through a straw to prevent staining his teeth.

▶ Tell the patient to report reactions, such as nausea, vomiting, diarrhea, constipation, fever, or severe stomach pain, which may require a dosage adjustment.

▶ If the patient receives I.V. iron, monitor the infusion rate carefully and observe for an allergic reaction. Stop the infusion and begin supportive treatment immediately if the patient shows signs of an adverse reaction. Monitor the patient for thrombophlebitis around the I.V. site and tell him to report any dizziness or headache.

Supportive management of patients with anemia

To meet the anemic patient's nutritional needs:
- If the patient is fatigued, urge him to eat small, frequent meals throughout the day.
- If the patient has oral lesions, suggest soft, cool, bland foods.
- If the patient has dyspepsia, eliminate spicy foods, and include milk and dairy products in his diet.
- If the patient is anorexic and irritable, encourage his family to bring his favorite foods from home (unless his diet is restricted) and to keep him company during meals, if possible.

To set limitations on activities:
- Assess the effect of a specific activity by monitoring pulse rate during the activity. If the patient's pulse accelerates rapidly and he develops hypotension with hyperpnea, diaphoresis, light-headedness, palpitations, shortness of breath, or weakness, the activity is too strenuous.
- Tell the patient to pace his activities and to allow for frequent rest periods.

To decrease susceptibility to infection:
- Use strict sterile technique.
- Isolate the patient from infectious persons.
- Instruct the patient to avoid crowds and other sources of infection. Encourage him to practice good hand-washing technique. Stress the importance of receiving necessary immunizations and prompt medical treatment for any sign of infection.

To prepare the patient for diagnostic testing:
- Explain erythropoiesis, the function of blood, and the purpose of diagnostic and therapeutic procedures.
- Tell the patient how he can participate in diagnostic testing. Give him an honest description of the pain or discomfort he will probably experience.
- If possible, schedule all tests to avoid disrupting the patient's meals, sleep, and visiting hours.

To prevent complications:
- Observe for signs of bleeding that may exacerbate anemia. Check stool for occult bleeding. Assess for ecchymoses, gingival bleeding, and hematuria. Monitor vital signs frequently.
- If the patient is confined to strict bed rest, assist with range-of-motion exercises and frequent turning, coughing, and deep breathing.
- If blood transfusions are needed for severe anemia (hemoglobin level less than 5 g/dl), give washed red blood cells, as ordered, in partial exchange if evidence of pump failure is present. Carefully monitor for signs of circulatory overload or transfusion reaction. Watch for a change in pulse rate, blood pressure, or respiratory rate, or onset of fever, chills, pruritus, or edema. If any of these signs develop, stop the transfusion and notify the physician.
- Warn the patient to move about or change positions slowly to minimize dizziness induced by cerebral hypoxia.

▶ Use the Z-track injection method when administering iron I.M. to prevent skin discoloration, scarring, and irritating iron deposits in the skin. (See *How to inject iron solutions.*)

▶ Because an iron deficiency may recur, advise regular checkups and blood studies.

Health professionals can play a vital role in preventing iron deficiency anemia by:

▶ teaching the basics of a nutritionally balanced diet—red meats, green vegetables, eggs, whole wheat products, and iron-fortified bread. (However, no food in itself contains enough iron to *treat* iron deficiency anemia; an average-sized person with anemia would have to eat at least 10 pounds of steak daily to receive therapeutic amounts of iron.)

▶ emphasizing the need for high-risk individuals—such as premature infants, children younger than age 2, and pregnant women—to receive prophylactic oral iron, as ordered by a physician. (Children younger than age 2 should also receive supplemental cereals and formulas high in iron. Maximum dosage of

How to inject iron solutions

For deep I.M. injections of iron solutions, use the Z-track technique to avoid subcutaneous irritation and discoloration from leaking medication.

Choose a 19G to 20G, 2″ to 3″ needle. After drawing up the solution, change to a fresh needle to avoid tracking the solution through to subcutaneous tissue. Draw 0.5 cc of air into the syringe as an "air lock."

Displace the skin and fat at the injection site (in the upper outer quadrant of the buttocks or the ventrogluteal site only) firmly to one side. Clean the area and insert the needle. Aspirate to check for entry into a blood vessel. Inject the solution slowly, followed by 0.5 cc of air in the syringe.

Wait 10 seconds, then pull the needle straight out, and release tissues.

Apply direct pressure to the site but don't massage it. Caution the patient against vigorous exercise for 15 to 30 minutes.

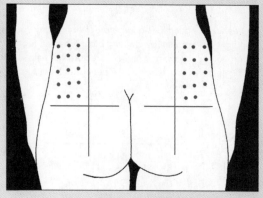

1. Displace tissues.   2. Inject solution.

3. Wait 10 seconds.   4. Release tissues.

---

iron for children younger than age 2 is 10 mg/day.)[4]

▶ assessing a family's dietary habits for iron intake and noting the influence of childhood eating patterns, cultural food preferences, and family income on adequate nutrition.

▶ encouraging families with deficient iron intake to eat meat, fish, or poultry; whole or enriched grain; and foods high in ascorbic acid. (See *Do bioengineered foods help prevent anemia?* page 330.)

▶ carefully assessing a patient's drug history because certain drugs, such as pancreatic enzymes and vitamin E, may interfere with iron metabolism and absorption and because aspirin, steroids, and other drugs may cause GI bleeding. (Teach patients who must take gastric irritants to take these medications with meals.)

Do bioengineered foods help prevent anemia?

Iron deficiency anemia is a large problem in many countries. Engineers are developing ways to help fight this problem by creating bioengineered food that's higher in iron content, lower in iron absorption inhibitors, and higher in factors that help increase iron absorption. While research is still being done to determine how beneficial these foods may be to preventing anemia, the early research is promising.[3]

REFERENCES

1. Wish, J.B. "Assessing Iron Status: Beyond Serum Ferritin and Transferrin Saturation," *Clinical Journal of the American Society of Nephrology* 1 Suppl 1:S4-8, September 2006.
2. Wall, G.C., and Pauly, R.A. "Evaluation of Total-Dose Iron Sucrose Infusions in Patients with Iron Deficiency Anemia" *American Journal of Health-System Pharmacy* 65(2):150-53, January 2008.
3. Cockell, K.A. "An Overview of Methods for Assessment of Iron Bioavailability from Foods Nutritionally Enhanced Through Biotechnology," *Journal of AOAC International* 90(5):1480-91, September-October 2007.
4. Milman, N. "Iron Prophylaxis in Pregnancy—General or Individual and in Which Dose?" *Annals of Hematology* 85(12):821-28, December 2006.

PLATELET FUNCTION DISORDERS

Platelet function disorders are similar to thrombocytopenia but result from platelet dysfunction rather than platelet deficiency. They characteristically cause defects in platelet adhesion or procoagulation activity (the ability to bind coagulation factors to their surface to form a stable fibrin clot). Such disorders may also create defects in platelet aggregation and thromboxane A_2 and may produce abnormalities by preventing the release of adenosine diphosphate (a defective platelet release reaction). The prognosis varies widely.

Causes

Abnormal platelet function disorders may be inherited (autosomal recessive) or acquired. Inherited disorders cause bone marrow production of platelets that are ineffective in the clotting mechanism. Acquired disorders result from the effects of such drugs as aspirin or carbenicillin; from such systemic diseases as uremia; or from other hematologic disorders.

Signs and symptoms

Generally, the sudden appearance of petechiae or purpura or excessive bruising and bleeding of the nose and gums are the first overt signs of platelet function disorders. More serious signs are external hemorrhage, internal hemorrhage into the muscles and visceral organs, or excessive bleeding during surgery.

Complications

▶ Hemorrhage

Diagnosis

Prolonged bleeding time in a patient with both a normal platelet count and normal clotting factors suggests this diagnosis. Determination of the defective mechanism requires a blood film and a platelet function test to measure platelet release reaction and aggregation. Depending on the type of

platelet dysfunction, some or all of the test results may be abnormal.

Other typical laboratory findings are poor clot retraction and decreased prothrombin conversion. Baseline testing includes complete blood count and differential and appropriate tests to determine hemorrhage sites. In platelet function disorders, plasma clotting factors, platelet counts, and prothrombin, partial thromboplastin, and thrombin times are usually normal.

Treatment
Platelet replacement is the only satisfactory treatment for inherited platelet dysfunction. However, acquired platelet function disorders respond to adequate treatment of the underlying disease or discontinuation of damaging drug therapy.[1] Plasmapheresis effectively controls bleeding caused by a plasma element that's inhibiting platelet function. During this procedure, one or more units of whole blood are removed from the patient; the plasma is removed from the whole blood and the remaining packed red blood cells are reinfused. (See *Facts about platelet concentrate*.)

Special considerations
▶ Obtain an accurate patient history, including onset of bleeding, use of drugs (especially aspirin), and family history of bleeding disorders.
▶ Watch closely for bleeding from skin, nose, gums, GI tract, or an injury site.
▶ Help the patient avoid unnecessary trauma. Advise him to tell his dentist about this condition before undergoing oral surgery. (Also stress the need for good oral hygiene to help prevent the need for such surgery.)
▶ Alert other care team members to the patient's hemorrhagic potential, especially before he undergoes diagnostic tests or surgery that may cause trauma and bleeding.
▶ Observe the patient undergoing plasmapheresis for hypovolemia, hypotension,

Facts about platelet concentrate

CONTENTS
● Platelets, white blood cells, some plasma
● Random platelets (ABO matched)
● Human leukocyte antigen (HLA) platelets (HLA-typed for multiple transfusions)

AMOUNT
● 30 to 50 ml per donor
● 4 to 8 donor units given each time (each unit should raise the platelet count by 5,000/μl)

SHELF LIFE
● 6 to 72 hours (best used within 24 hours)

HEPATITIS RISK
● Same as with whole blood

tachycardia, and other signs of volume depletion.
▶ If platelet dysfunction is inherited, help the patient and his family understand and accept the disorder's nature. Teach them how to manage potential bleeding episodes. Warn them that petechiae, ecchymoses, and bleeding from the nose, gums, and GI tract signal abnormal bleeding and should be reported immediately.
▶ Tell the patient with a known coagulopathy or hepatic disease to avoid aspirin, aspirin compounds, and other agents that impair coagulation.
▶ Advise the patient to wear a medical identification bracelet or to carry a card identifying him as a potential bleeder.

REFERENCES
1. Johns Hopkins Medicine International (2007). "Platelet Function Disorders" [Online]. Available at *www.jhintl.net/forpatients/search.aspx?id=1304*.

POLYCYTHEMIA VERA

Polycythemia vera is a chronic, myeloproliferative disorder characterized by increased red blood cell (RBC) mass, leukocytosis, thrombocytosis, and increased hemoglobin concentration, with normal or increased plasma volume. This disease is also known as *primary polycythemia, erythremia, polycythemia rubra vera, splenomegalic polycythemia,* and *Vaquez-Osler disease.*

The prognosis depends on the patient's age at diagnosis, the type of treatment used, and complications. Mortality is high if polycythemia is untreated or is associated with leukemia or myeloid metaplasia.

Causes and incidence

In polycythemia vera, uncontrolled and rapid cellular reproduction and maturation cause proliferation or hyperplasia of all bone marrow cells (panmyelosis). The cause of such uncontrolled cellular activity is unknown but it's probably due to a multipotential stem cell defect.

Polycythemia vera usually occurs between ages 50 and 70, with slightly more males than females affected.[1] It was previously thought to be more common in people of Jewish ancestry but studies show it occurs in all ethnic groups.[1] It's a rare disorder affecting 0.6 to 1.6 people per 1 million in the United States.[1]

Signs and symptoms

Increased RBC mass results in hyperviscosity and inhibits blood flow to microcirculation. Subsequently, increased viscosity, diminished velocity, and thrombocytosis promote intravascular thrombosis. In its early stages, polycythemia vera usually produces no symptoms. (Increased hematocrit [HCT] may be an incidental finding.) However, as altered circulation secondary to increased RBC mass produces hypervolemia and hyperviscosity, the patient may complain of a feeling of fullness in the head, headache,

dizziness, and other symptoms, depending on the body system affected. The patient may also complain of severe itching after a warm or hot shower. Hyperviscosity may lead to thrombosis of smaller vessels with ruddy cyanosis of the nose and clubbing of the digits. (See *Clinical features of polycythemia vera.*)

Complications

▶ Hemorrhage due to defective platelet function or to hyperviscosity and the local effects from excess RBCs exerting pressure on distended venous and capillary walls
▶ Splenomegaly
▶ Renal calculi
▶ Abdominal thrombosis
▶ Stroke
▶ Peptic ulcer disease

Diagnosis

Laboratory studies confirm polycythemia vera by showing increased RBC mass and normal arterial oxygen saturation in association with splenomegaly or two of the following: thrombocytosis, leukocytosis, elevated leukocyte alkaline phosphatase level, or elevated serum vitamin B_{12} level or unbound B_{12}-binding capacity.

Another common finding is increased uric acid production, leading to hyperuricemia and hyperuricuria. Other laboratory results include increased blood histamine levels, decreased serum iron concentration, and decreased or absent urinary erythropoietin. Bone marrow biopsy reveals panmyelosis.

Researchers have also recently discovered that the Janus kinase 2 mutation (JAK2) is present in almost all patients who have polycythemia vera.[2]

Treatment

Phlebotomy can reduce RBC mass promptly. The frequency of phlebotomy and the amount of blood removed each time depend on the patient's condition. Typically, 350 to 500 ml of blood can be removed every other

Clinical features of polycythemia vera

SIGNS AND SYMPTOMS	CAUSES
Eyes, ears, nose, and throat	
• Vision disturbances (blurring, diplopia, scotoma), engorged veins of the fundus and retina, and congestion of conjunctiva, retina, retinal veins, and oral mucous membrane	• Hypervolemia and hyperviscosity
• Epistaxis or gingival bleeding	• Engorgement of capillary beds
Central nervous system	
• Headache or fullness in the head, lethargy, weakness, fatigue, syncope, tinnitus, paresthesia of digits, and impaired mentation	• Hypervolemia and hyperviscosity
Cardiovascular system	
• Hypertension	• Hypervolemia and hyperviscosity
• Intermittent claudication, thrombosis and emboli, angina, thrombophlebitis	• Hypervolemia, thrombocytosis, and vascular disease
• Hemorrhage	• Engorgement of capillary beds
Skin	
• Pruritus (especially after hot bath)	• Basophilia (secondary histamine release)
• Urticaria	• Altered histamine metabolism
• Ruddy cyanosis	• Hypervolemia and hyperviscosity due to congested vessels, increased oxyhemoglobin, and reduced hemoglobin
• Night sweats	• Hypermetabolism
• Ecchymosis	• Hemorrhage
GI system	
• Epigastric distress	• Hypervolemia and hyperviscosity
• Early satiety and fullness	• Hepatosplenomegaly
• Peptic ulcer pain	• Gastric thrombosis and hemorrhage
• Hepatosplenomegaly	• Congestion, extramedullary hemopoiesis, and myeloid metaplasia
• Weight loss	• Hypermetabolism
Respiratory system	
• Dyspnea	• Hypervolemia and hyperviscosity
Musculoskeletal system	
• Joint symptoms	• Increased urate production secondary to nucleoprotein turnover

day until the HCT is reduced to the low-normal range. After repeated phlebotomies, the patient develops iron deficiency, which stabilizes RBC production and reduces the need for phlebotomy. Pheresis permits the return of plasma to the patient, diluting the blood and reducing hypovolemic symptoms.

Phlebotomy doesn't reduce the white blood cell or platelet count and won't control the hyperuricemia associated with marrow cell proliferation. For severe symptoms, myelosuppressive therapy may be used. Chemotherapeutic agents may be used to suppress the bone marrow. These agents may cause leukemia, however, and should be reserved for older patients and those with problems uncontrolled by phlebotomy. The current preferred myelosuppressive agent is hydroxyurea.[1] Hydroxyurea has been studied and although there's a question regarding the long-term risk of leukemia, the risk of thrombosis compared with phlebotomy alone is no greater.[1] Patients who have had previous thrombotic problems should be considered for myelosuppressive therapy. The use of antiplatelet therapy is controversial because it may cause gastric bleeding. Allopurinol may be given for hyperuricemia.

Researchers are hoping to build on the knowledge of the JAK2 mutation to develop gene-specific drugs to help prevent or reverse polycythemia vera.[3]

Special considerations

If the patient requires phlebotomy, explain the procedure, and reassure him that it will relieve distressing symptoms. Check his blood pressure, pulse rate, and respiratory rate. During phlebotomy, make sure the patient is lying down comfortably to prevent vertigo and syncope. Stay alert for tachycardia, clamminess, or complaints of vertigo. If these effects occur, the procedure should be stopped.

▶ Immediately after phlebotomy, check the patient's blood pressure and pulse rate. Have him sit up for about 5 minutes before allowing him to walk; this prevents vasovagal attack or orthostatic hypotension. Also, have him drink about 24 oz (710 ml) of juice or water.

▶ Tell the patient to watch for and report signs or symptoms of iron deficiency (pallor, weight loss, asthenia [weakness], and glossitis).

▶ Keep the patient active and ambulatory to prevent thrombosis. If bed rest is absolutely necessary, prescribe a daily program of both active and passive range-of-motion exercises.

▶ Watch for complications: hypervolemia, thrombocytosis, and signs or symptoms of an impending stroke (decreased sensation, numbness, transitory paralysis, fleeting blindness, headache, and epistaxis).

▶ Regularly examine the patient for bleeding. Tell him which are the most common bleeding sites (such as the nose, gingiva, and skin) so he can check for bleeding. Advise him to report any abnormal bleeding promptly.

▶ To compensate for increased uric acid production, give additional fluids, administer allopurinol, and alkalinize the urine to prevent uric acid calculi.

▶ If the patient has symptom-producing splenomegaly, suggest or provide small, frequent meals, followed by a rest period, to prevent nausea and vomiting.

▶ Report acute abdominal pain immediately; it may signal splenic infarction, renal calculi, or abdominal organ thrombosis.

During myelosuppressive treatment:

▶ Monitor the patient's complete blood count and platelet count before and during therapy. Warn the patient who develops leukopenia that his resistance to infection is low; advise him to avoid crowds and watch for the symptoms of infection. If leukopenia develops in a hospitalized patient who needs reverse isolation, follow hospital guidelines. If thrombocytopenia develops, tell the patient to watch for signs of bleeding (blood in urine, nosebleeds, and black stool).

▶ Tell the patient about possible reactions (nausea, vomiting, and risk of infection) to alkylating agents. Alopecia may follow the use of busulfan, cyclophosphamide, and uracil mustard; sterile hemorrhagic cystitis may follow the use of cyclophosphamide (forcing fluids can prevent it). Watch for and

report all reactions. If nausea and vomiting occur, begin antiemetic therapy and adjust the patient's diet.

REFERENCES

1. Besa, E.C., and Woermann, U. (2006, May 17). "Polycythemia Vera" [Online]. Available at *www.emedicine.com/MED/topic1864.htm.*
2. Tefferi, A., et al. "Proposals and Rationale for Revision of the World Health Organization Diagnostic Criteria for Polycythemia Vera, Essential Thrombocythemia, and Primary Myelofibrosis: Recommendations from an Ad Hoc International Expert Panel," *Blood* 110(4):1092-97, August 2007.
3. Finazzi, G., and Barbui, T. "How I Treat Patients with Polycythemia Vera," *Blood* 109(12):5104-11, June 2007.

SICKLE CELL ANEMIA

Sickle cell anemia, a congenital hemolytic anemia occurring primarily but not exclusively in blacks, results from a defective hemoglobin molecule (hemoglobin S or HbS) that causes red blood cells (RBCs) to roughen and become sickle-shaped. Such cells impair circulation, resulting in chronic ill health (fatigue, dyspnea on exertion, swollen joints), periodic crises, long-term complications, and premature death.

Penicillin prophylaxis can decrease morbidity and mortality from bacterial infections. One-half of the patients with sickle cell anemia die by their early twenties; few live to middle age.

Causes and incidence

Sickle cell anemia results from homozygous inheritance of the gene that produces HbS (chromosome 11). It's inherited as an autosomal recessive trait. Heterozygous inheritance of this gene results in sickle cell trait, a condition that usually produces no symptoms. (See *Sickle cell trait.*) Sickle cell anemia is most common in people whose relatives come from Africa, South and Central

Sickle cell trait

Sickle cell trait is a relatively benign condition that results from heterozygous inheritance of the abnormal hemoglobin (Hb)S-producing gene. Like sickle cell anemia, this condition is most common in blacks. Sickle cell trait *never* progresses to sickle cell anemia.

In persons with sickle cell trait (known as *carriers*), 20% to 40% of their total Hb is HbS; the rest is normal.

Such persons usually have no symptoms. They have normal Hb and hematocrit values and can expect a normal life span. Nevertheless, they must avoid situations that provoke hypoxia, which can occasionally cause a sickling crisis similar to that in sickle cell anemia.

Genetic counseling is essential for sickle cell carriers. If two sickle cell carriers produce offspring, each of their children has a 25% chance of inheriting sickle cell anemia.

America, Caribbean Islands, Mediterranean countries, India, and Saudi Arabia. About 1 in 12 Blacks carry the abnormal gene.[1] Sickle cell anemia affects about 1 in every 500 Black births and 1 in 1,000 to 1,400 Hispanic births in the United States.[1]

If two parents who are both carriers of sickle cell trait (or another hemoglobinopathy) have offspring, each child has a 25% chance of developing sickle cell anemia. (See *Inheritance patterns in sickle cell anemia, page 336.*) The abnormal HbS found in the RBCs of patients with sickle cell anemia become insoluble whenever hypoxia occurs. As a result, these RBCs become rigid, rough, and elongated, forming a crescent or sickle shape, and producing hemolysis (cell destruction). (See *Comparing normal and sickled red blood cells, page 337.*) In addition, these altered cells tend to pile up in capillaries and smaller blood vessels, making blood more viscous. Normal circulation is im-

Inheritance patterns in sickle cell anemia

When both parents are carriers of sickle cell trait, each child has a 25% chance of developing sickle cell anemia, a 25% chance of being a normal (unaffected) noncarrier, and a 50% chance of being a carrier of sickle cell trait.

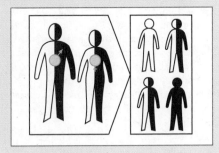

When one parent has sickle cell anemia and one is normal, all offspring will be carriers of sickle cell trait.

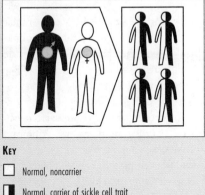

KEY

☐ Normal, noncarrier

◨ Normal, carrier of sickle cell trait

■ Sickle cell anemia (affected with sickle cell disease)

paired, causing pain, tissue infarctions, and swelling. Such blockage causes anoxic changes that lead to further sickling and obstruction.

Signs and symptoms

Characteristically, sickle cell anemia produces tachycardia, cardiomegaly, systolic and diastolic murmurs, pulmonary infarctions (which may result in cor pulmonale), chronic fatigue, unexplained dyspnea or dyspnea on exertion, hepatomegaly, jaundice, pallor, joint swelling, aching bones, chest pains, ischemic leg ulcers (especially around the ankles), and increased susceptibility to infection. Such symptoms usually don't develop until after age 6 months because large amounts of fetal Hb protect infants for the first few months after birth. Low socioeconomic status and related problems, such as poor education, may delay diagnosis and supportive treatment.

Infection, stress, dehydration, and conditions that provoke hypoxia—strenuous exercise, high altitude, unpressurized aircraft, cold, and vasoconstrictive drugs—may all provoke periodic crises. A painful crisis (vasoocclusive crisis, infarctive crisis), the most common crisis and the hallmark of the disease, usually appears periodically after age 5. It results from blood vessel obstruction by rigid, tangled sickle cells, which causes tissue anoxia and possible necrosis. This type of crisis is characterized by severe abdominal, thoracic, muscular, or bone pain and possibly worsening jaundice, dark urine, and a low-grade fever.

Autosplenectomy, in which splenic damage and scarring is so extensive that the spleen shrinks and becomes impalpable, occurs in patients with long-term disease. This can lead to increased susceptibility to *Streptococcus pneumoniae* sepsis, which can be fatal without prompt treatment. Infection may develop after the crisis subsides (in 4 days to several weeks), so watch for lethargy, sleepiness, fever, or apathy.

An aplastic crisis (megaloblastic crisis) results from bone marrow depression and usually is associated with viral infection. It's characterized by pallor, lethargy, sleepiness,

dyspnea, possible coma, markedly decreased bone marrow activity, and RBC hemolysis.

In infants between ages 8 months and 2 years, an acute sequestration crisis may cause sudden massive entrapment of RBCs in the spleen and liver. This rare crisis causes lethargy and pallor and, if untreated, commonly progresses to hypovolemic shock and death.

A hemolytic crisis is quite rare and usually occurs in patients who also have glucose-6-phosphate dehydrogenase deficiency. It probably results from complications of sickle cell anemia, such as infection, rather than from the disorder itself. Hemolytic crisis causes liver congestion and hepatomegaly as a result of degenerative changes. It worsens chronic jaundice, although increased jaundice doesn't always point to a hemolytic crisis.

Suspect any of these crises in a patient with sickle cell anemia who has pale lips, tongue, palms, or nail beds; lethargy; listlessness; sleepiness with difficulty awakening; irritability; severe pain; a fever over 104° F (40° C); or a fever of 100° F (37.8° C) that persists for 2 days.

Complications
▶ Delayed puberty
▶ If a child reaches adulthood, his body build tends to be spiderlike—narrow shoulders and hips, long extremities, curved spine, barrel chest, and elongated skull
▶ Chronic obstructive pulmonary disease
▶ Heart failure
▶ Organ infarction—retinopathy and nephropathy
▶ Splenic infarctions and splenomegaly
▶ Premature death
▶ Pulmonary hypertension[5]

Diagnosis
A positive family history and typical clinical features suggest sickle cell anemia. It can also be confirmed by hemoglobin electrophoresis showing HbS or other hemoglo-

Comparing normal and sickled red blood cells

When a person with sickle cell anemia develops hypoxia, the abnormal hemoglobin S found in his red blood cells (RBCs) becomes insoluble. This causes the RBCs to become rigid, rough, and elongated, forming the characteristic sickle shape.

NORMAL RBCs

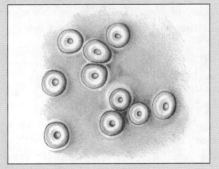

SICKLE CELLS

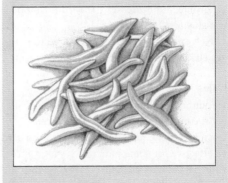

binopathies. Electrophoresis should be done on umbilical cord blood samples at birth to provide sickle cell disease screening for all neonates at risk.[3]

Additional laboratory studies may show a low RBC count, elevated white blood cell and platelet counts, decreased erythrocyte sedimentation rate, increased serum iron, decreased RBC survival, and reticulocytosis. Hb levels may be low or normal. During ear-

ly childhood, palpation may reveal spleno-megaly; however, as the child grows older, the spleen shrinks.

Treatment

Treatment begins before age 4 months with prophylactic penicillin. If the patient's hemo-globin level drops suddenly or if his condition deteriorates rapidly, he'll need to be hospitalized for a transfusion of packed RBCs. In a sequestration crisis, treatment may include sedation, administration of analgesics, blood transfusion, oxygen administration, and large amounts of oral or I.V. fluids.

Daily folic acid supplementation is recommended to prevent megaloblastic crisis. Hydroxyurea, which causes an increase in the synthesis of fetal hemoglobin and a significant reduction in crises, is being used for some patients with sickle cell anemia. Researchers have found it helpful for some patients because it reduces the frequency of painful crises and episodes of acute chest syndrome and decreases the need for blood transfusions.[2]

Newer drugs are being developed to manage sickle cell anemia. Some of these agents try to induce the body to produce more fetal hemoglobin, which helps decrease the amount of sickling. Others work by increasing the binding of oxygen to sickle cells. Currently, bone marrow transplantation can be effective for some patients. It's used for younger patients with severe disease and may be a risky procedure with serious side effects.[1] Gene therapy (replacing HbS with normal HbA) may be the ideal treatment, but it's difficult to perform and research continues on it.[2]

Special considerations

Supportive measures during crises and precautions to avoid them are important. Here are some actions you can take during a painful crisis:

▶ Apply warm compresses to painful areas, and cover the child with a blanket. (Never use cold compresses because they aggravate the condition.)

▶ Administer an analgesic-antipyretic, such as aspirin or acetaminophen. Additional pain relief may be required during an acute crisis. (See *Pain relief in sickle cell anemia*.)

▶ Encourage fluids and bed rest, and place the patient in a sitting position. If dehydration or severe pain occurs, hospitalization may be necessary.

▶ When cultures indicate infection, give antibiotics as ordered.

During remissions:

▶ Advise the patient to avoid tight clothing that restricts circulation.

▶ Warn against strenuous exercise, vasoconstricting medications, cold temperatures (including drinking large amounts of ice water and swimming), unpressurized aircraft, high altitude, and other conditions that provoke hypoxia.

HEALTH & SAFETY *Stress the importance of normal childhood immunizations, meticulous wound care, good oral hygiene, regular dental checkups, and a balanced diet as safeguards against infection.*

▶ Emphasize the need for prompt treatment of infection.

▶ Inform the patient of the need to increase fluid intake to prevent dehydration caused by an impaired ability to concentrate urine properly. Tell parents to encourage the child to drink more fluids, especially in the summer, by offering fluids such as milkshakes and ice pops.

During pregnancy or surgery:

▶ Warn women with sickle cell anemia that they may have increased obstetrical risks. However, the use of hormonal contraceptives may also be risky; refer them for birth control counseling to a qualified obstetric or gynecologic health care provider.[4]

Pain relief in sickle cell anemia

Question: *Do nurses adequately estimate pain in patients with sickle cell anemia?*

Research: Pain has long been accepted as part of life for patients with sickle cell anemia. Researchers are interested in finding out if nurses and other health-care professionals adequately estimate their patients' pain from sickle cell anemia. The researchers studied 223 patients age 16 and older. They had the participants complete a daily pain diary, which included recording their maximum pain level on a scale of 0 to 9, whether they were in a crisis, and if they required hospital, emergency, or unscheduled ambulatory care for pain management on the previous day.

Conclusion: Patients reported pain on 55% of the total days. Overall, more than 29% of patients stated that they had pain on more than 95% of the days recorded. The overall pain rating increased as the number of days with pain increased.

Application: Patients with sickle cell anemia have pain more frequently and higher pain levels than originally thought. When a patient with sickle cell anemia is admitted to the hospital, either due to a crisis or for other reasons, the nurse should be aware of the patient's pain level and be ready to treat the patient for higher levels of pain.

Source: Smith, W.R., et al. "Daily Assessment of Pain in Adults with Sickle Cell Disease," *Annals of Internal Medicine* 148(2):94-101, January 2008.

▶ If such women do become pregnant, they should maintain a balanced diet and take a folic acid supplement.

▶ During general anesthesia, a patient who has sickle cell anemia requires optimal ventilation to prevent hypoxic crisis. Make sure the surgeon and the anesthesiologist know that the patient has sickle cell anemia. Provide a preoperative transfusion of packed RBCs, as needed.

General tips:

▶ To encourage normal mental and social development, warn parents against being overprotective. Although the child must avoid strenuous exercise, he can enjoy most everyday activities.

▶ Refer parents of children with sickle cell anemia for genetic counseling to answer their questions about the risk to future offspring. Recommend screening of other family members to determine if they're heterozygote carriers. These parents may also need psychological counseling to cope with guilt feelings. In addition, suggest they join an appropriate community support group.

▶ Adolescents or adult males with sickle cell anemia may develop sudden, painful episodes of priapism. Such episodes are common and, if prolonged, can have serious reproductive consequences. Advise the patient to contact the physician when these episodes occur.

REFERENCES

1. National Heart Lung and Blood Institute (2007, November). "Sickle Cell Anemia" [Online]. Available at *www.nhlbi.nih.gov/health/dci/ Diseases/Sca/SCA_WhatIs.html.*

2. Sickle Cell Disease Association of America, Inc. "About Sickle Cell Disease" [Online]. Available at *www.sicklecelldisease.org/about_scd/ index.phtml.*

3. Anglin, S. "Sickle Cell and Thalassaemia Screening: Early Care," *Practising Midwife* 10(9):22-25, October 2007.

4. ACOG Committee on Practice Bulletins-Gynecology. "ACOG Practice Bulletin No. 73: Use of Hormonal Contraception in Women with Coexisting Medical Conditions," *Obstetrics and Gynecology* 107(6):1453-72, June 2006.

5. Barnett, C.F., et al. "Pulmonary Hypertension: An Increasingly Recognized Complication of Hereditary Hemolytic Anemias and HIV Infection," *JAMA* 299(3):324-31, January 2008.

THROMBOCYTOPENIA

The most common cause of hemorrhagic disorders, thrombocytopenia is characterized by deficiency of circulating platelets. Because platelets play a vital role in coagulation, this disease poses a serious threat to hemostasis. (See *What happens in thrombocytopenia*, pages 342 and 343.) The prognosis is excellent in drug-induced thrombocytopenia if the offending drug is withdrawn; in such cases, recovery may be immediate. In other types, the prognosis depends on the patient's response to treatment of the underlying cause.

Causes and incidence

Thrombocytopenia may be congenital or acquired; the acquired form is more common. In either case, it usually results from decreased or defective production of platelets in the bone marrow (such as occurs in leukemia, aplastic anemia, or toxicity with certain drugs) or from increased destruction outside the bone marrow caused by an underlying disorder (such as cirrhosis of the liver, disseminated intravascular coagulation, or severe infection). Less commonly, it results from sequestration (hypersplenism and hypothermia) or platelet loss. Acquired thrombocytopenia may result from certain drugs, such as quinidine, amiodarone, captopril, sulfonamides, glibenclamide, carbamazepine, ibuprofen, cimetidine, tamoxifen, ranitidine, phenytoin, vancomycin and piperacillin.[1] (See *Causes of decreased circulating platelets*.) Most frequently, patients receiving heparin will develop thrombocytopenia. New research has shown that patients who receive glycoprotein IIb/IIIa receptor agonists are also at risk for developing life-threatening thrombocytopenia.[2]

An idiopathic form of thrombocytopenia commonly occurs in children, and a transient form may follow viral infection (such as Epstein-Barr virus or infectious mononucleosis).

Signs and symptoms

Thrombocytopenia typically produces a sudden onset of petechiae or ecchymoses in the skin or bleeding into any mucous membrane. Nearly all patients are otherwise asymptomatic, although some may complain of malaise, fatigue, and general weakness. In adults, large, blood-filled bullae characteristically appear in the mouth. In severe thrombocytopenia, hemorrhage may lead to tachycardia, shortness of breath, loss of consciousness, and death.

Complications

▶ Acute hemorrhage of the brain and GI tract
▶ Intrapulmonary bleeding
▶ Cardiac tamponade

Diagnosis

Diagnosis is based on the results of the patient's history (especially the drug history), physical examination, and laboratory tests. Coagulation tests reveal a decreased platelet count, prolonged bleeding time, and normal prothrombin and partial thromboplastin times. Bleeding with minimal trauma may occur if platelet counts are below 50,000/ul. If increased destruction of platelets is causing thrombocytopenia, bone marrow studies will reveal a greater number of megakaryocytes (platelet precursors) and shortened platelet survival (several hours or days rather than the usual 7 to 10 days).

Treatment

Treatment varies with the underlying cause and may include corticosteroids or immune globulin to increase platelet production. The treatment of choice is removal of the offending agents in drug-induced thrombocytopenia or treatment of the underlying cause.[3] Platelet transfusions are helpful only in treating complications of severe hemorrhage.

Special considerations

When caring for the patient with thrombocytopenia, take every possible precaution against bleeding.

▶ Protect the patient from trauma. Keep the side rails up and pad them, if possible. Promote the use of an electric razor and a soft toothbrush. Avoid invasive procedures, such as venipuncture or urinary catheterization, if possible. When venipuncture is unavoidable, be sure to exert pressure on the puncture site for at least 20 minutes or until the bleeding stops.

▶ Monitor the patient's platelet count daily.

▶ Test the patient's stool for guaiac; dipstick urine and vomitus for blood.

▶ Observe for bleeding (petechiae, ecchymoses, surgical or GI bleeding, and menorrhagia).

▶ Warn the patient to avoid aspirin in any form and other drugs that impair coagulation. Teach him how to recognize aspirin or ibuprofen compounds on the labels of over-the-counter remedies.

▶ Advise the patient to avoid straining when defecating or coughing, as both can lead to increased intracranial pressure, possibly causing cerebral hemorrhage in the patient with thrombocytopenia. Provide a stool softener to avoid constipation.

▶ During periods of active bleeding, maintain the patient on strict bed rest if necessary.

▶ When administering platelet concentrate, remember that platelets are extremely fragile, so infuse them quickly. Don't give platelets to a patient with a fever.

Causes of decreased circulating platelets

DIMINISHED OR DEFECTIVE PLATELET PRODUCTION

Congenital
- Wiskott-Aldrich syndrome
- Maternal ingestion of thiazides
- Neonatal rubella

Acquired
- Aplastic anemia
- Marrow infiltration (acute and chronic leukemias, tumor)
- Nutritional deficiency (B_{12}, folic acid)
- Myelosuppressive agents
- Drugs that directly influence platelet production (thiazides, alcohol, hormones)
- Radiation
- Viral infections (measles, dengue)

INCREASED PERIPHERAL PLATELET DESTRUCTION

Congenital
- Nonimmune (prematurity, erythroblastosis fetalis, infection)
- Immune (drug sensitivity, maternal idiopathic thrombocytopenic purpura [ITP]).

Acquired
- Nonimmune (infection, disseminated intravascular coagulation, thrombotic thrombocytopenic purpura)
- Immune (drug-induced, especially with quinine and quinidine; post-transfusion purpura; acute and chronic ITP; sepsis; alcohol)
- Invasive lines and devices
- Intra-aortic balloon pump
- Prosthetic heart valves
- Heparin

PLATELET SEQUESTRATION
- Hypersplenism
- Hypothermia

PLATELET LOSS
- Hemorrhage
- Extracorporeal perfusion

What happens in thrombocytopenia

Thrombocytopenia is the most common cause of bleeding disorders and is characterized by a severe decrease in platelets. This platelet decrease can result from hematologic malignancy, radiation or drug therapy, idiopathic causes, blood transfusions, disseminated intravascular coagulation (DIC), or splenomegaly. Excessive hemorrhaging can lead to shock if interventions are delayed. This chart shows how these conditions and treatments develop into thrombocytopenic hemorrhage.

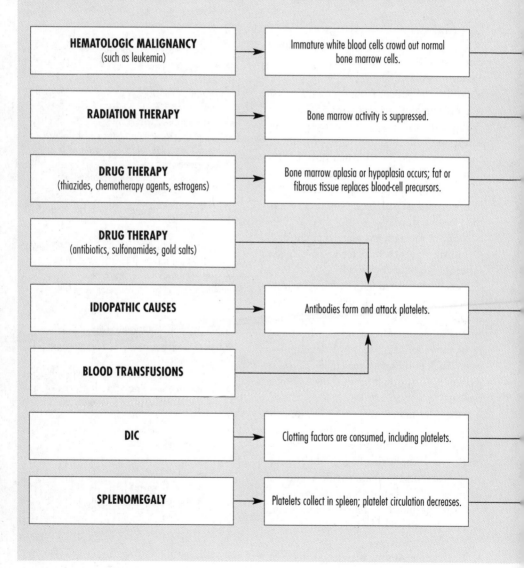

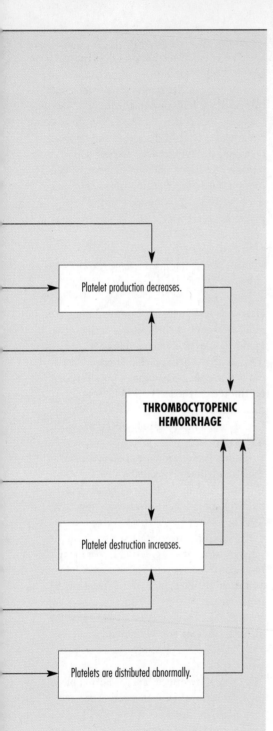

Platelet production decreases.

THROMBOCYTOPENIC HEMORRHAGE

Platelet destruction increases.

Platelets are distributed abnormally.

▶ During platelet transfusion, monitor for a febrile reaction (flushing, chills, fever, headache, tachycardia, and hypertension). Histocompatibility locus antigen-typed platelets may be ordered to prevent febrile reaction. A patient with a history of minor reactions may benefit from acetaminophen and diphenhydramine before transfusion.

▶ If thrombocytopenia is drug-induced, stress the importance of avoiding the offending drug.

▶ If the patient must receive long-term steroid therapy, teach him to watch for and report cushingoid signs (acne, moon face, hirsutism, buffalo hump, hypertension, girdle obesity, thinning arms and legs, glycosuria, and edema). Emphasize that steroid doses must be discontinued gradually. During steroid therapy, monitor fluid and electrolyte balance, and watch for infection, pathologic fractures, and mood changes.

▶ Advise the patient to avoid tattoos or body piercing.

▶ Advise the patient to avoid forceful nose blowing. If nosebleed occurs, teach him to apply pressure to the bridge of the nose and apply an ice pack.

REFERENCES

1. Thiagarajan, P. (2006, July 20). "Platelet Disorders" [Online]. Available at *www.emedicine.com/med/topic987.htm*.
2. Huxtable, L.M., et al. "Frequency and Management of Thrombocytopenia with the Glycoprotein IIb/IIIa Receptor Antagonists," *American Journal of Cardiology* 97(3):426-29, February 1, 2006.
3. Warkentin, T.E., and Greinacher, A. "Heparin-induced Thrombocytopenia: Recognition, Treatment, and Prevention: The Seventh ACCP Conference on Antithrombotic and Thrombolytic Therapy," *Chest* 126(3 Suppl):311S-37S, September 2004.

VON WILLEBRAND'S DISEASE

V on Willebrand's disease is a hereditary bleeding disorder characterized
by prolonged bleeding time; moderate deficiency of von Willebrand's factor
(vWF), clotting factor VIII (antihemophilic
factor) and, possibly, factor VIII coagulant
protein (VIII:C); and impaired platelet function. This disease commonly causes bleeding
from the skin or mucosal surfaces and, in females, excessive uterine bleeding. Bleeding
may range from mild, producing no symptoms, to severe. The prognosis, however, is
usually good.

Causes and incidence

Unlike hemophilia, von Willebrand's disease
is inherited as an autosomal dominant trait
that affects males and females equally. One
theory of pathophysiology holds that mild to
moderate deficiency of factor VIII and defective platelet adhesion prolong coagulation
time. Specifically, this results from a deficiency of the vWF, which stabilizes the factor
VIII molecule and is needed for proper
platelet function.

Defective platelet function is characterized
by:
▶ decreased agglutination and adhesion at
the bleeding site
▶ reduced platelet retention when filtered
through a column of packed glass beads
▶ diminished ristocetin-induced platelet aggregation.

Recently, an acquired form has been identified in patients with cancer and immune
disorders.

Von Willebrand's disease is the most common of all inherited bleeding disorders.[1] It
occurs in about 1 out of 100 to 1,000 people.[1] Von Willebrand's disease doesn't have
any racial or ethnic associations.[2]

Signs and symptoms

Von Willebrand's disease produces easy
bruising, epistaxis, and bleeding from the
gums. Petechiae are rarely seen. Women can
have increased menstrual bleeding.[2]

Severe forms of this disease may cause
hemorrhage after laceration or surgery, menorrhagia, and GI bleeding. Excessive postpartum bleeding is uncommon because factor VIII levels and bleeding time abnormalities become less pronounced during
pregnancy.

Complications
▶ Life-threatening hemorrhage (rare)

Diagnosis

Diagnosis is difficult because symptoms are
mild, laboratory values are borderline, and
factor VIII levels fluctuate. However, a positive family history and characteristic bleeding patterns and laboratory values help establish the diagnosis. Typical laboratory
data include:
▶ prolonged bleeding time (more than
6 minutes)
▶ slightly prolonged partial thromboplastin
time (more than 45 seconds)
▶ absent or reduced levels of factor VIII-
related antigens and low factor VIII activity
level
▶ defective in vitro platelet aggregation (using the ristocetin coagulation factor assay
test)
▶ normal platelet count and normal clot retraction.
Research is currently being done to develop
a genetic test for von Willebrand's disease.[3]

Treatment

The goals of treatment are to shorten bleeding time by local measures and to replace
factor VIII (and, consequently, vWF) by infusion of cryoprecipitate or blood fractions
that are rich in factor VIII. For excessive
bleeding, antihemophilic factor-von
Willebrand factor may be required.[2] During

bleeding and before surgery, I.V. infusion of cryoprecipitate or fresh frozen plasma (in quantities sufficient to raise factor VIII levels to 50% of normal) shortens bleeding time.[4] For mild bleeding, desmopressin given parenterally or intranasally is effective in raising serum levels of vWF.[2]

Special considerations
The care plan should include local measures to control bleeding and patient teaching to prevent bleeding, unnecessary trauma, and complications.

▶ After surgery, monitor bleeding time for 24 to 48 hours, and watch for signs of new bleeding.

▶ During a bleeding episode, elevate and apply cold compresses and gentle pressure to the bleeding site.

▶ Refer parents of affected children for genetic counseling.

▶ Advise the patient to consult the physician after even minor trauma and before all surgery to determine if replacement of blood components is necessary.

▶ Instruct the patient to watch for signs of hepatitis within 6 weeks to 6 months after transfusion.

▶ Warn the patient against using aspirin and other drugs that impair platelet function.

▶ Advise the patient who has a severe form to avoid contact sports.

REFERENCES

1. National Heart Lung and Blood Institute. "von Willebrand Disease" [Online]. Available at *www.nhlbi.nih.gov/health/dci/Diseases/vWD/vWD_Treatments.html.*
2. National Hemophilia Foundation (2006). "von Willebrand Disease" [Online]. Available at *www.hemophilia.org/NHFWeb/MainPgs/MainNHF.aspx?menuid=182&contentid=47&rptname=bleeding.*
3. Riddel, J.P. Jr, and Aouizerat, B.E. "Genetics of von Willebrand Disease Type 1," *Biological Research for Nursing* 8(2):147-56, October 2006.
4. "Practice Guidelines for Blood Component Therapy: A Report by the American Society of Anesthesiologists Task Force on Blood Component Therapy," *Anesthesiology* 84(3):732-47, March 1996.

Metabolic disorders

HYPERLIPOPROTEINEMIA

Hyperlipoproteinemia is characterized by increased plasma concentrations of one or more lipoproteins. It affects lipid transport in serum and produces various clinical changes, from relatively mild symptoms that can be corrected by dietary management to potentially fatal pancreatitis.

Causes and incidence

Primary hyperlipoproteinemia includes five distinct metabolic disorders—all of which may be inherited. Types I and III are transmitted as autosomal recessive traits; Types II, IV, and V are transmitted as autosomal dominant traits. (See *Types of hyperlipoproteinemia.*) Secondary hyperlipoproteinemia results from other metabolic disorders, such as diabetes, pancreatitis, hypothyroidism, or renal disease.

About one in five people with elevated plasma lipid and lipoprotein levels has hyperlipoproteinemia. People with an increased risk of hyperlipoproteinemia include those with relatives who have the disease, and people who are overweight, have a high fat diet, are physically inactive, and consume a moderate to excessive amount of alcohol. (See *Affective states and familial hypercholesterolemia,* page 348.)

Signs and symptoms

▶ *Type I:* recurrent attacks of severe abdominal pain similar to pancreatitis, usually preceded by fat intake; abdominal spasm, rigidity, or rebound tenderness; hepatosplenomegaly, with liver or spleen tenderness; papular or eruptive xanthomas (pinkish-yellow cutaneous deposits of fat) over pressure points and extensor surfaces; lipemia retinalis (reddish-white retinal vessels); malaise; anorexia; and fever
▶ *Type II:* tendinous xanthomas (firm masses) on the Achilles tendons and tendons of the hands and feet, tuberous xanthomas, xanthelasma, juvenile corneal arcus (opaque ring surrounding the corneal periphery), accelerated atherosclerosis and premature coronary artery disease (CAD), and recurrent polyarthritis and tenosynovitis
▶ *Type III:* peripheral vascular disease manifested by claudication or turboeruptive xanthomas (soft, inflamed, pedunculated lesions) over the elbows and knees; palmar xanthomas on the hands, particularly the fingertips; premature atherosclerosis
▶ *Type IV:* predisposition to atherosclerosis and early coronary artery disease, exacerbated by excessive calorie intake, obesity, diabetes, and hypertension
▶ *Type V:* abdominal pain (most common), pancreatitis, peripheral neuropathy, eruptive xanthomas on extensor surfaces of the arms

Types of hyperlipoproteinemia

TYPE	CAUSES AND INCIDENCE	DIAGNOSTIC FINDINGS
I (Frederickson's hyperlipoproteinemia, fat-induced hyperlipemia, idiopathic familial)	• Deficient or abnormal lipoprotein lipase, resulting in decreased or absent post-heparin lipolytic activity • Relatively rare • Present at birth	• Chylomicrons (very-low-density lipoprotein [VLDL], low-density lipoprotein [LDL], high-density lipoprotein), in plasma 14 hours or more after last meal • Highly elevated serum chylomicrons and triglyceride levels; slightly elevated serum cholesterol levels • Lower serum lipoprotein lipase levels • Leukocytosis
II (familial hyperbetalipoproteinemia, essential familial hypercholesterolemia)	• Deficient cell surface receptor that regulates LDL degradation and cholesterol synthesis, resulting in increased levels of plasma LDL over joints and pressure points • Onset between ages 10 and 30	• Increased plasma concentrations of LDL • Increased serum LDL and cholesterol levels • Amniocentesis shows increased LDL levels
III (familial broad-beta disease, dysbetalipoproteinemia, remnant removal disease, xanthoma tuberosum)	• Unknown underlying defect results in deficient conversion of triglyceride-rich VLDL to LDL • Uncommon; usually occurs after age 20 but can occur earlier in men	• Abnormal serum beta-lipoprotein • Elevated cholesterol and triglyceride levels • Slightly elevated glucose tolerance • Hyperuricemia
IV (endogenous hypertriglyceridemia, hyperbetalipoproteinemia)	• Usually occurs secondary to obesity, alcoholism, diabetes, or emotional disorders • Relatively common, especially in middle-age men	• Elevated VLDL levels • Abnormal levels of triglycerides in plasma; variable increase in serum • Normal or slightly elevated serum cholesterol levels • Mildly abnormal glucose tolerance • Family history • Early coronary artery disease
V (mixed hypertriglyceridemia, mixed hyperlipidemia)	• Defective triglyceride clearance causes pancreatitis; usually secondary to another disorder, such as obesity or nephrosis • Uncommon; onset usually occurs in late adolescence or early adulthood	• Chylomicrons in plasma • Elevated plasma VLDL levels • Elevated serum cholesterol and triglyceride levels

and legs, lipemia retinalis, and hepatosplenomegaly.

Complications

▶ CAD
▶ Pancreatitis

EVIDENCE-BASED PRACTICE

Affective states and familial hypercholesterolemia

Question: *Do patients with heterozygous familial hypercholesterolemia feel guilt or shame related to how they manage the condition?*

Research: During this study, 40 patients with heterozygous familial hypercholesterolemia were interviewed about their feelings of guilt and shame associated with how they managed the disorder. Systematic text condensation was used to analyze the data.

Conclusion: The study demonstrated that the participants experienced guilt or shame if they failed to follow their self-imposed dietary management of the disorder or if they received abnormal results of cholesterol testing; however, they were all aware that the condition was inherited and not caused by an unhealthy lifestyle. One group of study participants felt that healthcare professionals had humiliated them when providing counseling on lifestyle and diet; whereas a second group felt this to be the provider's concern for their welfare.

Application: Although the condition isn't caused by poor lifestyle and dietary choices, the nurse should be sensitive to the patient's feelings when discussing individual disease management with a patient who has familial hypercholesterolemia. Even an unintentional implication that the patient may be responsible for poor test results or inadequate dietary management can cause the patient to experience guilt or shame about his ability to manage the disease.

Source: Frich, J.C., et al. "Experiences of Guilt and Shame in Patients with Familial Hypercholesterolemia: A Qualitative Interview Study," *Patient Education and Counseling* 69(1-3):108-13, December 2007.

Diagnosis

Hyperlipoproteinemia is indicated by serum lipid profiles—elevated levels of total cholesterol, triglycerides, very-low density lipoproteins, low density lipoproteins (LDLs), or high density lipoproteins. (See *Types of hyperlipoproteinemia,* page 347, for more specifics.)

Treatment

The first goal of hyperlipoproteinemia treatment is to identify and treat any underlying problem such as diabetes. If no underlying problem exists, the primary treatment of Types II, III, and IV is dietary management (especially restriction of cholesterol intake) that's possibly supplemented by drug therapy to lower plasma triglyceride or cholesterol level when diet alone is ineffective. HMG-CoA reductase inhibitors reduce cholesterol and include the following drugs: pravastatin, lovastatin, simvastatin, rosuvastatin. Niacin is also effective in most cases of hyperlipidemia in lowering cholesterol and triglycerides.[2] Children with familial hyperlipoproteinemia should be started on HMG-CoA reductase inhibitors as early as possible to help decrease the risk of developing atherosclerosis in adolescence.[1]

Type I hyperlipoproteinemia requires long-term weight reduction, with fat intake restricted to less than 20 g/day. A 20- to 40-g/day medium-chain triglyceride diet may be ordered to supplement calorie intake. The patient should also avoid alcoholic beverages to decrease plasma triglyceride levels. The prognosis is good with treatment; without treatment, death can result from pancreatitis.

For Type II, dietary management to restore normal lipid levels and decrease the risk of atherosclerosis includes restriction of cholesterol intake to less than 300 mg/day for adults and less than 150 mg/day for children. Triglyceride intake must be restricted to less than 100 mg/day for children and adults and the diet should be high in polyunsaturated fats.

In familial hypercholesterolemia, nicotinic acid with a bile acid usually normalizes LDL levels.

For severely affected children, a portacaval shunt is a last resort to reduce plasma cholesterol levels. The prognosis remains poor regardless of treatment; in homozygotes, myocardial infarction usually causes death before age 30.

For Type III, dietary management includes restriction of cholesterol intake to less than 300 mg/day. Carbohydrates must be restricted, whereas polyunsaturated fats should be increased. Weight reduction is also helpful. Clofibrate and niacin may be given to help lower blood lipid levels. With strict adherence to the prescribed diet, the prognosis is good.

For Type IV, weight reduction may normalize blood lipid levels without additional treatment. Long-term dietary management includes restricted cholesterol intake, increased polyunsaturated fats, and avoidance of alcoholic beverages. Clofibrate and niacin may be given to help lower plasma lipid levels. The prognosis remains uncertain, however, because of the predisposition to premature CAD.

The most effective treatment for Type V is weight reduction and long-term maintenance of a low-fat diet. Alcoholic beverages must be avoided. Niacin, clofibrate, gemfibrozil, and a 20- to 40-g/day medium-chain triglyceride diet may prove helpful. The prognosis is uncertain because of the risk of pancreatitis. Increased fat intake may cause recurrent bouts of illness, possibly leading to pseudocyst formation, hemorrhage, and death.

Using bile acid sequestrants

Before giving the patient a bile acid sequestrant such as cholestyramine to lower cholesterol levels, make sure he isn't taking a drug or nutritional supplement, whose absorption is affected by bile acid sequestrants. For example, bile acid sequestrants decrease the absorption of diuretics such as chlorothiazide. Other drugs and supplements that are affected include:
- beta-adrenergic blockers
- digitoxin
- fat-soluble vitamins
- folic acid
- thiazides
- thyroxine
- warfarin.

Special considerations

Nursing care for hyperlipoproteinemia emphasizes careful monitoring for adverse drug effects and teaching the importance of long-term dietary management.

▶ Administer cholestyramine before meals or before bedtime. This drug must not be given with other medications. (See *Using bile acid sequestrants*.) Watch for adverse effects, such as nausea, vomiting, constipation, steatorrhea, rashes, and hyperchloremic acidosis.

▶ Give clofibrate as ordered. Watch for adverse effects, such as cholelithiasis, cardiac arrhythmias, intermittent claudication, thromboembolism, nausea, weight gain (from fluid retention), and myositis.

▶ Urge the patient to adhere to the ordered diet (usually 1,000 to 1,500 calories/day), to use polyunsaturated fats (vegetable oils) while minimizing the intake of saturated fats (higher in meats and coconut oil), to avoid excess sugar, and to follow the other recommendations specific for his type

▶ Instruct the patient, for the 2 weeks preceding serum cholesterol and serum triglyc-

eride tests, to maintain a steady weight and to adhere strictly to the prescribed diet. He should also fast for 12 hours preceding the test.

▶ Instruct women with elevated serum lipid levels to avoid hormonal contraceptives or drugs that contain estrogen.

REFERENCES

1. Rodenburg, J., et al. "Statin Treatment in Children with Familial Hypercholesterolemia: The Younger, the Better," *Circulation* 116(6): 664-68, August 2007.
2. Roy, H. (2007, August 14). "Hyperlipoproteinemia" [Online]. Available at *www.emedicine.com/OPH/topic505.htm.*

HYPOGLYCEMIA

Hypoglycemia is an abnormally low glucose level in the bloodstream. It occurs when glucose burns up too rapidly, when the glucose release rate falls behind tissue demands, or when excessive insulin enters the bloodstream.

Hypoglycemia is classified as reactive or fasting. *Reactive hypoglycemia* results from a reaction to the disposition of meals or the administration of excessive insulin. *Fasting hypoglycemia* causes discomfort during long periods of abstinence from food, for example, in the early morning before breakfast. Although hypoglycemia is a specific endocrine imbalance, its symptoms are often vague and depend on how quickly the patient's glucose levels drop. If not corrected, severe hypoglycemia may result in coma and irreversible brain damage.

Causes and incidence

Reactive hypoglycemia can take one of several forms. In a patient with diabetes, it may result from administration of too much insulin or, less commonly, too much oral antidiabetic medication. In a patient with mild diabetes (or one in the early stages of diabetes mellitus), reactive hypoglycemia may result from delayed and excessive insulin production after carbohydrate ingestion.

Similarly, a nondiabetic patient can suffer reactive hypoglycemia from a sharp increase in insulin output after a meal. Sometimes called *postprandial hypoglycemia,* this type of reactive hypoglycemia usually disappears when the patient eats something sweet. In some patients, reactive hypoglycemia has no known cause (idiopathic reactive) or it can result from gastric dumping syndrome or impaired glucose tolerance.

Fasting hypoglycemia usually results from an excess of insulin or insulin-like substance or from a decrease in counterregulatory hormones. It can be *exogenous,* resulting from such external factors as alcohol or drug ingestion, or *endogenous,* resulting from organic problems.

Endogenous hypoglycemia can result from tumors or liver disease. Insulinomas, small islet cell tumors in the pancreas, secrete excessive amounts of insulin, which inhibit hepatic glucose production. In most patients (90%), insulinomas are benign. Extrapancreatic tumors, though uncommon, can also cause hypoglycemia by increasing glucose utilization and inhibiting glucose output. Such tumors occur primarily in the mesenchyma, liver, adrenal cortex, GI system, and lymphatic system. They can be benign or malignant.

Among the nonendocrine causes of fasting hypoglycemia are severe liver diseases, including hepatitis, cancer, cirrhosis, and liver congestion associated with heart failure. All of these conditions reduce the uptake and release of glycogen from the liver.

Some endocrine causes of fasting hypoglycemia include adrenocortical insufficiency, which contributes to hypoglycemia by reducing the production of the cortisol and cortisone needed for gluconeogenesis; and pituitary insufficiency, which reduces corticotropin and growth hormone levels.

Usually, infants develop hypoglycemia because of an increased number of cells per unit of body weight and because of increased demands on stored liver glycogen to support respirations, thermoregulation, and muscular activity.

In full-term neonates, hypoglycemia may occur 24 to 72 hours after birth and is usually transient. In neonates who are premature or small for gestational age, the onset of hypoglycemia is much more rapid (it can occur as soon as 6 hours after birth) because of their small, immature livers, which produce much less glycogen.

Maternal disorders that can produce hypoglycemia in neonates within 24 hours after birth include diabetes mellitus, toxemia, erythroblastosis, and glycogen storage disease.[3]

The incidence of hypoglycemia in neonates is 1.3 to 3 per 1000 live births. It's greatest in high-risk neonatal groups.[1] In adults and children older than age 10, it's more commonly a side effect of diabetes.[2] As adults, females are affected more than males, and older adults are more likely to be affected.

Signs and symptoms

Signs and symptoms of hypoglycemia include fatigue, malaise, nervousness, irritability, trembling, tension, headache, hunger, cold sweats, and rapid heart rate. In addition, fasting hypoglycemia may also cause central nervous system (CNS) disturbances, such as blurry or double vision, confusion, motor weakness, hemiplegia, seizures, or coma.

In infants and children, signs and symptoms of hypoglycemia are vague. A neonate's refusal to feed may be the primary clue to underlying hypoglycemia. Associated CNS effects include tremors, twitching, weak or high-pitched cry, sweating, limpness, seizures, and coma.

Complications

Prolonged or severe hypoglycemia can cause:
▶ brain damage
▶ death.

Diagnosis

A blood glucose monitor and glucose reagent strips provide quick screening methods for determining the blood glucose level. A reading less than 45 mg/dl indicates the need for a venous blood sample.

Laboratory testing confirms the diagnosis. The following values indicate hypoglycemia:
▶ Full-term infants:
– less than 30 mg/dl before feeding
– less than 40 mg/dl after feeding
▶ Preterm infants:
– less than 20 mg/dl before feeding
– less than 30 mg/dl after feeding
▶ Children and adults:
– less than 40 mg/dl before a meal
– less than 50 mg/dl after a meal.

In addition, a 5-hour glucose tolerance test may be administered to provoke reactive hypoglycemia. Following a 12-hour fast, laboratory testing to detect plasma insulin and plasma glucose levels can identify fasting hypoglycemia. (See *Diagnosing hypoglycemia,* page 352.)

Treatment

Effective treatment of reactive hypoglycemia requires dietary modification to help delay glucose absorption and gastric emptying. Usually this includes small, frequent meals; ingestion of complex carbohydrates, fiber, and fat; and avoidance of simple sugars (including alcohol and fruit drinks).[2] The patient may also receive anticholinergic drugs to slow gastric emptying and intestinal motility, and to inhibit vagal stimulation of insulin release.

For fasting hypoglycemia, surgery and drug therapy are usually required. In patients with insulinoma, tumor removal is the treatment of choice. Drug therapy may include nondiuretic thiazides such as diazoxide

Diagnosing hypoglycemia

This flowchart lists possible diagnostic findings and interpretations to assist with treatment of the patient with hypoglycemia.

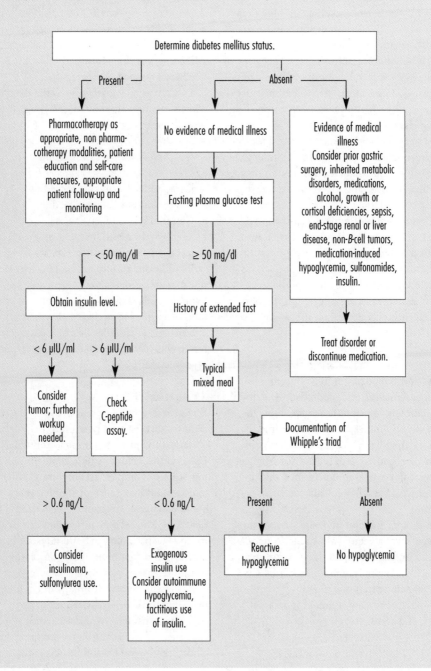

to inhibit insulin secretion; streptozocin; and hormones, such as glucocorticoids and long-acting glycogen.

Preventive measures are part of the therapy for neonates who have hypoglycemia or for those who are at risk for developing it. A hypertonic solution of 10% dextrose in water, calculated at 5 to 10 ml/kg of body weight, administered I.V. over 10 minutes and followed by 4 to 8 mg/kg/minute for maintenance, should correct a severe hypoglycemic state in neonates. To reduce the chance of hypoglycemia in high-risk neonates, they should receive feedings (either breast milk or a solution of 5% to 10% glucose and water) as soon after birth as possible.

Special considerations

▶ Watch for and report signs of hypoglycemia, such as poor feeding, in high-risk neonates.

▶ Monitor the infusion of hypertonic glucose in the neonate to avoid hyperglycemia, circulatory overload, and cellular dehydration. Terminate glucose solutions gradually to prevent hypoglycemia caused by hyperinsulinemia.

▶ Explain to the patient and his family the purpose and procedure for any diagnostic tests. Collect blood samples at the appropriate times, as ordered.

▶ Monitor the effects of drug therapy and watch for the development of any adverse effects.

▶ Teach the patient and his family which foods to include in his diet (complex carbohydrates, fiber, fat) and which foods to avoid (simple sugars, alcohol). Refer the patient and his family for dietary counseling as appropriate.

REFERENCES

1. Stotland, N.E., et al. "Gestational Weight Gain and Adverse Neonatal Outcome among Term Infants," *Obstetrics and Gynecology* 108(3 Pt 1):635-43, September 2006.

2. The National Diabetes Information Clearinghouse Publication No. 03–3926 (2003, March). "Hypoglycemia" [Online]. Available at *www.diabetes.niddk.nih.gov/dm/pubs/ hypoglycemia/index.htm.*

3. Ahlsson, F.S., et al. "Lipolysis and Insulin Sensitivity at Birth in Infants Who Are Large for Gestational Age," *Pediatrics* 120(5):958-65, November 2007.

METABOLIC SYNDROME

Metabolic syndrome—also called *syndrome X, insulin resistance syndrome, dysmetabolic syndrome,* and *multiple metabolic syndrome*—is a cluster of conditions that occur together, increasing an individual's risk of contracting heart disease, stroke, and type 2 diabetes. According to the American Heart Association and the National Heart, Lung, and Blood Institute, the diagnosis is indicated in patients who exhibit three or more of the following conditions:

▶ abdominal obesity (in men, greater than or equal to 40″ [101.6 cm] and in women greater than or equal to 35″ [88.9 cm])

▶ elevated fasting glucose level greater than or equal to 100 mg/dl

▶ elevated triglyceride level

▶ reduced high-density lipoprotein (HDL) cholesterol level (in men less than 40 mg/dl and women less than 50 mg/dl)

▶ high blood pressure greater than or equal to 130/85 mm Hg.[1]

In normal digestion, the intestines break down food into its basic components, one of which is glucose. Glucose is used to provide energy for cellular activity; any excess is stored in cells for future use. Insulin, a hormone secreted in the pancreas, guides glucose into the storage cells. In people with metabolic syndrome, however, the glucose resists prompting from the insulin so the pancreas produces even more insulin to overcome this resistance. This excess in insulin quantity and force damages the artery

Link between gestational diabetes and metabolic syndrome

Question: *Is there a link between gestational diabetes mellitus and the development of metabolic syndrome in women and their children?*

Research: Researchers conducted a review of multiple studies to determine the risk of obesity and metabolic syndrome in women with a history of gestational diabetes mellitus. They also examined the same risks in relation to the children of such mothers. The review compared the development of obesity, hypertension, metabolic abnormalities, metabolic syndrome, and type II diabetes in mothers with a history of gestational diabetes to control mothers and the children of these mothers to those of the control mothers.

Conclusion: The studies demonstrated that women with a prior history of gestational diabetes and obesity are at significantly greater risk for developing metabolic syndrome than mothers with no history of gestational diabetes or obesity. The researchers also found that the development of metabolic syndrome in children correlated to maternal gestational diabetes mellitus, maternal glycemia in the 3rd trimester, maternal obesity, neonatal macrosomia, and childhood obesity.

Application: With the number of adults and children with obesity steadily increasing, the risk of metabolic syndrome continues to rise. When providing teaching, especially to pregnant women or those anticipating pregnancy, the nurse should stress the importance of weight loss and the potential long-term effects of obesity and gestational diabetes on both the mother and the child.

Source: Vohr, B.R., and Boney, C.M. "Gestational Diabetes: The Forerunner for the Development of Maternal and Childhood Obesity and Metabolic Syndrome?" *Journal of Maternal-Fetal and Neonatal Medicine* 21(3): 149-57, March 2008.

linings, promotes fat storage deposits, and prevents fat breakdown. This can lead to diabetes, blood clots, and coronary events.

Causes and incidence

Abdominal obesity is a strong predictor of metabolic syndrome. Intra-abdominal fat tends to be more resistant to insulin than fat in other areas. Insulin is responsible for reducing the amount of fatty acids that reach the liver; when there's resistance, more fatty acids are released into the portal system and the liver. This leads to increased apolipoprotein B, low-density lipoprotein (LDL), and triglyceride levels and a decreased HDL level. These, in turn, increase the risk of cardiovascular disease.

Just as metabolic syndrome puts individuals at greater risk for type 2 diabetes, individuals who have been diagnosed with type 2 diabetes are at risk for metabolic syndrome. (As noted previously, one hallmark for metabolic syndrome is a fasting glucose greater than 100 mg/dl—which is also a measure of pre-diabetes.) Diabetes also puts individuals at risk for coronary heart disease as evidenced by people with diabetes developing atherosclerotic heart disease at a younger age than other people. They're also at increased risk for macrovascular disease (ischemic heart disease, stroke, and peripheral vascular disease).[4]

Insulin resistance and dyslipidemia are also risk factors because insulin resistance leads to hyperinsulinemia, hyperglycemia, abnormal glucose and lipid metabolism, damaged endothelium, and cardiovascular

disease. Dyslipidemia also leads to cardiovascular disease.

High blood pressure is a risk factor because the combination of insulin resistance, hyperinsulinemia, and abdominal obesity leads to hypertension and its harmful cardiovascular effects.[5]

Research indicates that there also may be a genetic predisposition to metabolic syndrome. (See *Link between gestational diabetes and metabolic syndrome.*)

Metabolic syndrome can be found in over 50 million Americans.[1] 60% of people who are obese have metabolic syndrome. Research has also shown that children who are overweight and have increased risk factors for metabolic syndrome are at a significantly increased risk for developing metabolic syndrome as an adult.[2]

Signs and symptoms

Assessment commonly reveals a history of hypertension, sedentary lifestyle, poor diet, and a family history of metabolic syndrome. Physical findings—as mentioned previously—include abdominal obesity, blood pressure 130/85 mm Hg or higher, and a fasting blood glucose level that's 100 mg/dl or higher. The patient may feel tired, especially after eating, and may have difficulty losing weight.

Complications

▶ Coronary artery disease[4]
▶ Diabetes
▶ Hyperlipidemia
▶ Premature death

Diagnosis

Blood studies commonly indicate elevated blood glucose levels, hyperinsulinemia, and elevated serum uric acid levels. Lipid profile studies reveal elevated LDL and triglyceride levels and low HDL levels. Further diagnostic procedures are nonspecific, but may be performed to detect hypertension, diabetes, hyperlipidemia, and hyperinsulinemia.

Treatment

Lifestyle modification, focusing on weight reduction through diet and exercise, is an important part of the treatment regimen. Modest weight reduction considerably improves hemoglobin A_{1C} levels, reduces insulin resistance, improves blood lipid levels, and decreases blood pressure.[5] For patients with impaired glucose tolerance, recent studies have shown that losing an average of 7% of body weight reduced the risk of developing Type 2 diabetes by 58%.

The best diet to improve cardiovascular health is rich in vegetables, fruits, whole grains, fish, and low-fat dairy products. Moreover, nutrient-dense, low-energy foods should replace low-nutrient, high-calorie foods. Meal replacements and shakes may also reduce risk factors for metabolic syndrome and improve weight loss. (See *Therapeutic lifestyle change diet,* page 356.)

Dietary modifications should be paired with a regular exercise program of moderate physical activity—defined by the Surgeon General's Report on Physical Activity and Health as a minimum of 30 minutes on most (if not all) days of the week.[3] This can promote weight loss, improve insulin sensitivity, and reduce blood glucose levels.[6] The selected exercise program should improve cardiovascular conditioning, increase strength through resistance training, and improve flexibility. [6]

Medications may be used to treat metabolic syndrome in patients who have a body mass index (BMI) of 27 kg/m[2] or greater in the presence of other risk factors (such as diabetes, hypertension, and hyperlipidemia); or for patients with a BMI of 30 kg/m[2] or greater without other risk factors. Weight loss medications may also be added to the treatment regimen if the patient hasn't achieved significant weight loss after 12 weeks.

Pharmacologic treatment can include the use of such drugs as phentermine, orlistat, and sibutramine. Phentermine is useful for

Therapeutic lifestyle change diet

The therapeutic lifestyle change diet is low in saturated fats and cholesterol to reduce blood cholesterol levels and prevent development of heart disease and its complications.

NUTRIENT	RECOMMENDED INTAKE
Saturated fat*	< 7% of total calories
Polyunsaturated fat	Up to 10% of total calories
Monounsaturated fat	Up to 20% of total calories
Total fat	25% to 35% of total calories
Carbohydrate**	50% to 60% of total calories
Fiber	20 to 30 gm/day
Protein	Approximately 15% of total calories
Cholesterol	< 200 mg/day
Total calories***	Balance energy intake and expenditure to maintain desirable body weight and prevent weight gain

*Trans fatty acids are another low-density lipoprotein-raising fat that should be kept at a low intake.
**Carbohydrates should be derived predominantly from foods rich in complex carbohydrates, including grains—especially whole grains, fruits, and vegetables.
***Daily expenditure should include at least moderate physical activity (contributing approximately 200 kcal/day).

Source: The National Heart, Blood, and Lung Institute. Available: www.nhlbi.nih.gov/cgi-bin/chd/step2intro.cgi

short-term treatment of obesity in conjunction with diet and exercise. Orlistat decreases the absorption of dietary fat by inhibiting pancreatic lipase, which is needed for fat breakdown and absorption. However, because orlistat may reduce the absorption of fat-soluble vitamins, the patient may require vitamin supplements. Studies show that obese patients who take orlistat in conjunction with dieting achieve greater weight loss and serum glucose control than by dieting alone. Sibutramine promotes weight loss by inhibiting the reuptake of serotonin, norepinephrine, and dopamine, and increases the satiety-producing effects of serotonin. It also reduces the drop in metabolic rate that commonly occurs with weight loss.

Surgical treatment of obesity, such as gastric bypass procedures, produces a greater degree and duration of weight loss than other therapies and improves or resolves most of the factors of metabolic syndrome. Candidates for surgical intervention include patients with a BMI greater than 40 kg/m² or those with a BMI greater than 35 kg/m² with obesity-related medical conditions. Gastric bypass procedures produce permanent weight loss in the majority of patients.

Special considerations

▶ Monitor the patient's blood pressure, blood glucose, blood cholesterol, and insulin levels.[5]
▶ Encourage patients with metabolic syndrome to begin an exercise and weight loss program with a friend or family member or, if that isn't feasible, support him in exploring other options. Research indicates that longer lifestyle modification programs are associated with improved weight loss maintenance.[6]
▶ To improve compliance, schedule frequent follow-up appointments with the patient. At that time, review his food diaries and exercise logs. Be positive and promote his active participation and partnership in his treatment plan.

REFERENCES

1. American Heart Association. "Metabolic Syndrome" [Online]. Available at *www. americanheart.org/presenter.jhtml?identifier=4756.*
2. Morrison, J.A., et al. "Metabolic Syndrome in Childhood Predicts Adult Metabolic Syndrome and Type 2 Diabetes Mellitus 25 to 30 Years Later," *Journal of Pediatrics* 152(2):201-206, February 2008.
3. National Center for Chronic Disease Prevention and Health Promotion (1999, November 16). "Physical Activity and Health, A Report of the Surgeon General" [Online]. Available at *www.cdc.gov/nccdphp/sgr/ adults.htm.*
4. Obunai, K., et al. "Cardiovascular Morbidity and Mortality of the Metabolic Syndrome," *The Medical Clinics of North America* 91(6):1169-84, November 2007.
5. Lann, D., and LeRoith, D. "Insulin Resistance as the Underlying Cause for the Metabolic Syndrome," *The Medical Clinics of North America* 91(6):1063-77, November 2007.
6. Johnson, J.L., et al. "Exercise Training Amount and Intensity Effects on Metabolic Syndrome (from Studies of a Targeted Risk Reduction Intervention through Defined Exercise)," *American Journal of Cardiology* 100(12):1759-66, December 2007.

OBESITY

O besity is an excess of body fat, generally 20% above ideal body weight. The prognosis for weight correction is poor. Fewer than 30% of patients succeed in losing 20 lb (9 kg), and only one-half of these maintain the loss over a prolonged period.

Causes and incidence

Obesity is the result of excessive calorie intake paired with an inadequate expenditure of energy. A number of theories have been proposed to explain this condition: they include abnormal absorption of nutrients, genetic predisposition, hypothalamic dysfunction of hunger and satiety centers, and im-

paired action of GI and growth hormones and hormonal regulators such as insulin. In women especially, an inverse relationship between socioeconomic status and the prevalence of obesity has been documented.

Obesity in parents increases the probability of obesity in children, through genetic or environmental factors such as activity levels and learned patterns of eating. Psychological factors, such as stress or emotional eating, may also contribute. There have been no significant changes in obesity prevalence among men and women since the 2003-2004 National Health and Nutrition Examination Survey; obesity rates are still high—34% of adults in the United States age 20 and older are considered obese.[1] According to that survey, an estimated 17% of children ages 2 to 19 are overweight. This number has increased from previous years.[2]

Complications
▶ Respiratory difficulties
▶ Hypertension
▶ Cardiovascular disease
▶ Diabetes mellitus
▶ Renal disease
▶ Gallbladder disease
▶ Psychosocial difficulties
▶ Premature death

Diagnosis
Body mass index (BMI) is used to determine whether an individual is overweight or obese.

BMI is a measure of body fat using height and weight measurements. In an adult, a BMI between 25 and 29.9 kg/m^2 is considered overweight and a BMI of greater than or equal to 30 kg/m^2 is considered obese.[3] In children, BMI compares height and weight against a growth chart that's adjusted for age and sex. BMI is reported as a BMI-for-age percentile. Children who are overweight have a BMI-for-age in the 95th percentile or greater.[3] Waist circumference is also measured to determine health risks related to

obesity. Risk for heart disease and type 2 diabetes is increased by a waist size greater than 35" (88.9 cm) for women and 40" (101.6 cm) for men.[3]

Measurement of the thickness of subcutaneous fat folds with calipers provides an approximation of total body fat. Although this measurement is reliable and isn't subject to daily fluctuations, it has little meaning for the patient in monitoring subsequent weight loss.

Treatment

To lose weight, the patient must decrease his daily calorie intake while increasing his activity level. Meals should be built around a balanced, low-calorie diet that eliminates foods high in fat or sugar.[4] Moderate intensity activity should be done for at least 30 minutes most days of the week to maintain overall health.[3] To lose weight, 60 to 90 minutes of moderate-intensity activity should be done daily.[3] Lifelong maintenance of these improved eating and exercise patterns is necessary to achieve long-term benefits.

The popular low-carbohydrate diets offer no long-term advantage; rapid early weight reduction is due to loss of water, not fat. These and other crash or fad diets have one huge drawback: they don't teach the patient how to modify eating patterns over the long term, and these diets often lead to the "yo-yo syndrome"—repeated episodes of weight loss followed by weight gain. This can be more detrimental than the obesity itself because of the severe stress this places on the body.[7]

Prolonged fasting and very-low-calorie diets have been associated with sudden death, possibly resulting from cardiac arrhythmias caused by electrolyte abnormalities. These methods also neglect patient re-education, which is necessary for long-term weight maintenance.

Comprehensive treatment may also include hypnosis and behavior modification techniques, which promote fundamental changes in eating habits and activity patterns. In addition, psychotherapy may be beneficial for some patients who tend to overeat in response to stress. Antidepressants are also helpful in weight loss for some patients.

Weight loss medications, such as sibutramine and orlistat, can be used along with diet and exercise to promote weight reduction.[3] A low-dose form of orlistat was approved for over-the-counter use in 2007.

Other medications not approved for weight loss may also be helpful. Topiramate and zonisamide, used to treat seizures, have been shown to promote weight loss and are being studied for effectiveness in the treatment of obesity.[3] Metformin, used to treat diabetes, may cause weight loss in people with obesity and diabetes, and has been shown to reduce hunger and food intake.[3]

As a last resort, morbid obesity, which is indicated by body weight that's 50% to 100% higher than ideal, body weight that's 100 pounds higher than ideal, or a BMI greater than 39 kg/m^2, may be treated surgically with a variety of restrictive procedures.[5] The two most popular bariatric surgeries are vertical-banded gastroplasty and gastric bypass surgery. These procedures decrease the volume of food that the stomach can hold or bypass the stomach, with the goal of producing satiety with a smaller intake. Bypassing the stomach also induces diarrhea when concentrated sweets are ingested. These techniques cause fewer complications than jejunoileal bypass, which induces a permanent malabsorption syndrome. Extended liquid diets are necessary adjuncts to surgery. Psychological counseling is also recommended.

Special considerations

▶ Obtain an accurate diet history to identify the patient's eating patterns and the importance of food to his lifestyle. Ask the patient to keep a careful record of what, where, and

when he eats to help identify situations that normally provoke overeating.[4]

▶ Explain the prescribed diet carefully, and encourage compliance to improve health status.

▶ Promote increased physical activity, including an exercise program, to increase calorie expenditure. Recommend varying activity levels according to the patient's general condition and cardiovascular status.

▶ Watch carefully for signs of dependence or abuse if the patient is taking appetite-suppressing drugs; also watch for adverse effects, such as insomnia, excitability, dry mouth, and GI disturbances.

▶ Teach the grossly obese patient the importance of good skin care to prevent breakdown in moist skin folds. Recommend the regular use of powder to keep skin dry.

▶ To help prevent obesity in children, teach parents to avoid overfeeding their infants and to familiarize themselves with actual nutritional needs and optimum growth rates. Discourage parents from using food to reward or console their children, from requiring children to eat everything on their plate, and from allowing children to eat to prevent hunger rather than to satisfy it.[6]

▶ Encourage physical activity and exercise, especially in children and young adults, to establish lifelong patterns. Suggest low-calorie snacks such as raw vegetables.

REFERENCES

1. National Center for Health Statistics (2007, November 28). "New CDC Study Finds No Increase in Obesity Among Adults; But Levels Still High" [Online]. Available at *www.cdc.gov/ nchs/pressroom/07newsreleases/obesity.htm.*

2. National Center for Health Statistics (2007, January 30). "Prevalence of Overweight Among Children and Adolescents: United States, 2003-2004" [Online]. Available at *www.cdc.gov/nchs/products/pubs/pubd/ hestats/overweight/overwght_child_03.htm.*

3. National Heart Lung and Blood Institute. "Overweight and Obesity" [Online]. Available

at *www.nhlbi.nih.gov/health/dci/Diseases/ obe/obe_diagnosis.html.*

4. Kris-Etherton, P.M., et al. "Position of the American Dietetic Association and Dietitians of Canada: Dietary Fatty Acids," *Journal of the American Dietetic Association* 107(9):1599-611, September 2007.

5. DeMaria, E.J., "Bariatric Surgery for Morbid Obesity," *New England Journal of Medicine* 356(21):2176-83, May 2007.

6. Joanna Briggs Institute. "Effective Dietary Interventions for Managing Overweight and Obesity in Children," *Nursing New Zealand* 13(5):30-31, June 2007.

7. Tay, J., et al. "Metabolic Effects of Weight Loss on a Very-low-carbohydrate Diet Compared with an Isocaloric High-carbohydrate Diet in Abdominally Obese Subjects," *Journal of the American College of Cardiology* 51(1):59-67, January 2008.

SYNDROME OF INAPPROPRIATE ANTIDIURETIC HORMONE

Syndrome of inappropriate antidiuretic hormone (SIADH), also known as *dilutional hyponatremia*, is marked by excessive release of antidiuretic hormone (ADH), which disturbs fluid and electrolyte balance. Such disturbances result from the inability to excrete dilute urine, free water retention, extracellular fluid volume expansion, and hyponatremia. SIADH occurs secondary to diseases that affect the osmoreceptors (supraoptic nucleus) of the hypothalamus. The prognosis depends on the underlying disorder and response to treatment.

Causes

Oat cell carcinoma of the lung, which secretes excessive ADH or vasopressor-like substances, can cause SIADH. Other neoplastic diseases, such as pancreatic and prostatic cancer, Hodgkin's disease, and thymoma, may also trigger SIADH.

Watch for signs of hyponatremia

Question: *Is hyponatremia a common electrolyte abnormality in critically ill patients?*

Research: This study of the diagnosis, pathophysiology, and management of hyponatremia among critically ill, hospitalized patients was performed through searches of English-language literature published between 1967 and 2006, by accessing MEDLINE and ScienceDirect, and reviewing meeting abstracts from scientific sessions and clinical trials of drugs.

Conclusion: Researchers concluded from their studies that hyponatremia is the most common electrolyte disorder found in critically ill, hospitalized patients. It can develop in patients with congestive heart failure and syndrome of inappropriate antidiuretic hormone secretion as well as many other conditions, regardless of whether the patient is hypervolemic, euvolemic, or hypovolemic. The results of the study suggest that delays in diagnosis and incorrect medical management may lead to increased morbidity and mortality from hyponatremia.

Application: Hyponatremia can be associated with significant morbidity and mortality in critically ill patients because it may not be diagnosed and treated in a timely and appropriate manner. The nurse caring for critically ill patients should be knowledgeable about the risk factors of hyponatremia and closely observe the patient for any related signs and symptoms. Laboratory test results should also be monitored closely. The physician must be notified immediately if hyponatremia is suspected so that appropriate treatment can be instituted.

Source: Patel, G.P., and Balk, R.A. "Recognition and Treatment of Hyponatremia in Acutely Ill Hospitalized Patients," *Clinical Therapeutics* 29(2):211-29, February 2007.

Less common causes include:
- central nervous system disorders: brain tumor or abscess, stroke, head injury, Guillain-Barré syndrome, and lupus erythematosus
- pulmonary disorders: pneumonia, tuberculosis, lung abscess, and positive-pressure ventilation
- drugs: chlorpropamide, vincristine, cyclophosphamide, carbamazepine, clofibrate, morphine, exogenous vasopressin, nonsteroidal anti-inflammatory drugs, nicotine, diuretics, tricyclic antidepressants, selective serotonin reuptake inhibitors, and thioridazine[2]
- miscellaneous conditions: myxedema and psychosis.

Signs and symptoms
SIADH may produce weight gain despite anorexia, nausea, vomiting, muscle weakness, restlessness and, possibly, coma and seizures. Edema is rare unless water overload exceeds 4 liters because much of the free water excess is within cellular boundaries.

Complications
- Water intoxication
- Cerebral edema
- Severe hyponatremia (see *Watch for signs of hyponatremia*)
- Coma and death

Diagnosis
A complete medical history revealing positive water balance may suggest SIADH. Serum osmolality less than 280 mOsm/kg of water and a serum sodium level below 123 mEq/L confirm the diagnosis (normal urine osmolality is 1½ times serum values).[1]

Supportive laboratory values include high urine sodium secretion (more than 20 mEq/L) without diuretics and high urine osmolality (greater than 100 mOsm/L).[1] In addition, diagnostic studies show normal renal function and no evidence of dehydration.

Treatment

Treatment for SIADH is symptomatic and begins with restricted water intake (500 to 1,000 ml/day). Some patients who continue to have symptoms are given a high-salt, high-protein diet or urea supplements to enhance water excretion. They may also receive demeclocycline or lithium to help block the renal response to ADH.[1] With severe water intoxication, administration of 200 to 300 ml of 5% saline solution may be necessary to raise the serum sodium level. When possible, treatment should include correction of the underlying cause of SIADH. If the disorder is due to cancer, success in alleviating water retention may be obtained by surgical resection, irradiation, or chemotherapy.

Special considerations

▶ Closely monitor and record intake and output, vital signs, and daily weight. Watch for hyponatremia.

▶ Observe for restlessness, irritability, seizures, heart failure, and unresponsiveness due to hyponatremia and water intoxication.

▶ To prevent water intoxication, explain to the patient and his family why he must restrict his intake.

REFERENCES

1. Ellison, D.H., and Berl, T. "Clinical Practice. The Syndrome of Inappropriate Antidiuresis," *New England Journal of Medicine* 356(20):2064-72, May 2007.
2. Rottmann, C.N. "SSRIs and the Syndrome of Inappropriate Antidiuretic Hormone Secretion," *AJN* 107(1):51-58, January 2007.

10

Endocrine disorders

ADRENAL HYPOFUNCTION

Primary adrenal hypofunction (also called *adrenal insufficiency* or *Addison's disease*) originates within the adrenal gland itself and is characterized by decreased mineralocorticoid, glucocorticoid, and androgen secretion. Adrenal hypofunction can also occur secondary to a disorder outside the gland (such as a pituitary tumor, with corticotropin deficiency), but aldosterone secretion frequently continues intact. Although it's a relatively uncommon disorder, primary adrenal hypofunction can occur at any age and in both sexes. Secondary adrenal hypofunction is more common and can occur when a patient abruptly stops taking long-term exogenous steroid therapy. With early diagnosis and adequate replacement therapy, the prognosis for adrenal hypofunction is good.

Adrenal crisis (addisonian crisis), a critical deficiency of mineralocorticoids and glucocorticoids, generally follows acute stress, sepsis, trauma, surgery, or omission of steroid therapy in patients who have chronic adrenal insufficiency. A medical emergency, adrenal crisis necessitates immediate, vigorous treatment.

Causes and incidence

Primary adrenal hypofunction occurs when more than 90% of both adrenal glands are destroyed, an occurrence that typically results from an autoimmune process in which circulating antibodies react specifically against the adrenal tissue. 70% of reported cases are caused by an autoimmune disorder.[1] Other causes include tuberculosis (once the chief cause; now responsible for less than 20% of cases,[1] bilateral adrenalectomy, hemorrhage into the adrenal gland, neoplasms, and infections (acquired immunodeficiency syndrome, histoplasmosis, and cytomegalovirus).[2] Rarely, a familial tendency to autoimmune disease predisposes the patient to adrenal hypofunction and other endocrinopathies.

Secondary adrenal hypofunction that results in glucocorticoid deficiency can stem from hypopituitarism (causing decreased corticotropin secretion), abrupt withdrawal of long-term corticosteroid therapy (long-term exogenous corticosteroid stimulation suppresses pituitary corticotropin secretion and results in adrenal gland atrophy), or removal of a nonendocrine, corticotropin-secreting tumor. Adrenal crisis follows when trauma, surgery, or other physiologic stress exhausts the body's stores of glucocorticoids in a person with adrenal hypofunction. Current research shows that the use of etomidate in trauma patients may increase the risk of developing adrenal hypofunction.[3]

In adults, it affects 1 in 100,000 people.[1] There's no racial predilection.

Signs and symptoms

Adrenal hypofunction typically produces such effects as weakness, fatigue, weight loss, and various GI disturbances, such as nausea, vomiting, anorexia, and chronic diarrhea. When primary, the disorder usually causes a conspicuous bronze coloration of the skin. The patient appears to be deeply suntanned, especially in the creases of the hands and over the metacarpophalangeal joints, the elbows, and the knees. He may also exhibit a darkening of scars, areas of vitiligo (absence of pigmentation), and increased pigmentation of the mucous membranes, especially the buccal mucosa. Abnormal skin and mucous membrane coloration results from decreased secretion of cortisol (one of the glucocorticoids), which causes the pituitary gland to simultaneously secrete excessive amounts of corticotropin and melanocyte-stimulating hormone (MSH).

Associated cardiovascular abnormalities in adrenal hypofunction include orthostatic hypotension, decreased cardiac size and output, and a weak, irregular pulse. Other clinical effects include decreased tolerance for even minor stress, poor coordination, fasting hypoglycemia (due to decreased gluconeogenesis), and a craving for salty food. Adrenal hypofunction may also retard axillary and pubic hair growth in females, decrease the libido (from decreased androgen production) and, in severe cases, cause amenorrhea.

Secondary adrenal hypofunction produces similar clinical effects but without hyperpigmentation because corticotropin and MSH levels are low. Because aldosterone secretion may continue at fairly normal levels in secondary adrenal hypofunction, this condition doesn't necessarily cause accompanying hypotension and electrolyte abnormalities.

Complications

▶ Adrenal crisis—profound weakness, fatigue, nausea, vomiting, hypotension, dehydration and, occasionally, high fever followed by hypothermia. If untreated, this condition can ultimately lead to vascular collapse, renal shutdown, coma, and death.

Diagnosis

Diagnosis requires demonstration of decreased corticosteroid concentrations in plasma and an accurate classification of adrenal hypofunction as primary or secondary. If secondary adrenal hypofunction is suspected, the metyrapone test is indicated. This test requires oral or I.V. administration of metyrapone, which blocks cortisol production and should stimulate the release of corticotropin from the hypothalamic-pituitary system. In adrenal hypofunction, the hypothalamic-pituitary system responds normally, and plasma reveals high levels of corticotropin; however, plasma levels of cortisol precursor and urinary concentrations of 17-hydroxycorticosteroids don't rise.

If either primary or secondary adrenal hypofunction is suspected, a short corticotropin stimulation test may be done. If both corticotropin and cortisol are low, the long corticotropin test may be done. The test requires I.V. administration of corticotropin over 6 to 8 hours, after samples have been obtained to determine baseline plasma cortisol and 24-hour urine cortisol levels. In adrenal hypofunction, plasma and urine cortisol levels fail to rise normally in response to corticotropin; in secondary hypofunction, repeated doses of corticotropin over successive days produce a gradual increase in cortisol levels until normal values are reached.

In a patient with typical addisonian symptoms, the following laboratory findings strongly suggest acute adrenal hypofunction:
▶ decreased cortisol levels in plasma (less than 10 mcg/dl in the morning, with lower levels in the evening); however, this test is time-consuming, and emergency therapy shouldn't be postponed for test results
▶ decreased serum sodium and fasting blood glucose levels

▶ increased serum potassium and blood urea nitrogen levels

▶ elevated hematocrit and lymphocyte and eosinophil counts

▶ X-rays showing a small heart and adrenal calcification.

Treatment

For all patients with primary or secondary adrenal hypofunction, corticosteroid replacement, usually with cortisone or hydrocortisone (both of which also have a mineralocorticoid effect) is the primary treatment and must continue throughout life. Adrenal hypofunction may also necessitate treatment with I.V. desoxycorticosterone, a pure mineralocorticoid, or oral fludrocortisone, a synthetic mineralocorticoid; both prevent dangerous dehydration and hypotension.

Adrenal crisis requires prompt I.V. bolus administration of hydrocortisone. Later, doses are given I.M. or are diluted with dextrose in saline solution and given I.V. until the patient's condition stabilizes.

With proper treatment, adrenal crisis usually subsides quickly; the patient's blood pressure should stabilize, and water and sodium levels should return to normal. After the crisis, maintenance doses of hydrocortisone preserve physiologic stability.[5]

Special considerations

In adrenal crisis, monitor vital signs carefully, especially for hypotension, volume depletion, and other signs of shock (decreased level of consciousness and urine output). Watch for hyperkalemia before treatment and for hypokalemia after treatment (from excessive mineralocorticoid effect).[4]

▶ If the patient also has diabetes, check blood glucose levels periodically because steroid replacement may require adjustment of insulin dosage.

▶ Record weight and intake and output carefully because the patient may have volume depletion. Until the onset of the mineralocorticoid effect, force fluids to replace excessive fluid loss.

To manage the patient receiving maintenance therapy:

▶ Arrange for a diet that maintains sodium and potassium balances.

▶ If the patient is anorectic, suggest six small meals a day to increase calorie intake. Ask the dietitian to provide a diet high in protein and carbohydrates. Keep a late-morning snack available in case the patient becomes hypoglycemic.[5]

▶ Observe the patient receiving steroids for cushingoid signs such as fluid retention around the eyes and face. Watch for fluid and electrolyte imbalance, especially if the patient is receiving mineralocorticoids. Monitor weight and check blood pressure to assess body fluid status. Remember, steroids administered in the late afternoon or evening may cause stimulation of the central nervous system and insomnia in some patients. Check for petechiae because the patient bruises easily.

▶ If the patient receives glucocorticoids alone, observe for orthostatic hypotension or electrolyte abnormalities, which may indicate a need for mineralocorticoid therapy.[5]

▶ Explain that lifelong steroid therapy is necessary.

▶ Teach the patient the symptoms of too great or too little a dose.[5]

▶ Tell the patient that the dosage may need to be increased during times of stress (when he has a cold for example).

▶ Warn that infection, injury, or profuse sweating in hot weather may precipitate adrenal crisis.

▶ Warn the patient that any stress may necessitate additional cortisone to prevent adrenal crisis.

▶ Instruct the patient to always carry a medical identification card stating that he takes a steroid and giving the name of the drug and the dosage.

▶ Tell the patient to keep an emergency kit available containing hydrocortisone in a prepared syringe for use in times of stress.
▶ Teach the patient how to give himself an injection of hydrocortisone.

REFERENCES

1. National Endocrine and Metabolic Diseases Information Service Publication No. 04–3054 (June, 2004). "Addison's Disease" [Online]. Available at *www.endocrine.niddk.nih.gov/pubs/addison/addison.htm.*
2. Alevritis, E.M., et al. "Infectious Causes of Adrenal Insufficiency," *Southern Medical Journal* 96(9):888-90, September 2003.
3. Cotton, B.A., et al. "Increased Risk of Adrenal Insufficiency Following Etomidate Exposure in Critically Injured Patients," *Archives of Surgery* 143(1):62-67, January 2008.
4. Pfadt, E., and Carlson, D.S. "Acute Adrenal Crisis," *Nursing* 36(8):80, August 2006.
5. Salvatori, R. "Adrenal Insufficiency" *JAMA* 294(19):2481-88, November 2005.

CUSHING'S SYNDROME

Cushing's syndrome is a cluster of clinical abnormalities caused by excessive levels of adrenocortical hormones (particularly cortisol) or related corticosteroids and, to a lesser extent, androgens and aldosterone. Its unmistakable signs include rapidly developing adiposity of the face (moon face), neck, and trunk and purple striae on the skin. (See *Symptoms of cushingoid syndrome,* page 366.) The prognosis depends on the underlying cause; it's poor in untreated people and in those with untreatable ectopic corticotropin-producing carcinoma.

Causes and incidence

In approximately 70% of patients, Cushing's syndrome results from excessive production of corticotropin and consequent hyperplasia of the adrenal cortex. Overproduction of corticotropin may stem from pituitary hypersecretion (Cushing's disease), a corticotropin-producing tumor in another organ (particularly bronchogenic or pancreatic cancer), or excessive administration of exogenous glucocorticoids.

In the remaining 30% of patients, Cushing's syndrome results from a cortisol-secreting adrenal tumor, which is usually benign. In infants, the usual cause of Cushing's syndrome is adrenal carcinoma.

Cushing's syndrome affects 10 to 15 of every 1 million people.[1] It's more common in females than in males and occurs primarily between ages 25 and 40.

Signs and symptoms

Like other endocrine disorders, Cushing's syndrome induces changes in multiple body systems, depending on the adrenocortical hormone involved. Clinical effects may include the following:
▶ *Endocrine and metabolic systems:* diabetes mellitus, with decreased glucose tolerance, fasting hyperglycemia, and glycosuria
▶ *Musculoskeletal system:* muscle weakness due to hypokalemia or to loss of muscle mass from increased catabolism, pathologic fractures due to decreased bone mineral, and skeletal growth retardation in children
▶ *Skin:* purplish striae; fat pads above the clavicles, over the upper back (buffalo hump), on the face (moon face), and throughout the trunk, with slender arms and legs; little or no scar formation; poor wound healing; acne and hirsutism in females
▶ *GI system:* peptic ulcer, resulting from increased gastric secretions and pepsin production, and decreased gastric mucus
▶ *Central nervous system (CNS):* irritability and emotional lability, ranging from euphoric behavior to depression or psychosis; insomnia
▶ *Cardiovascular system:* hypertension due to sodium and water retention; left ventricular hypertrophy; capillary weakness due to protein loss, which leads to bleeding, petechiae, and ecchymosis

Symptoms of cushingoid syndrome

Chronic depression, alcoholism, and long-term treatment with corticosteroids may produce an adverse effect called *cushingoid syndrome*—a condition marked by obvious fat deposits between the shoulders and around the waist and widespread systemic abnormalities.

Differentiating between cushingoid syndrome and Cushing's syndrome can be difficult, so in addition to the symptoms shown in the illustration at right, observe for signs of hypertension, renal disorders, hyperglycemia, tissue wasting, muscle weakness, and labile emotional state. The patient may also have amenorrhea and glycosuria.

Resolution of the underlying disorder results in disappearance of cushingoid symptoms.

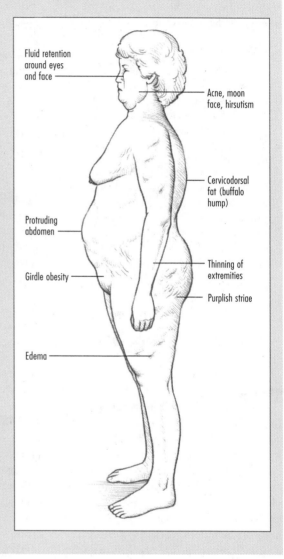

Fluid retention around eyes and face

Acne, moon face, hirsutism

Cervicodorsal fat (buffalo hump)

Protruding abdomen

Girdle obesity

Thinning of extremities

Purplish striae

Edema

▶ *Immune system:* increased susceptibility to infection due to decreased lymphocyte production and suppressed antibody formation; decreased resistance to stress (suppressed inflammatory response may mask even a severe infection)

▶ *Renal and urologic systems:* sodium and secondary fluid retention, increased potassium excretion, inhibited antidiuretic hormone secretion, ureteral calculi from increased bone demineralization with hypercalciuria

▶ *Reproductive system:* increased androgen production with clitoral hypertrophy, mild virilism, and amenorrhea or oligomenorrhea in females; sexual dysfunction also occurs.

Complications

▶ Osteoporosis and pathologic fractures
▶ Peptic ulcer
▶ Dyslipidosis
▶ Impaired glucose tolerance
▶ Diabetes mellitus
▶ Frequent infections
▶ Hypertension
▶ Menstrual disturbances
▶ Psychiatric problems

Diagnosis

Initially, diagnosis of Cushing's syndrome requires determination of plasma steroid levels. In people with normal hormone balance, plasma cortisol levels are higher in the morning and decrease gradually throughout the day (diurnal variation). In patients with Cushing's syndrome, cortisol levels don't fluctuate and typically remain consistently elevated; 24-hour urine sample demonstrates elevated free cortisol levels.

A low-dose dexamethasone suppression test confirms the diagnosis of Cushing's syndrome. Salivary cortisol levels collected at midnight (usually performed on an outpatient basis) are elevated and are the most sensitive confirmatory test.[2] (See *Diagnosing Cushing's syndrome,* page 368.)

A high-dose dexamethasone suppression test can determine if Cushing's syndrome results from pituitary dysfunction (Cushing's disease). In this test, dexamethasone suppresses plasma cortisol levels, and urinary 17-hydroxycorticosteroid (17-OHCS) and 17-ketogenic steroid levels fall to 50% or less of basal levels. Failure to suppress these levels indicates that the syndrome results from an adrenal tumor or a nonendocrine, corticotropin-secreting tumor. This test can produce false-positive results.[4]

In a stimulation test, administration of metyrapone, which blocks cortisol production by the adrenal glands, tests the ability of the pituitary gland and the hypothalamus to detect and correct low levels of plasma cortisol by increasing corticotropin production.

The patient with Cushing's disease reacts to this stimulus by secreting an excess of plasma corticotropin as measured by levels of urinary 17-OHCS. If the patient has an adrenal or a nonendocrine corticotropin-secreting tumor, the pituitary gland—which is suppressed by the high cortisol levels—can't respond normally, so steroid levels remain stable or fall.

Ultrasound, computed tomography (CT) scan, or angiography localizes adrenal tumors; CT scan and magnetic resonance imaging of the head may identify pituitary tumors.

Treatment

Treatment to restore hormone balance and reverse Cushing's syndrome may necessitate radiation, drug therapy, or surgery. For example, pituitary-dependent Cushing's syndrome with adrenal hyperplasia and severe cushingoid symptoms (such as psychosis, poorly controlled diabetes mellitus, osteoporosis, and severe pathologic fractures) may require partial or complete hypophysectomy or pituitary irradiation. If the patient fails to respond, bilateral adrenalectomy may be performed.[3] Nonendocrine corticotropin-producing tumors require excision of the tumor, followed by drug therapy (for example, with mitotane, metyrapone, or aminoglutethimide) to decrease cortisol levels if symptoms persist.[3]

Aminoglutethimide and ketoconazole decrease cortisol levels and have been beneficial for many cushingoid patients but must be used with caution and monitoring. Aminoglutethimide alone, or in combination with metyrapone, may also be useful in metastatic adrenal carcinoma.

Before surgery, the patient with cushingoid symptoms should have special management to control hypertension, edema, diabetes, and cardiovascular manifestations and to prevent infection. Glucocorticoid administration on the morning of surgery can help

Diagnosing Cushing's syndrome

The flowchart below aids in differential diagnosis of Cushing's syndrome.

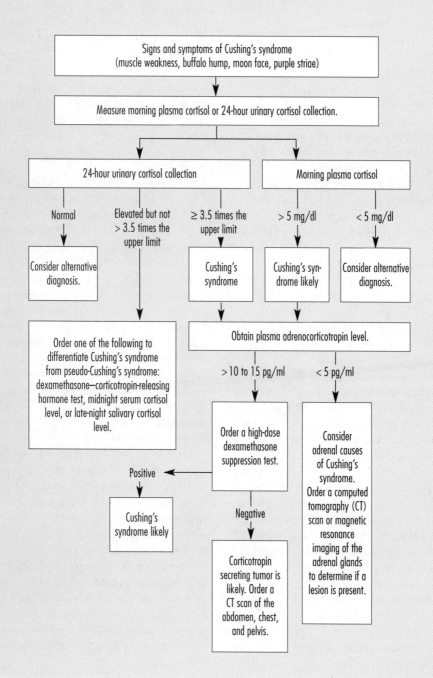

prevent acute adrenal hypofunction during surgery.[3]

Cortisol therapy is essential during and after surgery, to help the patient tolerate the physiologic stress imposed by removal of the pituitary or adrenals. If normal cortisol production resumes, steroid therapy may be gradually tapered and eventually discontinued. However, bilateral adrenalectomy or total hypophysectomy mandates lifelong steroid replacement therapy to correct hormonal deficiencies.

Special considerations

Patients with Cushing's syndrome require painstaking assessment and vigorous supportive care:
▶ Frequently monitor vital signs, especially blood pressure. Carefully observe the hypertensive patient who also has cardiac disease.
▶ Check laboratory reports for hypernatremia, hypokalemia, hyperglycemia, and glycosuria.
▶ Because the cushingoid patient is likely to retain sodium and water, check for edema, and monitor daily weight and intake and output carefully. To minimize weight gain, edema, and hypertension, ask the dietary department to provide a diet that's high in protein and potassium but low in calories, carbohydrates, and sodium.
▶ Watch for infection—a particular problem in Cushing's syndrome.
▶ If the patient has osteoporosis and is bedridden, perform passive range-of-motion exercises carefully because of the severe risk of pathologic fractures.
▶ Remember, Cushing's syndrome produces emotional lability. Record incidents that upset the patient, and try to prevent such situations from occurring if possible. Help him get the physical and mental rest he needs—by sedation if necessary. Offer support to the emotionally labile patient throughout the difficult testing period.

After bilateral adrenalectomy and pituitary surgery:
▶ Report wound drainage or temperature elevation to the patient's physician immediately. Use strict sterile technique in changing the patient's dressings.
▶ Administer analgesics and replacement steroids, as ordered.
▶ Monitor urine output and check vital signs carefully, watching for signs of shock (decreased blood pressure, increased pulse rate, pallor, and cold, clammy skin). To counteract shock, give vasopressors and increase the rate of I.V. fluids, as ordered. Because mitotane, aminoglutethimide, and metyrapone decrease mental alertness and produce physical weakness, assess neurologic and behavioral status, and warn the patient of adverse CNS effects. Also watch for severe nausea, vomiting, and diarrhea.
▶ Check laboratory reports for hypoglycemia due to removal of the source of cortisol, a hormone that maintains blood glucose levels.
▶ Check for abdominal distention and return of bowel sounds after adrenalectomy.
▶ Check regularly for signs of adrenal hypofunction—orthostatic hypotension, apathy, weakness, and fatigue—indicators that steroid replacement is inadequate.
▶ In the patient undergoing pituitary surgery, check for and immediately report signs of increased intracranial pressure (confusion, agitation, changes in level of consciousness, nausea, and vomiting). Watch for hypopituitarism.[3]

Provide comprehensive teaching to help the patient cope with lifelong treatment:
▶ Advise the patient to take replacement steroids with antacids or meals, to minimize gastric irritation. (Usually it's helpful to take two-thirds of the dosage in the morning and the remaining one-third in the early afternoon to mimic diurnal adrenal secretion.)
▶ Tell the patient to carry a medical identification card and to immediately report physiologically stressful situations such as infections, which necessitate increased dosage.

▶ Instruct the patient to watch closely for signs of inadequate steroid dosage (fatigue, weakness, dizziness) and of overdosage (severe edema, weight gain). Emphatically warn against abrupt discontinuation of steroid dosage because this may produce a fatal adrenal crisis.

REFERENCES

1. National Endocrine and Metabolic Diseases Information Service Publication No. 02-3007 (June, 2002). "Cushing's Syndrome" [Online]. Available at *www.endocrine.niddk.nih.gov/pubs/cushings/cushings.htm#introduction*.
2. Gatta, B., et al. "Reevaluation of the Combined Dexamethasone Suppression-corticotropin-releasing Hormone Test for Differentiation of Mild Cushing's Disease from Pseudo-Cushing's Syndrome," *Journal of Clinical Endocrinology and Metabolism* 92(11):4290-93, November 2007.
3. Jagannathan, J., et al. "Gamma Knife Surgery for Cushing's Disease," *Journal of Neurosurgery* 106(6):980-87, June 2007.
4. Erickson, D., et al. "Dexamethasone-suppressed Corticotropin-releasing Hormone Stimulation Test for Diagnosis of Mild Hypercortisolism," *Journal of Clinical Endocrinology and Metabolism* 92(8):2972-76, August 2007.

DIABETES INSIPIDUS

Diabetes insipidus (DI) is a disorder of water metabolism resulting from a deficiency of circulating vasopressin (also called *antidiuretic hormone* [ADH]). It's characterized by excessive fluid intake and hypotonic polyuria. In uncomplicated diabetes insipidus, the prognosis is good with adequate water replacement and replacement of ADH by tablet or nasal spray, and patients usually lead normal lives.

Diabetes insipidus is divided into four types: pituitary DI (also called *central DI* and *neurogenic DI*), gestational DI, nephrogenic DI, and dipsogenic DI.[1]

Causes and incidence

Pituitary diabetes insipidus is the most common type.[1] It results centrally from intracranial neoplastic or metastatic lesions, hypophysectomy or other neurosurgery, a skull fracture, or head trauma that damages the neurohypophyseal structures. It can also result nephrogenically from infection, granulomatous disease, and vascular lesions; it may be idiopathic and, rarely, familial.

Normally, the hypothalamus synthesizes vasopressin. The posterior pituitary gland (or neurohypophysis) stores vasopressin and releases it into general circulation, where it causes the kidneys to reabsorb water by making the distal tubules and collecting duct cells water-permeable. The absence of vasopressin in diabetes insipidus allows the filtered water to be excreted in the urine instead of being reabsorbed.

Nephrogenic diabetes insipidus involves a defect in the parts of the kidneys that reabsorb water back into the bloodstream. It occurs less commonly than central diabetes insipidus. Nephrogenic diabetes insipidus may occur as an inherited disorder in which male children receive the abnormal gene that causes the disease on the X chromosome from their mothers. Nephrogenic diabetes insipidus may also be caused by diseases of the kidney (such as polycystic kidney disease) and the effects of certain drugs (such as lithium and amphotericin B).

Diabetes insipidus is rare, affecting 1 in 25,000 people. Males and females are affected equally.

Signs and symptoms

The patient's history typically shows an abrupt onset of extreme polyuria (usually 4 to 16 L/day of dilute urine but sometimes as much as 30 L/day). As a result, the patient is extremely thirsty and drinks great quantities of water to compensate for the body's water loss. This disorder may also result in nocturia. In severe cases, it may lead to extreme

fatigue from inadequate rest caused by frequent voiding and excessive thirst.

Other characteristic features of diabetes insipidus include signs and symptoms of dehydration (poor tissue turgor, dry mucous membranes, constipation, muscle weakness, dizziness, and hypotension). These symptoms usually begin abruptly, commonly appearing within 1 to 2 days after a basal skull fracture, a stroke, or surgery. Relieving cerebral edema or increased intracranial pressure may cause all of these symptoms to subside just as rapidly as they began.

Complications

▶ Hypovolemia
▶ Hyperosmolality
▶ Circulatory collapse
▶ Loss of consciousness
▶ Central nervous system damage
▶ Bladder distention
▶ Enlarged caliceal
▶ Hydroureter
▶ Hydronephrosis

Diagnosis

Urinalysis reveals almost colorless urine of low osmolality (less than 200 mOsm/kg, less than that of plasma) and low specific gravity (less than 1.005).

Diagnosis requires evidence of vasopressin deficiency, resulting in the kidneys' inability to concentrate urine during a water deprivation test.

In this test, after baseline vital signs, weight, and urine and plasma osmolalities are obtained, the patient is deprived of fluids and observed to make sure he doesn't drink anything surreptitiously. Measurements are taken hourly to record the total volume of urine output, body weight, urine osmolality or specific gravity, and plasma osmolality. Throughout the test, blood pressure and pulse rate must be monitored for signs of orthostatic hypotension. Fluid deprivation continues until the patient loses 3% of his body weight (indicating severe dehydration).

When urine osmolality stops increasing in three consecutive hourly specimens, patients receive 5 units of aqueous vasopressin subcutaneously (subQ).

Hourly measurements of urine volume and specific gravity continue after injection of aqueous vasopressin. Patients with pituitary diabetes insipidus respond to exogenous vasopressin with decreased urine output and increased specific gravity. Patients with nephrogenic diabetes insipidus show no response to vasopressin.

Treatment

Mild cases require no treatment other than fluid intake to replace fluid lost. Until the cause of more severe cases of diabetes insipidus can be identified and eliminated, administration of various forms of vasopressin or of a vasopressin stimulant can control fluid balance and prevent dehydration.[4] Vasopressin injection is an aqueous preparation that's administered subQ or I.M. several times per day because it's effective for only 2 to 6 hours; this form of the drug is used in acute disease and as a diagnostic agent.

Desmopressin acetate can be given by nasal spray that's absorbed through the mucous membranes or by injection given subQ or I.V.; this drug is effective for 8 to 20 hours, depending on the dosage. It's also available in tablet form, to be given at bedtime or in divided doses.[2]

Hydrochlorothiazide can be used in both central and nephrogenic diabetes insipidus.[4] Indomethacin and amiloride are also used for nephrogenic diabetes insipidus. If nephrogenic diabetes insipidus is caused by medication (such as lithium), stopping the medicine leads to kidney recovery.

Special considerations

Patient care includes monitoring symptoms to ensure that fluid balance is restored and maintained.
▶ Record fluid intake and output carefully. Maintain fluid intake that's adequate to pre-

vent severe dehydration. Watch for signs of hypovolemic shock and monitor blood pressure and heart and respiratory rates regularly, especially during the water deprivation test. Check the patient's weight daily.

▶ If the patient is dizzy or has muscle weakness, keep the side rails up and assist him with walking.

▶ Monitor urine specific gravity between doses. Watch for a decrease in specific gravity accompanied by increasing urine output, indicating the recurrence of polyuria and necessitating administration of the next dose of medication or a dosage increase.[4]

▶ Institute safety precautions for the patient who's dizzy or who has muscle weakness.

▶ If constipation develops, add more high-fiber foods and fruit juices to the patient's diet. If necessary, obtain an order for a mild laxative such as milk of magnesia.

▶ Provide meticulous skin and mouth care; apply petroleum jelly, as needed, to cracked or sore lips.

▶ Before discharge, teach the patient how to monitor intake and output.

▶ Instruct the patient to administer desmopressin by nasal spray only after the onset of polyuria—not before—to prevent excess fluid retention and water intoxication.[4]

▶ Tell the patient to report weight gain, which may indicate that his medication dosage is too high. Recurrence of polyuria, as reflected on the intake and output sheet, indicates that the dosage is too low.

▶ Teach the parents of a child with diabetes insipidus about normal growth and development. Discuss how their child may differ from others at his developmental stage.[3]

▶ Encourage the parents to help identify the child's strengths and to use them in developing coping strategies.[3]

▶ Refer the family for counseling if necessary.

▶ Advise the patient with diabetes insipidus to wear a medical identification bracelet and to carry his medication with him at all times.

REFERENCES

1. Robertson, G.L. (2006, December). "What is Diabetes Insipidus?" [Online]. Available at *www.diabetesinsipidus.org/whatisdi.htm*.
2. Gaines, K.K., "Desmopressin (DDAVP) for Enuresis, Diabetes Insipidus, and...," *Urology Nursing* 24(6):520-23, December 2004.
3. Trimarchi, T., "Endocrine Problems in Critically Ill Children: An Overview," *AACN Clinical Issues* 17(1):66-78, January-March 2006.
4. Innis, J., "Treating Nephrogenic Diabetes Insipidus: A Case Study," *Dimensions of Critical Care Nursing* 21(3):98-99, May-June 2002.

DIABETES MELLITUS

Diabetes mellitus (DM) is a chronic disease of absolute or relative insulin deficiency or resistance characterized by disturbances in carbohydrate, protein, and fat metabolism. A leading cause of death by disease in the United States, this syndrome is a contributing factor in about 50% of myocardial infarctions and about 75% of strokes as well as in renal failure and peripheral vascular disease. About 65% of people with DM die of some form of heart or blood vessel disease. It's also the leading cause of new blindness.

DM occurs in four forms classified by etiology: type 1, type 2, other specific types, and gestational diabetes mellitus (GDM). Type 1 is further subdivided into immune-mediated diabetes and idiopathic diabetes. Children and adolescents with type 1 immune-mediated diabetes rapidly develop ketoacidosis, but most adults with this type experience only modest fasting hyperglycemia unless they develop an infection or experience another stressor. Patients with type 1 idiopathic diabetes are prone to ketoacidosis.

Most patients with type 2 diabetes are obese. The "other specific types" category includes people who have diabetes as a result

of a genetic defect, endocrinopathies, or exposure to certain drugs or chemicals. GDM occurs during pregnancy. In this type of diabetes, glucose tolerance levels usually return to normal after delivery.

Causes and incidence

DM affects 20 million children and adults, an estimated 7% of the population of the United State and about one-third of whom are undiagnosed.[2] Incidence is greater in females and rises with age.[2] The incidence in American Indians, Alaska Natives, non-Hispanic Blacks, and Hispanic or Latino Americans is higher than in non-Hispanic Whites.[2] Type I diabetes in children is found in one in every 400 to 600 children.[2] Type 2 accounts for 90% to 95% of cases of diabetes and Type 1 accounts for 5% to 10% of all diagnosed cases.[3]

In type 1 diabetes, pancreatic beta-cell destruction or a primary defect in beta-cell function results in failure to release insulin and ineffective glucose transport. Type 1 immune-mediated diabetes is caused by cell-mediated destruction of pancreatic beta cells. The rate of beta-cell destruction is usually higher in children than in adults.[4] The idiopathic form of type 1 diabetes has no known cause. Patients with this form have no evidence of autoimmunity and don't produce insulin. This form is inherited.[4]

In type 2 diabetes, beta cells release insulin, but receptors are insulin-resistant and glucose transport is variable and ineffective. Risk factors for type 2 diabetes include:
▶ obesity (even an increased percentage of body fat primarily in the abdominal region); risk decreases with weight and drug therapy
▶ lack of physical activity
▶ history of GDM
▶ hypertension
▶ Black, Hispanic, Pacific Islander, Asian American, Native American origin
▶ strong family history of diabetes
▶ older than age 45

▶ high-density lipoprotein cholesterol level less than 35 mg/dl or triglyceride level greater than 250 mg/dl
▶ seriously impaired glucose tolerance test.

The "other specific types" of DM result from various conditions (such as a genetic defect of the beta cells or endocrinopathies) or from the use of or exposure to certain drugs or chemicals. GDM is considered present whenever a patient has any degree of abnormal glucose during pregnancy. This form may result from weight gain and increased levels of estrogen and placental hormones, which antagonize insulin.

Insulin transports glucose into the cell for use as energy and storage as glycogen. It also stimulates protein synthesis and free fatty acid storage in the fat deposits. Insulin deficiency compromises the body tissues' access to essential nutrients for fuel and storage.

Signs and symptoms

Diabetes may begin dramatically with ketoacidosis or insidiously. Its most common symptom is fatigue from energy deficiency and a catabolic state. Insulin deficiency causes hyperglycemia, which pulls fluid from body tissues, causing osmotic diuresis, polyuria, dehydration, polydipsia, dry mucous membranes, poor skin turgor and, in most patients, unexplained weight loss.

In ketoacidosis and hyperosmolar hyperglycemic nonketotic syndrome, dehydration may cause hypovolemia and shock. Wasting of glucose in the urine usually produces weight loss and hunger in type 1 diabetes, even if the patient eats voraciously.

Long-term effects of diabetes may include retinopathy, nephropathy, atherosclerosis, and peripheral and autonomic neuropathy. Peripheral neuropathy usually affects the hands and feet and may cause numbness or pain. Autonomic neuropathy may manifest itself in several ways, including gastroparesis (leading to delayed gastric emptying and a feeling of nausea and fullness after meals),

Classifying fasting blood glucose levels

The American Diabetes Association classifies fasting blood glucose levels as follows:
- Normal: < 100 mg/dl
- Prediabetes: 100 to 125 mg/dl
- Diabetes: ≥ 126 mg/dl

nocturnal diarrhea, impotence, and orthostatic hypotension.

Because hyperglycemia impairs the patient's resistance to infection, diabetes may result in skin and urinary tract infections (UTIs) and vaginitis. Glucose content of the epidermis and urine encourages bacterial growth.

Complications
- Ketoacidosis
- Hyperosmolar coma
- Cardiovascular disease
- Peripheral vascular disease
- Retinopathy
- Nephropathy
- Diabetic dermopathy
- Peripheral and autonomic neuropathy
- Renal failure
- Blindness
- Cognitive depression

Diagnosis
According to the American Diabetes Association (ADA), DM can be diagnosed if any of the following exist:
- symptoms of diabetes (polyuria, polydipsia, and unexplained weight loss) plus a random (non-fasting) blood glucose level greater than or equal to 200 mg/dl accompanied by symptoms of diabetes
- a fasting blood glucose level (no caloric intake for at least 8 hours) greater than or equal to 126 mg/dl

- a plasma glucose value in the 2-hour sample of the oral glucose tolerance test greater than or equal to 200 mg/dl. This test should be performed after a glucose load dose of 75 g of anhydrous glucose.

If results are questionable, the diagnosis should be confirmed by a repeat test on a different day. The ADA also recommends the following testing guidelines:
- Test every 3 years: people age 45 or older without symptoms
- Test immediately: people with the classic symptoms
- High-risk groups should be tested frequently: Individuals with impaired glucose tolerance usually have normal blood levels unless challenged by a glucose load, such as a piece of pie or glass of orange juice. Two hours after a glucose load, the glucose level ranges from 140 to 199 mg/dl. These individuals have an abnormal fasting glucose level between 110 and 125 mg/dl. Because the fasting plasma glucose test is sufficient to make the diagnosis of diabetes, it replaces the oral glucose tolerance test. (See *Classifying fasting blood glucose levels.*)

An ophthalmologic examination may show diabetic retinopathy. Other diagnostic and monitoring tests include urinalysis for acetone and blood testing for glycosylated hemoglobin, which reflects recent glucose cortisol.[1]

Treatment
Effective treatment normalizes blood glucose and decreases complications using insulin replacement, diet, and exercise. Current forms of insulin replacement include single-dose, mixed-dose, split-mixed dose, and multiple-dose regimens. The multiple-dose regimens may use an insulin pump. Insulin may be rapid acting, intermediate acting, long acting, or a combination of rapid acting and intermediate acting; it may be standard or purified, and it may be derived from beef, pork, or human sources. Purified human insulin is used commonly today. Pancreas

transplantation is experimental and requires chronic immunosuppression.

Successful treatment requires extensive dietary education. The patient's diet is specifically tailored to include the right amount and combination of foods. Almost all foods may be eaten occasionally. The diet should address dietary prescriptions as well as personal and cultural preferences to improve adherence and control. For the obese patient with type 2 diabetes, weight reduction is a goal.[7] In type 1 diabetes, the calorie allotment may be high, depending on growth stage and activity level.

Type 2 diabetes may require oral antidiabetic drugs to stimulate endogenous insulin production, increase insulin sensitivity at the cellular level, and suppress hepatic gluconeogenesis.[7]

Five classes of drugs are used to treat diabetes. Sulfonylureas stimulate pancreatic insulin release, increase tissue sensitivity to insulin, and require insulin's presence to work. Meglitinides cause immediate, brief release of insulin and are taken immediately before meals. Biguanides decrease hepatic glucose production and increase tissue sensitivity to insulin. Alpha-glucosidase inhibitors slow the breakdown of glucose and decrease postprandial glucose peaks. The thiazolidinediones enhance the action of insulin; however, insulin must be present for them to work. These drugs also reduce insulin resistance by decreasing hepatic glucose production and increasing glucose uptake. They have also been shown to lower blood pressure in diabetic hypertensive patients. Cholesterol and triglyceride levels may also be reduced. Dipeptidyl peptidase 4 (DPP-4) is a new class of drug for DM.[5] It interferes with the process that breaks down glucagon-like peptide 1, which reduces blood glucose levels in the body. DPP-4 inhibitors don't cause weight gain and have a neutral or positive effect on cholesterol levels.[5]

Treatment of long-term diabetic complications may include transplantation or dialysis for renal failure, photocoagulation for retinopathy, and vascular surgery for large-vessel disease. Meticulous blood glucose control is essential.

Keeping glucose at near-normal levels for 5 years or more reduces both the onset and progression of retinopathy, nephropathy, and neuropathy. In type 2 diabetes, blood pressure control as well as smoking cessation reduces the onset and progression of complications, including cardiovascular disease.[6]

Special considerations

Stress the importance of complying with the prescribed treatment program. Tailor your teaching to the patient's needs, abilities, and developmental stage. (See *Diabetes knowledge among nurses,* page 376.) Include diet; purpose, administration, and possible adverse effects of medication; exercise; monitoring; hygiene; and the prevention and recognition of hypoglycemia and hyperglycemia. Stress the effect of blood glucose control on long-term health.[6]

▶ Watch for acute complications of diabetic therapy, especially hypoglycemia (vagueness, slow cerebration, dizziness, weakness, pallor, tachycardia, diaphoresis, seizures, and coma); immediately give carbohydrates, ideally in the form of fruit juice, glucose tablets, honey or, if the patient is unconscious, glucagon or dextrose I.V.

▶ Be alert for signs of ketoacidosis (acetone breath, dehydration, weak and rapid pulse, and Kussmaul's respirations) and hyperosmolar coma (polyuria, thirst, neurologic abnormalities, and stupor). These hyperglycemic crises require I.V. fluids, insulin and, usually, potassium replacement.

▶ Monitor diabetes control by obtaining blood glucose, glycohemoglobulin, lipid levels, and blood pressure measurements regularly.[1]

▶ Watch for diabetic effects on the cardiovascular system, such as cerebrovascular, coronary artery, and peripheral vascular impairment, and on the peripheral and auto-

EVIDENCE-BASED PRACTICE

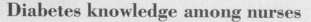

Diabetes knowledge among nurses

Question: *Do nurses require ongoing diabetes management education?*

Research: To determine and compare the diabetes knowledge of nurses and residents in surgical, internal medicine, and family practice, researchers developed and administered a 21-question survey based on current diabetes standards of care. The survey was completed by 52 internal medicine residents, 21 family practice residents, 42 surgical residents, and 48 registered nurses (which included a subgroup of 13 nurses with additional diabetes training). The survey results were stratified by type of participant and analyzed statistically.

Conclusion: The survey showed that the internal medicine and family practice residents and nurses have similar but insufficient levels of knowledge about diabetes, achieving scores of 69%, 64%, and 66% respectively. Surgical residents scored the lowest at 44%; the nurses with extra diabetes training the highest, at 82%. The nurses showed greater knowledge than the residents on questions regarding insulin prepara-

tion, treatment of hypoglycemia, and perioperative insulin management.

Application: To be able to provide optimal care to patients with diabetes, nurses must seek additional and ongoing education in diabetes management, regardless of their area of practice. Nurses caring for patients with diabetes should be prepared to accurately answer the patients' questions and provide teaching about diabetes medications, cardiovascular risk reduction, foot care, nutrition and specialized diets, and physical activity guidelines as well as the prevention of complications, such as hypertension, nephropathy, retinopathy, neuropathy, and periodontal disease.

Source: Rubin, D.J., et al. "Diabetes Knowledge: Are Resident Physicians and Nurses Adequately Prepared to Manage Diabetes?" *Endocrine Practice* 13(1):17-21, January-February 2007.

nomic nervous systems. Treat all injuries, cuts, and blisters (particularly on the legs or feet) meticulously. Be alert for signs of UTI and renal disease.[8]
▶ Urge regular ophthalmologic examinations to detect diabetic retinopathy.
▶ Assess for signs of diabetic neuropathy (numbness or pain in hands and feet, footdrop, neurogenic bladder). Stress the need for personal safety precautions because decreased sensation can mask injuries. Minimize complications by maintaining strict blood glucose control.[8]
▶ Teach the patient to care for his feet by washing them daily, drying carefully between toes, and inspecting for corns, calluses, redness, swelling, bruises, and breaks in the skin. Urge him to report changes to the physician. Advise him to wear nonconstrict-

ing shoes and to avoid walking barefoot. Instruct him to use over-the-counter athlete's foot remedies and seek professional care should athlete's foot not improve.[6]
▶ Teach the patient how to manage his diabetes when he has a minor illness, such as a cold, flu, or upset stomach.[6]
▶ To delay the clinical onset of diabetes, teach people at high risk to avoid risk factors. Advise genetic counseling for young adult diabetics who are planning families.
▶ Further information may be obtained from the Juvenile Diabetes Foundation, the ADA, and the American Association of Diabetes Educators.

REFERENCES

1. Qaseem, A., et al. "Glycemic Control and Type 2 Diabetes Mellitus: The Optimal Hemoglobin

A_{1C} Targets. A Guidance Statement from the American College of Physicians," *Annals of Internal Medicine* 147(6):417-22, September 2007.

2. American Diabetes Association. "Total Prevalence of Diabetes and Pre-diabetes" [Online]. Available at *www.diabetes.org/diabetes-statistics/prevalence.jsp*.

3. Centers for Disease Control and Prevention (2005). "National Diabetes Fact Sheet" [Online]. Available at *www.cdc.gov/diabetes/pubs/pdf/ndfs_2005.pdf*.

4. The American Diabetes Association. "Diagnosis and Classification of Diabetes Mellitus," *Diabetes Care* 31(Suppl 1):S55-60, January 2008.

5. American Diabetes Association. "Other Diabetes Medications" [Online]. Available at *www.diabetes.org/type-2-diabetes/oral-medications.jsp*.

6. Seley, J.J., and Weinger, K. "Executive Summary. The State of the Science on Nursing Best Practices for Diabetes Self-Management," *AJN* 107(6):73-78, June 2007.

7. Meneghini, L., et al. "Appropriate Advancement of Type 2 Diabetes Therapy," *Journal of Family Practice* 56(10 Suppl A):19A-29A, October 2007.

8. Brem, H., et al. "Evidence-based Protocol for Diabetic Foot Ulcers," *Plastic and Reconstructive Surgery* 117(7 Suppl):193S-209S, June 2006.

HYPERALDOSTERONISM

In hyperaldosteronism (Conn's syndrome), hypersecretion of the mineralocorticoid aldosterone by the adrenal cortex causes excessive reabsorption of sodium and water, and excessive renal excretion of potassium.

Causes and incidence

Hyperaldosteronism may be primary (uncommon) or secondary. In 70% of patients, hyperaldosteronism results from a benign aldosterone-producing adrenal adenoma. In 15% to 30% of patients, the cause is unknown; rarely, the cause is bilateral adrenocortical hyperplasia (in children) or carcinoma. Incidence is higher in females than in males (ratio 2:1) and is highest between ages 30 and 50.

In primary hyperaldosteronism, chronic aldosterone excess is independent of the renin-angiotensin system and, in fact, suppresses plasma renin activity. This aldosterone excess enhances sodium reabsorption by the kidneys, which leads to mild hypernatremia and, simultaneously, hypokalemia and increased extracellular fluid (ECF) volume. Expansion of intravascular fluid volume also occurs and results in volume-dependent hypertension and increased cardiac output. Excessive ingestion of English black licorice or licorice-like substances can produce a syndrome similar to primary hyperaldosteronism due to the mineralocorticoid action of glycyrrhizic acid.

Secondary hyperaldosteronism results from an extra-adrenal abnormality that stimulates the adrenal gland to increase production of aldosterone. For example, conditions that reduce renal blood flow (renal artery stenosis) and ECF volume or produce a sodium deficit activate the renin-angiotensin system and, subsequently, increase aldosterone secretion. Thus, secondary hyperaldosteronism may result from conditions that induce hypertension through increased renin production (such as Wilms' tumor), ingestion of hormonal contraceptives, and pregnancy.

However, secondary hyperaldosteronism may also result from disorders unrelated to hypertension, which may or may not cause edema. For example, nephrotic syndrome, hepatic cirrhosis with ascites, and heart failure commonly induce edema, whereas Bartter's syndrome and salt-losing nephritis don't.

Signs and symptoms

Most clinical effects of hyperaldosteronism result from hypokalemia, which increases neuromuscular irritability and produces

muscle weakness; intermittent, flaccid paralysis; fatigue; headaches; paresthesia; and, possibly, tetany (resulting from metabolic alkalosis), which can lead to hypocalcemia.

Diabetes mellitus is common, perhaps because hypokalemia interferes with normal insulin secretion.[3] Hypertension and its accompanying complications are also common.[1] Other characteristic findings include vision disturbances and loss of renal concentrating ability, resulting in nocturnal polyuria and polydipsia. Azotemia indicates chronic potassium depletion nephropathy.

Complications
- Neuromuscular irritability
- Tetany
- Paresthesia
- Seizures
- Arrhythmias
- Ischemic heart disease
- Left ventricular hypertrophy
- Heart failure
- Death
- Metabolic alkalosis
- Nephropathy
- Azotemia

Diagnosis
Persistently low serum potassium levels in a nonedematous patient who isn't taking diuretics, who doesn't have obvious GI losses (from vomiting or diarrhea), and who has a normal sodium intake, suggest hyperaldosteronism. If hypokalemia develops in a hypertensive patient shortly after starting treatment with potassium-wasting diuretics (such as thiazides) and if it persists after the diuretic has been discontinued and potassium replacement therapy has been instituted, evaluation for hyperaldosteronism is necessary.

A low plasma renin level that fails to increase appropriately during volume depletion (upright posture, sodium depletion) and a high plasma aldosterone level during volume expansion by salt loading confirm primary hyperaldosteronism in a hypertensive patient without edema.

The serum bicarbonate level is often elevated, with ensuing alkalosis due to hydrogen and potassium ion loss in the distal renal tubules. Other tests show markedly increased urinary aldosterone levels, increased plasma aldosterone levels and, in secondary hyperaldosteronism, increased plasma renin levels.[4]

A suppression test is useful to differentiate between primary and secondary hyperaldosteronism. During this test, the patient receives oral desoxycorticosterone for 3 days while plasma aldosterone levels and urinary metabolites are continuously measured. These levels decrease in secondary hyperaldosteronism but remain the same in primary hyperaldosteronism. Simultaneously, renin levels are low in primary hyperaldosteronism and high in secondary hyperaldosteronism.

Other helpful diagnostic evidence includes an increase in plasma volume of 30% to 50% above normal, electrocardiogram signs of hypokalemia (ST-segment depression and U waves), chest X-ray showing left ventricular hypertrophy from chronic hypertension, and localization of the tumor by adrenal angiography or computed tomography scan.

Treatment
Although treatment of primary hyperaldosteronism may include unilateral adrenalectomy, administration of a potassium-sparing diuretic—spironolactone—and sodium restriction may control hyperaldosteronism without surgery.[2] For bilateral adrenal hyperplasia, spironolactone is the drug of choice. Treatment of secondary hyperaldosteronism must include correction of the underlying cause.

Special considerations
Patient care includes careful monitoring and recording of urine output, blood pressure, weight, and serum potassium levels.

▶ Watch for signs of tetany (muscle twitching, Chvostek's sign) and for hypokalemia-induced cardiac arrhythmias, paresthesia, or weakness. Give potassium replacement, as ordered, and keep calcium gluconate I.V. available.

▶ Ask the dietitian to provide a low-sodium, high-potassium diet.

▶ After adrenalectomy, watch for weakness, hyponatremia, rising serum potassium levels, and signs of adrenal hypofunction, especially hypotension.

▶ If the patient is taking spironolactone, advise him to watch for signs of hyperkalemia. Tell him that impotence and gynecomastia may follow long-term use.

▶ Tell the patient who must take steroid hormone replacement to wear a medical identification bracelet.

REFERENCES

1. Rossi, G.P., et al. "A Prospective Study of the Prevalence of Primary Aldosteronism in 1,125 Hypertensive Patients," *Journal of the American College of Cardiology* 48(11):2293-300, December 2006.
2. Medline Plus (2006, February 27). "Hyperaldosteronism-Primary and Secondary" [Online]. Available at *www.nlm.nih.gov/ medlineplus/ency/article/000330.htm#Treatment.*
3. Catena, C., et al. "Insulin Sensitivity in Patients with Primary Aldosteronism: A Follow-up Study," *Journal of Clinical Endocrinology and Metabolism* 91(9):3457-63, September 2006.
4. Al Fehaily, M., and Duh, Q.Y. "Clinical Manifestation of Aldosteronoma" *Surgical Clinics of North America* 84(3):887-905, June 2004.

HYPERPARATHYROIDISM

Hyperparathyroidism is characterized by overactivity of one or more of the four parathyroid glands, resulting in excessive secretion of parathyroid hormone (PTH). Hypersecretion of PTH promotes bone resorption and leads to hypercalcemia and hypophosphatemia, which in turn results in increased renal and GI absorption of calcium.

Causes and incidence

Hyperparathyroidism may be primary or secondary. In primary hyperparathyroidism, one or more of the parathyroid glands enlarges, increasing PTH secretion and elevating serum calcium levels. The most common cause (85% of cases) is a single adenoma which has formed on one of the parathyroid glands, causing it to become overactive.[1] Other causes include a genetic disorder or multiple endocrine neoplasia. Primary hyperparathyroidism is rare in children. It usually occurs after age 40 and is much more prevalent in women than in men, by an incidence rate of 2:1. Two out of 1,000 women older than age 60 will develop it each year.[1] The overall estimated incidence is 1 out of 500 to 1,000 people.

In secondary hyperparathyroidism, excessive compensatory production of PTH stems from a hypocalcemia-producing abnormality outside the parathyroid gland, which causes a resistance to the metabolic action of PTH. Some hypocalcemia-producing abnormalities are chronic renal failure, renal absorption disorders, vitamin D deficiency (especially in the housebound elderly), or osteomalacia due to phenytoin or laxative abuse.

Signs and symptoms

Clinical effects of primary hyperparathyroidism result from hypercalcemia and are typically present in several body systems:

▶ *Renal system:* nephrocalcinosis due to elevated levels of calcium and, possibly, recurring nephrolithiasis, which may lead to renal insufficiency. Renal manifestations, including polyuria, are the most common effects of hyperparathyroidism.

▶ *Skeletal and articular system:* chronic low back pain and easy fracturing due to bone degeneration, bone tenderness, chondrocalcinosis, occasional severe osteopenia (especial-

Bone resorption in primary hyperparathyroidism

Erosion and demineraliza-
tion, which occur with hyperparathyroidism, are illustrated
at right.

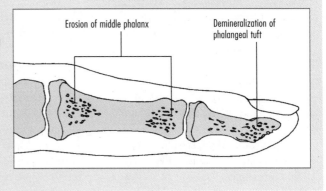

Erosion of middle phalanx

Demineralization of
phalangeal tuft

ly on the vertebrae), erosions of the juxta-
articular surface, subchondral fractures,
traumatic synovitis, and pseudogout
▶ *GI system:* pancreatitis, causing constant,
severe epigastric pain radiating to the back;
peptic ulcers, causing abdominal pain,
anorexia, nausea, and vomiting
▶ *Neuromuscular system:* marked muscle
weakness and atrophy, particularly in the
legs
▶ *Central nervous system:* psychomotor and
personality disturbances, depression, overt
psychosis, stupor and, possibly, coma
▶ *Other:* skin necrosis, cataracts, calcium
microthrombi to lungs and pancreas, polyuria, anemia, and subcutaneous calcification.
   Similarly, in secondary hyperparathyroidism, decreased serum calcium levels may
produce the same features of calcium imbalance, with skeletal deformities of the long
bones (rickets, for example) as well as symptoms of the underlying disease.

Complications
▶ Nephrolithiasis-most frequent complica-
tion occurring in 20% of patients with pri-
mary hyperparathyroidism
▶ Cardiac arrhythmias
▶ Vascular damage
▶ Heart failure

▶ Parathyroid poisoning

Diagnosis
In primary disease, a high concentration of
serum PTH on radioimmunoassay with accompanying hypercalcemia confirms the diagnosis.[2]
   In addition, X-rays may show diffuse
demineralization of bones, bone cysts, outer
cortical bone absorption, and subperiosteal
erosion of the phalanges and distal clavicles.
(See *Bone resorption in primary hyperparathyroidism.*) Microscopic examination of the
bone with tests such as X-ray spectropho-
tometry typically demonstrates increased
bone turnover. Reduced bone mineral density, particularly of the forearm, is seen on
bone densitometry.
   Laboratory tests reveal elevated urine and
serum calcium, chloride, and alkaline phosphatase levels and decreased serum phosphorus levels. Hyperparathyroidism may also
raise uric acid and creatinine levels and increase basal acid secretion and serum im-
munoreactive gastrin. Increased serum amylase levels may indicate acute pancreatitis.
   Laboratory findings in secondary hyperparathyroidism show normal or slightly decreased serum calcium levels and variable
serum phosphorus levels. Phosphorus can be

significantly elevated, especially in osteomalacia or renal disease. Patient history may reveal familial renal disease, seizure disorders, or drug ingestion. Other laboratory values and physical examination findings identify the cause of secondary hyperparathyroidism.

Treatment

Treatment varies, depending on the cause of the disease. Treatment of primary hyperparathyroidism may include surgery to remove the adenoma or, depending on the extent of hyperplasia, all but one-half of one gland (the remaining part of the gland is necessary to maintain normal PTH levels).[2] Surgery may relieve bone pain within 3 days. However, renal damage may be irreversible.

Preoperatively—or if surgery isn't feasible or necessary—other treatments can decrease calcium levels. These include forcing fluids; limiting dietary intake of calcium; promoting sodium and calcium excretion through forced diuresis using normal saline solution (up to 6 liters in life-threatening circumstances), furosemide, or ethacrynic acid; and administering oral sodium or potassium phosphate, subcutaneous calcitonin, I.V. plicamycin, or I.V. bisphosphonates.[3, 4]

Therapy for potential postoperative magnesium and phosphate deficiencies includes I.V. administration of magnesium and phosphate, or sodium phosphate solution given orally or by retention enema. In addition, during the first 4 to 5 days after surgery, when serum calcium falls to low normal levels, supplemental calcium may be necessary; vitamin D or calcitriol may also be used to raise serum calcium levels.[3]

Treatment of secondary hyperparathyroidism must correct the underlying cause of parathyroid hypertrophy. Vitamin D therapy or, in the patient with renal disease, administration of an oral calcium preparation (calcium acetate, if possible) for hyperphosphatemia, are typically used, although surgical excision may be necessary. In the patient with renal failure, dialysis is necessary to lower calcium levels and may have to continue for the remainder of the patient's life. In the patient with chronic secondary hyperparathyroidism, the enlarged glands may not revert to normal size and function even after calcium levels have been controlled.

Special considerations

Care emphasizes prevention of complications from the underlying disease and its treatment.

▶ Obtain pretreatment baseline serum potassium, calcium, phosphate, and magnesium levels because these values may change abruptly during treatment.

▶ During hydration to reduce serum calcium level, record intake and output accurately. Strain urine to check for calculi. Provide at least 3 qt (3 L) of fluid a day, including cranberry or prune juice to increase urine acidity and help prevent calculus formation. As ordered, obtain blood and urine samples to measure sodium, potassium, and magnesium levels, especially for the patient taking furosemide.

▶ Auscultate for breath sounds often. Listen for signs of pulmonary edema in the patient receiving large amounts of normal saline solution I.V., especially if he has pulmonary or cardiac disease. Monitor the patient on cardiac glycosides carefully because elevated calcium levels can rapidly produce toxic effects.

▶ Because the patient is predisposed to pathologic fractures, take safety precautions to minimize the risk of injury. Assist him with walking, keep the bed at its lowest position, and raise the side rails. Lift the immobilized patient carefully to minimize bone stress. Schedule care to allow the patient with muscle weakness as much rest as possible.

▶ Watch for signs of peptic ulcer and administer antacids, as appropriate.

After parathyroidectomy:

▶ Check frequently for respiratory distress, and keep a tracheotomy tray at the bedside.

Watch for postoperative complications, such as laryngeal nerve damage or, rarely, hemorrhage. Monitor intake and output carefully.

▶ Check for swelling at the operative site. Place the patient in semi-Fowler's position, and support his head and neck with sandbags to decrease edema, which may cause pressure on the trachea.

▶ Watch for signs of mild tetany, such as complaints of tingling in the hands and around the mouth. These symptoms should subside quickly but may be prodromal signs of tetany, so keep calcium gluconate or calcium chloride I.V. available for emergency administration. Watch for increased neuromuscular irritability and other signs of severe tetany, and report them immediately. Ambulate the patient as soon as possible postoperatively, even though he may find this uncomfortable, because pressure on bones speeds up bone recalcification.

▶ Check laboratory results for low serum calcium and magnesium levels.

▶ Monitor mental status and watch for listlessness. In the patient with persistent hypercalcemia, check for muscle weakness and psychiatric symptoms.

▶ Before discharge, advise the patient of the possible adverse effects of drug therapy. Emphasize the need for periodic follow-up through laboratory blood tests. If hyperparathyroidism wasn't corrected surgically, warn the patient to avoid calcium-containing antacids and thiazide diuretics.

REFERENCES

1. National Endocrine and Metabolic Disease Information Services Publication No. 6-3425 (2006, May). "Hyperparathyroidism" [Online]. Available at *www.endocrine.niddk.nih.gov/pubs/hyper/hyper.htm.*
2. Ambrogini, E., et al. "Surgery or Surveillance for Mild Asymptomatic Primary Hyperparathyroidism: A Prospective, Randomized Clinical Trial," *Journal of Clinical Endocrinology and Metabolism* 92(8):3114-21, August 2007.
3. Farford, B., et al. "Nonsurgical Management of Primary Hyperparathyroidism," *Mayo Clinic Proceedings* 82(3):351-55, March 2007.
4. Khan, A.A., et al. "Alendronate in Primary Hyperparathyroidism: A Double-blind, Randomized, Placebo-controlled Trial," *Journal of Clinical Endocrinology and Metabolism* 89(7):3319-25, July 2004.

HYPERTHYROIDISM

Hyperthyroidism is a metabolic imbalance that results from thyroid hormone overproduction. The most common form of hyperthyroidism, Graves' disease, increases thyroxine (T_4) production and enlarges the thyroid gland.[1]

With treatment, most patients can lead normal lives. However, *thyroid storm*—an acute exacerbation of hyperthyroidism—is a medical emergency that may lead to life-threatening cardiac, hepatic, or renal failure.

Causes and incidence

Hyperthyroidism may result from both genetic and immunologic factors. Graves' disease is an autoimmune disease in which autoantibodies are directed against thyroid stimulating hormone (TSH), which results in an increase in thyroid hormone production.[1] Graves disease is associated with a family history of hyperparathyroidism or autoimmune disorders, high iodine intake, stress, use of sex steroids, and smoking.[1]

In latent hyperthyroidism, excessive dietary intake of iodine and, possibly, stress can precipitate clinical hyperthyroidism. In a person with inadequately treated hyperthyroidism, stress—including surgery, infection, or trauma—can precipitate thyroid storm.[1] (See *Other forms of hyperthyroidism.*)

The overall incidence of hyperthyroidism is about .05 to 1.3%. [1] Whites and Hispanics have a slightly higher prevalence than Blacks and it's more common in females.[1] The incidence of Graves' disease is highest in individuals between ages 20 and

Other forms of hyperthyroidism

• *Toxic adenoma*—a small, benign nodule in the thyroid gland that secretes thyroid hormone—is the second most common cause of hyperthyroidism. The cause of toxic adenoma is unknown; incidence is highest in elderly people. Clinical effects are essentially similar to those of Graves' disease, except that toxic adenoma doesn't induce ophthalmopathy, pretibial myxedema, or acropachy. Presence of adenoma is confirmed by radioactive iodine (^{131}I) uptake and thyroid scan, which show a single hyperfunctioning nodule suppressing the rest of the gland. Treatment includes ^{131}I therapy or surgery to remove the adenoma after antithyroid drugs achieve a euthyroid state.

• *Thyrotoxicosis factitia* results from chronic ingestion of thyroid hormone for thyrotropin suppression in patients with thyroid carcinoma or from thyroid hormone abuse by people who are trying to lose weight.

• *Functioning metastatic thyroid carcinoma* is a rare disease that causes excess production of thyroid hormone.

• *Thyroid-stimulating hormone-secreting pituitary tumor* causes overproduction of thyroid hormone.

• *Subacute thyroiditis* is a virus-induced granulomatous inflammation of the thyroid, producing transient hyperthyroidism associated with fever, pain, pharyngitis, and tenderness in the thyroid gland.

• *Silent thyroiditis* is a self-limiting, transient form of hyperthyroidism, with histologic thyroiditis but no inflammatory symptoms.

40,[1] especially in those with family histories of thyroid abnormalities.

Signs and symptoms

The classic features of hyperthyroidism are an enlarged thyroid (goiter), nervousness, heat intolerance, weight loss despite increased appetite, sweating, diarrhea, tremor, and palpitations. Exophthalmos is considered most characteristic but is absent in many patients with hyperthyroidism.

Many other symptoms are common because hyperthyroidism profoundly affects virtually every body system:

▶ *Central nervous system:* difficulty in concentrating because increased T_4 secretion accelerates cerebral function; excitability or nervousness due to increased basal metabolic rate; fine tremor, shaky handwriting, and clumsiness from increased activity in the spinal cord area that controls muscle tone; emotional instability and mood swings, ranging from occasional outbursts to overt psychosis

▶ *Skin, hair, and nails:* smooth, warm, flushed skin (patient sleeps with minimal covers and little clothing); fine, soft hair; premature graying and increased hair loss in both sexes; friable nails and onycholysis (distal nail separated from the bed); pretibial myxedema (dermopathy), producing thickened skin, accentuated hair follicles, raised red patches of skin that are itchy and sometimes painful, with occasional nodule formation (Microscopic examination shows increased mucin deposits.)

▶ *Cardiovascular system:* tachycardia; full, bounding pulse; wide pulse pressure; cardiomegaly; increased cardiac output and blood volume; visible point of maximal impulse; paroxysmal supraventricular tachycardia and atrial fibrillation (especially in the elderly); and occasionally, systolic murmur at the left sternal border

▶ *Respiratory system:* dyspnea on exertion and at rest, possibly from cardiac decompensation and increased cellular oxygen utilization

▶ *GI system:* possible anorexia; nausea and vomiting due to increased GI mobility and peristalsis; increased defecation; soft stools

or, with severe disease, diarrhea; and liver enlargement

▶ *Musculoskeletal system:* weakness, fatigue, and muscle atrophy; rare coexistence with myasthenia gravis; possible generalized or localized paralysis associated with hypokalemia; and occasional acropachy—soft-tissue swelling, accompanied by underlying bone changes where new bone formation occurs

▶ *Reproductive system:* in females, oligomenorrhea or amenorrhea, decreased fertility, higher incidence of spontaneous abortions; in males, gynecomastia due to increased estrogen levels; in both sexes, diminished libido

▶ *Eyes:* exophthalmos (from the combined effects of accumulation of mucopolysaccharides and fluids in the retro-orbital tissues that force the eyeball outward, and of lid retraction that produces the characteristic staring gaze); occasional inflammation of conjunctivae, corneas, or eye muscles; diplopia; and increased tearing

When hyperthyroidism escalates to thyroid storm, these symptoms can be accompanied by extreme irritability, hypertension, tachycardia, vomiting, temperature up to 106° F (41.1° C), delirium, and coma.

Complications
▶ Cardiovascular complications
▶ Osteoporosis
▶ Paralysis
▶ Vitiligo and skin hyperpigmentation
▶ Corneal ulcers
▶ Myasthenia gravis
▶ Impaired fertility
▶ Decreased libido
▶ Gynecomastia

Diagnosis
The diagnosis of hyperthyroidism is usually straightforward and depends on a careful clinical history and physical examination, a high index of suspicion, and routine hormone determinations.

The following tests confirm the disorder:
▶ Radioimmunoassay shows increased serum T_4 and triiodothyronine (T_3) concentrations.[3]
▶ Thyroid scan reveals increased uptake of radioactive iodine (^{131}I). This test is contraindicated if the patient is pregnant.
▶ TSH levels are decreased.[3]
▶ Ultrasonography confirms subclinical ophthalmopathy.
▶ Antithyroglobulin antibody is positive in Grave's disease.

Treatment
A number of approaches are used to treat hyperthyroidism, primarily antithyroid drugs, ^{131}I, and surgery. Appropriate treatment depends on the size of the goiter, the causes, the patient's age and parity, and how long surgery will be delayed (if the patient is an appropriate candidate for surgery).

Antithyroid drug therapy is used for children, young adults, pregnant females, and patients who refuse surgery or ^{131}I treatment.[2] Thyroid hormone antagonists are given to block thyroid hormone synthesis. Drugs available in the United States include methimazole and propylthiouracil. Although hypermetabolic symptoms subside within 4 to 8 weeks after such therapy begins, the patient must continue the medication for 6 months to 2 years, depending on the clinical circumstances. Approximately 40% to 70% of patient's with Graves' disease may go into remission and, with continued monitoring (to watch for relapse), their medication can be stopped. Beta-adrenergic blockers may be given concomitantly to manage tachycardia and other peripheral effects of excessive hypersympathetic activity.[3]

During pregnancy, antithyroid medication should be kept at the minimum dosage required to keep maternal thyroid function within the high-normal range until delivery and to minimize the risk of fetal hypothyroidism—even though most infants of hyperthyroid mothers are born with mild and

transient hyperthyroidism.[2] (Neonatal hyperthyroidism may even necessitate treatment with antithyroid medications and propranolol for 2 to 3 months.) Because hyperthyroidism is sometimes exacerbated in the puerperal period, continuous control of maternal thyroid function is essential.[2]

Approximately 3 to 6 months postpartum, antithyroid drug administration can be gradually tapered and thyroid function reassessed. The mother receiving low-dose antithyroid treatment may breast-feed as long as the infant's thyroid function is checked periodically. Small amounts of the drug can be found in breast milk.[2]

A single oral dose of ^{131}I is the treatment of choice for patients who aren't pregnant or breast-feeding.[3] Patients of reproductive age must wait 8 to 12 weeks after treatment before becoming pregnant. During treatment with ^{131}I, the thyroid gland picks up the radioactive element as it would regular iodine. Subsequently, the radioactivity destroys some of the cells that normally concentrate iodine and produce T_4, thus decreasing thyroid hormone production and normalizing thyroid size and function. In most patients, hypermetabolic symptoms diminish from 6 to 8 weeks after such treatment. However, some patients may require a second dose.

Subtotal (partial) thyroidectomy, which decreases the thyroid gland's capacity for hormone production, is indicated for patients with a large goiter whose hyperthyroidism has repeatedly relapsed after drug therapy or patients who refuse or aren't candidates for ^{131}I treatment. [3] Preoperatively, the patient may receive iodides (Lugol's solution or saturated solution of potassium iodide), antithyroid drugs, or high doses of propranolol, to help prevent thyroid storm. If euthyroidism isn't achieved, surgery should be delayed and propranolol administered to decrease the systemic effects (cardiac arrhythmias) caused by hyperthyroidism. After ablative treatment with ^{131}I or surgery, patients require regular medical supervision

for the rest of their lives because they usually develop hypothyroidism, sometimes as long as several years after treatment.

Therapy for hyperthyroid ophthalmopathy includes local applications of topical medications but may require high doses of corticosteroids. A patient with severe exophthalmos that causes pressure on the optic nerve may require external beam radiation therapy or surgical decompression to lessen pressure on the orbital contents.

Treatment of thyroid storm includes administration of an antithyroid drug, propranolol I.V. to block sympathetic effects, a corticosteroid to inhibit the conversion of T_4 to T_3 and replace depleted cortisol levels, and an iodide to block the release of thyroid hormone. Supportive measures include administration of nutrients, vitamins, fluids, and sedatives.

Special considerations

Patients with hyperthyroidism require vigilant care to prevent acute exacerbations and complications.[3]

▶ Record vital signs and weight.

▶ Monitor serum electrolyte levels, and check periodically for hyperglycemia and glycosuria.

▶ Carefully monitor cardiac function if the patient is elderly or has coronary artery disease. If the heart rate is more than 100 beats/minute, check blood pressure and pulse rate often.

▶ Check level of consciousness and urine output.

▶ If the patient is pregnant, tell her to watch closely during the first trimester for signs of spontaneous abortion and to report such signs immediately.[2]

▶ Encourage bed rest, and keep the patient's room cool, quiet, and dark. The patient with dyspnea will be most comfortable sitting upright or in high Fowler's position.

▶ Remember, extreme nervousness may produce bizarre behavior. Reassure the patient and his family that such behavior will prob-

ably subside with treatment. Provide sedatives as necessary.

▶ To promote weight gain, provide a balanced diet, with six meals a day. If the patient has edema, suggest a low-sodium diet.

▶ If iodide is part of the treatment, mix it with milk, juice, or water to prevent GI distress, and administer it through a straw to prevent tooth discoloration.

▶ Check intake and output carefully to ensure adequate hydration and fluid balance.

▶ Closely monitor blood pressure, cardiac rate and rhythm, and temperature. If the patient has a high fever, reduce it with appropriate hypothermic measures. Maintain an I.V. line and give drugs, as ordered.

▶ If the patient has exophthalmos or other ophthalmopathy, suggest sunglasses or eye patches to protect his eyes from light. Moisten the conjunctivae often with isotonic eye drops. Warn the patient with severe lid retraction to avoid sudden physical movements that might cause the lid to slip behind the eyeball. He should avoid cigarette smoke.

▶ Avoid excessive palpation of the thyroid to avoid precipitating thyroid storm.

Thyroidectomy necessitates meticulous postoperative care to prevent complications:

▶ Watch for evidence of hemorrhage into the neck, such as a tight dressing with no blood on it. Change dressings and perform wound care, as ordered; check the *back* of the dressing for drainage. Keep the patient in semi-Fowler's position, and support his head and neck with sandbags to ease tension on the incision.

▶ Check for dysphagia or hoarseness from possible laryngeal nerve injury.

▶ Watch for signs of hypoparathyroidism (tetany, numbness), a complication that results from accidental removal of the parathyroid glands during surgery.

▶ Stress the importance of regular medical follow-up after discharge because hypothyroidism may develop from 2 to 4 weeks postoperatively.

Drug therapy and ^{131}I therapy require careful monitoring and comprehensive patient teaching:

▶ After ^{131}I therapy, tell the patient not to expectorate or cough freely because his saliva will be radioactive for 24 hours. Stress the need for repeated measurement of serum T_4 levels.

▶ If the patient is taking propylthiouracil and methimazole, monitor complete blood count periodically to detect leukopenia, thrombocytopenia, and agranulocytosis. Instruct him to take these medications with meals to minimize GI distress and to avoid over-the-counter cough preparations because many contain iodine.

▶ Tell him to report fever, enlarged cervical lymph nodes, sore throat, mouth sores, and other signs of blood dyscrasias and any rash or skin eruptions—signs of hypersensitivity.

▶ Watch the patient taking propranolol for signs of hypotension (dizziness, decreased urine output). Tell him to rise slowly after sitting or lying down to prevent orthostatic syncope.

▶ Instruct the patient receiving antithyroid drugs or ^{131}I therapy to report any symptoms of hypothyroidism.

REFERENCES

1. Schraga, E.D. (2006, May 24). "Hyperthyroidism, Thyroid Storm, and Graves Disease" [Online]. Available at *www.emedicine.com/EMERG/topic269.htm.*
2. Abalovich, M., et al. "Management of Thyroid Dysfunction during Pregnancy and Postpartum: An Endocrine Society Clinical Practice Guideline," *The Journal of Clinical Endocrinology and Metabolism* 92(8 Suppl):S1-47, August 2007.
3. American Association of Clinical Endocrinologists. "American Association of Clinical Endocrinologists Medical Guidelines for Clinical Practice for the Evaluation and Treatment of Hyperthyroidism and Hypothyroidism," *Endocrine Practice* 8(6):457-69, November-December 2002.

HYPOPARATHYROIDISM

Hypoparathyroidism is a deficiency of parathyroid hormone (PTH) caused by disease, injury (usually surgical), or congenital malfunction of the parathyroid glands. Because the parathyroid glands primarily regulate calcium balance, hypoparathyroidism causes hypocalcemia, producing neuromuscular symptoms ranging from paresthesia to tetany. The clinical effects of hypoparathyroidism are usually correctable with replacement therapy. However, some complications of this disorder, such as cataracts and basal ganglion calcifications, are irreversible.

Causes and incidence

Hypoparathyroidism may be acute or chronic and is classified as idiopathic or acquired. The acquired form may also be reversible. *Idiopathic hypoparathyroidism* may result from an autoimmune genetic disorder or the congenital absence of the parathyroid glands. *Acquired hypoparathyroidism* commonly results from accidental removal of, or injury to, one or more parathyroid glands during thyroidectomy or other neck surgery.[1] Rarely, it results from massive thyroid irradiation. It may also result from ischemic infarction of the parathyroids during surgery or from hemochromatosis, sarcoidosis, amyloidosis, tuberculosis, neoplasms, or trauma. An *acquired, reversible hypoparathyroidism* may result from suppression of normal gland function due to hypercalcemia, from hypomagnesemia-induced impairment of hormone synthesis, or from delayed maturation of parathyroid function. (See *What happens in acute hypoparathyroidism,* page 388.)

PTH isn't regulated by the pituitary or hypothalamus. It normally maintains blood calcium levels by increasing bone resorption and GI absorption of calcium. It also maintains an inverse relationship between serum calcium and phosphate levels by inhibiting phosphate reabsorption in the renal tubules. Abnormal PTH production disrupts this balance. The incidence of hypoparathyroidism hasn't been determined in the United States. It is affects males and females equally.

Signs and symptoms

Although mild hypoparathyroidism may not produce symptoms, it usually produces hypocalcemia and high serum phosphate levels that affect the central nervous system (CNS) as well as other body systems. Chronic hypoparathyroidism typically causes neuromuscular irritability, increased deep tendon reflexes, Chvostek's sign (hyperirritability of the facial nerve, producing a characteristic spasm when it's tapped), dysphagia, organic mental syndrome, psychosis, mental deficiency in children, and tetany.

Acute (overt) tetany begins with a tingling in the fingertips, around the mouth and, occasionally, in the feet. This tingling spreads and becomes more severe, producing muscle tension and spasms and consequent adduction of the thumbs, wrists, and elbows. Pain varies with the degree of muscle tension but seldom affects the face, legs, and feet. Chronic tetany is usually unilateral and less severe; it may cause difficulty in walking and a tendency to fall. Both forms of tetany can lead to laryngospasm, stridor and, eventually, cyanosis. They may also cause seizures. These CNS abnormalities tend to be exaggerated during hyperventilation, pregnancy, infection, withdrawal of thyroid hormone, therapy with diuretics, and before menstruation.

Other clinical effects include abdominal pain; dry, lusterless hair; spontaneous hair loss; brittle fingernails that develop ridges or fall out; dry, scaly skin; cataracts; and weakened tooth enamel, which causes teeth to stain, crack, and decay easily. Hypocalcemia may induce cardiac arrhythmias and may eventually lead to heart failure.

What happens in acute hypoparathyroidism

Causes of acute hypoparathyroidism include injury to the glands, accidental removal of the parathyroid glands during thyroidectomy or other neck surgery, autoimmune disease, tumor, tuberculosis (TB), sarcoidosis, hemochromatosis, and severe magnesium deficiency associated with alcoholism and intestinal malabsorption. These disorders and conditions cause a cascade of effects that result in severe hypocalcemia and hyperphosphatemia, which can lead to seizures, tetany, laryngospasm, and central nervous system (CNS) abnormalities, as shown in the flowchart below.

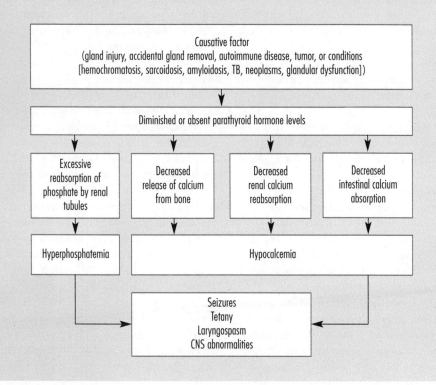

Complications
▶ Hypercholesterolemia with arteriosclerosis and ischemic heart disease
▶ Poor peripheral circulation
▶ Heart enlargement
▶ Heart failure
▶ Pleural and pericardial effusions
▶ Achlorhydria
▶ Pernicious anemia
▶ Adynamic colon, megacolon, and intestinal obstruction

▶ Iron deficiency anemia
▶ Bleeding tendencies
▶ Deafness
▶ Psychiatric disturbances
▶ Carpal tunnel syndrome
▶ Benign intracranial hypertension
▶ Impaired fertility

Diagnosis
The following test results confirm the diagnosis of hypoparathyroidism:

▶ Radioimmunoassay for PTH: decreased PTH concentration

▶ Serum calcium: decreased

▶ Serum phosphorus: increased

▶ Electrocardiogram (ECG): prolonged QT and ST intervals due to hypocalcemia.

Inflating a blood pressure cuff on the upper arm to between diastolic and systolic blood pressure and maintaining this inflation for 3 minutes elicits Trousseau's sign (carpal spasm), thereby provoking clinical evidence of hypoparathyroidism.

Treatment

Because calcium absorption from the small intestine requires the presence of vitamin D, treatment includes vitamin D and calcium supplements. Therapy is usually lifelong, except for the reversible form of the disease. If the patient can't tolerate the pure form of vitamin D, alternatives include dihydrotachysterol, if hepatic and renal function is adequate, and calcitriol, if it's severely compromised. In patients with preexisting hypomagnesemia, this condition must be corrected to treat the resulting hypocalcemia. A high-calcium, low-phosphorous diet is recommended.

Acute life-threatening tetany requires immediate I.V. administration of calcium to raise serum calcium levels. The patient who's awake and able to cooperate can help raise serum calcium levels by breathing into a paper bag and then inhaling his own carbon dioxide; this produces hypoventilation and mild respiratory acidosis. Sedatives and anticonvulsants may control spasms until calcium levels rise. Chronic tetany requires maintenance therapy with oral calcium and vitamin D supplements.

Special considerations

While awaiting diagnosis of hypoparathyroidism in a patient with a history of tetany, maintain a patent I.V. line and keep I.V. calcium available. Because the patient is vulnerable to seizures, maintain seizure precau-

tions. Also, keep a tracheotomy tray and endotracheal tube at the bedside because laryngospasm may result from hypocalcemia.

▶ Instruct the patient to follow a diet with adequate calcium and Vitamin D intake.

▶ When caring for the patient with chronic disease, particularly a child, stay alert for minor muscle twitching and for signs of laryngospasm because these effects may signal the onset of tetany.

▶ For the patient on drug therapy, emphasize the importance of checking serum calcium levels at least three times a year. Instruct the patient to watch for signs of hypercalcemia and to keep medications away from light and heat.

▶ Dental changes, cataracts, and brain calcifications are permanent. These can be prevented with early detection and periodic calcium determinations.

▶ Because the patient with chronic disease has prolonged QT intervals on ECG, watch for heart block and signs of decreasing cardiac output. Because calcium potentiates the effect of cardiac glycosides, closely monitor the patient receiving both a cardiac glycoside and calcium. Stay alert for signs of digoxin toxicity, such as arrhythmias, nausea, fatigue, vision changes.

▶ Instruct the patient with scaly skin to use creams to soften his skin. Also, tell him to keep his nails trimmed to prevent them from splitting.

▶ Hyperventilation or recent blood transfusions may worsen tetany. (Anticoagulant in stored blood binds calcium.)

▶ For the patient with tetany, administer 10% calcium gluconate by slow I.V. infusion (1 ml/minute), and maintain a patent airway. The patient may also require intubation and sedation. Monitor vital signs often after administering sedation to make certain that blood pressure and heart rate return to normal.

REFERENCES

1. National Institute of Child Health and Human Development (2007, March 22). "Hypoparathyroidism" [Online]. Available at *www.nichd. nih.gov/health/topics/hypoparathyroidism.cfm.*

HYPOPITUITARISM

Hypopituitarism, which includes panhypopituitarism or dwarfism, is a complex syndrome marked by metabolic dysfunction, sexual immaturity, and growth retardation (when it occurs in childhood), resulting from a deficiency of the hormones secreted by the anterior pituitary gland. Panhypopituitarism refers to a generalized condition caused by partial or total failure of the anterior pituitary's vital hormones—corticotropin, thyroid-stimulating hormone (TSH), luteinizing hormone (LH), follicle-stimulating hormone (FSH), human growth hormone (hGH), and prolactin—plus the posterior pituitary hormone, antidiuretic hormone. Partial hypopituitarism and complete hypopituitarism occur in adults and children; in children, these diseases may cause dwarfism and delayed puberty. The prognosis may be good with adequate replacement therapy and correction of the underlying causes.

Causes

The most common cause of primary hypopituitarism in adults is a tumor.[1] Other causes include congenital defects (hypoplasia or aplasia of the pituitary gland); pituitary infarction (most often from postpartum hemorrhage); partial or total hypophysectomy by surgery, irradiation, or chemical agents; and, rarely, granulomatous disease (tuberculosis, for example). Occasionally, hypopituitarism may have no identifiable cause or it may be related to autoimmune destruction of the gland. Secondary hypopituitarism stems from a deficiency of releasing hormones produced by the hypothalamus—either idiopathic or possibly resulting from infection, trauma, or a tumor.

Primary hypopituitarism usually develops in a predictable pattern of hormonal failures. It generally starts with hypogonadism from gonadotropin failure (decreased FSH and LH levels). In adults, it causes cessation of menses in females and impotence in men. Growth hormone (GH) deficiency follows; in children, this causes short stature, delayed growth, and delayed puberty. In adults, it causes osteoporosis, decreased lean-to-fat body mass index, adverse lipid changes, and subtle emotional dysphoria and lethargy. Subsequent failure of thyrotropin (decreased TSH levels) causes hypothyroidism; finally, adrenocorticotropic failure (decreased corticotropin levels) results in adrenal insufficiency. However, when hypopituitarism follows surgical ablation or trauma, the pattern of hormonal events may not necessarily follow this sequence. Sometimes, damage to the hypothalamus or neurohypophysis from one of the above leads to diabetes insipidus. The incidence of hypopituitarism is 2 to 8 per 100,000 persons and it affects men and woman equally.[1]

Signs and symptoms

Clinical features of hypopituitarism develop slowly and vary with the severity of the disorder and the number of deficient hormones. Signs and symptoms of hypopituitarism in adults may include gonadal failure (secondary amenorrhea, impotence, infertility, decreased libido), diabetes insipidus, hypothyroidism (fatigue, lethargy, sensitivity to cold, menstrual disturbances), and adrenocortical insufficiency (hypoglycemia, anorexia, nausea, abdominal pain, orthostatic hypotension). Cardiovascular disease is higher among hypopituitary patients.[1]

Postpartum necrosis of the pituitary gland (Sheehan's syndrome) characteristically causes failure of lactation, menstruation, and

growth of pubic and axillary hair and symptoms of thyroid and adrenocortical failure.

In children, hypopituitarism causes retarded growth or delayed puberty. Dwarfism usually isn't apparent at birth. Early signs begin to appear during the first few months of life, and by age 6 months, growth retardation is obvious. Although these children generally enjoy good health, pituitary dwarfism may cause chubbiness due to fat deposits in the lower trunk, delayed secondary tooth eruption and, possibly, hypoglycemia. Growth continues at less than one-half the normal rate—sometimes extending into the patient's 20s or 30s—to an average height of 48" (122 cm), with normal proportions.

When hypopituitarism strikes before puberty, it prevents development of secondary sex characteristics (including facial and body hair). In males, it produces undersized testes, penis, and prostate gland; absent or minimal libido; and the inability to initiate and maintain an erection. In females, it usually causes immature development of the breasts, sparse or absent pubic and axillary hair, and primary amenorrhea.

Panhypopituitarism may induce a host of mental and physiologic abnormalities, including lethargy, psychosis, orthostatic hypotension, bradycardia, anemia, and anorexia. However, clinical manifestations of hormonal deficiencies resulting from pituitary destruction don't become apparent until 75% of the gland is destroyed. Total loss of all hormones released by the anterior pituitary is fatal unless treated.

Neurologic signs associated with hypopituitarism and produced by pituitary tumors include headache, bilateral temporal hemianopia, loss of visual acuity and, possibly, blindness. Acute hypopituitarism resulting from surgery or infection is often associated with fever, hypotension, vomiting, and hypoglycemia—all characteristic of adrenal insufficiency.

Complications
▶ Pituitary apoplexy
▶ Inability to cope with minor stressors can lead to fever, shock, coma, and death
▶ Secondary hypopituitarism can lead to diabetes insipidus

Diagnosis

In suspected hypopituitarism, evaluation must confirm hormonal deficiency due to impairment or destruction of the anterior pituitary gland and rule out disease of the target organs (adrenals, gonads, and thyroid) or the hypothalamus. Low serum levels of thyroxine (T_4), for example, indicate diminished thyroid gland function, but further tests are necessary to identify the source of this dysfunction as the thyroid, pituitary, or hypothalamus.[3] (See *Thyroid function tests diagnosing hypopituitarism,* page 392.)

Serum insulin–like growth factor 1 (IGF-1) is decreased. Cranial computed tomography (CT) scan or magnetic resonance imaging (MRI) may reveal a tumor or abnormal mass in the pituitary gland of the hypothalamus. Radioimmunoassay showing decreased plasma levels of some or all pituitary hormones, accompanied by end-organ hypofunction, suggests pituitary failure, and eliminates target gland disease. Failure of thyrotropin-releasing hormone administration to increase TSH or prolactin concentrations rules out hypothalamic dysfunction as the cause of hormonal deficiency.

Provocative tests are helpful in pinpointing the source of low cortisol levels. Oral metyrapone blocks cortisol synthesis, which should stimulate pituitary secretion of corticotropin and the adrenal precursors of cortisol, measured in urine as hydroxycorticosteroids.[3] Insulin-induced hypoglycemia also stimulates corticotropin secretion. Persistently low levels of corticotropin indicate pituitary or hypothalamic failure. These tests require careful medical supervision because they may precipitate an adrenal crisis.

Thyroid function tests in diagnosing hypopituitarism

Question: *Are thyroid function tests alone sufficient to rule out a diagnosis of hypopituitarism?*

Research: A previous study was conducted, using the thyroid function test (TFT) values of thyroid-stimulating hormone (TSH) and free thyroxine (T_4) or total T_4, to arrive at a hypopituitarism incidence rate of 3.2 cases/100,000/year in a Scottish population. The aim of the researchers in this study was to verify the results of the previous study and determine the incidence of unsuspected hypopituitarism in the same group of people. To do this, they used reflective testing that consisted of free T_4 (repeat analysis following assay recalibration), total T_3, testosterone (males), luteinizing hormone, follicle-stimulating hormone, prolactin, and cortisol levels.

Conclusion: As a result of this study, researchers identified an additional 10 cases of hypopituitarism, making the incidence rate approximately 4 cases/100,000/year. In addition, pituitary imaging performed on eight of these patients was abnormal in five cases, showing two large pituitary tumors, one macroadenoma, and two empty sellae. The results of this study showed that a significant number of cases of unsuspected hypopituitarism can be diagnosed by reflective testing on appropriate samples.

Application: When a patient presents with a clinical picture suggestive of hypopituitarism he should receive a broad range of tests to confirm or rule-out the disease. Early identification and treatment with replacement therapy, surgery, or radiation, depending on the cause of the hypopituitarism and the patient's condition, can produce a favorable prognosis.

Source: Preiss, D., et al. "Diagnosing Unsuspected Hypopituitarism in Adults from Suggestive Thyroid Function Test Results," *Annals of Clinical Biochemistry* 45(Pt 1):70-75, January 2008.

Diagnosis of hypopituitarism requires measurement of GH levels in the blood after administration of regular insulin (inducing hypoglycemia) or levodopa (causing hypotension). These drugs should provoke increased secretion of GH. Persistently low GH levels, despite provocative testing, confirm GH deficiency.[3] CT scan, MRI, or cerebral angiography confirms the presence of intrasellar or extrasellar tumors.

Treatment

Surgery to remove the tumor causing hypopituitarism is done when possible. Radiation therapy can be used for large tumors. Replacement of hormones secreted by the target glands is used if the cause can't be treated. Hormone replacement therapy includes cortisol, T_4, and androgen or cyclic estrogen.[2] Prolactin need not be replaced. The patient of reproductive age may benefit from administration of FSH and human chorionic gonadotropin to boost fertility. GH replacement is recommended for adults as well as children. Replacement is done by administering daily subcutaneous injections of one of two recombinant deoxyribonucleic acid (DNA) GHs, accompanied by follow-up of serum IGF-1 levels. Lean body mass increases, whereas adipose tissue—particularly in the abdomen—decreases. Risk of cardiovascular disease and osteoporosis also decrease with treatment. Many patients also notice an improved sense of well-being.

Somatrem, which is identical to hGH but is the product of recombinant DNA technol-

ogy, has replaced GHs derived from human sources. It's effective for treating dwarfism and stimulates growth increases as great as 4" to 6" (10 to 15 cm) in the first year of treatment.[4] The growth rate tapers off in subsequent years.[4] After pubertal changes have occurred, the effects of somatrem therapy are limited. Occasionally, a child becomes unresponsive to somatrem therapy, even with larger doses, perhaps because antibodies have formed against it. In such refractory patients, small doses of androgen may again stimulate growth but extreme caution is necessary to prevent premature closure of the epiphyses. Children with hypopituitarism may also need replacement of adrenal and thyroid hormones and, as they approach puberty, sex hormones.

Special considerations

Caring for patients with hypopituitarism requires an understanding of hormonal effects and skilled physical and psychological support.

▶ Monitor the results of all laboratory tests for hormonal deficiencies, and know what they mean. Until hormone replacement therapy is complete, check for signs of thyroid deficiency (increasing lethargy), adrenal deficiency (weakness, orthostatic hypotension, hypoglycemia, fatigue, and weight loss), and gonadotropin deficiency (decreased libido, lethargy, and apathy).

▶ Watch for anorexia in the patient with panhypopituitarism. Help plan a menu containing favorite foods—ideally, high-calorie foods. Monitor for weight loss or gain.

▶ If the patient has trouble sleeping, encourage exercise during the day.

▶ Record temperature, blood pressure, and heart rate every 4 to 8 hours. Check eyelids, nail beds, and skin for pallor, which indicates anemia.

▶ Prevent infection by giving meticulous skin care. Because the patient's skin is probably dry, use oil or lotion instead of soap. If body temperature is low, provide additional clothing and covers, as needed, to keep the patient warm.

▶ Darken the room if the patient has a tumor that's causing headaches and vision disturbances. Help with any activity that requires good vision such as reading the menu. The patient with bilateral hemianopia has impaired peripheral vision, so be sure to stand where he can see you and advise the family to do the same.

▶ During insulin testing, monitor the patient closely for signs of hypoglycemia (initially, slow cerebration, tachycardia, diaphoresis, and nervousness, progressing to seizures). Keep dextrose 50% in water available for I.V. administration to correct hypoglycemia rapidly.

▶ To prevent orthostatic hypotension, be sure to keep the patient supine during levodopa testing.

▶ Instruct the patient to wear a medical identification bracelet. Teach him and his family members how to administer steroids parenterally in case of an emergency.

▶ Refer the family of a child with dwarfism to the appropriate community resources for psychological counseling because the emotional stress caused by this disorder increases as the child becomes more aware of his condition.

REFERENCES

1. Naradzay, J., and Brilliant, S.A. (2006, November 9). "Hypopituitarism" [Online]. Available at *www.emedicine.com/EMERG/topic277.htm.*
2. Wierman, M.E., et al. "Androgen Therapy in Women: An Endocrine Society Clinical Practice Guideline," *Journal of Clinical Endocrinology and Metabolism* 91(10):3697-710, October 2006.
3. Schneider, H.J., et al. "Hypopituitarism," *Lancet* 369(9571):1461-70, April 2007.
4. de Ridder, M.A., et al. "Prediction of Adult Height in Growth-hormone-treated Children with Growth Hormone Deficiency," *Journal of Clinical Endocrinology and Metabolism* 92(3):925-31, March 2007.

HYPOTHYROIDISM

Hypothyroidism, a state of low serum thyroid hormone, results from hypothalamic, pituitary, or thyroid insufficiency. The disorder can progress to life-threatening myxedema coma.

Causes and incidence

Hypothyroidism results from inadequate production of thyroid hormone, most commonly caused by chronic autoimmune thyroiditis (Hashimoto's disease) in the United States. Other causes include dysfunction of the thyroid gland due to surgery (thyroidectomy), irradiation therapy (particularly with radioactive iodine, inflammation or, rarely, such conditions as amyloidosis and sarcoidosis). It may also result from pituitary failure to produce thyroid-stimulating hormone (TSH), hypothalamic failure to produce thyrotropin-releasing hormone, inborn errors of thyroid hormone synthesis, the inability to synthesize thyroid hormone because of iodine deficiency (usually dietary), or the use of antithyroid medications such as propylthiouracil. Other medications that may cause hypothyroidism include methimazole, lithium and amiodarone. In patients with hypothyroidism, infection, exposure to cold, and sedatives may precipitate myxedema coma.

According to the National Health and Nutrition Examination Survey III, hypothyroidism affects 4.6% of the population. It's more prevalent in females with small body size at birth and low body mass during childhood and it's two to eight times more prevalent in females than males. Frequency increases with age.

Signs and symptoms

Typically, the early clinical features of hypothyroidism are vague: fatigue, menstrual changes, hypercholesterolemia, forgetfulness, sensitivity to cold, unexplained weight gain, and constipation. As the disorder progresses, characteristic myxedematous signs and symptoms appear: decreasing mental stability; dry, flaky, inelastic skin; puffy face, hands, and feet; hoarseness; periorbital edema; upper eyelid droop; dry, sparse hair; and thick, brittle nails. (See *Facial signs of myxedema*.)

Cardiovascular involvement leads to decreased cardiac output, slow pulse rate, signs of poor peripheral circulation and, occasionally, an enlarged heart. Other common effects include anorexia, abdominal distention, menorrhagia, decreased libido, infertility, ataxia, intention tremor, and nystagmus. Reflexes show delayed relaxation time (especially in the Achilles tendon).

Progression to myxedema coma is usually gradual but when stress (such as hip fracture, infection, or myocardial infarction) aggravates severe or prolonged hypothyroidism, coma may develop abruptly. Clinical effects include progressive stupor, hypoventilation, hypoglycemia, hyponatremia, hypotension, and hypothermia.

Complications

▶ Cardiac complications, which include hypercholesterolemia, arteriosclerosis, ischemic heart disease, poor peripheral circulation, heart enlargement, heart failure, and pleural and pericardial effusions
▶ GI complications, which include achlorhydria, pernicious anemia, adynamic colon, megacolon, and intestinal obstruction
▶ Anemia and bleeding tendencies
▶ Conductive or sensorineural deafness
▶ Psychiatric disturbances
▶ Carpal tunnel syndrome
▶ Benign intracranial hypertension
▶ Impaired fertility

Diagnosis

Radioimmunoassay confirms hypothyroidism with low triiodothyronine (T_3) and thyroxine (T_4) levels.[1]

Supportive laboratory findings include:
▶ increased TSH level when hypothyroidism is due to thyroid insufficiency; decreased TSH level when hypothyroidism is due to hypothalamic or pituitary insufficiency[1]
▶ elevated levels of serum cholesterol, alkaline phosphatase, and triglycerides
▶ normocytic normochromic anemia.

In myxedema coma, laboratory tests may also show low serum sodium levels as well as decreased pH and increased partial pressure of carbon dioxide, which indicate respiratory acidosis.

Treatment
Therapy for hypothyroidism consists of gradual thyroid replacement with levothyroxine (for low T_4 levels) and, occasionally, liothyronine (for inadequate T_3 levels).[1] T_4 replacement is preferred as T_4 is readily converted to T_3 naturally in the blood stream.[1]

During myxedema coma, effective treatment supports vital functions while restoring euthyroidism. To support blood pressure and pulse rate, treatment includes I.V. administration of levothyroxine and hydrocortisone to correct possible pituitary or adrenal insufficiency. Hypoventilation requires oxygenation and respiratory support. Other supportive measures include fluid replacement and antibiotics for infection.

Special considerations
To manage the hypothyroid patient:
▶ Provide a high-bulk, low-calorie diet and encourage activity to combat constipation and promote weight loss. Administer cathartics and stool softeners, as needed.
▶ After thyroid replacement therapy begins, watch for symptoms of hyperthyroidism, such as restlessness, sweating, and excessive weight loss.[2]
▶ Tell the patient to report any signs of aggravated cardiovascular disease, such as chest pain and tachycardia.

Facial signs of myxedema

Characteristic myxedematous signs in adults include dry, flaky, inelastic skin; puffy face; and upper eyelid droop.

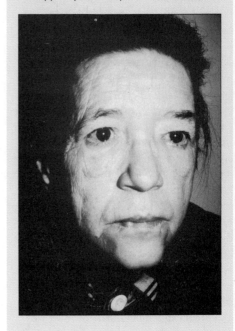

▶ To prevent myxedema coma, tell the patient to continue his course of thyroid medication even if his symptoms subside.
▶ Warn the patient to report infection immediately and to make sure any physician who prescribes drugs for him knows about the underlying hypothyroidism.

Treatment of myxedema coma requires supportive care:
▶ Check frequently for signs of decreasing cardiac output such as falling urine output.
▶ Monitor the patient's temperature until stable. Provide extra blankets and clothing and a warm room to compensate for hypothermia. Rapid rewarming may cause vasodilation and vascular collapse.[2]

▶ Record intake and output and daily weight. As treatment begins, urine output should increase and body weight decrease; if not, report this immediately.

▶ Turn the edematous bedridden patient every 2 hours and provide skin care, particularly around bony prominences.

▶ Avoid sedation when possible or reduce dosage because hypothyroidism delays metabolism of many drugs.

▶ Maintain a patent I.V. line. Monitor serum electrolyte levels carefully when administering I.V. fluids.

HEALTH & SAFETY *Monitor vital signs carefully when administering levothyroxine because rapid correction of hypothyroidism can cause adverse cardiac effects. Report chest pain or tachycardia immediately. Watch for hypertension and heart failure in the elderly patient.*

▶ Check arterial blood gas values for hypercapnia and hypoxia to determine whether the patient who's severely myxedematous requires ventilatory assistance.

▶ Because myxedema coma may have been precipitated by an infection, check possible sources of infection, such as blood or urine, and obtain sputum cultures.

REFERENCES

1. American Association of Clinical Endocrinologists. "American Association of Clinical Endocrinologists Medical Guidelines for Clinical Practice for the Evaluation and Treatment of Hyperthyroidism and Hypothyroidism," *Endocrine Practice* 8(6):457-69, November-December 2002.

2. Liles, A.M., and Harrell, K. "Common Thyroid Disorders. A Review of Therapies," *Advance for Nurse Practitioners* 14(1):29-32, January 2006.

PHEOCHROMOCYTOMA

Pheochromocytoma is a chromaffin-cell tumor of the adrenal medulla that secretes an excess of the catecholamines epinephrine and norepinephrine, resulting in severe hypertension, increased metabolism, and hyperglycemia. This disorder is potentially fatal but the prognosis is generally good with treatment. However, pheochromocytoma-induced kidney damage is irreversible.

Causes and incidence

A pheochromocytoma may result from an inherited autosomal dominant trait. While this tumor is usually benign, it may be malignant in as many as 10% of patients with this kind of tumor. According to some estimates, about 0.05% to 0.2% of patients with hypertension have pheochromocytoma.[1] It affects all races and both sexes, occurring primarily between ages 30 and 50.[1]

Signs and symptoms

The cardinal sign of pheochromocytoma is persistent or paroxysmal hypertension. Common clinical effects include palpitations, tachycardia, headache, diaphoresis, pallor, warmth or flushing, paresthesia, tremor, excitation, fright, nervousness, feelings of impending doom, abdominal pain, tachypnea, nausea, and vomiting. Orthostatic hypotension and paradoxical response to antihypertensive drugs are common, as are associated glycosuria, hyperglycemia, and hypermetabolism. Patients with hypermetabolism may show marked weight loss but some patients with pheochromocytomas are obese.

Symptomatic episodes may recur as seldom as once every 2 months or as often as 25 times a day. They may occur spontaneously or may follow certain precipitating events, such as postural change, exercise, laughing, smoking, induction of anesthesia, urination, or a change in environmental or body temperature.

Pheochromocytoma is commonly diagnosed during pregnancy, when uterine pressure on the tumor induces more frequent attacks; such attacks can prove fatal for both mother and fetus as a result of a stroke, acute pulmonary edema, cardiac arrhythmias, or hypoxia. In such patients, the risk of spontaneous abortion is high but most fetal deaths occur during labor or immediately after birth.

Complications

- ▶ Stroke
- ▶ Retinopathy
- ▶ Heart disease
- ▶ Irreversible kidney damage

Diagnosis

The most common presentation for pheochromocytoma is continuous hypertension with or without orthostatic hypotension. A history of acute episodes of hypertension, headache, sweating, and tachycardia—particularly in a patient with hyperglycemia, glycosuria, and hypermetabolism—strongly suggests pheochromocytoma. A patient who has intermittent attacks may have no symptoms during a latent phase. The tumor is rarely palpable; when it is, palpation of the surrounding area may induce an acute attack and help confirm the diagnosis. Generally, diagnosis depends on laboratory findings.

Increased urinary excretion of total free catecholamines and their metabolites, vanillylmandelic acid (VMA) and metanephrine, as measured by analysis of a 24-hour urine specimen, confirms pheochromocytoma.[4]

Labile blood pressure necessitates urine collection during a hypertensive episode and comparison of this specimen with a baseline specimen. Direct assay of total plasma catecholamines shows levels 10 to 50 times higher than normal.

Provocative tests with glucagon and phentolamine suggest the diagnosis; however, because they may precipitate a hypertensive crisis or induce a false-positive or false-

negative result, they're seldom used. The clonidine suppression test will cause decreased plasma catecholamine levels in normal patients but no change in those with pheochromocytoma. After demonstrating biochemical evidence of pheochromocytoma, a computed tomography scan or magnetic resonance imaging of the abdomen (where 95% of pheochromocytomas are located) is warranted. If a tumor isn't located—or if there's more than one—a radioactive iodine metaiodobenzylguanidine scintiscan or nuclear scan usually confirms the diagnosis in unclear cases. Angiography and excretory urography are no longer used; adrenal venography is used, but rarely.

IN THE NEWS *Research is being done to determine if there are genetic markers for pheochromocytoma malignancy.[3] (See Children with pheochromocytoma, page 398.)*

Treatment

Surgical removal of the tumor is the treatment of choice.[2] To decrease blood pressure, an alpha-adrenergic blocker or metyrosine is given from 1 to 2 weeks before surgery.[2] A beta-adrenergic blocker (propranolol) may also be used after achieving alpha blockade. Postoperatively, I.V. fluids, plasma volume expanders, vasopressors and, possibly, transfusions may be required for hypotension. Persistent hypertension can occur in the immediate postoperative period. If surgery isn't feasible, alpha- and beta-adrenergic blockers—such as phenoxybenzamine and propranolol, respectively—are beneficial in controlling catecholamine effects and preventing attacks. Management of an acute attack or hypertensive crisis requires I.V. phentolamine (push or drip) or nitroprusside to normalize blood pressure.

Special considerations

To ensure the reliability of urine catecholamine measurements, make sure the patient avoids foods high in vanillin (such as coffee,

EVIDENCE-BASED PRACTICE

Children with pheochromocytoma

Question: *Do children with pheochromocytoma present with the same symptoms as adults?*

Research: The characteristics of pheochromocytoma in children vary from those of adults with the disease. To identify these characteristics, researchers reviewed the records of 21 children with pheochromocytoma who were diagnosed clinically with confirmation by biochemical testing. Several factors were noted in performing the study, including the child's age, sex, presentation, associated conditions, diagnostic tests used, preoperative preparation, operative details, and outcome.

Conclusion: Of the 21 patients studied, 17 had adrenal tumors and 4 had extra-adrenal tumors; 17 had sporadic pheochromocytoma and 4 had the familial type; 2 patients (1 of each type) had malignant pheochromocytoma. The presenting symptoms varied from child to child; however, the children with the sporadic type all displayed hypertension and vision disturbances. All of the patients in the study had surgery to remove the tumors but only 17 re-

ceived alpha-adrenergic blockers preoperatively. Following treatment, 1 child with malignant pheochromocytoma died, 2 children continued to have significant vision disturbances, and 1 had ongoing neurologic deficits.

Application: Pheochromocytoma is rare in children and presents with characteristics that may be attributed to other disorders. Because early diagnosis and surgical removal are the most important aspects of treatment, the nurse should pay special attention to children who exhibit such symptoms as hypertension, headaches, and vision disturbances and refer them for additional evaluation to rule out an organic etiology.

Source: Bissada, N.K., et al. "Pheochromocytoma in Children and Adolescents: A Clinical Spectrum," *Journal of Pediatric Surgery* 43(3):540-43, March 2008.

nuts, chocolate, and bananas) for 2 days before urine collection of VMA. Also, be aware of possible drug therapy that may interfere with the accurate determination of VMA (such as guaifenesin and salicylates). Collect the urine in a special container, with hydrochloric acid, that has been prepared by the laboratory.[4]

▶ Obtain blood pressure readings often because transient hypertensive attacks are possible. Tell the patient to report headaches, palpitations, nervousness, or other symptoms of an acute attack. If hypertensive crisis develops, monitor blood pressure and heart rate every 2 to 5 minutes until blood pressure stabilizes at an acceptable level.[5]

▶ Check blood for glucose and watch for weight loss from hypermetabolism.

▶ After surgery, blood pressure may rise or fall sharply. Keep the patient quiet; provide a private room, if possible, because excitement may trigger a hypertensive episode. Postoperative hypertension is common because the stress of surgery and manipulation of the adrenal gland stimulate secretion of catecholamines. Because this excess secretion causes profuse sweating, keep the room cool, and change the patient's clothing and bedding often. If the patient receives phentolamine, monitor blood pressure closely. Observe and record adverse effects: dizziness, hypotension, and tachycardia. The first 24 to 48 hours immediately after surgery are the most critical because blood pressure can drop drastically.[5]

▶ If the patient is receiving vasopressors I.V., check blood pressure as per facility pro-

tocol or every 15 minutes while titrating, and regulate the drip to maintain a safe pressure. Arterial pressure lines facilitate constant monitoring.

▶ Watch for abdominal distention and return of bowel sounds.

▶ Give analgesics for pain, as ordered, but monitor blood pressure carefully because many analgesics, especially meperidine, can cause hypotension.

▶ If autosomal dominant transmission of pheochromocytoma is suspected, the patient's family should also be evaluated for this condition.

REFERENCES

1. Sweeney, A., et al (2007, September 11). "Pheochromocytoma" [Online]. Available at *www.emedicine.com/med/topic1816.htm.*
2. Pacak, K. "Preoperative Management of the Pheochromocytoma Patient," *Journal of Clinical Endocrinology and Metabolism* 92(11):4069-79, November 2007.
3. Thouënnon, E., et al. "Identification of Potential Gene Markers and Insights into the Pathophysiology of Pheochromocytoma Malignancy," *Journal of Clinical Endocrinology and Metabolism* 92(12):4865-72, December 2007.
4. Boyle, J.G., et al. "Comparison of Diagnostic Accuracy of Urinary Free Metanephrines, Vanillyl Mandelic Acid, and Catecholamines and Plasma Catecholamines for Diagnosis of Pheochromocytoma," *Journal of Clinical Endocrinology and Metabolism* 92(12):4602-08, December 2007.
5. Daub, K.F. "Pheochromocytoma: Challenges in Diagnosis and Nursing Care," *Nursing Clinics of North America* 42(1):101-11, March 2007.

THYROIDITIS

Inflammation of the thyroid gland occurs as autoimmune thyroiditis (long-term inflammatory disease), subacute granulomatous thyroiditis (self-limiting inflammation), Riedel's thyroiditis (rare, invasive fibrotic process), and miscellaneous thyroiditis (acute suppurative, chronic infective, and chronic noninfective).

Causes and incidence

Autoimmune thyroiditis is due to antibodies formed in response to thyroid antigens in the blood. The condition may cause inflammation and lymphocytic infiltration (Hashimoto's thyroiditis). It's the most common cause of hypothyroidism in the United States.[1] Glandular atrophy (myxedema) and Graves' disease are linked to autoimmune thyroiditis.

Subacute granulomatous thyroiditis usually follows mumps, influenza, coxsackievirus, or adenovirus infection. Riedel's thyroiditis is a rare condition of unknown etiology.

Miscellaneous thyroiditis results from bacterial invasion of the gland in acute suppurative thyroiditis; tuberculosis (TB), syphilis, actinomycosis, or other infectious agents in the chronic infective form; and sarcoidosis and amyloidosis in chronic noninfective thyroiditis. Postpartum thyroiditis (silent thyroiditis) is another autoimmune disorder associated with transient thyroiditis in females within 1 year after delivery.

Autoimmune thyroiditis is most prevalent among people ages 30 to 50 and is more common in females than in males (95% of cases occur in women).[2]

Signs and symptoms

Autoimmune thyroiditis usually produces no symptoms and commonly occurs in females, with peak incidence in middle age. It's the most prevalent cause of spontaneous hypothyroidism.

In subacute granulomatous thyroiditis, moderate thyroid enlargement may follow an upper respiratory tract infection or a sore throat. The thyroid may be painful and tender and dysphagia may occur.

In Riedel's thyroiditis, the gland enlarges slowly as it's replaced by hard, fibrous tissues. This fibrosis may compress the trachea

or the esophagus. The thyroid feels firm. Clinical effects of miscellaneous thyroiditis are characteristic of pyogenic infection: fever, pain, tenderness, and reddened skin over the gland.

Diagnosis

Precise diagnosis depends on the type of thyroiditis:

▶ *Autoimmune:* high titers of thyroglobulin and microsomal antibodies present in serum

▶ *Subacute granulomatous:* elevated erythrocyte sedimentation rate, increased thyroid hormone levels, decreased thyroidal radioiodine uptake

▶ *Chronic infective and noninfective:* varied findings, depending on underlying infection or other disease.

Treatment

Appropriate treatment varies with the type of thyroiditis. Drug therapy includes levothyroxine for accompanying hypothyroidism, propranolol for transient hyperthyroidism, and steroids for severe episodes of acute inflammation.[3] Analgesics and nonsteroidal anti-inflammatory drugs are used for mild subacute granulomatous thyroiditis and corticosteroids for more severe cases. Suppurative thyroiditis requires antibiotic therapy. A partial thyroidectomy may be necessary to relieve tracheal or esophageal compression in Riedel's thyroiditis.

Special considerations

Before treatment, obtain a patient history to identify underlying diseases that may cause thyroiditis, such as TB or a recent viral infection.

▶ Check the patient's vital signs, and examine her neck for unusual swelling, enlargement, or redness. Provide a liquid diet if she has difficulty swallowing, especially when due to fibrosis. If the neck is swollen, measure and record the circumference daily to monitor progressive enlargement.

▶ Administer antibiotics as ordered and report and record elevations in temperature.

▶ Instruct the patient to watch for and report signs of hypothyroidism (lethargy, restlessness, sensitivity to cold, forgetfulness, and dry skin), especially if she has Hashimoto's thyroiditis, which often causes hypothyroidism.

▶ Check for signs of hyperthyroidism (nervousness, tachycardia, tremor, and weakness), which commonly occurs in subacute thyroiditis.[3]

▶ After thyroidectomy, check vital signs every 15 to 30 minutes until the patient's condition stabilizes. Stay alert for signs of tetany secondary to accidental parathyroid injury during surgery. Keep 10% calcium gluconate available for I.V. use if needed. Assess dressings frequently for excessive bleeding. Watch for signs of airway obstruction, such as difficulty in talking or increased swallowing; keep tracheotomy equipment handy.

▶ Explain to the patient that she'll need lifelong thyroid hormone replacement therapy if hypothyroidism occurs. Tell her to watch for signs of overdosage, such as nervousness and palpitations, and to promptly report them to the prescriber.

REFERENCES

1. Mathur, R. (2007, August 9). "Hashimoto's Thyroiditis" [Online]. Available at *www.medicinenet.com/hashimotos_thyroiditis/article.htm.*
2. Slatosky, J., et al. "Thyroiditis: Differential Diagnosis and Management," *American Family Physician* 61(4):1047, February 2000.
3. American Association of Clinical Endocrinologists, "American Association of Clinical Endocrinologists Medical Guidelines for Clinical Practice for the Evaluation and Treatment of Hyperthyroidism and Hypothyroidism," *Endocrine Practice* 8(6):457-69, November-December 2002.

11

Sensory disorders

AGE-RELATED MACULAR DEGENERATION

Macular degeneration is the atrophy or degeneration of the macular region of the retina. Two types of age-related macular degeneration occur. The dry or atrophic form is the most common, characterized by atrophic pigment epithelial changes. It is most often associated with slow, progressive, and mild vision loss. The wet, exudative form causes progressive visual distortion leading to vision loss. It's characterized by subretinal neovascularization that causes leakage, hemorrhage, and fibrovascular scar formation, which produce significant loss of central vision.

Causes and incidence

Age-related macular degeneration (AMD) results from underlying pathologic changes that occur primarily at the level of the retinal pigment epithelium, Bruch's membrane, and the choriocapillaris in the macular region. Drusen (bumps), which are common in elderly people, appear as yellow deposits beneath the pigment epithelium and may be prominent in the macula. No predisposing conditions have been identified; however, some forms of the disorder are hereditary.

Macular degeneration is the most common cause of legal blindness in adults, accounting for about 12% of cases in the United States and about 17% of new blindness cases. It is estimated that by the year 2030, macular degeneration will cause more blindness in the U.S. than any of the other age-related diseases combined.[1] It's also one of the causes of severe irreversible loss of central vision in elderly people—by age 75, almost 15% of people have this condition. Whites have the highest incidence. Other risk factors are family history and cigarette smoking. Smoking may be associated with the progression of AMD and may increase the risk for the early onset of AMD.[2]

HEALTH & SAFETY *Quitting smoking may decrease the risk for early incidence of AMD.*

Signs and symptoms

The patient notices a change in central vision. Initially, straight lines (for example, of buildings) become distorted; later, a blank area appears in the center of a printed page (central scotoma).

Complications
- Bilateral macular lesions
- Nystagmus
- Blindness

Diagnosis

▶ Indirect ophthalmoscopy—fundus examination through a dilated pupil may reveal gross macular changes.

▶ I.V. fluorescein angiography—sequential photographs may show leaking vessels as fluorescein dye flows into the tissues from the subretinal neovascular net.

▶ Amsler's grid—used to monitor visual field loss.

Treatment

Treatment options are available for wet macular degeneration, but they are aimed at stopping the further progression of the disease. The damage already caused by macular degeneration cannot be reversed.[3] There is no treatment available for dry macular degeneration. However, there is an ongoing national study to determine the effectiveness of laser photocoagulation in patients with dry macular degeneration associated with drusen.[3]

Laser photocoagulation reduces the incidence of severe vision loss in the patient with subretinal neovascularization, turning serous age-related macular degeneration to the dry form.

Photodynamic therapy, which can be performed in a physician's office, is an option for the patient with wet macular degeneration. In this procedure, verteporfin (a light-sensitive medication) is injected into a vein in the patient's arm and allowed to circulate to the eyes. The physician then shines a laser into the eyes, and the verteporfin produces a chemical reaction that destroys abnormal blood vessels. If the vessels regrow, the procedure can be repeated. Antivascular endothelial growth factor medications (injections into the eye) are the newest treatment for AMD. Clinical trials are being done with future treatments such as kenalog (steroid injections), rheophoresis (blood filtering), and implantable optical devices.[3]

Special considerations

▶ Inform the patient with bilateral central vision loss of the visual rehabilitation services available to him.

▶ Special devices such as low-vision optical aids are available to improve the quality of life in the patient with good peripheral vision.

REFERENCES

1. Centers for Disease Control and Prevention (2001 March). "Trends in Vision and Hearing Among Older Americans" [Online]. Available at *www.cdc.gov/nchs/data/ahcd/agingtrends/02vision.pdf.*
2. Klein, R., et al. "Further Observations on the Association between Smoking and the Long-Term Incidence and Progression of Age-Related Macular Degeneration," *Archives of Ophthalmology* 126(1):115–21, January 2008.
3. Mayo Clinic (2008 March 27). "Macular Degeneration" [Online]. Available at *www.mayoclinic.com/health/macular-degeneration/DS00284.*

● CATARACT

The most common cause of correctable vision loss, a cataract is a gradually developing opacity of the lens or lens capsule of the eye. Cataracts commonly occur bilaterally, with each progressing independently. Exceptions are traumatic cataracts, which are usually unilateral, and congenital cataracts, which may remain stationary. The prognosis is generally good; surgery improves vision in 95% of people who undergo cataract surgery. Identified risk factors associated with cataracts include diabetes mellitus, hypertension, and high body mass index.[1]

Causes and incidence

Cataracts have various causes:

▶ Senile cataracts develop in elderly patients, probably because of degenerative changes in the chemical state of lens proteins.

▶ Congenital cataracts occur in neonates as genetic defects or as a sequela of maternal rubella during the first trimester. They acquire them through autosomal dominant inheritance, which will occur even if only one parent passes it along. Fifty percent of children in such families are affected.

▶ Traumatic cataracts may occur years after the injury.[2] They develop after a foreign body injures the lens with sufficient force to allow aqueous or vitreous humor to enter the lens capsule. Trauma may also dislocate the lens.

▶ Complicated cataracts develop as secondary effects in patients with uveitis, glaucoma, or retinitis pigmentosa, or in the course of a systemic disease, such as diabetes, hypoparathyroidism, or atopic dermatitis. They can also result from exposure to ionizing radiation or infrared rays.

▶ Toxic cataracts result from drug or chemical toxicity with prednisone, ergot alkaloids, dinitrophenol, naphthalene, phenothiazines, or pilocarpine, or from extended exposure to ultraviolet rays.

Cataracts occur as part of the aging process and are most prevalent in people older than age 70.

Signs and symptoms

Characteristically, a patient with a cataract experiences painless, gradual blurring and loss of vision. As the cataract progresses, the normally black pupil appears hazy, and when a mature cataract develops, the white lens may be seen through the pupil. Some patients complain of blinding glare from headlights when they drive at night; others complain of poor reading vision and an unpleasant glare and poor vision in bright sunlight. Patients with central opacities report better vision in dim light than in bright light because the cataract is nuclear and, as the pupils dilate, patients can see around the lens opacity.

Complications

▶ Complete vision loss (without corrective surgery)

Diagnosis

On examination, visual acuity is decreased, and the lens opacity remains unnoticeable until the cataract is advanced.

Ophthalmoscopy or slit-lamp examination confirms the diagnosis by revealing a dark area in the normally homogeneous red reflex.

Treatment

Treatment consists of surgical extraction of the cataractous lens opacity and intraoperative correction of visual deficits. Bilateral cataract surgery is scheduled on separate dates in order to give each eye a chance to heal.[3] The current trend is to perform the surgery as a same-day procedure. Surgical procedures include the following:

▶ Extracapsular cataract extraction (ECCE) removes the anterior lens capsule and cortex, leaving the posterior capsule intact. With this procedure, a posterior chamber intraocular lens (IOL) is implanted where the patient's own lens used to be. (A posterior chamber IOL is currently the most common type of lens used in the United States.) This procedure is appropriate for use in patients of all ages.

▶ Phacoemulsification uses ultrasonic vibrations to fragment and then emulsify the lens, which is then aspirated through a small incision.

▶ Intracapsular cataract extraction removes the entire lens within the intact capsule. This procedure is seldom performed today. ECCE with phacoemulsification has replaced it as the most commonly performed procedure.

▶ Discission and aspiration can still be used for children with soft cataracts, but this procedure has largely been replaced by phacoemulsification.

Infection is the most serious complication of intraocular surgery. Wound dehiscence can occur but is seldom a complication because of the small incision and minute sutures that are used. Hyphema, pupillary block glaucoma, and retinal detachment still occasionally occur.

The patient with an IOL implant may experience improved vision shortly after surgery if there's no corneal or retinal pathology. Most IOLs correct for distance vision, but new IOLs are multifocal. However, the majority of patients will need either corrective reading glasses or a corrective contact lens, which will be fitted sometime between 4 and 6 weeks after surgery.

Where no IOL has been implanted, the patient may be given temporary aphakic cataract glasses; in about 4 to 8 weeks, he'll be refracted for his own glasses.

Some patients who have an extracapsular cataract extraction develop a secondary membrane in the posterior lens capsule (which has been left intact), which causes decreased visual acuity. This membrane can be removed by the Nd:YAG laser, which cuts an area out of the center of the membrane, thereby restoring vision. Laser therapy isn't used to remove a cataract. Although cataract development prevention is not known, limiting the following may delay the occurrence of cataracts: cigarette smoking, ultraviolet light exposure, and alcohol consumption.[1]

Posterior capsular opacification occurs in approximately 15% to 20% of all patients within 2 years after cataract surgery.

Special considerations

After surgery to extract a cataract:

▶ Because the patient will be discharged after he recovers from anesthesia, remind him to return for a checkup the next day, and warn him to avoid activities that increase intraocular pressure such as straining at stool.

▶ Urge the patient to protect the eye from accidental injury at night by wearing a plastic or metal shield with perforations; a shield or glasses should be worn for protection during the day.

▶ Before discharge, teach the patient to administer antibiotic ointment or drops to prevent infection and steroids to reduce inflammation. Combination steroid-antibiotic eyedrops can also be used.

▶ Advise the patient to watch for the development of complications, such as a sharp pain in the eye that is not reduced by analgesics (the likely cause: hyphema) or clouding in the anterior chamber (which may herald an infection). The patient should report these developments immediately.

▶ Caution the patient about activity restrictions, and advise him that it will take several weeks for him to receive his corrective reading glasses or lenses.

REFERENCES

1. World Health Organization. "Prevention of Blindness and Visual Impairment: Cataract" [Online]. Available at *www.who.int/blindness/causes/priority/en/index1.html.*
2. National Eye Institute. "Cataract" [Online]. Available at *www.nei.nih.gov/health/cataract/cataract_facts.asp.*
3. Mayo Clinic (2008 March 27). "Cataract Surgery" [Online]. Available at *www.mayoclinic.com/health/cataract-surgery/EY00014.*

CORNEAL ULCERS

A major cause of blindness worldwide, ulcers produce corneal scarring or perforation. They occur in the central or marginal areas of the cornea, vary in shape and size, and may be singular or multiple. Marginal ulcers are the most common form. Prompt treatment (within hours of onset) can prevent visual impairment.

Causes

Corneal ulcers generally result from protozoan, bacterial, viral, or fungal infections. Common bacterial sources include *Staphylococcus aureus, Pseudomonas aeruginosa, Streptococcus viridans, Streptococcus (Diplococcus) pneumoniae,* and *Moraxella liquefaciens;* viral sources comprise *Herpes simplex* type 1, *Variola, Vaccinia,* and *Varicella zoster* viruses; and

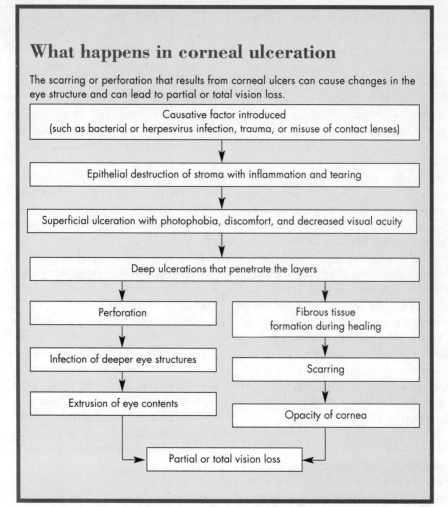

What happens in corneal ulceration

The scarring or perforation that results from corneal ulcers can cause changes in the eye structure and can lead to partial or total vision loss.

Causative factor introduced
(such as bacterial or herpesvirus infection, trauma, or misuse of contact lenses)

↓

Epithelial destruction of stroma with inflammation and tearing

↓

Superficial ulceration with photophobia, discomfort, and decreased visual acuity

↓

Deep ulcerations that penetrate the layers

Perforation	Fibrous tissue formation during healing
↓	↓
Infection of deeper eye structures	Scarring
↓	↓
Extrusion of eye contents	Opacity of cornea

Partial or total vision loss

common fungal sources are *Candida, Fusarium,* and *Cephalosporium.*

Other causes include trauma, exposure, reactions to bacterial infections, toxins, trichiasis, entropion, allergens, and wearing of contact lenses. (See *What happens in corneal ulceration.*) Tuberculoprotein causes a classic phlyctenular keratoconjunctivitis, vitamin A deficiency results in xerophthalmia, and fifth cranial nerve lesions lead to neurotropic ulcers. Another cause that's on the rise—poor hygiene habits regarding the care of contact lens by wearers of contact lenses. Those who use the continuous

wear and overnight type of lenses are at greater risk.[1]

HEALTH & SAFETY *Proper contact lens care and wearing schedules are essential to reducing the risks of developing corneal ulcers. Between 46% and 57% of patients are noncompliant with recommended contact lens care guidelines.[1]*

Signs and symptoms

Typically, corneal ulceration begins with pain (aggravated by blinking) and photophobia, followed by increased tearing. Eventually, central corneal ulceration pro-

duces pronounced visual blurring. The eye may appear infected. If a bacterial ulcer is present, purulent discharge is possible.

Complications
▶ Eye tic (involuntary eye blinking)
▶ Corneal infiltrates
▶ Vision loss

Diagnosis
A history of trauma or use of contact lenses and flashlight examination that reveals irregular corneal surface suggest corneal ulcer. Exudate may be present on the cornea, and a hypopyon (accumulation of white cells in the anterior chamber) may appear as a white crescent moon that moves when the head is tilted. A slit lamp microscope is used. Fluorescein dye, instilled in the conjunctival sac, stains the outline of the ulcer and also confirms the diagnosis. A visual acuity test, refraction test, and a tear test are additional diagnostic methods.[2]

Culture and sensitivity testing of corneal scrapings may identify the causative bacteria or fungus and may indicate appropriate antibiotic or antifungal therapy.

Treatment
Prompt treatment is essential for all forms of corneal ulcer to prevent complications and permanent visual impairment. Treatment usually consists of systemic and topical broad-spectrum antibiotics until culture results identify the causative organism. The goals of treatment are to eliminate the underlying cause of the ulcer, relieve pain, and restore vision:
▶ Fungi—topical instillation of natamycin for *Fusarium, Cephalosporium,* and *Candida.*
▶ Herpes simplex type 1 virus—topical application of trifluridine drops or vidarabine ointment. Corneal ulcers resulting from a viral infection often recur, requiring further treatment with trifluridine.
▶ Hypovitaminosis A—correction of dietary deficiency or GI malabsorption of vitamin A.

▶ Infection by *P. aeruginosa*—polymyxin B and gentamicin, administered topically and by subconjunctival injection, or carbenicillin and tobramycin I.V. Because this type of corneal ulcer spreads so rapidly, it can cause corneal perforation and loss of the eye within 48 hours. Immediate treatment and isolation of hospitalized patients are required. Sometimes corneal implant surgery is needed to restore vision.[3]

Treatment for a corneal ulcer due to bacterial infection should never include an eye patch because patching creates the dark, warm, moist environment ideal for bacterial growth.
▶ Neurotropic ulcers or exposure keratitis—frequent instillation of artificial tears or lubricating ointments and use of a plastic bubble eye shield.
▶ *Varicella zoster* virus—topical sulfonamide ointment applied three to four times daily to prevent secondary infection. These lesions are unilateral, following the pathway of the fifth cranial nerve, and are typically quite painful. Give analgesics as ordered. Associated anterior uveitis requires cycloplegic eyedrops. Watch for signs of secondary glaucoma (transient vision loss and halos around lights).

Special considerations
▶ Keep the room darkened, and orient the patient as necessary.
▶ Teach the patient how to properly clean and wear his contact lenses to prevent a recurrence.

REFERENCES
1. Jeng, B. H. "Corneal Infections: Epidemiology, Prevention," *Review of Ophthalmology* 13:07, July 10, 2006.
2. Georgetown University Hospital (2006 September 1). "Corneal Ulcers and Infections" [Online]..Available at *www.georgetown universityhospital.org/body.cfm?id=555563& action=articleDetail&AEProductID=Adam 2004_1&AEArticleID=001032.*

3. Mayo Clinic (2007 February). "Cornea
Transplants: Restoring Sight with Donor
Tissue" [Online]. Available at *www.mayoclinic.
com/health/cornea-transplant/EY00004*.

GLAUCOMA

Glaucoma is a group of disorders characterized by an abnormally high intraocular pressure (IOP), which can damage the optic nerve. IOP changes are an important predictor of glaucoma progression.[1] If untreated, glaucoma can lead to gradual peripheral vision loss and, ultimately, blindness. (See *Blindness*.) Glaucoma occurs in several forms: chronic open-angle (primary), acute angle-closure, congenital (inherited as an autosomal recessive trait), and secondary to other causes. The prognosis for maintaining vision is good with early treatment.

Blindness

Blindness affects 28 million people worldwide. In the United States, blindness is legally defined as optimal visual acuity of 20/200 or less in the better eye after best correction, or a visual field of 20 degrees or less in the better eye.

According to the World Health Organization, the most common causes of preventable blindness worldwide are trachoma, cataracts, onchocerciasis (microfilarial infection transmitted by a blackfly and other species of *Simulium*), and xerophthalmia (dryness of conjunctiva and cornea from vitamin A deficiency).

In the United States, the most common causes of acquired blindness are glaucoma, age-related macular degeneration, and diabetic retinopathy. However, the incidence of blindness from glaucoma is decreasing owing to early detection and treatment. Rarer causes of acquired blindness include herpes simplex keratitis, cataracts, and retinal detachment.

Causes and incidence

Glaucoma affects approximately 2.5 million people in the United States and is expected to increase to 60.5 million people worldwide by 2010.[2]

Chronic open-angle glaucoma results from overproduction of aqueous humor or obstruction to its outflow through the trabecular meshwork or the canal of Schlemm. (See *Normal flow of aqueous humor.*) This form of glaucoma, which is estimated to be present in 1% to 2% of people older than age 40, is frequently familial in origin and affects 90% of all patients with glaucoma. Diabetes and systemic hypertension have also been associated with this form of glaucoma.

Acute angle-closure (narrow-angle) glaucoma results from obstruction to the outflow of aqueous humor due to anatomically narrow angles between the anterior iris and the posterior corneal surface, shallow anterior chambers, a thickened iris that causes angle closure on pupil dilation, or a bulging iris that presses on the trabeculae, closing the angle (peripheral anterior synechiae).

Blacks are four times more likely to have this disorder than Whites, and people with a family history of open-angle glaucoma are twice as likely to develop it as people without a family history of this disorder. The use of systemic anticholinergic medications, such as atropine or eye dilation drops, in a person who is already at high-risk for acute glaucoma increases the risk. Other risk factors include farsightedness and age-related changes that create an increase in intraocular pressure.

Congenital glaucoma occurs when there is an abnormal fluid drainage angle of the eye. It may be caused by congenital infections such as the TORCH virus (toxoplasmosis, other [*Varicella*, mumps, parvovirus, human immunodeficiency virus], rubella, cytomegalovirus, and herpes), Sturge-Weber syndrome, or retinopathy of prematurity.

Secondary glaucoma can result from uveitis, trauma, or drugs (such as steroids).

Neovascularization in the angle of the anterior chamber can result from vein occlusion or diabetes.

Signs and symptoms

IN THE NEWS *Glaucoma has no symptoms in its early stages and up to 40% of useful sight can be lost before a person realizes he has the condition.[3] Chronic open-angle glaucoma is usually bilateral, with insidious onset and a slowly progressive course. Symptoms appear late in the disease and include mild aching in the eyes, loss of peripheral vision, seeing halos around lights, and reduced visual acuity (especially at night) that isn't correctable with glasses.*

Acute angle-closure glaucoma typically has a rapid onset, constituting an ophthalmic emergency. Symptoms include acute pain in a unilaterally inflamed eye, with pressure over the eye, moderate pupil dilation that is nonreactive to light, a cloudy cornea, blurring and decreased visual acuity, photophobia, and seeing halos around lights. Increased IOP may induce nausea and vomiting, which may cause glaucoma to be misinterpreted as GI distress. Unless treated

Normal flow of aqueous humor

Aqueous humor, a plasma-like fluid produced by the ciliary epithelium of the ciliary body, flows from the posterior chamber to the anterior chamber through the pupil. Here it flows peripherally and filters through the trabecular meshwork to the canal of Schlemm, through which the fluid ultimately enters venous circulation.

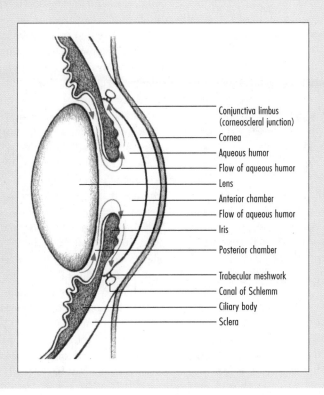

- Conjunctiva limbus (corneoscleral junction)
- Cornea
- Aqueous humor
- Flow of aqueous humor
- Lens
- Anterior chamber
- Flow of aqueous humor
- Iris
- Posterior chamber
- Trabecular meshwork
- Canal of Schlemm
- Ciliary body
- Sclera

promptly, this acute form of glaucoma produces blindness in 3 to 5 days.

Complications of untreated glaucoma

▶ Gradual vision loss
▶ Blindness

Diagnosis

Loss of peripheral vision and disk changes confirm that glaucoma is present. Diagnosis is made by:

▶ testing IOP
▶ measuring the visual field and noting changes, such as an enlarged blind spot and loss of peripheral vision field
▶ observing changes in the cup/disk ratio of the optic nerve head.

Relevant diagnostic tests include:

▶ Tonometry (using an applanation Tonopen or air puff tonometer)—This test measures the IOP and provides a baseline for reference. Normal IOP ranges from 8 to 21 mm Hg. However, patients who fall within this normal range can develop signs and symptoms of glaucoma, and patients who have abnormally high pressure may have no clinical effects. Fingertip tension is another way to measure IOP. On gentle palpation of closed eyelids, one eye feels harder than the other in acute angle-closure glaucoma.
▶ Slit-lamp examination—The slit lamp facilitates examination of the anterior structures of the eye: the cornea, iris, and lens.
▶ Gonioscopy—By determining the angle of the anterior chamber of the eye, this test enables differentiation between chronic open-angle glaucoma and acute angle-closure glaucoma. The angle is normal in chronic open-angle glaucoma. However, in older patients, partial closure of the angle may occur, so that two forms of glaucoma may co-exist.
▶ Ophthalmoscopy—This test enables the examiner to look at the fundus to establish if there are any cup/disk ratio changes. These changes appear later in chronic glaucoma if the disease isn't brought under control.

▶ Fundus photography—Pictures of the optic nerve head are made to track changes.
▶ Perimetry or visual field tests—These reveal the extent of damage to the optic neurons, signaled by an enlarged blind spot and loss of peripheral vision.
▶ Pachymetry—Numbing drops are applied, and an ultrasound wave instrument is used to measure corneal thickness.

Treatment

For chronic open-angle glaucoma, treatment initially decreases IOP through the use of an alpha antagonist, brimonidine tartrate (Alphagan or Iopidine), and then beta-adrenergic blockers, such as timolol (contraindicated for asthmatics or patients with bradycardia) or betaxolol (Betoptic) to reduce aqueous humor production. A topical anhydrase inhibitor is used in preference to a systemic anhydrase inhibitor such as acetazolamide. A tubo-plast or tube shunt or valve may also be used. Miotic eyedrops, such as pilocarpine, facilitate the outflow of aqueous humor.

Patients who are unresponsive to drug therapy may be candidates for argon laser trabeculoplasty (ALT) or a surgical filtering procedure called trabeculectomy, which creates an opening for aqueous outflow. In ALT, an argon laser beam is focused on the trabecular meshwork of an open angle. This produces a thermal burn that changes the surface of the meshwork and increases the outflow of aqueous humor. In trabeculectomy, a flap of sclera is dissected free to expose the trabecular meshwork. Then this discrete tissue block is removed, and a peripheral iridectomy is performed. This produces an opening for aqueous outflow under the conjunctiva, creating a filtering bleb. In chronic refractory glaucoma, a turboplast or tube shunt or valve is used to keep IOP within normal limits.

Acute angle-closure glaucoma is an ocular emergency requiring immediate treatment to lower the high IOP. Preoperative drug therapy

lowers IOP with I.V. acetazolamide, plus pilocarpine (which constricts the pupil, forcing the iris away from the trabeculae, allowing fluid to escape), timolol, and a topical steroid to quiet the inflammatory response, along with I.V. mannitol (20%) or oral glycerin (50%) to force fluid from the eye by making the blood hypertonic. Latanoprost is a topical medication that helps drain the aqueous outflow from the eye and lower the IOP. Oral medication or topical drops may be prescribed separately or in combination. Severe pain may necessitate administration of opioid analgesics. If pressure doesn't decrease with drug therapy, laser iridotomy or surgical peripheral iridectomy must be performed promptly to save the patient's vision. Iridectomy relieves pressure by excising part of the iris to reestablish aqueous humor outflow. A prophylactic iridectomy is performed a few days later on the other eye to prevent an acute episode of glaucoma in the normal eye.

Special considerations

▶ Stress the importance of meticulous compliance with prescribed drug therapy to prevent an increase in IOP, resulting in disk changes and loss of vision.

▶ For the patient with acute angle-closure glaucoma, give medications as ordered, and prepare him physically and psychologically for laser iridotomy or surgery.

▶ Postoperative care after peripheral iridectomy includes cycloplegic eyedrops to relax the ciliary muscle and to decrease inflammation, thus preventing adhesions.

HEALTH & SAFETY *Cycloplegics must be used only in the affected eye. The use of these drops in the normal eye may precipitate an attack of acute angle-closure glaucoma in this eye, threatening the patient's residual vision.*

▶ Encourage ambulation immediately after surgery.

▶ Following surgical filtering, postoperative care includes dilation and topical steroids to rest the pupil.

▶ Stress the importance of glaucoma screening for early detection and prevention. All people older than age 35, especially those with family histories of glaucoma, should have an annual tonometric examination.

REFERENCES

1. Lee, P. P., et al. "Association between Intraocular Pressure Variation and Glaucoma Progression: Data from a United States Chart Review," *American Journal of Ophthalmology* 144(6):901–907, December 2007.
2. Goldberg, Lawrence D. "Disease Management Programs for Glaucoma: Has the Vision Become a Reality?," *Disease Management & Health Outcomes* 15(4):199–205, 2007.
3. Royal National Institute of Blind People (2008 July 3). "Glaucoma Awareness Campaign" [Online]. Available at *www.rnib.org/xpedio/ groups/public/documents/publicwebsite/ public_glaucomacampaign.hcsp.*

MÉNIÈRE'S DISEASE

Ménière's disease, a labyrinthine dysfunction also known as endolymphatic hydrops, produces severe vertigo, sensorineural hearing loss, and tinnitus. After multiple attacks over several years, this disorder leads to residual tinnitus and hearing loss. Usually, only one ear is involved. Ninety-three percent of primary care patients with vertigo may have Ménière's disease.[1]

Causes and incidence

The exact cause of Ménière's disease is unknown. It may result from overproduction or decreased absorption of endolymph, which causes endolymphatic hydrops or endolymphatic hypertension, with consequent degeneration of the vestibular and cochlear hair cells. This condition may also stem from autonomic nervous system dysfunction that produces a temporary constriction of blood vessels supplying the inner ear. In some cases, Ménière's disease may be related to otitis

media, syphilis, or head injury. Risk factors include recent viral illness, respiratory infection, stress, fatigue, use of prescription or nonprescription drugs (such as aspirin), and a history of allergies, smoking, and alcohol use. There also may be genetic risk factors: In some women, premenstrual edema may precipitate attacks of Ménière's disease. There is strong evidence that Ménière's disease may have a familial component as well. About one in three patients with Ménière's disease has a first-degree relative with the disease.[2]

Signs and symptoms

Ménière's disease produces three characteristic effects: severe episodic vertigo, tinnitus, and sensorineural hearing loss. A feeling of fullness or blockage in the ear is also common. Violent paroxysmal attacks last from 10 minutes to several hours. During an acute attack, other symptoms include severe nausea, vomiting, sweating, giddiness, and nystagmus. Vertigo may cause loss of balance and falling to the affected side. Symptoms tend to wax and wane as the endolymphatic pressure rises and falls. To lessen these symptoms, the patient may assume a characteristic posture—lying on the side of the unaffected ear and looking in the direction of the affected ear.

Initially, the patient may be asymptomatic between attacks, except for residual tinnitus that worsens during an attack. Such attacks may occur several times a year, or remissions may last as long as several years. These attacks become less frequent as hearing loss progresses (usually unilaterally); they may cease when hearing loss is total. All symptoms are aggravated by motion.

Complications

▶ Residual tinnitus
▶ Partial to total hearing loss
▶ Permanent balance disability
▶ Trauma from falling

▶ Dehydration
▶ Reduced quality of life

Diagnosis

Presence of all three typical symptoms suggests Ménière's disease. Audiometric studies indicate a sensorineural hearing loss and loss of discrimination and recruitment. Selected studies such as electronystagmography, electrocochleography, computed tomography scan, magnetic resonance imaging, or X-rays of the internal meatus may be necessary for differential diagnosis.

Laboratory studies, including thyroid and lipid studies, may be performed to rule out other conditions such as *Treponema pallidum.*

Caloric testing may reveal loss or impairment of thermally induced nystagmus on the involved side. However, it's important not to overlook an acoustic tumor, which produces an identical clinical picture.

Treatment

Treatment with atropine may stop an attack in 20 to 30 minutes. Epinephrine or diphenhydramine may be necessary in a severe attack; dimenhydrinate, meclizine, diphenhydramine, or diazepam may be effective in a milder attack.

Long-term management includes use of a diuretic or vasodilator and restricted sodium intake (less than 2 g/day). A typical diuretic regimen is hydrochlorothiazide 100 to 500 mg daily. Prophylactic antihistamines or mild sedatives (phenobarbital, diazepam) may also be helpful. If Ménière's disease persists after 2 years of treatment, produces incapacitating vertigo, or resists medical management, surgery may be necessary. In 2002, the Food and Drug Administration approved the Meniette device as a noninvasive treatment of Ménière's disease. It is a pressure-emitting instrument that is used as an alternative to surgery or with the placement of a standard myringotomy tube for patients who fail conventional treatment.[3]

Destruction of the affected labyrinth permanently relieves symptoms but results in irreversible hearing loss. Systemic streptomycin is reserved for the patient with bilateral disease for whom no other treatment can be considered. If a patient fails medical therapy and remains disabled by his vertigo, surgical decompression of the endolymphatic sac may bring relief.

Special considerations

If the patient is in the hospital during an attack of Ménière's disease:
▶ Advise him against reading and exposure to glaring lights to reduce dizziness.
▶ Keep the side rails of the patient's bed up to prevent falls. Tell him not to get out of bed or walk without assistance.
▶ Instruct the patient to avoid sudden position changes and any tasks that vertigo makes hazardous because an attack can begin quite rapidly. Hazardous activities, such as driving and climbing, should be avoided until one week after symptoms disappear.
▶ Before surgery, if the patient is vomiting, record fluid intake and output and characteristics of vomitus. Administer antiemetics as needed, and give small amounts of fluid frequently.
▶ After surgery, record intake and output carefully. Tell the patient to expect dizziness and nausea for 1 to 2 days after surgery. Give prophylactic antibiotics and antiemetics, as ordered.

REFERENCES
1. Labuguen, R. H. "Initial Evaluation of Vertigo," *American Family Physician* 73(2):244–51, January 2006.
2. Arevalo, J. D. "Ménière's Disease: A Diagnosis of Exclusion with Controversial Therapies," *ENToday* 3(1):12–14, 16, January 2008.
3. Mattox, Douglas E., Reichert, Mary. "Meniett Device for Meniere's Disease: Use and Compliance at 3 to 5 Years," *Otology & Neurotology* 29(1):29–32, January 2008.

OTITIS EXTERNA

Otitis externa, inflammation of the skin of the external ear canal and auricle, may be acute or chronic. Also known as external otitis and swimmer's ear, it is most common in the summer. With treatment, acute otitis externa usually subsides within 7 days, but it can last for several weeks. It may become chronic, and it tends to recur. The unique structure of the external auditory canal contributes to the development of otitis externa. The external auditory canal is warm, dark, and prone to becoming moist, making it an excellent environment for bacterial and fungal growth.[1]

Causes and incidence

Otitis externa usually results from bacteria, such as *Pseudomonas, Proteus vulgaris, Staphylococcus aureus,* and *streptococci* and, sometimes, from fungi, such as *Aspergillus niger* and *Candida albicans* (fungal otitis externa is most common in tropical regions). Acute otitis externa is unilateral in 90% of patients; it peaks in people ages 7 to 12 and declines after age 50.[2] Occasionally, chronic otitis externa results from dermatologic conditions, such as seborrhea or psoriasis. It affects 3% to 5% of the population.[2] Allergic reactions stemming from nickel or chromium earrings, chemicals in hair spray, cosmetics, hearing aids, and medications (such as sulfonamide and neomycin, which is commonly used to treat otitis externa) can also cause otitis externa.

Annually, otitis externa affects 4 in 1,000 persons in the United States.[2]

Predisposing factors include:
▶ Swimming in contaminated water; cerumen creates a culture medium for the waterborne organism.
▶ Cleaning the ear canal with a cotton swab, bobby pin, finger, or other foreign object; this irritates the ear canal and, possibly, introduces the infecting microorganism.

▶ Exposure to dust or hair care products (such as hair spray or other irritants), which causes the patient to scratch his ear, excoriating the auricle and canal.

▶ Regular use of earphones, earplugs, or earmuffs, which trap moisture in the ear canal, creating a culture medium for infection (especially if earplugs don't fit properly).

▶ Chronic drainage due to a perforated tympanic membrane.

▶ Use of perfumes or self-administered eardrops.

Signs and symptoms

Acute otitis externa characteristically produces moderate to severe pain that's exacerbated by manipulating the auricle or tragus, clenching the teeth, opening the mouth, or chewing. Its other clinical effects may include fever, foul-smelling discharge, crusting in the external ear, regional cellulitis, partial hearing loss, and itching. It's usually difficult to view the tympanic membrane because of pain in the external canal. Hearing acuity is normal unless complete occlusion has occurred.

Fungal otitis externa may be asymptomatic, although *A. niger* produces a black or gray, blotting, paperlike growth in the ear canal. In chronic otitis externa, pruritus replaces pain, and scratching may lead to scaling and skin thickening. Aural discharge may also occur.

Complications

▶ Complete closure of ear canal
▶ Significant hearing loss
▶ Middle ear infection (otitis media)
▶ Cellulitis
▶ Abscesses
▶ Decolorization
▶ Disfigurement of the pinna
▶ Lymphadenopathy
▶ Ostitis
▶ Septicemia
▶ Stenosis

Diagnosis

Physical examination confirms otitis externa. In acute otitis externa, otoscopy reveals a swollen external ear canal (sometimes to the point of complete closure), periauricular lymphadenopathy (tender nodes anterior to the tragus, posterior to the ear, or in the upper neck) and, occasionally, regional cellulitis.

In fungal otitis externa, removal of the growth reveals thick red epithelium. Microscopic examination or culture and sensitivity tests can identify the causative organism and determine antibiotic treatment. Pain on palpation of the tragus or auricle distinguishes acute otitis externa from acute otitis media. (See *Differentiating acute otitis externa from acute otitis media,* page 415.)

In chronic otitis externa, physical examination reveals thick red epithelium in the ear canal. Severe chronic otitis externa may reflect underlying diabetes mellitus, hypothyroidism, or nephritis. Microscopic examination or culture and sensitivity tests can identify the causative organism and help in the determination of antibiotic treatment.

Treatment

To relieve the pain of acute otitis externa, treatment includes heat therapy to the periauricular region (heat lamp; hot, damp compresses; or a heating pad), aspirin or acetaminophen, and codeine. Instillation of antibiotic eardrops (with or without hydrocortisone) follows cleaning of the ear and removal of debris. However, a corticosteroid helps reduce the inflammatory response. If fever persists or regional cellulitis or tender postauricular adenopathy develops, a systemic antibiotic is necessary.

If the ear canal is too edematous for the instillation of eardrops, an ear wick may be used for the first few days.

Topical treatment is generally required for otitis externa, as systemic antibiotics alone aren't sufficient. Analgesics, such as aceta-

minophen or ibuprofen, may be required temporarily.

As with other forms of this disorder, fungal otitis externa necessitates careful cleaning of the ear. Application of a keratolytic or 2% salicylic acid in cream containing nystatin may help treat otitis externa resulting from candidal organisms. Instillation of slightly acidic eardrops creates an unfavorable environment in the ear canal for most fungi as well as Pseudomonas. No specific treatment exists for otitis externa caused by *A. niger,* except repeated cleaning of the ear canal with baby oil.

In chronic otitis externa, primary treatment consists of cleaning the ear and removing debris. Supplemental therapy includes instillation of antibiotic eardrops or application of antibiotic ointment or cream (neomycin, bacitracin, or polymyxin B, possibly combined with hydrocortisone). Another ointment contains phenol, salicylic acid, precipitated sulfur, and petroleum jelly and produces exfoliative and antipruritic effects.

For mild chronic otitis externa, treatment may include instillation of antibiotic eardrops once or twice weekly and wearing of specially fitted earplugs while the patient is showering, shampooing, or swimming.

Special considerations

If the patient has acute otitis externa:
▶ The patient shouldn't participate in any swimming activity.
▶ Have the patient return to the clinic in 1 week for evaluation of the external auditory canal and integrity of the tympanic membrane.
▶ Monitor vital signs, particularly temperature. Watch for and record the type and amount of aural drainage.
▶ Remove debris and gently clean the ear canal with mild Burow's solution (aluminum acetate). Place a wisp of cotton soaked with solution into the ear, and apply a saturated compress directly to the auricle. Afterward, dry the ear gently but thoroughly. (In severe otitis externa, such cleaning may be delayed until after initial treatment with antibiotic eardrops.)
▶ To instill eardrops in an adult, grasp the helix and pull upward and backward to straighten the canal. To instill eardrops in a child, pull the earlobe downward and backward. To ensure that the drops reach the epithelium, insert a wisp of cotton moistened with eardrops.
▶ Tell the patient to notify the physician if he develops an allergic reaction to the antibiotic drops or ointment, which may be indicated by increased swelling, hives and discomfort of the area and worsening of other symptoms.

If the patient has chronic otitis externa, clean the ear thoroughly. Use wet soaks intermittently on oozing or infected skin. If the patient has a chronic fungal infection, clean the ear canal well, then apply an exfoliative ointment.

To prevent otitis externa:
▶ Suggest using lamb's wool earplugs coated with petroleum jelly to keep water out of the ears when showering or shampooing.
▶ Tell the patient to wear earplugs or to keep his head above water when swimming and to instill two or three drops of 3% boric acid solution in 70% alcohol into his ear before and after swimming to toughen the skin of the external ear canal.
▶ Do not use cotton swabs or other objects to clean the ear canals.
▶ If the patient is an elderly person or diabetic, evaluate him for malignant otitis externa.
▶ Urge prompt treatment for otitis media to prevent perforation of the tympanic membrane.
▶ Children who have an intact tympanic membrane but are predisposed to otitis externa from swimming should place 2 or 3 drops of a mixture of vinegar, isopropyl

Differentiating acute otitis externa from acute otitis media

Use the assessment findings shown below to help differentiate acute otitis externa from acute otitis media.

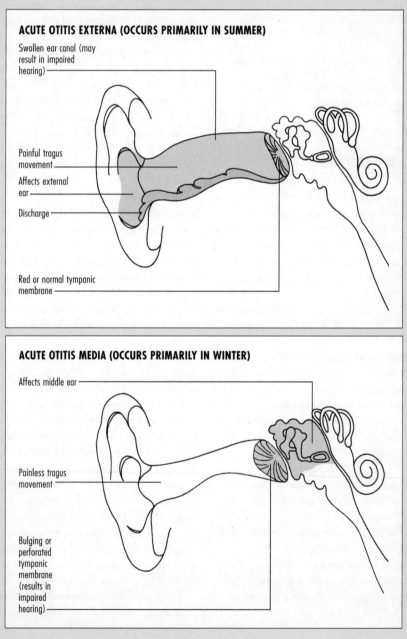

ACUTE OTITIS EXTERNA (OCCURS PRIMARILY IN SUMMER)

Swollen ear canal (may result in impaired hearing)

Painful tragus movement

Affects external ear

Discharge

Red or normal tympanic membrane

ACUTE OTITIS MEDIA (OCCURS PRIMARILY IN WINTER)

Affects middle ear

Painless tragus movement

Bulging or perforated tympanic membrane (results in impaired hearing)

alcohol, and water into their ears after their ears come in contact with water.[3]

REFERENCES
1. Sander, R. "Otitis Externa: A Practical Guide to Treatment and Prevention," *American Family Physician* 63(5):927–36, 941–2, March 2001.
2. Osguthorpe, D. J., et al. "Otitis Externa: Review and Clinical Update," *American Family Physician* 74(9):1510–6, November 2006.
3. Children's Hospital Boston. "Otitis Externa (Swimmer's Ear)" [Online]. Available at *www.childrenshospital.org/az/Site1398/mainpageS1398P0.html.*

OTITIS MEDIA

There are two types of otitis media: acute otitis media, a middle ear infection that occurs abruptly, causing swelling and redness; and otitis media with effusion, when mucus continues to accumulate in the middle ear after an initial infection subsides.[2]

Further categorized, otitis media, inflammation of the middle ear, may be suppurative or secretory, persistent, unresponsive, or chronic. With prompt treatment, the prognosis for acute otitis media is excellent; however, prolonged accumulation of fluid within the middle ear cavity causes chronic otitis media and, possibly, perforation of the tympanic membrane. (See *Site of otitis media.*)

Chronic suppurative otitis media may lead to scarring, adhesions, and severe structural or functional ear damage. Chronic secretory otitis media, with its persistent inflammation and pressure, may cause conductive hearing loss.

Recurrent otitis media is defined as three or more acute otitis media episodes within 6 months or four episodes of acute otitis media within 1 year.

Otitis media with complications involves damage to middle ear structures (such as adhesions, retraction, pockets, cholesteatoma, and intratemporal and intracranial complications).

Causes and incidence

Otitis media results from disruption of eustachian tube patency. In the suppurative form, respiratory tract infection, allergic reaction, nasotracheal intubation, or positional changes allow nasopharyngeal flora to reflux through the eustachian tube and colonize the middle ear. Suppurative otitis media usually results from bacterial infection with *pneumococcus, Haemophilus influenzae* (the most common cause in children younger than age 6), *Moraxella catarrhalis, beta-hemolytic streptococci, staphylococci* (most common cause in children age 6 or older), or gram-negative bacteria. Predisposing factors include the normally wider, shorter, more horizontal eustachian tubes and increased lymphoid tissue in children, as well as anatomic anomalies. Chronic suppurative otitis media results from inadequate treatment for acute otitis episodes or from infection by resistant strains of bacteria or, rarely, tuberculosis.

Secretory otitis media results from obstruction of the eustachian tube. This causes a buildup of negative pressure in the middle ear that promotes transudation of sterile serous fluid from blood vessels in the membrane of the middle ear. Such effusion may be secondary to eustachian tube dysfunction from viral infection or allergy. It may also follow barotrauma (pressure injury caused by the inability to equalize pressures between the environment and the middle ear), as occurs during rapid aircraft descent in a person with an upper respiratory tract infection or during rapid underwater ascent in scuba diving (barotitis media).

Chronic secretory otitis media follows persistent eustachian tube dysfunction from mechanical obstruction (adenoidal tissue

Site of otitis media

The common site of otitis media is shown below.

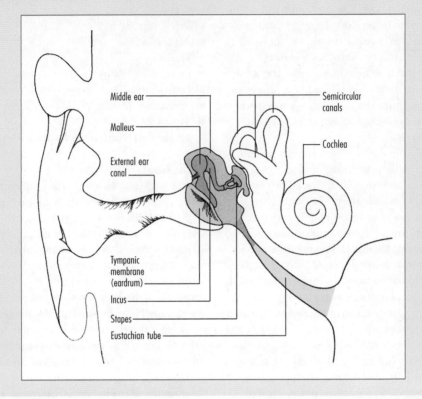

Middle ear

Malleus

External ear canal

Tympanic membrane (eardrum)

Incus

Stapes

Eustachian tube

Semicircular canals

Cochlea

overgrowth or tumors), edema (allergic rhinitis or chronic sinus infection), or inadequate treatment for acute suppurative otitis media.

Acute otitis media is common in children; its incidence rises during the winter months, paralleling the seasonal rise in nonbacterial respiratory tract infections.

Acute otitis media is the most commonly treated bacterial infection in children. Treatment of this infection accounts for greater than 50% of pediatric antibiotic prescriptions and as much as $5 billion annually in cost.[2]

Chronic secretory otitis media most commonly occurs in children with tympanostomy tubes or those with a perforated tympanic membrane.

Signs and symptoms

Clinical features of acute suppurative otitis media can range from a mild feeling of "water in my ear" to severe, deep, throbbing pain (from pressure behind the tympanic membrane); signs of upper respiratory tract infection (sneezing or coughing); mild to very high fever; hearing loss (usually mild and conductive); tinnitus; dizziness; nausea; and vomiting. Other possible effects include bulging of the tympanic membrane, with concomitant erythema, and purulent drainage in the ear canal from tympanic

membrane rupture. However, many patients are asymptomatic.

Acute secretory otitis media produces a severe conductive hearing loss—which varies from 15 to 35 dB, depending on the thickness and amount of fluid in the middle ear cavity. In the early stages, popping or cracking may occur as fluid buildup and Eustachian tube dysfunction increase and as the Eustachian tube returns to normal function. Accumulation of fluid may also cause the patient to hear an echo when he speaks and to experience a vague feeling of top-heaviness.

The cumulative effects of chronic otitis media include thickening and scarring of the tympanic membrane, decreased or absent tympanic membrane mobility, cholesteatoma (a cyst-like mass in the middle ear) and, in chronic suppurative otitis media, a painless, purulent discharge. The extent of associated conductive hearing loss varies with the size and type of tympanic membrane perforation and ossicular destruction.

If the tympanic membrane has ruptured, the patient may state that the pain has suddenly stopped. A purulent discharge may be visible. Complications may include mastoiditis, abscesses (brain, subperiosteal, and epidural), sigmoid sinus or jugular vein thrombosis, septicemia, meningitis, suppurative labyrinthitis, facial paralysis, and otitis externa.

The following factors increase a child's risk of developing otitis media:
▶ acute otitis media in the first year of life (recurrent otitis media)
▶ day care
▶ family history of middle ear disease
▶ formula feeding
▶ male gender
▶ sibling history of otitis media
▶ smoking in the household
▶ environmental allergens.

Acute otitis media may not produce any symptoms in the first few months of life; irritability may be the only indication of earache.

Complications
▶ Spontaneous rupture of tympanic membrane
▶ Chronic otitis media
▶ Mastoiditis
▶ Meningitis
▶ Cholesteatomas
▶ Septicemia
▶ Abscesses
▶ Vertigo
▶ Lymphadenopathy
▶ Leukocytosis
▶ Permanent hearing loss
▶ Tympanosclerosis
▶ Speech and language problems

Diagnosis
In acute suppurative otitis media, otoscopy reveals obscured or distorted bony landmarks of the tympanic membrane and an opaque tympanic membrane with fluid ranging from white to brown to red. Pneumatoscopy can show decreased tympanic membrane mobility to no mobility. This procedure is painful with an obviously bulging, erythematous tympanic membrane. The pain pattern is diagnostically significant: For example, in acute suppurative otitis media, pulling the auricle doesn't exacerbate the pain. A culture of the ear drainage identifies the causative organism.

In acute secretory otitis media, otoscopic examination reveals tympanic membrane retraction, which causes the bony landmarks to appear more prominent.

Examination also detects clear or amber fluid behind the tympanic membrane. If hemorrhage into the middle ear has occurred, as in barotrauma, the tympanic membrane appears blue-black.

In chronic otitis media, patient history discloses recurrent or unresolved otitis media. Otoscopy shows thickening, sometimes scarring, and decreased mobility of the tympanic membrane; pneumatoscopy shows decreased or absent tympanic membrane movement. A history of recent air travel or scuba diving suggests barotitis media.

Tympanocentesis for microbiologic diagnosis is recommended for treatment failures and may be followed by myringotomy. Tympanometry, acoustic reflex measurement, or acoustic reflexometry may be needed to document the presence of fluid in the middle ear. White blood cell count is higher in bacterial otitis media than in sterile otitis media. Mastoid X-rays or computed tomography scan of the head or mastoids may show the spreading of the infection beyond the middle ear.

Treatment

The American Academy of Pediatrics and the American Academy of Family Physicians recommend a wait-and-see approach for the first 72 hours for children who are older than age 6 months, are otherwise healthy, and have mild signs and symptoms or an uncertain diagnosis. Most ear infections clear on their own in just a few days.[3]

In acute suppurative otitis media, antibiotic therapy includes amoxicillin. In areas with a high incidence of beta-lactamase producing *H. influenzae* and in patients who aren't responding to ampicillin or amoxicillin, amoxicillin/clavulanate potassium may be used. For those who are allergic to penicillin derivatives, therapy may include cefaclor or trimethoprim-sulfamethoxazole. Severe, painful bulging of the tympanic membrane usually necessitates myringotomy. Broad-spectrum antibiotics can help prevent acute suppurative otitis media in high-risk patients. A single dose of ceftriaxone 50 mg/kg is effective against major pathogens but is expensive and is reserved for very sick infants. In the patient with recurring otitis media, antibiotics must be used with discretion to prevent development of resistant strains of bacteria.

In acute secretory otitis media, inflation of the eustachian tube using Valsalva's maneuver several times a day may be the only treatment required. Otherwise, nasopharyngeal decongestant therapy may be helpful. It should continue for at least 2 weeks and, sometimes, indefinitely, with periodic evaluation. Care should be given not to hyperextend the tympanic membrane. If decongestant therapy fails, myringotomy and aspiration of middle ear fluid are necessary. This is followed by the insertion of a polyethylene tube into the tympanic membrane for immediate and prolonged equalization of pressure. The tube falls out spontaneously after 6 to 12 months. Concomitant treatment for the underlying cause (such as elimination of allergens, or adenoidectomy for hypertrophied adenoids) may also be helpful in correcting this disorder.

Treatment for chronic otitis media includes broad-spectrum antibiotics (such as amoxicillin/clavulanate potassium or cefuroxime) for exacerbations of acute otitis media, elimination of eustachian tube obstruction, treatment for otitis externa, myringoplasty and tympanoplasty to reconstruct middle ear structures when thickening and scarring are present and, possibly, mastoidectomy. Cholesteatoma requires excision.

Special considerations

▶ Explain all diagnostic tests and procedures. After myringotomy, maintain drainage flow. Don't place cotton or plugs deeply into the ear canal; however, sterile cotton may be placed loosely in the external ear to absorb drainage. To prevent infection, change the cotton whenever it gets damp, and wash hands before and after giving ear care. Watch for and report headache, fever, severe pain, or disorientation.

▶ After tympanoplasty, reinforce dressings, and observe for excessive bleeding from the ear canal. Administer analgesics as needed. Warn the patient against blowing his nose or getting the ear wet when bathing.

▶ Encourage the patient to complete the prescribed course of antibiotic treatment. If nasopharyngeal decongestants are ordered, teach correct instillation.

▶ Suggest application of heat to the ear to relieve pain.

▶ Advise the patient with acute secretory otitis media to watch for and immediately report pain and fever—signs of secondary infection.

To prevent otitis media:

▶ Teach the patient how to recognize upper respiratory tract infections, and encourage early treatment.

▶ Instruct the parents not to feed the infant in a supine position or put him to bed with a bottle. This prevents reflux of nasopharyngeal flora.

▶ To promote eustachian tube patency, instruct the patient to perform Valsalva's maneuver several times daily.

▶ Identify and treat allergies.

REFERENCES

1. Children's Hospital Boston. "Otitis Media (Middle Ear Infection)" [Online]. Available at *www.childrenshospital.org/az/Site1399/ mainpageS1399P0.html.*
2. Varrasso, D. A. "Otitis Media: The Need for a New Paradigm in Medical Education," *Pediatrics* 118(4):1731–33, October 2006.
3. Mayo Clinic (2007 January 26) "Ear Infection, Middle Ear" [Online]. Available at *www. mayoclinic.com/health/ear-infections/DS00303.*

RETINAL DETACHMENT

Retinal detachment, also referred to as retinal tear, occurs when the outer retinal pigment epithelium splits from the neural retina, creating subretinal space. This space then fills with fluid, called subretinal fluid. Retinal detachment usually involves only one eye but may later involve the other eye. Surgical reattachment is usually successful. However, the prognosis for good vision depends on which area of the retina has been affected.

Causes and incidence

Any retinal tear or hole allows the liquid vitreous to seep between the retinal layers, separating the retina from its choroidal blood supply. Predisposing factors include myopia, intraocular surgery, and trauma. In adults, retinal detachment usually results from degenerative changes of aging, which cause a spontaneous retinal hole. Peripheral retinal lesions are also associated with causes of retinal detachment. The type of retinal lesion determines if prophylactic treatment to prevent retinal detachment is necessary.[1]

Perhaps the influence of trauma explains why retinal detachment is twice as common in males. Retinal detachment may also result from seepage of fluid into the subretinal space (because of inflammation, tumors, or systemic diseases) or from traction that's placed on the retina by vitreous bands or membranes (due to proliferative diabetic retinopathy, posterior uveitis, or a traumatic intraocular foreign body). A retinal detachment can occur at any age, but it is more common in people older than age 40. It affects males more than females and Whites more than Blacks.[2]

Retinal detachment is rare in children, but occasionally can develop as a result of retinopathy of prematurity, tumors (retinoblastomas), trauma, or myopia (which tends to run in families).

Nontraumatic retinal detachment occurs in approximately 1 in 10,000 people per year.[3]

Signs and symptoms

Initially, the patient may complain of floating spots and recurrent flashes of light (photopsia). However, as detachment progresses, gradual, painless vision loss may be described as a veil, curtain, or cobweb that eliminates a portion of the visual field. A retinal detachment is a medical emergency.[3]

Complications

▶ Severe vision impairment
▶ Blindness
▶ Future retinal detachment

Diagnosis

Diagnosis depends on ophthalmoscopy after full pupil dilation. Examination shows the usually transparent retina as gray and opaque; in severe detachment, it reveals folds in the retina and ballooning out of the area. Indirect ophthalmoscopy is used to search for retinal tears. Ultrasound is performed if the lens is opaque.

Treatment

Treatment depends on the location and severity of the detachment and the type of peripheral retinal lesion if this is the underlying cause. However, surgery is the only method to repair a retinal detachment. Restriction of eye movements and complete bed rest may be ordered until surgical reattachment is done.

Scleral buckling surgery, pneumatic retinopexy, and vitrectomy are the most common methods of repairing a retinal detachment; laser photocoagulation and cryopexy are the most common methods of repairing a retinal tear.[4]

In the scleral buckling procedure, a piece of silicone sponge, rubber, or semi-hard plastic is placed on the outer layer of the eye and sewn in place. This relieves traction on the retina, preventing tears from getting worse, and holds the layers of the retina together.[4]

With the pneumatic retinopexy procedure, a gas bubble is injected in the eye, and the patient's head is positioned to facilitate retina reattachment. This procedure can be performed under local anesthesia. The bubble floats to the detached area and presses lightly against the tear, closing the tear and flattening the retina so that no fluid can build up under it.[4]

In a vitrectomy, removal of the vitreous gel from the eye is done to gain better access to the retina, to repair holes, and to close very large tears. Basic salt solution is used to keep the retina in place while the vitreous is removed.[4]

In laser photocoagulation, an intense beam of light is passed through the eye, and tiny burns are formed around the retinal tear, which form scar tissue and seal the tear.

Cryopexy, freezing, is done by inserting a probe or a laser beam into the eye to seal the retina around the tear.[4] Research is being done to determine the effectiveness of prophylactic laser surgery treatment against peripheral retinal lesions to prevent retinal detachment.[1]

Special considerations

▶ Provide emotional support because the patient may be understandably distraught about his loss of vision.
▶ During transportation, position the patient's head so that the detached portion of the retina will fall back with the aid of gravity.
▶ To prepare for surgery, wash the patient's face with no-tears shampoo. Give antibiotics and cycloplegic-mydriatic eyedrops.
▶ Postoperatively, position the patient face-down on his right or left side and with the head of the bed raised. Discourage straining at stool, bending down, hard coughing, or sneezing, and ask the patient to guard against vomiting, all of which can raise intraocular pressure. Antiemetics may be indicated.
▶ Protect the patient's eye with a shield or glasses.
▶ To reduce edema and discomfort, apply ice packs as ordered. Administer pain medication, as ordered, for eye pain.
▶ After removing the eye shield, gently clean the eye with cycloplegic eyedrops, and administer steroid-antibiotic eyedrops,

as ordered. Use cold compresses to decrease swelling and pain.

▶ Administer analgesics as needed, and report persistent pain. Teach the patient how to properly instill eyedrops, and emphasize compliance and follow-up care. Suggest dark glasses to compensate for light sensitivity caused by cycloplegia.

REFERENCES

1. Kreis, A. J. "Prophylaxis for Retinal Detachment: Evidence or Eminence Based?," *Retina* 27(4):468–472, April/May 2007.
2. National Eye Institute (2008 February). "Retinal Detachment" [Online]. Available at *www.nei.nih.gov/health/retinaldetach/index.asp*.
3. Soni, M., et al. "Prophylaxis of Retinal Detachment," *Comprehensive Ophthalmology Update* 4(6):179–183, April–May 2005.
4. Billings Clinic (2005 September 29). "Retinal Detachment" [Online]. Available at *www.billingsclinic.com/body.cfm?id=416&action=detail&aeproductid=HW_Knowledgebase&aearticleid=hw187829*.

SINUSITIS

Sinusitis—inflammation of the paranasal sinuses—may be acute, subacute, chronic, allergic, or hyperplastic. Acute sinusitis usually results from the common cold and lingers in subacute form in only about 10% of patients. Chronic sinusitis follows persistent bacterial infection; allergic sinusitis accompanies allergic rhinitis; hyperplastic sinusitis is a combination of purulent acute sinusitis and allergic sinusitis or rhinitis. The prognosis is good for all types.

Causes and incidence

Sinusitis usually results from viral or bacterial infection. The bacteria responsible for acute sinusitis are usually pneumococci, other streptococci, *Haemophilus influenzae*, and *Moraxella catarrhalis*. Staphylococci and gram-negative bacteria are more likely to cause sinusitis in chronic cases or in intensive care patients. A recent study showed that staphylococcus aureus may be a major pathogen in acute bacterial sinusitis, yet increasing trends in drug-resistant strains may make it difficult to select the appropriate antibiotic.[1]

Predisposing factors include any condition that interferes with drainage and ventilation of the sinuses, such as chronic nasal edema, deviated septum, viscous mucus, nasal polyps, allergic rhinitis, nasal intubation or debilitation due to chemotherapy, malnutrition, diabetes, blood dyscrasias, cystic fibrosis, human immunodeficiency virus or other immunodeficiency disorders, or chronic use of steroids. Bacterial invasion commonly occurs as a result of the conditions listed above or after a viral infection. It may also result from swimming in contaminated water.

Other risk factors for developing sinusitis include a history of asthma; overuse of nasal decongestants; presence of a foreign body in the nose; frequent swimming or diving; dental work; pregnancy; changes in altitude (flying or climbing); air pollution and smoke; gastroesophageal reflux disease; and having a deviated nasal septum, nasal bone spur, or polyp.

Each year, more than 30 million adults and children get sinusitis.

The incidence of both acute and chronic sinusitis increases in later childhood. Sinusitis may be more prevalent in children who have had tonsils and adenoids removed.

Signs and symptoms

The primary indication of acute sinusitis is nasal congestion, followed by a gradual buildup of pressure in the affected sinus. For 24 to 48 hours after onset, nasal discharge may be present and later may become purulent. Associated symptoms include malaise, sore throat, headache,

and low-grade fever of 99° to 99.5° F [37.2° to 37.5° C]).

Characteristic pain depends on the affected sinus: maxillary sinusitis causes pain over the cheeks and upper teeth; ethmoid sinusitis, pain over the eyes; frontal sinusitis, pain over the eyebrows; and sphenoid sinusitis (rare), pain behind the eyes.

Purulent nasal drainage that continues for longer than 3 weeks after an acute infection subsides suggests subacute sinusitis. Other clinical features of the subacute form include nasal congestion, vague facial discomfort, fatigue, and a nonproductive cough.

The effects of chronic sinusitis are similar to those of acute sinusitis, but the chronic form causes continuous mucopurulent discharge.

The effects of allergic sinusitis are the same as those of allergic rhinitis. In both conditions, the prominent symptoms are sneezing, frontal headache, watery nasal discharge, and a stuffy, burning, itchy nose.

In hyperplastic sinusitis, bacterial growth on the diseased tissue causes pronounced tissue edema; thickening of the mucosal lining and the development of mucosal polyps combine to produce chronic stuffiness of the nose in addition to headaches.

Complications

▶ Meningitis
▶ Cavernous sinus thrombosis syndrome
▶ Bacteremia or septicemia
▶ Brain abscess
▶ Frontal lobe abscess
▶ Osteomyelitis
▶ Mucocele
▶ Orbital cellulitis

Diagnosis

The following measures are useful:
▶ Antral puncture promotes drainage of purulent material. It may also be used to provide a specimen for culture and sensitivity testing of the infecting organism, but it's seldom performed.
▶ Nasal examination reveals inflammation and pus.
▶ Sinus X-rays reveal cloudiness in the affected sinus, air and fluid, and any thickening of the mucosal lining.
▶ Transillumination is a simple diagnostic tool that involves shining a light into the patient's mouth with his lips closed around the diagnostic tool. Infected sinuses look dark, and normal sinuses transilluminate.
▶ Ultrasound, computed tomography scan, magnetic resonance imaging, and X-rays aid in diagnosing suspected complications.

Treatment

Local decongestants usually are tried before systemic decongestants; steam inhalation may also be helpful. Antibiotics are necessary to combat purulent or persistent bacterial infections usually lasting longer than 7 days. High doses of amoxicillin and amoxicillin/clavulanate potassium are usually the antibiotics of choice. Other possible therapy includes cefixime for responsive infections or if beta-lactamase–producing bacteria are present. Because sinusitis is a deep-seated infection, antibiotics should be given for 10 days, with the exception of azithromycin, which is given for 5 days. Local applications of heat may help to relieve pain and congestion. In subacute sinusitis, antibiotics, decongestants, and saline nasal spray may be helpful.

Treatment for allergic sinusitis must include treatment for allergic rhinitis. Nasal corticosteroids such as Flonase, Beconase, or Nasacort are used to help reduce swelling for severe inflammation of the sinuses.[2] Identification of allergens by skin testing and desensitization by immunotherapy should be done also. In both chronic sinusitis and hyperplastic sinusitis, using antihistamines, antibiotics, and a steroid nasal spray may relieve pain and conges-

tion. However, chronic sinusitis is an inflammatory disease and contrary to common practice, long-term antibiotics are likely not useful.[3] If subacute infection persists, the sinuses may be irrigated. If irrigation fails to relieve symptoms, endoscopic sinus surgery may be required to obtain a histologic diagnosis, remove polyps, and provide adequate ventilation of the infected sinuses. Partial or total resection of the middle turbinate as well as more radical procedures such as total sphenoethmoidectomy may be performed.

Special considerations

▶ Enforce bed rest, and encourage the patient to drink plenty of fluids to promote drainage. Don't elevate the head of the bed more than 30 degrees.

▶ To relieve pain and promote drainage, apply warm compresses continuously, or four times daily for 2-hour intervals. Also, give analgesics and antihistamines as needed.

▶ Watch for and report complications, such as vomiting, chills, fever, edema of the forehead or eyelids, blurred or double vision, and personality changes.

▶ If surgery is necessary, tell the patient what to expect postoperatively: nasal packing will be in place for 12 to 24 hours following surgery; he'll have to breathe through his mouth and won't be able to blow his nose. After surgery, monitor for excessive drainage or bleeding, and watch for complications.

▶ To prevent edema and promote drainage, place the patient in semi-Fowler's position. To relieve edema and pain and to minimize bleeding, apply ice compresses or a rubber glove filled with ice chips over the nose, and iced saline gauze over the eyes. Continue these measures for 24 hours.

▶ Frequently change the mustache dressing or drip pad, and record the consistency, amount, and color of drainage (expect scant, bright red, and clotty drainage).

▶ Because the patient will be breathing through his mouth, provide meticulous mouth care.

▶ Tell the patient that even after the packing is removed, nose blowing may cause bleeding and swelling. If the patient is a smoker, instruct him not to smoke for at least 2 to 3 days after surgery.

▶ Tell the patient to finish the prescribed antibiotics, even if his symptoms disappear.

REFERENCES

1. Spencer C. P., et al. "*Staphylococcus aureus* is a Major Pathogen in Acute Bacterial Rhinosinusitis: A Meta-Analysis," *Clinical Infectious Diseases* 45:122–127, November 2007.
2. Mayo Clinic (2006 October 13). "Chronic Sinusitis" [Online]. Available at *www.mayo clinic.com/health/chronic-sinusitis/DS00232.*
3. Leung, R. S., and Katial, R. "The Diagnosis and Management of Acute and Chronic Sinusitis," *Primary Care: Clinics in Office Practice* 35(1):11–24, March 2008.

12

Infections

ANTHRAX

nthrax is an acute bacterial infection that most commonly occurs in grazing animals, such as cattle, sheep, goats, and horses. It can also affect people who come in contact with contaminated animals or their hides, bones, fur, hair, or wool. It's also used as an agent for bioterrorism and biological warfare.

Anthrax occurs worldwide but is most common in developing countries. In humans, anthrax occurs in three forms, depending on the mode of transmission: cutaneous, inhalational, and GI.

Causes and incidence

Anthrax is caused by the bacteria *Bacillus anthracis,* which exists in the soil as spores that can live for years. Transmission to humans usually occurs through exposure to, or handling of, infected animals or animal products. Anthrax spores can enter the body through abraded or broken skin (cutaneous anthrax), by inhalation (inhalational anthrax), or through ingestion of undercooked meat from an infected animal (GI anthrax). Anthrax isn't known to spread from person to person. It can also be spread deliberately through biological weapon use. Twenty-two cases of anthrax infection occurred in the United States in 2001 when someone deliberately placed the anthrax powder in postal letters.[1]

Signs and symptoms

From the time of exposure, signs and symptoms of infection usually occur within 1 to 7 days for all three types but may take as long as 60 days to appear. The signs and symptoms of anthrax depend on the form acquired:

▶ Cutaneous anthrax: This is the most common form of anthrax with 95% infection rate occurring when the bacterium enters a cut in the skin. Skin infection may begin as a small, elevated, itchy lesion that resembles an insect bite, develops into a vesicle in 1 to 2 days, and finally becomes a small, painless ulcer with a necrotic center. Enlarged lymph glands in the surrounding area are common. It is also the least severe form: mortality is a mere 1% for those treated for it, and 20% for those who go without treatment.

▶ Inhalational anthrax: Symptoms can appear within a week or can take up to 42 days to appear. The patient may initially report common cold or flulike signs and symptoms, such as malaise, fever, headache, myalgia, and chills. These mild signs and symptoms may progress to severe respiratory difficulties, such as dyspnea, stridor, chest pain, and cyanosis, followed by the onset of shock. Even with treatment, inhalation anthrax is often fatal.

▶ GI anthrax: Ingestion of anthrax spores typically occurs from eating contaminated meat and can cause acute inflammation of the intestinal tract. The patient may present with nausea, vomiting, decreased appetite, and fever, which then progress to abdominal pain, vomiting blood, and severe diarrhea. As with inhalation anthrax, treatment does not ensure survival. Death occurs in 25% to 60% of cases in which patients have received treatment.

Complications
▶ Septicemia
▶ Death

Diagnosis
Anthrax can be diagnosed through cultures of the blood, skin lesions, or sputum of an exposed patient. If B. anthracis is isolated, the diagnosis is confirmed. Additionally, specific antibodies may be detected in the blood. Malign pustule is a black necrotic eschar tissue that is characteristic of cutaneous anthrax.[2]

Treatment
Treatment varies and is different for a person who is exposed to anthrax but is not yet sick. Penicillin remains the drug of choice, yet other antibiotics such as ciprofloxacin, doxycycline, and levofloxacin are given in combination with the anthrax vaccine to prevent anthrax infection.

Treatment for exposure to anthrax with symptoms includes a 60-day course of antibiotics. The success of treatment depends on the type of anthrax and how soon treatment begins. As stated above, treatment has a greater chance of success in patients with cutaneous anthrax and is no guarantee of survival for patients with inhalational or GI anthrax.

The anthrax vaccine is administered in six doses at 0, 2, and 4 weeks followed by booster immunizations at 6, 12, and 18 months. Subsequent boosters are given annually. Because of the continued threat of anthrax use as a biological weapon in warfare, the U.S. government is actively researching ways to improve the vaccine.[3]

Special considerations
▶ Any case of anthrax in either livestock or a person must be reported to the appropriate public health department.
▶ Supportive measures are geared toward the type of anthrax exposure.
▶ An anthrax vaccine is available and is recommended for people working directly with the Bacillus microbe in a laboratory, people who work with imported animal hides or furs in areas of substandard conditions, military personnel sent to areas designated a high risk, and veterinarians who work or travel to high-incidence countries.
▶ Anthrax vaccine isn't available for routine civilian use.

REFERENCES
1. Centers for Disease Control and Prevention. (2006 February 22). "Anthrax: What You Need to Know." [Online]. Available at *http://emergency.cdc.gov/agent/anthrax/need toknow.asp.*
2. Artac, H., et al. "A Rare Cause of Preseptal Cellulitis: Anthrax," *Pediatric Dermatology* 24(3): 330–1, May–June 2007.
3. World Health Organization. "WHO Guidance for the Surveillance and Control of Anthrax in Humans and Animals." Available at *www.who. int/csr/resources/publications/anthrax/WHO_ EMC_ZDI_98_6/en/index.html.*

BOTULISM

Botulism, a life-threatening paralytic illness, results from an exotoxin produced by the gram-positive, anaerobic bacillus Clostridium botulinum. It occurs with botulism food poisoning, wound botulism, and infant botulism. The mortality from botulism is about 25%; death is usually

caused by respiratory failure during the first week of illness.

Causes and incidence

Botulism is usually the result of ingesting inadequately cooked contaminated foods, especially those with low acid content, such as home-canned fruits and vegetables, sausages, and smoked or preserved fish or meat. Rarely, it results from wound infection with *C. botulinum*. It can also be contracted through exposure to bioterrorism agents (e.g. inhalational botulism).[1]

Botulism occurs worldwide and affects more adults than children. Recently, findings have shown that an infant's GI tract can become colonized with *C. botulinum* from some unknown source, and then the exotoxin is produced within the infant's intestine. Infant botulism is usually attributed to the ingestion of honey or corn syrup. Incidence had been declining, but the current trend toward home canning has resulted in an upswing (approximately 250 cases per year in the United States) in recent years.

Signs and symptoms

Symptoms generally begin within 6 hours to 2 weeks after exposure (often within 12 to 36 hours) after the ingestion of contaminated food.[2] Severity varies with the amount of toxin ingested and the patient's degree of immunocompetence. Generally, early onset (within 24 hours) signals critical and potentially fatal illness. Initial signs and symptoms include dry mouth, sore throat, weakness, dizziness, vomiting, and diarrhea. The cardinal sign of botulism, though, is acute symmetrical cranial nerve impairment (ptosis, diplopia, and dysarthria), followed by descending weakness or paralysis of muscles in the extremities or trunk, and dyspnea from respiratory muscle paralysis. Such impairment doesn't affect mental or sensory processes and isn't associated with fever.

Infant botulism usually afflicts infants between 3 and 20 weeks of age and can produce hypotonic (floppy) infant syndrome. Signs and symptoms are constipation, feeble cry, depressed gag reflex, and inability to suck. Cranial nerve deficits also occur in infants and are manifested by a flaccid facial expression, ptosis, and ophthalmoplegia. Infants also develop generalized muscle weakness, hypotonia, and areflexia. Loss of head control may be striking. Respiratory arrest is likely.

Complications

▶ Respiratory failure
▶ Paralytic ileus
▶ Death
▶ Chronic fatigue
▶ Long-term shortness of breath

Diagnosis

Identification of the offending toxin in the patient's serum, stool, gastric content, or the suspected food, or wound confirms the diagnosis. An electromyogram showing diminished muscle action potential after a single supramaximal nerve stimulus is also diagnostic.

Diagnosis also must rule out other diseases commonly confused with botulism, such as Guillain-Barré syndrome, myasthenia gravis, stroke, staphylococcal food poisoning, tick paralysis, chemical intoxications, carbon monoxide poisoning, fish poisoning, trichinosis, and diphtheria.

Treatment

Treatment consists of I.V. or I.M. administration of botulinus antitoxin (available through the Centers for Disease Control and Prevention and through the state health department). If breathing difficulty develops, intubation and mechanical ventilation may be required. I.V. fluids can be given if there are swallowing problems, and a nasogastric tube can also be ordered. Human botulism immune globulin, a human antitoxin, is available for botulism treatment in infants.

It can be obtained by contacting the California Department of Public Health.[3]

A recent study concluded that the use of Botulism Immune Globulin Intravenous significantly decreased overall hospital length of stay and length of mechanical ventilation in children with infant botulism.[4]

Special considerations

If you suspect ingestion of contaminated food:

▶ Obtain a careful history of the patient's food intake for the past several days. See if other family members or acquaintances who have shared meals or have a similar food history exhibit similar symptoms.

▶ Observe carefully for abnormal neurologic signs. Tell the patient's family to watch for signs of weakness, blurred vision, and slurred speech after he has returned home. If such signs appear, the patient must return to the hospital immediately.

▶ If ingestion has occurred within several hours, induce vomiting, begin gastric lavage, and give a high enema to purge any unabsorbed toxins from the bowel.

If clinical signs of botulism appear:

▶ Admit the patient to the intensive care unit, and monitor cardiac and respiratory functions carefully.

▶ Administer botulinus antitoxin as ordered to neutralize any circulating toxin. Before giving the antitoxin, be sure to obtain an accurate patient history of allergies, especially to horses, and perform a skin test. Afterward, watch for anaphylaxis or other hypersensitivity and serum sickness. Keep epinephrine 1:1,000 (for subcutaneous administration) and emergency airway equipment available.

▶ Assess respiratory function every 4 hours. Report decreased vital capacity on inspiratory effort and any signs of respiratory distress.

▶ Closely assess and accurately record neurologic function, including bilateral motor status (reflexes, ability to move arms and legs).

▶ Give I.V. fluids as ordered. Turn the patient often, and encourage deep-breathing exercises. Isolation isn't required.

▶ Because botulism is sometimes fatal, keep the patient and his family informed regarding the course of the disease.

▶ Immediately report all cases of botulism to local public health authorities.

▶ To help prevent botulism, encourage patients to observe proper techniques in processing and preserving foods. Warn them to avoid even tasting food from a bulging can or one with a peculiar odor and to sterilize by boiling any utensil that comes in contact with suspected food. Ingestion of even a small amount of food contaminated with botulism toxin can prove fatal.

REFERENCES

1. Jones, R., et al. "A Review of WHO International Standards for Botulinum Antitoxins," *Biologicals* 34(3):223–26, September 2006.
2. Centers for Disease Control and Prevention. (2006 April 19). "Botulism Facts for Health Care Providers" [Online]. Available at *www.bt.cdc.gov/agent/botulism/hcpfacts.asp.*
3. Koirala, J., and Basnet, S. "Botulism, Botulinum Toxin, and Bioterrorism: Review and Update," *Infections in Medicine* 21(6):284–290, June 2004.
4. Underwood, K. "Infant Botulism: A 30-Year Experience Spanning the Introduction of Botulism Immune Globulin Intravenous in the Intensive Care Unit at Children's Hospital Los Angeles," *Pediatrics* 120(6):1380–1385, December 2007.

CANDIDIASIS

Candidiasis (also called candidosis or moniliasis) is usually a mild, superficial fungal infection caused by the genus *Candida*. It usually infects the nails (onychomycosis), skin (diaper rash), or mucous membranes, especially the oropharynx (thrush), vagina (moniliasis), esophagus, and

GI tract. Rarely, these fungi enter the blood-stream and invade the kidneys, lungs, endo-cardium, brain, or other structures, causing serious infections. Such systemic infection is most prevalent among drug abusers and pa-tients already hospitalized, particularly dia-betics, immunosuppressed patients, or pa-tients receiving broad-spectrum antibiotics. The prognosis varies, depending on the patient's resistance.

Causes and incidence

Most cases of *Candida* infection result from *C. albicans.* Other infective strains include *C. parapsilosis, C. tropicalis, C. glabrata,* and *C. guilliermondii.* These fungi are part of the normal flora of the GI tract, mouth, vagina, and skin. They cause infection when some change in the body permits their sudden proli-feration (such as rising glucose levels from dia-betes mellitus; or lowered resistance from an immunosuppressive drug, radiation, aging, or disease); or when they are introduced systemi-cally by I.V. or urinary catheters, drug abuse, hyperalimentation, or surgery. However, the most common predisposing factor remains the use of broad-spectrum antibiotics, which de-crease the number of normal flora and permit an increasing number of candidal organisms to proliferate. The infant of a mother with vaginal candidiasis can contract oral thrush while passing through the birth canal. Thrush is also found in many infants who are breast-fed. A mother who is breast-feeding may also need to be treated if she has a fungal infection on her breasts. This will help decrease the chance of reinfecting the infant.[1] The inci-dence of candidiasis is rising because of wider use of I.V. therapy and a greater number of immunocompromised patients, especially those with HIV infection.

Also of concern is the potential spread of fungal infections through both artificial nails and infected natural fingernails while caring for susceptible patients in the clinical setting.[2] Underneath the nail bed and within the layers of the nail is the perfect reservoir for

the dark, moist conditions needed to sustain the fungal infection.

Signs and symptoms

Symptoms of superficial candidiasis cor-respond to the site of infection:
▶ skin—scaly, erythematous, papular rash, sometimes covered with exudate, appearing below the breast, between fingers, and at the axillae, groin, and umbilicus; in diaper rash, papules at the edges of the rash
▶ nails—red, swollen, darkened nail bed; occasionally, purulent discharge and the sep-aration of a pruritic nail from the nail bed
▶ oropharyngeal mucosa (thrush)—cream-colored or bluish white curdlike patches of ex-udate on the tongue, mouth, or pharynx that reveal bloody engorgement when scraped. They may swell, causing respiratory distress in infants, or they may be painful or cause a burning sensation in the throats and mouths of adults. (See *Recognizing candidiasis*)

Recognizing candidiasis

Candidiasis of the oropharyngeal mucosa (thrush) causes cream-colored or bluish white pseudomembranous patches on the tongue, mouth, or pharynx. Fungal invasion may extend to circumoral tissues.

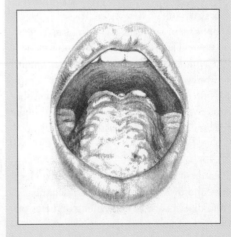

▶ esophageal mucosa—dysphagia, retrosternal pain, regurgitation and, occasionally, scales in the mouth and throat

▶ vaginal mucosa—white or yellow discharge, with pruritus and local excoriation; white or gray raised patches on vaginal walls, with local inflammation; dyspareunia

Systemic infection produces chills; high, spiking fever; hypotension; prostration; myalgias; arthralgias; and a rash. Specific signs and symptoms depend on the site of infection:

▶ pulmonary—hemoptysis, cough, fever

▶ renal—fever, flank pain, dysuria, hematuria, pyuria, cloudy urine

▶ brain—headache, nuchal rigidity, seizures, focal neurologic deficits

▶ endocardium—systolic or diastolic murmur, fever, chest pain, embolic phenomena

▶ eye—endophthalmitis, blurred vision, orbital or periorbital pain, scotoma, and exudate.

Complications

Candidiasis dissemination with organ failure of the:

▶ Kidneys

▶ Brain

▶ GI tract

▶ Eyes

▶ Lungs

▶ Heart

Diagnosis

Diagnosis of superficial candidiasis depends on clinical signs and symptoms plus evidence of *Candida* on a Gram stain of skin, vaginal scrapings, pus, or sputum or on skin scrapings prepared in potassium hydroxide solution. Systemic infections require obtaining a specimen for blood or tissue culture.

Treatment

Treatment first aims to improve the underlying condition that predisposes the patient to candidiasis, such as controlling diabetes or discontinuing antibiotic therapy and catheterization, if possible.

Nystatin is an effective antifungal for superficial candidiasis. Clotrimazole, fluconazole, ketoconazole, and miconazole are effective in mucous-membrane and vaginal candidal infections. Ketoconazole or fluconazole is the treatment of choice for chronic candidiasis of the mucous membranes. Treatment for systemic infection consists of I.V. amphotericin B or fluconazole.

Special considerations

▶ Instruct the patient using nystatin solution to swish it around in his mouth for several minutes before he swallows it.

▶ Nystatin oral lozenges should be dissolved in the mouth, not chewed.

▶ Swab nystatin on the oral mucosa of an infant with thrush. Treat the infant after a feeding because feedings will wash the medication away. The infant's mother should also be treated to prevent the infection from being passed back and forth.

▶ Provide the patient with a nonirritating mouthwash to loosen tenacious secretions and a soft toothbrush to avoid irritation.

▶ Relieve the patient's mouth discomfort with a topical anesthetic, such as lidocaine, at least 1 hour before meals. (It may suppress the gag reflex and cause aspiration.)

▶ Provide a soft diet for the patient with severe dysphagia. Tell the patient with mild dysphagia to chew food thoroughly, and make sure he doesn't choke.

▶ Use dry padding in intertriginous areas of obese patients to prevent irritation.

▶ Note dates of insertion of I.V. catheters, and replace them according to your hospital's policy to prevent phlebitis.

▶ Assess the patient with candidiasis for underlying causes such as diabetes mellitus. If the patient is receiving amphotericin B for systemic candidiasis, he may have severe chills, fever, anorexia, nausea, and vomiting. Premedicate with acetamino-

phen, antihistamines, or antiemetics to help reduce adverse effects.

▶ Frequently check vital signs of patients with systemic infections. Provide appropriate supportive care. In patients with renal involvement, carefully monitor intake and output, and urine blood and protein levels.

▶ Check high-risk patients daily, especially those receiving antibiotics, for patchy areas, irritation, sore throat, bleeding of the mouth or gums, or other signs of superinfection. Check for vaginal discharge; record color and amount.

▶ Encourage women in their third trimester of pregnancy to be examined for vaginal candidiasis to protect their neonate from infection at birth.

REFERENCES

1. Children's Hospital of Boston. (2005–2006). "Infants: Feeding Guide" [Online]. Available at *www.childrenshospital.org/az/Site1147/mainpageS1147P0.html.*
2. Parry, M. F., et al. "Candida Osteomyelitis and Diskitis After Spinal Surgery: An Outbreak that Implicates Artificial Nail Use," *Clinical Infectious Diseases* 32 (3):352–7, Feb. 2001.

COMMON COLD

The common cold (also known as acute coryza and viral rhinitis) is an acute, usually afebrile viral infection that causes inflammation of the upper respiratory tract. It's the most common infectious disease, accounting for more time lost from school or work than any other cause. Although a cold is benign and self-limiting, it can lead to secondary bacterial infections.

Causes and incidence

About 90% of colds stem from a viral infection of the upper respiratory passages and consequent mucous membrane inflammation; occasionally, colds result from a myco-plasmal infection. (See *What happens in the common cold,* page 432.)

More than a hundred viruses can cause the common cold. Major offenders include rhinoviruses, coronaviruses, myxoviruses, adenoviruses, coxsackie viruses, and echoviruses.

Transmission occurs through airborne respiratory droplets, contact with contaminated objects, and hand-to-hand transmission. Children acquire new strains from their schoolmates and pass them on to family members. Immunosuppression, physical and emotional stress, and fatigue increase susceptibility.

The common cold is more prevalent in children than in adults, in adolescent boys than in girls, and in females than in males. In temperate zones, it's more common in the colder months; in the tropics, during the rainy season.

Signs and symptoms

After a 1- to 4-day incubation period, the common cold produces pharyngitis; nasal congestion; coryza; headache; and burning, watery eyes. Additional effects may include fever (in children); chills; myalgia; arthralgia; malaise; lethargy; and a hacking, nonproductive, or nocturnal cough.

As the cold progresses, clinical features develop more fully. After a day, symptoms include a feeling of fullness with a copious nasal discharge that commonly irritates the nose, adding to discomfort. About 3 days after onset, major signs diminish, but the "stuffed up" feeling generally persists for about a week. Reinfection (with productive cough) is common, but complications (sinusitis, otitis media, pharyngitis, and lower respiratory tract infection) may occur. A secondary bacterial infection may develop and require antibiotics. Symptoms include an elevated temperature (100° F [37.8° C]) or higher; purulent drainage; chills; red, swollen throat. Symptoms usually occur approximately 6 to 7 days after initial onset of symptoms.[1] A cold is communicable for 2 to 3 days after the

What happens in the common cold

Virus-infected droplets enter the body and attack the cells lining the throat and nose. The virus particles then multiply rapidly.

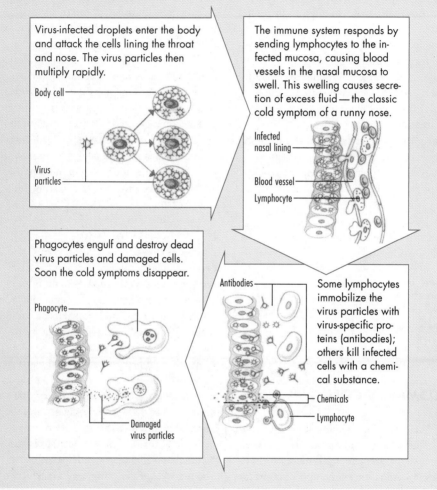

Virus-infected droplets enter the body and attack the cells lining the throat and nose. The virus particles then multiply rapidly.

Body cell

Virus particles

The immune system responds by sending lymphocytes to the infected mucosa, causing blood vessels in the nasal mucosa to swell. This swelling causes secretion of excess fluid — the classic cold symptom of a runny nose.

Infected nasal lining

Blood vessel

Lymphocyte

Phagocytes engulf and destroy dead virus particles and damaged cells. Soon the cold symptoms disappear.

Phagocyte

Damaged virus particles

Antibodies

Some lymphocytes immobilize the virus particles with virus-specific proteins (antibodies); others kill infected cells with a chemical substance.

Chemicals

Lymphocyte

onset of symptoms. The virus can live on inanimate objects for up to 3 days.[1]

Complications

▶ Secondary bacterial infection
▶ Sinusitis
▶ Otitis media
▶ Pharyngitis
▶ Lower respiratory tract infection

Diagnosis

No explicit diagnostic test exists to isolate the specific organism responsible for the common cold. Consequently, diagnosis rests on the typically mild, localized, and afebrile upper respiratory symptoms. Despite infection, white blood cell counts and differential are within normal limits. Diagnosis must rule out allergic rhinitis, measles, rubella,

and other disorders that produce similar early symptoms. A temperature higher than 100° F (37.8° C), severe malaise, anorexia, tachycardia, exudate on the tonsils or throat, petechiae, and tender lymph glands may point to more serious disorders and require additional diagnostic tests.

Treatment

The primary treatments—aspirin, acetaminophen or ibuprofen, fluids, and rest—are purely symptomatic because the common cold has no cure. Aspirin eases myalgia and headache, fluids help loosen accumulated respiratory secretions and maintain hydration, and rest combats fatigue and weakness. In a child with a fever, acetaminophen is the drug of choice.

Decongestants can relieve congestion, and throat lozenges relieve soreness. Steam encourages expectoration. Nasal douching, sinus drainage, and antibiotics aren't necessary except in complications or chronic illness. Pure antitussives relieve severe coughs but are contraindicated in productive coughs and in children under 2 years of age, and when cough suppression is harmful.

HEALTH & SAFETY *The Food and Drug Administration recommends that over-the-counter cough and cold medicines not be given to children under 2 years of age because of their potentially life-threatening side effects.*[2]

The role of vitamin C remains controversial. However, the outcome of recent research was promising. Vitamin C used prophylactically prior to extreme physical exertion or exposure to significant cold stress proved to be beneficial.[3] In infants, saline nose drops and mucus aspiration with a bulb syringe may be beneficial.

Special considerations

▶ Emphasize that antibiotics don't cure the common cold.
▶ Tell the patient to maintain bed rest during the first few days, to use a lubricant on his nostrils to decrease irritation, to relieve throat irritation with hard candy or cough drops, to increase fluid intake, and to eat light meals.
▶ Warm baths or heating pads can reduce aches and pains but won't hasten a cure. Suggest hot- or cold-steam vaporizers. Commercial expectorants may be used.
▶ Advise against overuse of nose drops or sprays because they may cause rebound congestion.
▶ To help prevent colds, warn the patient to minimize contact with people who have colds. To avoid spreading colds, teach the patient to wash his hands often and before touching his eyes, to cover coughs and sneezes, and to avoid sharing towels and drinking glasses.

REFERENCES

1. Pratter, M. R. "Cough and the Common Cold: ACCP Evidence-Based Clinical Practice Guidelines," *Chest* 129 (1 Suppl):72S–74S, January 2006.
2. U.S. Food and Drug Administration. (2008 January 17). "Public Health Advisory: Nonprescription Cough and Cold Medicine Use in Children—FDA Recommends That Over-the-Counter (OTC) Cough and Cold Products Not be Used for Infants and Children Under 2 Years of Age" [Online]. Available at *www.fda.gov/cder/drug/advisory/cough_cold_2008.htm.*
3. Douglas, R. M., et al. "Vitamin C for Preventing and Treating the Common Cold," *Cochrane Database of Systematic Reviews* (2):CD000980, 1998, updated 2007.

CYTOMEGALOVIRUS INFECTION

Cytomegalovirus (CMV) infection is caused by the cytomegalovirus, a deoxyribonucleic acid, ether-sensitive virus belonging to the herpes family. Also known as generalized salivary gland disease or cytomegalic inclusion disease, CMV infection occurs worldwide and is transmitted by human contact.

Causes and incidence

CMV infection is very common. Approximately 50% to 85% of people in the United States have had a CMV infection by the time they are 40 years old.[1] In most of these people, the disease is so mild that it's overlooked. It is estimated that approximately 8,000 children each year suffer permanent disabilities caused by CMV. Congenital CMV–related illness causes as many serious disabilities as does Down syndrome, fetal alcohol syndrome, and neural tube defects.[1]

CMV has been found in the saliva, urine, semen, breast milk, feces, blood, and vaginal and cervical secretions of infected people. The virus is usually transmitted through contact with these infected secretions, which can harbor the virus for months or even years. It may be transmitted by sexual contact and can travel across the placenta, causing a congenital infection. Immunosuppressed patients, especially those who have received transplanted organs, run a 90% chance of contracting CMV infection. Recipients of blood transfusions from donors with positive CMV antibodies are at some risk.

CMV infection during pregnancy can be hazardous to the fetus, possibly leading to stillbirth, brain damage, and other birth defects or to severe neonatal illness. About 1% of all neonates have CMV.

Signs and symptoms

CMV probably spreads through the body in lymphocytes or mononuclear cells to the lungs, liver, GI tract, eyes, and central nervous system, where it commonly produces inflammatory reactions.

Most patients with CMV infection have mild, nonspecific complaints or none at all, even though antibody titers indicate infection. In these patients, the disease usually runs a self-limiting course. However, immunodeficient patients and those receiving immunosuppressants may develop pneumonia or other secondary infections. In patients with acquired immunodeficiency syndrome, disseminated CMV infection may cause CMV–related retinitis (resulting in blindness), colitis, encephalitis, abdominal pain, diarrhea, or weight loss. CMV retinitis in immunosuppressed patients occurred in approximately one-third of patients with autoimmune deficiency syndrome, and accounted for more than 90% of cases of human immunodeficiency virus-related blindness prior to the use of highly active antiretroviral therapy. In developing countries, CMV retinitis is a neglected disease, largely undiagnosed and untreated.[2]

Infected infants ages 3 to 6 months usually appear asymptomatic but may develop hepatic dysfunction, hepatosplenomegaly, spider angiomas, pneumonitis, and lymphadenopathy.

Congenital CMV infection is seldom apparent at birth, although the neonate's urine contains the virus. CMV can cause brain damage that may not show up for months after birth. It also can produce a rapidly fatal neonatal illness characterized by jaundice, petechial rash, hepatosplenomegaly, thrombocytopenia, hemolytic anemia, microcephaly, psychomotor retardation, mental deficiency, and hearing loss. Occasionally, this form is rapidly fatal.

In some adults, CMV may cause cytomegalovirus mononucleosis, with 3 weeks or more of irregular, high fever. Other findings may include a normal or elevated white blood cell (WBC) count, lymphocytosis, and increased atypical lymphocytes.

Complications

▶ Opportunistic infections (immunosuppressed patients)
▶ Pneumonia
▶ Hepatitis
▶ Ulceration of the GI tract
▶ Retinitis
▶ Encephalopathy
  Congenital CMV may lead to:
▶ Stillbirth
▶ Neonatal retinitis

▶ Microcephaly
▶ Mental retardation
▶ Seizures
▶ Hearing loss
▶ Thrombocytopenia
▶ Hemolytic anemia

Diagnosis

Although virus isolation in urine is the most sensitive laboratory method, diagnosis can also be made with virus isolated from saliva, throat, cervix, WBCs, or biopsy specimens.

Other laboratory tests supporting the diagnosis include complement fixation studies, hemagglutination inhibition antibody tests and, for congenital infections, indirect immunofluorescent tests for CMV immunoglobulin M antibody.

Treatment

Treatment aims to relieve symptoms and prevent complications. In the immunosuppressed patient, and in some special cases of infants with congenital CMV, treatment with acyclovir, ganciclovir, valganciclovir, cidofovir and, possibly, foscarnet may be used. However, these drugs have serious side effects and should be prescribed on a case-by-case basis.[1] Most important, parents of children with severe congenital CMV infection need support and counseling to help them cope with the possibility of brain damage or death. Presently, there is no vaccine to prevent congenital CMV, but more research is being done. This research is considered high priority given the epidemiology of the disease.[1]

Special considerations

To help prevent CMV infection:
▶ Maintain standard precautions at all times, keeping in mind that many patients who excrete CMV are asymptomatic.
▶ Warn immunosuppressed patients and pregnant women to avoid exposure to individuals with confirmed or suspected CMV infection. (Maternal CMV infection can cause fetal abnormalities: hydrocephaly,

microphthalmia, seizures, encephalitis, hepatosplenomegaly, hematologic changes, microcephaly, and blindness.)
▶ Urge patients with CMV infection to use good hand hygiene to prevent spreading it. Stress this particularly with young children.
▶ Be sure to observe standard precautions when handling body secretions.

REFERENCES

1. Centers for Disease Control and Prevention. (2006 February 6). "Cytomegalovirus (CMV)" [Online]. Available at *www.cdc.gov/cmv/facts.htm.*
2. PLoS Medicine, Heiden, D., et al. "Cytomegalovirus Retinitis: The Neglected Disease of the AIDS Pandemic." [Online]. Available at *www.pubmedcentral.nih.gov/articlerender.fcgi?artid=2100142.*

DIPHTHERIA

There are two types of diphtheria: respiratory diphtheria and cutaneous diphtheria. Diphtheria is an acute, highly contagious toxin-mediated infection caused by *Corynebacterium diphtheriae*, a gram-positive rod. It usually infects the respiratory tract, primarily the tonsils, nasopharynx, and larynx. Diphtheria causes a thick covering in the back of the throat. It can lead to breathing problems, paralysis, heart failure, and even death.[1] The GI and urinary tracts, conjunctivae, and ears are rarely involved.

Causes and incidence

Transmission usually occurs through intimate contact or by airborne respiratory droplets from asymptomatic carriers or convalescing patients. Many more people carry this disease than contract active infection. Diphtheria is more prevalent during the colder months because of closer person-to-person indoor contact, however it may be contracted at any time during the year.

Thanks to effective immunization, diphtheria is rare in many parts of the world, including the United States. Before vaccines and medications were available to prevent and treat the disease, nearly 1 out of 10 people died. Diphtheria was the leading cause of death among children.[2]

Since 1972, the incidence of cutaneous diphtheria has been increasing, especially in the Pacific Northwest and the Southwest, in areas where crowding and poor hygienic conditions prevail. Most victims are children younger than age 15; about 10% of patients die.

Signs and symptoms

Most infections go unrecognized, especially in partially immunized individuals. After an incubation period of less than a week, clinical cases of diphtheria characteristically show a thick, patchy, grayish green membrane over the mucous membranes of the pharynx, larynx, tonsils, soft palate, and nose; fever; sore throat; and a rasping cough, hoarseness, and other symptoms similar to croup. Attempts to remove the membrane usually cause bleeding, which is highly characteristic of diphtheria. If this membrane causes airway obstruction (particularly likely in laryngeal diphtheria), and the condition is left untreated, it could lead to tachypnea, stridor, possibly cyanosis, suprasternal retractions, and suffocation. Adenopathy and cervical swelling can occur. In cutaneous diphtheria, skin lesions resemble impetigo.

Complications

▶ Respiratory obstruction
▶ Myocarditis
▶ Polyneuritis (affecting motor and sensory fibers)
▶ Encephalitis
▶ Cerebral infarction
▶ Bacteremia
▶ Renal failure
▶ Pulmonary emboli
▶ Bronchopneumonia
▶ Serum sickness
▶ Thrombocytopenia

Diagnosis

Examination showing the characteristic membrane and a throat culture, or culture of other suspect lesions growing C. *diphtheriae,* confirm this diagnosis.

Treatment

Treatment must not wait for confirmation by culture. Treatment includes diphtheria antitoxin (DAT) administered I.M. or I.V. However, DAT is not licensed by the Food and Drug Administration for use in the United States. Physicians must special order DAT from the Centers for Disease Control and Prevention.[3] Antibiotics, such as penicillin or erythromycin, are used to eliminate the organisms from the upper respiratory tract and other sites, to terminate the carrier state, to prevent complications such as airway obstruction, and to prevent a tracheotomy. DAT is used prophylactically only under exceptional circumstances involving known or suspected exposure to toxigenic *Corynebacteria.*[3]

Diphtheria vaccines (combination vaccines) are available for children, teenagers, and adults as a preventive measure against diphtheria. The recommended vaccination schedules are as follows: children should be vaccinated at ages 2, 4, 6, and 15 to 18 months, again between 4 and 6 years of age followed by booster shots every 10 years. Adolescents should receive immunization at age 11 to 12 years and at age 15 years before entering high school. Adults under age 65 years should receive immunization every 10 years.[4]

Special considerations

Diphtheria requires comprehensive supportive care with psychological support.
▶ To prevent the spread of this disease, stress the need for droplet precautions. Teach proper disposal of nasopharyngeal secretions. Maintain infection precautions

until after two consecutive negative naso-pharyngeal cultures—at least 1 week after discontinuing drug therapy. Treatment of exposed individuals with antitoxin remains controversial. Suggest that the patient's family receive diphtheria toxoid if they haven't been immunized.

▶ Give drugs as ordered. Although time-consuming and risky, desensitization should be attempted if tests are positive, because diphtheria antitoxin is the only specific treatment available. If sensitivity tests are negative, the antitoxin is given before laboratory confirmation, because mortality increases directly with any delay in antitoxin administration. Before giving diphtheria antitoxin, which is made from horse serum, obtain eye and skin tests to determine sensitivity. After giving antitoxin or penicillin, be alert for anaphylaxis; keep epinephrine 1:1,000 and resuscitation equipment handy. In patients who receive erythromycin, watch for thrombophlebitis.

▶ Monitor respirations carefully, especially in laryngeal diphtheria (usually, such patients are in a high-humidity environment). Watch for signs of airway obstruction, and be ready to give immediate life support, including intubation and tracheotomy.

▶ Watch for signs of shock, which can develop suddenly.

▶ Obtain cultures as ordered.

▶ If neuritis develops, tell the patient it's usually transient. Be aware that peripheral neuritis may not develop until 2 to 3 months after the onset of illness.

▶ Be alert for signs of myocarditis, such as the development of heart murmurs or electro-cardiogram changes. Ventricular fibrillation is a common cause of sudden death in patients with diphtheria.

▶ Stress the need for childhood immunizations to all parents. Protective immunity doesn't last longer than 10 years after the last vaccination, so it's important to get tetanus-diphtheria boosters every 10 years.

▶ Report all cases to local public health authorities.

REFERENCES

1. Centers for Disease Control and Prevention. (2008 February 12). "Diphtheria Vaccination" [Online]. Available at *www.cdc.gov/vaccines/vpd-vac/diphtheria*.
2. University of Pittsburgh Medical Center. (2008 February 12). "Diphtheria" [Online]. Available at *www.upmc.com/HealthManagement/ManagingYourHealth/HealthReference/Diseases/?chunkiid=96791*.
3. Centers for Disease Control and Prevention. (2007 July 7). "Diphtheria Antitoxin" [Online]. *www.cdc.gov/vaccines/vpd-vac/diphtheria/dat/dat-main.htm*.
4. Pennsylvania Department of Health. (2007 November 19). "Communicable Diseases Fact Sheet: Diphtheria" [Online]. Available at *www.dsf.health.state.pa.us/health/cwp/view.asp?A=171&Q=235532*.

ESCHERICHIA COLI AND OTHER ENTEROBACTERIACEAE INFECTIONS

The Enterobacteriaceae—a group of mostly aerobic, gram-negative bacilli—cause local and systemic infections, including an invasive diarrhea resembling shigella and, more commonly, a noninvasive toxin-mediated diarrhea resembling cholera. With other Enterobacteriaceae, *Escherichia coli* causes most nosocomial infections. Noninvasive, enterotoxin-producing *E. coli* infections may be a major cause of diarrheal illness in children in the United States. (See *Enterobacterial infections,* page 438.)

The prognosis in mild to moderate infection is good. Severe infection requires immediate fluid and electrolyte replacement to avoid fatal dehydration, especially among children, in whom mortality may be quite high.

Enterobacterial infections

The Enterobacteriaceae include *Escherichia coli, Arizona, Citrobacter, Enterobacter, Erwinia, Hafnia, Klebsiella, Morganella, Proteus, Providencia, Salmonella, Serratia, Shigella,* and *Yersinia.*

Enterobacterial infections are exogenous (from other people or the environment), endogenous (from one part of the body to another), or a combination of both. Enterobacteriaceae infections may cause any of a long list of bacterial diseases: bacterial (gram-negative) pneumonia, empyema, endocarditis, osteomyelitis, septic arthritis, urethritis, cystitis, bacterial prostatitis, urinary tract infection, pyelonephritis, perinephric abscess, abdominal abscesses, cellulitis, skin ulcers, appendicitis, gastroenterocolitis, diverticulitis, eyelid and periorbital cellulitis, corneal conjunctivitis, meningitis, bacteremia, and intracranial abscesses.

Appropriate antibiotic therapy depends on the results of culture and sensitivity tests. Generally, the aminoglycosides, cephalosporins, and penicillins—such as ampicillin and piperacillin—are most effective. Cefepime and quinones are also effective for some infections.

Causes and incidence

Although some strains of *E. coli* exist as part of the normal GI flora, infection usually results from certain nonindigenous strains. For example, noninvasive diarrhea results from two toxins produced by strains called enterotoxic or enteropathogenic *E. coli.* Enteropathogenic *E. coli* serotype 0157:H7 is the most well-known strain in the United States. These toxins interact with intestinal juices and promote excessive loss of chloride and water. In the invasive form, *E. coli* directly invades the intestinal mucosa without producing enterotoxins, thereby causing local irritation, inflammation, and diarrhea.

Normal strains can cause infection in immunocompromised patients.

Transmission can occur directly from an infected person or indirectly by ingestion of contaminated substances, such as meat that is not thoroughly cooked, lettuce, spinach, sprouts, unpasteurized milk and juice, and water; or by contact with contaminated utensils. Incubation takes 12 to 72 hours.

In developing nations, annually *E. coli* causes between 280 and 400 million diarrheal episodes in children under 5 years old and an additional 100 million episodes in children 5 to 14 years old. Another estimated 400 million cases occur in people over 15 years old, causing substantial disease.[1] Because of the epidemiology of *E. coli* in developing nations, World Health Organization researchers are developing a vaccine as a protective role for antibody responses.[1]

Incidence of *E. coli* infection is highest among travelers returning from other countries, particularly Mexico, Southeast Asia, and South America. *E. coli* infection also induces other diseases, especially in people whose resistance is low. The strain *E. coli* 0157:H7 has been associated with undercooked hamburger and with animals and petting zoos. Ensuring that meats are safe for human consumption is the goal of the U.S. Department of Agriculture. Research is being done to reduce *E. coli* prevalence in naturally infected livestock through preharvest control. This simply means that the research effort is to determine how to control the prevalence of pathogens in livestock before they are harvested for human consumption.[2]

Signs and symptoms

Effects of noninvasive diarrhea depend on the causative toxin but may include the abrupt onset of watery diarrhea with cramping abdominal pain and, in severe illness, acidosis. Invasive infection produces chills,

abdominal cramps, and diarrheal stools containing blood and pus. Infantile diarrhea from an *E. coli* infection is usually noninvasive; it begins with loose, watery stools that change from yellow to green and contain little mucus or blood. Vomiting, listlessness, irritability, and anorexia commonly precede diarrhea. This condition can progress to fever, severe dehydration, acidosis, and shock. Bloody diarrhea may occur from infection with *E. coli* 0157:H7, which has also been associated with hemolytic uremic syndrome in children.

Complications

▶ Bacteremia
▶ Severe dehydration
▶ Life-threatening electrolyte disturbances
▶ Acidosis
▶ Shock

Diagnosis

Because certain strains of *E. coli* normally reside in the GI tract, culturing is of little value; a working diagnosis depends on clinical observation. However, if *E. coli* 0157:H7 is suspected, notify the laboratory so that appropriate testing of stool specimens can be performed.

A firm diagnosis requires sophisticated identification procedures, such as bioassays, that are expensive, time-consuming and, consequently, not widely available. Diagnosis must rule out salmonellosis and shigellosis, other common infections that produce similar signs and symptoms. Although *E. coli* 0157:H7 is the most well-known strain in the United States, and is routinely tested for, researchers suggest that other *E. coli* strains may be attributable to diarrheal infections. They recommend that commercial diagnostic tests be developed to assess the prevalence more broadly.[3]

Treatment

Treatment consists of correction of fluid and electrolyte imbalances. For an infant or immunocompromised patient, I.V. antibiotics based on the organism's drug sensitivity are administered, as well as salicylates or opium tincture for cramping and diarrhea.

Special considerations

▶ Keep accurate intake and output records. Measure stool volume, and note the presence of blood or pus. Replace fluids and electrolytes as needed, monitoring for decreased serum sodium and chloride levels and signs of gram-negative shock. Watch for signs of dehydration, such as poor skin turgor and dry mouth.

▶ For infants, use contact precautions, give nothing by mouth, administer antibiotics as ordered, and maintain body warmth.

To prevent spread of this infection:

▶ Prevent direct patient contact during epidemics. Report cases to local public health authorities. *E. coli* 0157:H7 is a reportable disease.

▶ Use proper hand-hygiene technique. Teach health care personnel, patients, and their families to do the same.

▶ Follow standard precautions. Provide the patient with a private room, wear protective clothing as necessary, such as when handling feces or soiled linens, and perform scrupulous hand hygiene before entering and after leaving the patient's room.

▶ Advise travelers to foreign countries to avoid unbottled water and uncooked fruits and vegetables.

REFERENCES

1. World Health Organization. (2006 March 17). "Weekly Epidemiological Record: Future Directions for Research on Enterotoxigenic *Escherichia Coli* Vaccines for Developing Countries" [Online]. Available at *http://whqlibdoc.who.int/wer/WHO_WER_2006/81_97-104(no11).pdf*.
2. U.S. Department of Agriculture. (2008 February 6). "Research Project: Prevention and Control of Shiga-Toxigenic Escherichia Coli in Livestock. (2006 Annual Report)." [Online]. Available at *www.ars.usda.gov/*

*research/projects/projects.htm?ACCN_
NO=410408.*

3. Dershewitz, R. A. "Unrecognized Diarrheagenic
E. coli in U.S. Children," *Journal Watch
General Medicine,* February 15, 2005.

HAEMOPHILUS INFLUENZAE INFECTION

Haemophilus influenzae is a small
gram-negative pleomazic coccobacil-
lus. It is a nonmotile, nonspore-
forming, fastidious, facultative anaerobe.
There are six different types (a-f). Some
strains have a polysaccharide capsule. The
most virulent strain is *H. influenzae* type b
(Hib). *Haemophilus influenzae* causes diseases in many organ systems but usually
attacks the respiratory system. It's a common cause of epiglottitis, laryngotracheo-
bronchitis, pneumonia, bronchiolitis, otitis
media, and meningitis. Less commonly,
it causes bacterial endocarditis, conjunctivitis, facial cellulitis, septic arthritis, and
osteomyelitis.

Causes and incidence

Transmission occurs by direct contact with
secretions or by respiratory droplets. From
1980 to 1990, incidence was 40 to 100 per
100,000 children older than 5 years old in
the United States. Due to routine use of the
Hib conjugate vaccine since 1990, the incidence of invasive Hib disease has decreased
to 1.3 per 100,000 children. However, Hib
remains a major cause of lower respiratory
tract infections in infants and children in developing countries where the vaccine is not
widely used.[1] In rare cases, children may still
develop *H. influenzae* type b infections if the
series of immunizations is not completed, or
in older children who did not receive the
vaccine as infants.[2]

Signs and symptoms

H. influenzae provokes a characteristic tissue
response: acute suppurative inflammation.
When *H. influenzae* infects the larynx, trachea, or bronchial tree, it leads to irritable
cough; dyspnea; mucosal edema; and thick,
purulent exudate. When it invades the lungs, it
leads to bronchopneumonia. In the pharynx,
H. influenzae usually produces no remarkable
changes, except when it causes epiglottitis,
which generally affects both the laryngeal and
pharyngeal surfaces. The pharyngeal mucosa
may be reddened, rarely with soft yellow exudate. Usually, though, it appears normal or
shows only slight diffuse redness, even while
severe pain makes swallowing difficult or
impossible. *H. influenzae* infections typically
cause high fever and generalized malaise.
Meningitis, the most serious infection caused
by *H. influenzae,* is indicated by fever and altered mental status. In young children, nuchal
rigidity may be absent.

Complications

▶ Subdural effusions
▶ Permanent neurologic sequelae from
meningitis
▶ Complete upper airway obstruction from
epiglottitis
▶ Cellulitis
▶ Pericarditis
▶ Pleural effusion
▶ Respiratory failure from pneumonia

Diagnosis

Specific tests will depend on the location of
the infection. In some cases, the physician
may take a culture of fluid from the eye, ear,
throat, or spinal fluid. Other diagnostic tests
may include chest or neck X-ray.[2]

Direct isolation of the organism, usually
with a blood culture, confirms the diagnosis
of *H. influenzae* infection.

Other laboratory findings include:
▶ polymorphonuclear leukocytosis (15,000
to 30,000/μl)

▶ leukopenia (2,000 to 3,000/μl) in young children with severe infection

▶ *H. influenzae* bacteremia, found in many patients with meningitis.

Treatment

H. influenzae infections usually respond to a course of ampicillin, cefotaxime, gatifloxacin, moxifloxacin, or ceftriaxone as an initial treatment, although resistant strains are becoming more common. As an alternative, a combination of chloramphenicol and ampicillin is prescribed. If the strain proves susceptible to ampicillin, chloramphenicol is discontinued. All children under 5 should be vaccinated against *H. influenzae*. The vaccine (Hib) is administered as an injection at 2 and 4 months. Depending on the vaccination preparation, a third in the series is administered at 6 months. A booster is required at some time between 12 and 15 months of age.[3]

Special considerations

▶ Maintain adequate respiratory function through proper positioning, humidification (croup tent) in children, and suctioning, as needed. Monitor rate and type of respirations. Watch for signs of cyanosis and dyspnea, which require intubation or a tracheotomy. Monitor the patient's level of consciousness (LOC); decreased LOC may indicate hypoxemia. For home treatment, suggest using a room humidifier or breathing moist air from a shower or bath, as necessary.

▶ Check the patient's history for drug allergies before administering antibiotics. Monitor his complete blood count for signs of bone marrow depression when therapy includes ampicillin or chloramphenicol.

▶ Monitor the patient's intake (including I.V. infusions) and output. Watch for signs of dehydration, such as decreased skin turgor, parched lips, concentrated urine, decreased urine output, and increased pulse rate.

▶ Organize your physical care measures beforehand, and do them quickly so as not to disrupt the patient's rest.

▶ Take preventive measures, such as vaccinating infants, maintaining droplet precautions, using proper hand-hygiene technique, properly disposing of respiratory secretions, placing soiled tissues in a plastic bag, and decontaminating all equipment.

REFERENCES

1. Centers for Disease Control and Prevention. (2005 October 11). "*Haemophilus Influenzae* Serotype b (Hib) Disease." [Online]. Available at *www.cdc.gov/ncidod/dbmd/diseaseinfo/haeminfluserob_t.htm*.
2. Children's Hospital of Philadelphia. "*Haemophilus Influenzae* Infections." [Online]. Available at *www.chop.edu/consumer/your_child/condition_section_index.jsp?id=-9194*.
3. University of Maryland Medical Center. (2007 February 14). "*Immunizations.*" [Online]. Available at *www.umm.edu/ency/article/002024.htm*.

HISTOPLASMOSIS

Histoplasmosis is a fungal infection caused by *Histoplasma capsulatum*. This disease may also be called Ohio Valley, Central Mississippi Valley, Appalachian Mountain, or Darling's disease. In the United States, it occurs in three forms: primary acute histoplasmosis, progressive disseminated histoplasmosis (acute disseminated or chronic disseminated disease), and chronic pulmonary (cavitary) histoplasmosis, which produces cavitations in the lung similar to those in pulmonary tuberculosis.

A fourth form, African histoplasmosis, occurs only in Africa and is caused by the fungus *Histoplasma capsulatum duboisii*.

The prognosis varies with each form. The primary acute disease is benign, the progressive disseminated disease is fatal in approximately 90% of patients and, without proper chemotherapy, chronic pulmonary histo-

plasmosis is fatal in 50% of patients within 5 years.

Causes and incidence

H. capsulatum is found in the feces of birds and bats or in soil contaminated by their feces, such as near roosts, chicken coops, barns or caves, or underneath bridges. Transmission occurs through inhalation of *H. capsulatum* or *H. duboisii* spores or through the invasion of spores after minor skin trauma. Possibly, oral ingestion of spores may cause the disease.

The incubation period is from 5 to 18 days, although chronic pulmonary histoplasmosis may progress slowly for many years. Probably because of occupational exposure, histoplasmosis is more common in adult males. Fatal disseminated disease, however, is more common in infants and elderly males.

Histoplasmosis occurs worldwide, especially in the temperate areas of Asia, Africa, Europe, and North and South America. It has not been reported on the continent of Antarctica.[1] In the United States, it's most prevalent in the central and southeastern states, especially in the Mississippi and Ohio River valleys.

Signs and symptoms

Symptoms vary with each form of this disease. Primary acute histoplasmosis may be asymptomatic or may cause symptoms of a mild respiratory illness similar to a severe cold or influenza. Typical clinical effects may include fever, malaise, headache, myalgia, anorexia, cough, chest pain, anemia, leukopenia, thrombocytopenia, and oropharyngeal ulcers.

Progressive disseminated histoplasmosis causes hepatosplenomegaly, general lymphadenopathy, anorexia, weight loss, fever and, possibly, ulceration of the tongue, palate, epiglottis, and larynx, with resulting pain, hoarseness, and dysphagia. It may also cause endocarditis, meningitis, pericarditis, and adrenal insufficiency.

Chronic pulmonary histoplasmosis mimics pulmonary tuberculosis and causes a productive cough, dyspnea, and occasional hemoptysis. Eventually, it produces weight loss, extreme weakness, breathlessness, and cyanosis.

African histoplasmosis produces cutaneous nodules, papules, and ulcers; lesions of the skull and long bones; lymphadenopathy; and visceral involvement without pulmonary lesions.

Complications

▶ Vascular obstruction
▶ Bronchial obstruction
▶ Acute pericarditis
▶ Pleural effusion
▶ Mediastinal fibrosis
▶ Granuloma
▶ Intestinal ulceration
▶ Addison's disease
▶ Endocarditis
▶ Meningitis

Diagnosis

The ultimate confirming diagnosis is a culture of *H. capsulatum* from sputum in acute primary and chronic pulmonary histoplasmosis, and from bone marrow, lymph node, blood, and infection sites in disseminated histoplasmosis. However, cultures take several weeks to grow these organisms, and faster diagnosis is possible with stained biopsies. Also available is a deoxyribonucleic acid probe for histoplasma that can be used for difficult isolates.

Indications of exposure include a history of exposure to contaminated soil in an endemic area, miliary calcification in the lung or spleen, a positive histoplasmin skin test, a positive urine antigen test, or rising complement fixation and agglutination titers (more than 1:32).

Diagnostic precision has improved greatly with the use of an assay for Histoplasma antigen in the urine.[2]

Findings must rule out tuberculosis and other diseases that produce similar symptoms. In a recent case, physicians were surprised to see signs and symptoms of disseminated histoplasmosis present as a chest wall mass in a patient.[3] The diagnosis of histoplasmosis caused by *H. duboisii* necessitates examination of tissue biopsy and culture of the affected site.

Treatment

Treatment consists of antifungal therapy, surgery, and supportive care. Antifungal treatment is not usually indicated for healthy, nonimmunocompromised persons with acute histoplasmosis, localized pulmonary infection, and the African form because these forms of the disease are self-limited, often resolving within 3 weeks.[1] Persons with persistent symptoms beyond 1 month and with severe disease, including diffuse pulmonary and disseminated histoplasmosis, can be treated with either itraconazole or amphotericin B.[1]

Other azoles may be used for refractory disease.[1] However, amphotericin B is indicated for pregnant women, not an azole antifungal. Consult an infectious disease specialist.

Supportive care usually includes oxygen for respiratory distress, glucocorticoids for adrenal insufficiency, and parenteral fluids for dysphagia due to oral or laryngeal ulcerations. Histoplasmosis doesn't require isolation.

Special considerations

Patient care is primarily supportive.
▶ Give medications as ordered, and teach patients about possible adverse effects. Because amphotericin B may cause chills, fever, nausea, and vomiting, give appropriate antipyretics and antiemetics as ordered.
▶ Patients with chronic pulmonary or disseminated histoplasmosis also need psychological support because of long-term hospitalization. As needed, refer the patient to a social worker or occupational therapist. Help the parents of children with this disease arrange for a visiting teacher.
▶ To help prevent histoplasmosis, teach people in endemic areas to watch for early signs and to seek treatment promptly. Instruct those who risk occupational exposure to contaminated soil to wear face masks.

REFERENCES

1. Centers for Disease Control and Prevention. (2008 February 15). "Prevention of Specific Infectious Diseases: Histoplasmosis" [Online]. Available at *wwwn.cdc.gov/travel/yellow BookCh4-Histoplasmosis.aspx*.
2. Kauffman, C. A. "Histoplasmosis: A Clinical and Laboratory Update," *Clinical Microbiology Reviews*, 20(1):115–32, January 2007.
3. Koo, H. L., et al. "Disseminated Histoplasmosis Manifesting as a Soft-Tissue Chest Wall Mass in a Heart Transplant Recipient," *Transplant Infectious Disease*, January 2008.

INFLUENZA

Influenza (also called the *grippe* or the *flu*), an acute, highly contagious infection of the respiratory tract, results from three different types of *Myxovirus influenzae*. It occurs sporadically or in epidemics (usually during the colder months). Epidemics tend to peak within 2 to 3 weeks after initial cases and subside within a month.

Although influenza affects all age groups, its incidence is highest in schoolchildren. However, its effects are most severe in persons who are young, elderly, or suffering from chronic disease. In these groups, influenza may even lead to death. The catastrophic pandemic of 1918 was responsible for an estimated 20 million deaths. The most recent pandemics (in 1957, 1968, and 1977) began in mainland China.

Causes and incidence

Transmission of influenza occurs through inhalation of a respiratory droplet from an infected person or by indirect contact with a contaminated object, such as a drinking glass or other items contaminated with respiratory secretions. The influenza virus then invades the epithelium of the respiratory tract, causing inflammation and desquamation.

One of the remarkable features of the influenza virus is its capacity for antigenic variation into numerous distinct strains, allowing it to infect new populations that have little or no immunologic resistance. Antigenic variation is characterized as antigenic drift (minor changes that occur yearly or every few years) and antigenic shift (major changes that lead to pandemics). Influenza viruses are classified into three groups:

▶ Type A, the most prevalent, strikes every year, with new serotypes causing epidemics every 3 years.

▶ Type B also strikes annually but causes epidemics only every 4 to 6 years.

▶ Type C is endemic and causes only sporadic cases.

Each year, tens of millions of people in the United States get the flu; about 114,000 people get sick enough to be hospitalized, and about 36,000 people die.

HEALTH & SAFETY *According to the Centers for Disease Control and Prevention, only 42% of health care professionals received immunizations against the flu virus in 2007. Because influenza annually leads to 200,000 hospitalizations, resulting from complications, and 36,000 deaths each year, nurses who are vaccinated against the virus not only safeguard themselves, but also help protect their patients, families, and communities.[1]*

Signs and symptoms

After an incubation period of 24 to 48 hours, flu symptoms begin to appear: sudden onset of chills, temperature of 101° to 104° F (38.3° to 40° C), headache, malaise, myalgia (particularly in the back and limbs), a nonproductive cough and, occasionally, laryngitis, hoarseness, conjunctivitis, rhinitis, and rhinorrhea. These symptoms usually subside in 3 to 5 days, but cough and weakness may persist. Fever is usually higher in children than in adults. Also, cervical adenopathy and croup are likely to be associated with influenza in children. In some patients (especially elderly patients), lack of energy and easy fatigability may persist for several weeks.

Fever that persists longer than 3 to 5 days signals the onset of complications. The most common is pneumonia, which occurs as primary influenza virus pneumonia or secondary to bacterial infection. Influenza may also cause myositis, exacerbation of chronic obstructive pulmonary disease, Reye's syndrome and, rarely, myocarditis, pericarditis, transverse myelitis, and encephalitis.

Complications

▶ Pneumonia (viral or bacterial)
▶ Myositis
▶ Exacerbation of chronic obstructive pulmonary disease
▶ Reye's syndrome
▶ Myocarditis (rare)
▶ Pericarditis
▶ Transverse myelitis
▶ Encephalitis

Diagnosis

At the beginning of an influenza epidemic, early cases are usually mistaken for other respiratory disorders. Because signs and symptoms of influenza aren't pathognomonic, isolation of *M. influenzae* through nose and throat cultures and increased serum antibody titers help confirm this diagnosis. After these measures confirm an influenza epidem-

ic, diagnosis requires only observation of clinical signs and symptoms. Making a reliable, rapid clinical diagnosis is essential to appropriate patient management. This may be especially important during shortages of antiviral agents when they are in high demand.[2] Uncomplicated cases show a decreased white blood cell count with an increase in lymphocytes.

Treatment

Treatment of uncomplicated influenza includes bed rest, adequate fluid intake, aspirin or acetaminophen (in children) to relieve fever and muscle pain, and dextromethorphan or another antitussive to relieve nonproductive coughing. Prophylactic antibiotics aren't recommended because they have no effect on the influenza virus.

Antiviral drugs used for chemoprophylaxis or treatment of influenza are adjuncts to vaccine but are not substitutes for annual vaccination.[1]

Amantadine and rimantadine (antiviral agents) have proven to be effective in reducing the duration of signs and symptoms of influenza A infection. Oseltamivir and zanamivir are effective against influenza A and B infection. In influenza complicated by pneumonia, supportive care (fluid and electrolyte supplements, oxygen, and assisted ventilation) and treatment of bacterial superinfection with appropriate antibiotics are necessary. No specific therapy exists for cardiac, central nervous system, or other complications.

Special considerations

Unless complications occur, influenza doesn't require hospitalization; patient care focuses on relief of symptoms:

▶ Advise the patient to increase his fluid intake. Warm baths or heating pads may relieve myalgia. Give him nonopioid analgesics-antipyretics as ordered.

▶ Screen visitors to protect the patient from bacterial infection and the visitors from influenza. Use droplet precautions.

▶ Teach the patient proper disposal of tissues and proper hand-hygiene technique to prevent the virus from spreading.

▶ Watch for signs and symptoms of developing pneumonia, such as crackles, another temperature rise, or coughing accompanied by purulent or bloody sputum. Assist the patient to gradually resume his normal activities.

▶ Educate patients about influenza immunizations. For high-risk patients and health care personnel, suggest annual inoculations at the start of the flu season (late autumn). Remember, however, that such vaccines are made from chicken embryos and must not be given to people who are hypersensitive to eggs. (For people who are hypersensitive to eggs, amantadine is an effective alternative to the vaccine; however, it must be started before the flu season and continued throughout the season.) The vaccine administered is based on the previous year's virus and is usually about 75% effective.

▶ Inform people receiving the vaccine of possible adverse effects (discomfort at the vaccination site, fever, malaise and, rarely, Guillain-Barré syndrome). Guillain-Barré syndrome has an annual incidence of 10 to 20 cases per 1 million adults.[1] Influenza vaccine (inactivated) is recommended for women who are pregnant and who will be in the second or third trimester during influenza season.

▶ Live-attenuated influenza vaccine is now available as a nasal spray. Criteria and contraindications for use vary from the inactivated, injectable vaccine. Recipients of live-attenuated influenza vaccine may shed influenza virus for up to 21 days postimmunization.

REFERENCES

1. Centers for Disease Control and Prevention. (2007 July 13). "Prevention and Control of

Influenza Recommendations of the Advisory Committee on Immunization Practices (ACIP)." [Online]. Available at *www.cdc.gov/flu/ professionals/acip/*.

2. Call, S. A., et al. "Does This Patient Have Influenza?" *JAMA* 293(8): 987–97, February 2005.

LYME DISEASE

A multisystemic disorder, Lyme disease is caused by the spirochete *Borrelia burgdorferi*, which is carried by *Ixodes dammini*, *Ixodes Pacificus*, and other ticks in the Ixodidae family. It commonly begins in the summer after a tick bite with a macule or papule that becomes red and warm but isn't painful. The lesion increases in diameter to form a large lesion with reddened borders with central clearing. This classic skin lesion is called erythema chronicum migrans (ECM), which may be confused with a similar rash caused by Southern tick-associated rash illness. (See *Southern tick-associated rash illness*.) Weeks or months later, cardiac or neurologic abnormalities sometimes develop, possibly followed by arthritis of the large joints. Chronic Lyme disease is a term sometimes used interchangeably with late Lyme disease. It is thought that patients with chronic Lyme disease have persistent *B. burgdorferi* infection and require long-term antibiotic treatment and may even be incurable. It is the latest in a series of syndromes that have been hypothesized in an attempt to attribute medically unexplained symptoms to particular infections.[1]

Causes and incidence

Lyme disease occurs when a tick injects spirochete-laden saliva into the bloodstream. After incubating for 3 to 32 days, the spirochetes migrate out to the skin, causing ECM. Then they disseminate to other skin sites or organs via the bloodstream or lymph system.

Southern tick-associated rash illness

Southern tick-associated rash illness (STARI) is a newly recognized tick-borne disease that produces a rash similar to the rash caused by Lyme disease. STARI is associated with the bite of the lone star tick, *Amblyomma americanum*, and occurs primarily in the southeastern and south-central states of the United States. Deoxyribonucleic acid analysis of the spirochetes found in the *A. americanum* tick has indicated that they are not *Borrelia burgdorferi*, the agent of Lyme disease, but are a different, newly recognized species, *Borrelia lonestari*.

Individuals living or traveling to southeastern or south-central states who develop a red, expanding rash with central clearing following a tick bite should see a physician. Mild illness, characterized by such signs and symptoms as fatigue, headache, stiff neck and, occasionally, fever, may accompany the rash.

Currently, there's no specific diagnostic test for STARI. It is suspected if diagnostic tests rule out Lyme disease, the patient's travel history is as indicated above and a known lone star tick bite has been reported, or the patient has participated in activities that may have resulted in exposure to a tick.

There are no current recommendations for treating STARI, but the rash and other accompanying signs and symptoms usually resolve with doxycycline therapy.

They may survive for years in the joints, or they may trigger an inflammatory response in the host and then die.

Initially, Lyme disease was identified in a group of children in Lyme, Connecticut. Now it's known to occur primarily in three parts of the United States: in the northeast, from Massachusetts to Maryland; in the Midwest, in Wisconsin and Minnesota; and in the west, in California and Oregon. Most patient reports of illness onset associated

with Lyme disease occur in the months of May, June, July, and August. Fewer than 8% of cases were reported with illness onset during the period of December to March.[2]

During the past 10 years, 90% of reported cases occurred in New York, Connecticut, Pennsylvania, New Jersey, Wisconsin, Rhode Island, Maryland, Massachusetts, Minnesota, and Delaware. With more than 15,000 cases reported annually, Lyme disease is the most common tickborne infectious illness in the United States.[3]

Although it's endemic to these areas, cases have been reported in all 50 states and in 20 other countries, including Germany, Switzerland, France, and Australia.

Signs and symptoms

Typically, Lyme disease has three stages. ECM heralds stage one with a red macule or papule, commonly at the site of a tick bite. This lesion typically feels hot and itchy and may grow to over 20 inches (50.8 cm) in diameter; it resembles a bull's eye or target. Within a few days, more lesions may erupt, and a migratory, ringlike rash, conjunctivitis, or diffuse urticaria occurs. In 3 to 4 weeks, lesions are replaced by small red blotches, which persist for several more weeks. Malaise and fatigue are constant, but other findings are intermittent: headache, neck stiffness, fever, chills, achiness, and regional lymphadenopathy. Less common effects are meningeal irritation, mild encephalopathy, migrating musculoskeletal pain, hepatitis, and splenomegaly. A persistent sore throat and dry cough may appear several days before ECM.

Weeks to months later, the second stage (disseminated infection) begins, and patients may develop additional symptoms depending on the system affected. Neurologic abnormalities—fluctuating meningo-encephalitis with peripheral and cranial neuropathy—usually resolve after days or months. Facial palsy is especially noticeable. Cardiac abnormalities, such as a brief, fluc-tuating atrioventricular heart block, left ventricular dysfunction, or cardiomegaly, may also develop. Cardiac involvement lasts only a few weeks but can be fatal.

Stage three (persistent infection) usually begins weeks or years later and is characterized by arthritis in about 80% of patients. Migrating musculoskeletal pain leads to frank arthritis with marked swelling, especially in the large joints. Recurrent attacks may precede chronic arthritis with severe cartilage and bone erosion.

Complications

▶ Myocarditis
▶ Pericarditis
▶ Arrhythmias
▶ Heart block
▶ Meningitis
▶ Encephalitis
▶ Cranial or peripheral neuropathies
▶ Arthritis

Diagnosis

Because isolation of *B. burgdorferi* is difficult in humans, and serologic testing isn't standardized, diagnosis is usually based on the characteristic ECM lesion and related clinical findings, especially in endemic areas. Antibodies to *B. burgdorferi* are identified by immunofluorescence or enzyme-linked immunosorbent assay (ELISA). ELISAs are confirmed with Western blot tests. Mild anemia and an elevated erythrocyte sedimentation rate, leukocyte count, serum immunoglobulin M, and aspartate aminotransferase levels support the diagnosis.

Clinicians must differentiate between Lyme disease and arthritis, encephalopathy, or polyneuropathy.

Treatment

Fourteen to 21 days of an antibiotic such as doxycycline is the treatment of choice for nonpregnant adults. Oral penicillin is usually prescribed for children and pregnant patients. Alternatives include tetracycline,

cefuroxime, and ceftriaxone. When given in the early stages, these drugs can minimize later complications. When given during the late stages, high-dose I.V. ceftriaxone may be successful.

Special considerations

▶ Take a detailed patient history, asking about travel to endemic areas and exposure to ticks.
▶ Check for drug allergies, and administer antibiotics carefully.
▶ For a patient with arthritis, help with range-of-motion and strengthening exercises, but avoid overexertion. Ibuprofen helps relieve joint stiffness.
▶ Assess the patient's neurologic function and level of consciousness frequently. Watch for signs of increased intracranial pressure and cranial nerve involvement, such as ptosis, strabismus, and diplopia. Also check for cardiac abnormalities, such as arrhythmias and heart block.

REFERENCES

1. Feder, Jr, H. M., et al. "A Critical Appraisal of Chronic Lyme Disease," *New England Journal of Medicine* 14(357):1422–1430, October 2007.
2. Centers for Disease Control and Prevention. *Morbidity and Mortality Weekly Report,* "Lyme Disease—United States, 2003–2005" [Online]. Available at *www.cdc.gov/mmwr/ preview/mmwrhtml/mm5623a1.htm.*
3. HealthCare Review, Northeast Network. (2004 July 26). "It's Prime Time for Lyme Disease, Apic Cautions." [Online]. Available at *http:// healthcarereview.com/index.php?src=directory &srctype=display&id=769&view=back_issues_ detail&PHPSESSID=.*

MALARIA

Malaria, an acute infectious disease, is caused by protozoa of the genus Plasmodium: *P. falciparum, P. vivax, P. malariae,* and *P. ovale,* all of which are transmitted to humans by mosquito vectors.

Falciparum malaria is the most severe form of the disease. When treated, malaria is rarely fatal; untreated, it's fatal in 10% of victims, usually as a result of complications such as disseminated intravascular coagulation.

Untreated primary attacks last from a week to a month, or longer. Relapses are common and can recur sporadically for several years. Susceptibility to the disease is universal.

Causes and incidence

Malaria literally means "bad air" and for centuries was thought to result from the inhalation of swamp vapors. It's now known that malaria is transmitted by the bite of female Anopheles mosquitoes, which abound in humid, swampy areas. When an infected mosquito bites, it injects Plasmodium sporozoites into the wound. The infective sporozoites migrate by blood circulation to parenchymal cells of the liver; there they form cystlike structures containing thousands of merozoites.

Upon release, each merozoite invades an erythrocyte and feeds on hemoglobin. Eventually, the erythrocyte ruptures, releasing heme (malaria pigment), cell debris, and more merozoites, which, unless destroyed by phagocytes, enter other erythrocytes. (See *What happens in malaria.*) At this point, the infected person becomes a reservoir of malaria who infects any mosquito that feeds on him, thus beginning a new cycle of transmission. Hepatic parasites (*P. vivax, P. ovale,* and *P. malariae*) may persist for years in the liver. These parasites are responsible for the chronic carrier state. Because blood transfusions and street-drug paraphernalia can also spread malaria, drug addicts have a higher incidence of the disease. Malaria is a worldwide health problem that continues to impede the development of many countries.

Malaria is a tropical and subtropical disease. It's most prevalent in Asia, Africa, and Latin America. The Centers for Disease Control and Prevention (CDC) estimates 300 to 500 million cases occur each year,

What happens in malaria

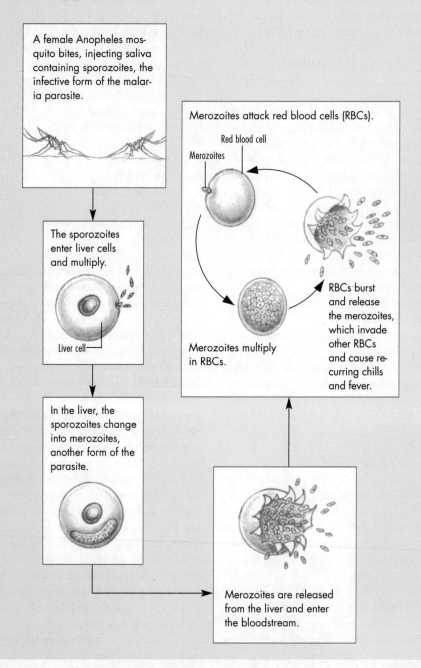

A female Anopheles mosquito bites, injecting saliva containing sporozoites, the infective form of the malaria parasite.

The sporozoites enter liver cells and multiply.

Liver cell

In the liver, the sporozoites change into merozoites, another form of the parasite.

Merozoites are released from the liver and enter the bloodstream.

Merozoites attack red blood cells (RBCs).

Red blood cell

Merozoites

Merozoites multiply in RBCs.

RBCs burst and release the merozoites, which invade other RBCs and cause recurring chills and fever.

with more than 1 million resulting in death. It's the greatest disease hazard for travelers in warm climates. Although malaria has been eliminated in the United States, it is estimated that approximately 1,200 U.S. residents per year traveling abroad have become infected, of whom 13 have died.[1]

Signs and symptoms

After an incubation period of 12 to 30 days, malaria produces chills, fever, headache, and myalgia, interspersed with periods of well-being (the hallmark of the benign form of malaria). Acute attacks (paroxysms) occur when erythrocytes rupture. There are three stages:
▶ cold stage, lasting 1 to 2 hours, ranging from chills to extreme shaking
▶ hot stage, lasting 3 to 4 hours, characterized by a high fever (up to 107° F [41.7° C])
▶ wet stage, lasting 2 to 4 hours and characterized by profuse sweating.

Paroxysms occur every 48 to 72 hours when malaria is caused by *P. malariae* and every 42 to 50 hours when malaria is caused by *P. vivax* or *P. ovale*. All three types have low levels of parasitosis and are self-limiting as a result of early acquired immunity.

P. vivax and *P. ovale* also produce hepatosplenomegaly. Hemolytic anemia is present in all but the mildest infections.

The most severe and only life-threatening form of malaria is caused by *P. falciparum*. This species produces persistent high fever, orthostatic hypotension, and red blood cell (RBC) sludging that leads to capillary obstruction at various sites. Signs and symptoms of obstruction include:
▶ cerebral—hemiplegia, seizures, delirium, and coma
▶ pulmonary—coughing and hemoptysis
▶ splanchnic—vomiting, abdominal pain, diarrhea, and melena
▶ renal—oliguria, anuria, and uremia.

During blackwater fever (a complication of *P. falciparum* infection), massive intravascular hemolysis causes jaundice, hemoglobinuria, a tender and enlarged spleen, acute renal failure, and uremia. This complication is fatal in about 20% of patients.

Complications
▶ Renal failure
▶ Liver failure
▶ Heart failure
▶ Pulmonary edema
▶ Disseminated intravascular coagulation (DIC)
▶ Circulatory collapse
▶ Severe normocytic anemia
▶ Seizures
▶ Hypoglycemia
▶ Splenic rupture
▶ Cerebral dysfunction
▶ Death

Diagnosis

Light microscopy of Giemsa-stained blood smears is the accepted standard for malaria diagnosis. If the initial blood smear is negative and malaria remains a possible diagnosis, the smear should be repeated every 12 hours until a diagnosis of malaria is made or ruled out.[2] In addition, a history showing travel to endemic areas, recent blood transfusion, or drug abuse in a person with high fever of unknown origin strongly suggests malaria. However, because symptoms of malaria mimic other diseases, unequivocal diagnosis depends on laboratory identification of the parasites in RBCs of peripheral blood smears.

The CDC can identify donors responsible for transfusion malaria through indirect fluorescent serum antibody tests. These tests are unreliable in the acute phase because antibodies can be undetectable for 2 weeks after onset.

Supplementary laboratory values that support this diagnosis include decreased hemoglobin levels, normal to decreased leukocyte count (as low as 3,000/µl), and protein and leukocytes in urine sediment. In falciparum malaria, serum values reflect DIC: reduced number of platelets (20,000 to 50,000/µl), prolonged prothrombin time (18 to 20 seconds), prolonged partial thromboplastin

time (60 to 100 seconds), and decreased plasma fibrinogen.

Treatment

Malaria is best treated with oral chloroquine in all forms except chloroquine-resistant *P. falciparum*. Symptoms and parasitemia decrease within 24 hours after such therapy begins, and the patient usually recovers within 3 to 4 days. If the patient is comatose or vomiting frequently, chloroquine is given I.M.

Malaria caused by *P. falciparum*, which is resistant to chloroquine, requires treatment with oral quinine given concurrently with pyrimethamine and a sulfonamide such as sulfadiazine. Mefloquine can also be used for resistant *P. falciparum*. Relapses require the same treatment, or quinine alone, followed by tetracycline.

The only drug that's available in the United States that is effective against the hepatic stage of the disease is primaquine. This drug can induce hemolytic anemia, especially in patients with glucose-6-phosphate dehydrogenase deficiency. (See *Special considerations for antimalarial drugs.*)

Before traveling and starting a prophylactic drug regimen to prevent contracting malaria, first confirm whether there is a risk of acquiring malaria. If so, do some research to find out if area health officials report any antimalaria drug resistance. Resistance to antimalarial drugs has developed in many regions of the world.[1]

As a preventive measure against malaria, the CDC recommends chemoprophylaxis. This is the strategy that uses medications before, during, and after the exposure period to prevent the disease caused by malaria parasites. CDC officials recommend the following chemoprophylaxis for travelers to malarious regions: oral mefloquine or chloroquine should begin 1 to 2 weeks before travel; prophylaxis with doxycycline, atovaquone/proguanil, or primaquine can begin 1 to

Special considerations for antimalarial drugs

CHLOROQUINE
- Perform baseline and periodic ophthalmologic examinations, and report blurred vision, increased sensitivity to light, and muscle weakness to the physician.
- Consult with the physician about altering therapy if muscle weakness appears in a patient on long-term therapy.
- Monitor the patient for tinnitus and other signs of ototoxicity, such as nerve deafness and vertigo.
- Caution the patient to avoid excessive exposure to the sun to prevent exacerbating drug-induced dermatoses.

PRIMAQUINE
- Give with meals or antacids.
- Halt administration if you observe a sudden fall in hemoglobin concentration or in erythrocyte or leukocyte count, or marked darkening of the urine, suggesting impending hemolytic reaction.

PYRIMETHAMINE
- Administer with meals to minimize GI distress.
- Check blood counts (including platelets) twice per week. If signs of folic or folinic acid deficiency develop, reduce or discontinue dosage while the patient receives parenteral folinic acid until blood counts become normal.

QUININE
- Use with caution in patients with cardiovascular conditions. Discontinue dosage if you see any signs of idiosyncrasy or toxicity, such as headache, epigastric distress, diarrhea, rashes, and pruritus, in a mild reaction; or delirium, seizures, blindness, cardiovascular collapse, asthma, hemolytic anemia, and granulocytosis, in a severe reaction.
- Monitor blood pressure frequently while administering quinine I.V. infusion. Rapid administration causes marked hypotension.

2 days before travel. Beginning the drug before travel allows the antimalarial agent to be in the blood before the traveler is exposed to malaria parasites.[1] (See *How to prevent malaria*.) Any traveler who develops an acute febrile illness should seek prompt medical attention, regardless of the prophylaxis taken. Ongoing research (through the Special Program for Research and Training in Tropical Disease Research at the World Health Organization), continues on ways to control malaria in malaria-endemic countries and the development of new programs aimed at acquiring additional research funding, publishing high-quality scientific publications, and training the next generation of malaria researchers.[3]

Special considerations

▶ Obtain a detailed patient history, noting any recent travel, foreign residence, blood transfusion, or drug addiction. Record symptom pattern, fever, type of malaria, and any systemic signs.

▶ Assess the patient on admission and daily thereafter for fatigue, fever, orthostatic hypotension, disorientation, myalgia, and arthralgia. Enforce bed rest during periods of acute illness.

▶ Protect the patient from secondary bacterial infection by following proper hand-hygiene and sterile techniques.

▶ Protect yourself by wearing gloves when handling blood or body fluids.

▶ Activate safety devices, and use safety syringes in practice.

▶ Discard needles and syringes in an impervious container designated for incineration.

▶ Handle bed linens according to standard precautions.

▶ To reduce fever, administer antipyretics as ordered. Document onset, duration, and symptoms before and after episodes.

▶ Fluid balance is fragile, so keep a strict record of intake and output. Monitor I.V. fluids closely. Avoid fluid overload (especially in *P. falciparum*), because it can lead to

---

How to prevent malaria

● Drain, fill, and eliminate breeding areas of the *Anopheles* mosquito.
● Install screens in living and sleeping quarters in endemic areas.
● Use a residual insecticide on clothing and skin to prevent mosquito bites.
● Seek treatment for known cases.
● Question blood donors about a history of malaria or possible exposure to malaria. They *may* give blood if:
– they haven't taken any antimalarial drugs and are asymptomatic after 6 months outside an endemic area
– they were asymptomatic after treatment for malaria more than 3 years ago
– they were asymptomatic after receiving malaria prophylaxis more than 3 years ago.
● Seek prophylactic drug therapy before traveling to an endemic area. Agents include mefloquine, doxycycline, chloroquine, hydroxychloroquine, or malarone (a combination of atovaquone and proguanil). They're usually started 2 weeks before visiting the endemic area and continue for 6 weeks after leaving the area.
● Use insect repellants containing 50% DEET.

---

pulmonary edema and aggravate cerebral symptoms. Observe blood chemistry levels for hyponatremia and increased blood urea nitrogen, creatinine, and bilirubin levels. Monitor urine output hourly, and maintain it at 40 to 60 ml/hour for an adult and at 15 to 30 ml/hour for a child. Immediately report any decrease in urine output or the onset of hematuria as a possible sign of renal failure; be prepared to perform peritoneal dialysis for uremia caused by renal failure.

▶ Slowly administer packed RBCs or whole blood while checking for crackles, tachycardia, and shortness of breath.

▶ If humidified oxygen is ordered, note the patient's response, particularly any changes in rate or character of respira-

tions, or any improvement in mucous membrane color.

▶ Watch for and immediately report signs of internal bleeding, such as tachycardia, hypotension, and pallor.

▶ Encourage frequent coughing and deep breathing, especially if the patient is on bed rest or has pulmonary complications. Record the amount and color of sputum.

▶ Watch for adverse effects of drug therapy, and take measures to relieve them.

▶ If the patient is comatose, make frequent, gentle changes in his position, and give passive range-of-motion exercises every 3 to 4 hours. If the patient is unconscious or disoriented, use restraints as needed, and keep an airway available as appropriate.

▶ Provide emotional support and reassurance, especially in critical illness. Explain the procedures and treatment to the patient and his family. Suggest that other family members be tested for malaria. Emphasize the need for follow-up care to check the effectiveness of treatment and to manage residual problems.

▶ Report all cases of malaria to local public health authorities.

REFERENCES

1. Centers for Disease Control and Prevention. (2008 February 15). "Prevention of Specific Infectious Diseases: Malaria." [Online]. Available at *www.cdc.gov/travel/yellowBookCh4-Malaria.aspx.*

2. Glikman, D., et al. "Clinical Malaria and Sickle Cell Disease among Multiple Family Members in Chicago, Illinois," *Pediatrics* 120(3):745–48, September 2007.

3. Nantulya, F. N., et al. "Research Themes and Advances in Malaria Research Capacity Made by the Multilateral Initiative on Malaria," *The Journal of Tropical Medicine and Hygiene,* 77(6_Suppl): 303–313, 2007.

METHICILLIN-RESISTANT *STAPHYLOCOCCUS AUREUS* INFECTION

Methicillin-resistant *Staphylococcus aureus* (MRSA) is a mutation of a very common bacterium spread easily by direct person-to-person contact. Once limited to large teaching hospitals and tertiary care centers, MRSA infection is now endemic in nursing homes, long-term care facilities, and community hospitals. It's also seen in patients who haven't been hospitalized, as community-acquired MRSA infections are increasing.

Patients most at risk for MRSA infection include immunosuppressed patients, burn patients, intubated patients, and those with central venous catheters, surgical wounds, or dermatitis. Others at risk include those with prosthetic devices, heart valves, and postoperative wound infections. Other risk factors include prolonged hospital stays, extended therapy with multiple or broad-spectrum antibiotics, and close proximity to those colonized or infected with MRSA. Also at risk are patients with acute endocarditis, bacteremia, cervicitis, meningitis, pericarditis, and pneumonia. MRSA infections can be fatal.[1]

Causes and incidence

MRSA enters health care facilities through an infected or colonized patient or a colonized health care worker. Although MRSA has been recovered from environmental surfaces, it's transmitted mainly by health care workers' hands. Healthy people can be colonized with MRSA and become silent carriers having no ill effects. They can pass the germ to others.[1] MRSA remains viable on surfaces for days.

The most frequent site of colonization is the anterior nares (40% of adults and most children become transient nasal carriers). Other less-common sites are the groin, axilla, and gut. Typically, MRSA colonization is diagnosed by isolating bacteria from nasal secretions.

In individuals where the natural defense system breaks down, such as after an invasive procedure, trauma, or chemotherapy, the normally benign bacteria can invade tissue, proliferate, and cause infection.

In a recent study at Texas Children's Hospital, the number of patients who have become severely ill because of community-acquired staph infections has risen since 2002, and 70% of the infections are caused by MRSA.[2]

MRSA infection has become prevalent with the overuse of antibiotics. Over the years, this has given once-susceptible bacteria the chance to develop defenses against antibiotics. This new capability allows resistant strains to flourish when antibiotics kill their more-sensitive cousins.

Signs and symptoms

Staph infections such as MRSA generally present as small red bumps that resemble pimples, boils, or spider bites. They can then advance to deep, painful abscesses that require surgical draining. Sometimes the bacteria can remain confined to the skin. However, they can also burrow deep into the body and cause potentially life-threatening infections in other areas such as bones, joints, surgical wounds, the bloodstream, heart valves, and lungs.[1] Often, there are no signs and symptoms with MRSA infections. It's often found incidentally during culture.

Complications

▶ Sepsis
▶ Death

Diagnosis

MRSA can be cultured from the suspected site with the appropriate method. For example, a wound can be swabbed for culture. Cultures of blood, urine, and sputum specimens will reveal sources of MRSA. However, cultures can take about 48 hours for the bacteria to grow. Newer tests that can detect staph deoxyribonucleic acid in hours are now becoming more widely available.[1] Many laboratories use oxacillin disks to check for staphylococcus sensitivity when testing culture specimens; resistance to oxacillin indicates MRSA.

Treatment

To eradicate MRSA colonization in the nares, the physician may order topical mupirocin to be applied inside the nostrils. Other protocols involve combining a topical agent and an oral antibiotic. Most facilities keep patients in isolation until surveillance cultures are negative.

To attack MRSA infection, vancomycin is the drug of choice. (See *Vancomycin-resistant infections.*) However, some hospitals report seeing MRSA that is resistant to vancomycin.[1] A serious adverse effect of vancomycin (mostly caused by histamine release) is itching, which can progress to anaphylaxis. Some physicians also add rifampin, but whether rifampin acts synergistically or antagonistically when given with vancomycin is controversial. Linezolid and clindamycin may be used. New evidence has surfaced of a multi-drug-resistant, community-acquired MRSA in San Francisco among populations of males who have sex with males. Further research needs to be done to determine if the route of transmission is through sex.[3]

Special considerations

▶ People in contact with the patient should perform hand hygiene before and after patient care.
▶ Good hand hygiene is the most effective way to prevent MRSA infection from spreading.
▶ Use an antiseptic soap such as chlorhexidine. Bacteria have been cultured from workers' hands washed with milder soap. One study showed that without proper hand hygiene, MRSA could survive on health care workers' hands for up to 3 hours. Chlorhexidine has a residual antimicrobial effect on the skin.
▶ Contact isolation precautions should be used when in contact with the patient. A dis-

Vancomycin-resistant infections

Some *Staphylococcus aureus* organisms have developed resistance to vancomycin. In some cases, the resistance is considered intermediate-strength resistance and is known as vancomycin-intermediate *S. aureus* (VISA). Another mutation, vancomycin-resistant *S. aureus* (VRSA), is fully resistant to vancomycin.

Researchers believe VISA and VRSA enter health care facilities through an infected or colonized patient or a colonized health care worker. They spread through direct contact between the patient and caregiver or between patients. They may also be spread through patient contact with contaminated surfaces.

Patients with laboratory-confirmed VISA or VRSA must be placed in a single room on contact precautions, and the number of health care workers involved in patient care should be limited. Other patients who shared the patient's room should be checked for VISA or VRSA colonization using an anterior nares culture. (Notify the laboratory to look specifically for *S. aureus* and to check sensitivity).

People involved in direct care of the patient before the initiation of contact precautions should be interviewed regarding the extent of their interactions. Those with extensive interaction should have an anterior nares culture. The local health department should be notified immediately. Antimicrobial treatment may include an increased dosage of vancomycin (for VISA only) and linezolid, quinupristin and dalfopristin, or a combination of other antimicrobials, according to the sensitivity pattern of the organism.

infected private room should be made available with dedicated equipment.

▶ Change gloves when contaminated or when moving from a "dirty" area of the body to a clean one.

▶ Instruct the patient's family and friends to wear protective clothing when they visit him, and show them how to dispose of it.

▶ Provide teaching and emotional support to the patient and his family members.

▶ Consider grouping infected patients together and having the same nursing staff care for them.

▶ Don't lay equipment used on the patient on the bed or bed stand. Be sure to wipe it with appropriate disinfectant before leaving the room.

▶ Ensure judicious and careful use of antibiotics. Encourage physicians to limit their use.

▶ Instruct the patient to take antibiotics for the full period prescribed, even if he begins to feel better.

REFERENCES

1. Mayo Clinic (2008 April 1). "MRSA Infection." [Online]. Available at *www.mayoclinic.com/health/mrsa/DS00735*.

2. Gonzalez, Blanca E. MD, et al. "Severe Staphylococcal Sepsis in Adolescents in the Era of Community-Acquired Methicillin-Resistant *Staphylococcus aureus*," *Pediatrics* 115(3): 642–8, March 2005.

3. Diep, A. B., et al. "Emergence of Multidrug-Resistant, Community-Associated, Methicillin-Resistant *Staphylococcus aureus* Clone USA300 in Men Who Have Sex with Men," *Annals of Internal Medicine*, 148(4), February 2008.

MUMPS

Mumps, also known as infectious or epidemic parotitis, is an acute viral disease caused by a paramyxovirus. It causes painful enlargement of the salivary or parotid glands. It may also infect other organs, such as the testes, the central nervous system, and the pancreas. The prognosis for complete recovery is good, although mumps sometimes causes complications.

Causes and incidence

The mumps paramyxovirus is found in the saliva of an infected person and is transmitted by droplets or by direct contact. The virus is present in the saliva 6 days before to 9 days

after onset of parotid gland swelling; the 48-hour period immediately preceding onset of swelling is probably the time of highest communicability. The incubation period ranges from 14 to 25 days (the average is 18). One attack of mumps (even if unilateral) almost always confers lifelong immunity. Yet researchers in a recent study concluded that reinfection with mumps is not as rare as it is believed to be. They report that several outpatient cases of suspected reinfection with mumps were confirmed through a method noted as reverse transcription loop-mediated isothermal amplification and an IgG avidity test.[1]

Mumps is most prevalent in children between ages 6 and 8. Infants younger than age 1 seldom get this disease because of the passive immunity received from maternal antibodies. Peak incidence occurs during late winter and early spring.

Signs and symptoms

The clinical features of mumps vary widely. An estimated 30% of susceptible people have subclinical illness.

Mumps usually begins with prodromal symptoms that last for 24 hours and include myalgia, anorexia, malaise, headache, and low-grade fever followed by an earache that's aggravated by chewing, parotid gland tenderness and swelling, a temperature of 101° to 104° F (38.3° to 40° C), and pain when chewing or drinking sour or acidic liquids. Simultaneously with the swelling of the parotid gland or several days later, one or more of the other salivary glands may become swollen.

Complications can include epididymoorchitis and mumps meningitis. In approximately 25% of postpubertal males who contract mumps, epididymoorchitis occurs and produces abrupt onset of testicular swelling and tenderness, scrotal erythema, lower abdominal pain, nausea, vomiting, fever, and chills. Swelling and tenderness may last for several weeks; epididymitis may precede or accompany the orchitis. In 50% of men with

mumps-induced orchitis, the testicles show some atrophy, but sterility is extremely rare.

Mumps meningitis complicates the disease in 10% of patients and affects three to five times more males than females. Signs and symptoms include fever, meningeal irritation (nuchal rigidity, headache, and irritability), vomiting, drowsiness, and a cerebrospinal fluid lymphocyte count ranging from 500 to 2,000/μl. Recovery is usually complete. Less-common effects are pancreatitis, deafness, arthritis, myocarditis, encephalitis, pericarditis, oophoritis, and nephritis.

Complications

▶ Epididymoorchitis
▶ Testicular swelling
▶ Tenderness
▶ Scrotal erythema
▶ Lower abdominal pain
▶ Nausea
▶ Vomiting
▶ Fever
▶ Chills
▶ Testicular atrophy
▶ Sterility

Mumps meningitis

▶ Fever
▶ Meningeal irritation (nuchal rigidity, headaches, and irritability)
▶ Vomiting
▶ Drowsiness
▶ Cerebral spinal lymphocytic fluid count from 500 to 2,000/ul

Less common

▶ Pancreatitis
▶ Transient sensineural hearing loss
▶ Transverse myelitis
▶ Arthritis
▶ Myocarditis
▶ Pericarditis
▶ Oophoritis
▶ Diabetes mellitus
▶ Thyroiditis
▶ Nephritis

Diagnosis

The clinical case definition of mumps, according to the Centers for Disease Control and Prevention, is an illness with acute onset of unilateral or bilateral tender, self-limited swelling of the parotid or other salivary gland lasting 2 or more days, and without other apparent cause. Since the clinical diagnosis of mumps may be unreliable, suspected cases of mumps should be laboratory confirmed combined with signs and symptoms.[2] Anyone with a history of exposure to mumps should also be considered. A buccal swab, serum samples, and a mumps viral specimen should be collected. The presence of serum mumps immunoglobulin M (IgM), a fourfold rise in serum mumps immunoglobulin G (IgG) titer between acute and convalescent phase serum specimens, positive mumps virus culture, or detection of viral ribonucleic acid by reverse transcription-polymerase chain reaction (RT-PCR) confirms the diagnosis.[2] Serologic antibody testing can verify the diagnosis when parotid or other salivary gland enlargement is absent. If comparison between a blood specimen obtained during the acute phase of illness and another specimen obtained 3 weeks later shows a fourfold rise in antibody titer, the patient most likely had mumps.

Treatment

Treatment includes analgesics for pain, antipyretics for fever, and adequate fluid intake to prevent dehydration from fever and anorexia. Aspirin is not recommended because of the risk of Reye's syndrome. If the patient can't swallow, consider I.V. fluid replacement. Warm saltwater gargles, soft foods, and extra fluids also may help relieve symptoms.

Special considerations

▶ Stress the need for bed rest during the febrile period. Give analgesics, and apply warm or cool compresses to the neck to relieve pain. Give antipyretics and tepid sponge baths for fever. To prevent dehydration, encourage the patient to drink fluids; to minimize pain and anorexia, advise him to avoid spicy, irritating, acidic foods and drinks and those that require a lot of chewing. Offer a soft, bland diet to decrease the amount of chewing.

▶ During the acute phase, observe the patient closely for signs of central nervous system involvement, such as altered level of consciousness and nuchal rigidity.

▶ Because the mumps virus is present in the saliva throughout the course of the disease, follow droplet precautions until symptoms subside.

▶ Emphasize the importance of routine immunization with live attenuated mumps virus (paramyxovirus) at age 15 months and for susceptible patients (especially males) who are approaching or are past puberty. Remember, immunization within 24 hours of exposure may prevent or attenuate the actual disease. Immunity against mumps lasts at least 12 years.

▶ Report all cases of mumps to local public health authorities.

REFERENCES

1. Centers for Disease Control and Prevention (2007). "Mumps." [Online]. Available at *www.cdc.gov/vaccines/pubs/pinkbook/downloads/mumps.pdf.*
2. Yoshida, N., et al. "Mumps Virus Reinfection Is Not a Rare Event Confirmed by Reverse Transcription Loop-Mediated Isothermal Amplification," *Journal of Medical Virology* 80(3):517–23, March 2008.

PNEUMOCYSTIS CARINII PNEUMONIA

Because of its association with human immunodeficiency virus (HIV) infection, *Pneumocystis carinii* pneumonia (PCP), an opportunistic infection, has increased in incidence since the 1980s. Before the advent of PCP prophylaxis, this disease

provided the first clue in about 60% of patients that HIV infection was present.

PCP was the leading cause of death in these patients. Prophylactic therapy with co-trimoxazole in HIV patients with low immune function has prevented PCP from higher mortality rates. Disseminated infection doesn't occur.

PCP is also associated with other immuno-compromising conditions, including organ transplantation, leukemia, lymphoma, and steroid use. Peak incidence in the United States is among 20- to 40-year-olds, but it is also seen in children less than 2 years of age.

Causes and incidence

P. carinii, the cause of PCP, usually is classified as a protozoan, although some investigators consider it more closely related to fungi. The organism exists as a saprophyte in the lungs of humans and various animals as part of the normal flora in most healthy people. It becomes an aggressive pathogen in the immunocompromised patient. Impaired cell-mediated (T-cell) immunity is thought to be more important than impaired humoral (B-cell) immunity in predisposing the patient to PCP, but the immune defects involved are poorly understood. *P. carinii* becomes activated in immunocompromised patients when the CD4+ T-cell count falls below 200/µl. *P. carinii* invades the lungs bilaterally and multiplies extracellularly. As the infestation grows, alveoli fill with organisms and exudate, impairing gas exchange. The alveoli hypertrophy and thicken progressively, eventually leading to extensive consolidation. HIV infected patients who use tobacco are at a higher risk for developing PCP infection.[1] The primary transmission route for *P. carinii* seems to be air, although the organism is already present in most people. The incubation period probably lasts for 4 to 8 weeks.

Signs and symptoms

The patient typically has a history of an immunocompromising illness (such as HIV infection, leukemia, or lymphoma) or procedure (such as organ transplantation).

PCP begins insidiously with increasing shortness of breath, fever and a nonproductive cough. Anorexia, generalized fatigue, and weight loss may follow. Although the patient may have hypoxemia and hypercapnia, he may not exhibit significant symptoms. He may, however, have a low-grade, intermittent fever.

Other signs and symptoms include tachypnea, dyspnea, accessory muscle use for breathing, crackles (in about one-third of patients), marked pallor, and decreased breath sounds (in advanced pneumonia). Cyanosis may appear with acute illness; pulmonary consolidation develops later.

Complications

▶ Pulmonary insufficiency
▶ Death (untreated)
▶ Disseminated infection

Diagnosis

The diagnosis of PCP is difficult because it requires microscopic examination to identify Pneumocystis. Histologic studies confirm *P. carinii* in all patients through one of the following methods: fiber-optic bronchoscopy, induced sputum, bronchoalveolar lavage (BAL), transbronchial biopsy and open-lung biopsy. Fiber optics remains the most commonly used study to confirm PCP. Induced sputum is the quickest and least-invasive method to identify the organism. This is achieved by having the patient inhale a hypertonic saline solution. BAL is a more invasive procedure. Sometimes a transbronchial biopsy may be performed in conjunction with BAL. An open-lung biopsy is performed less commonly.

In patients with HIV infection, initial examination of a first-morning sputum specimen (induced by inhaling an ultrasonically dispersed saline mist) may be sufficient; however, this technique usually is ineffective in patients without HIV infection.

Chest X-rays may show slowly progressing, fluffy infiltrates and, occasionally, nodular lesions or a spontaneous pneumothorax, but these findings must be differentiated from findings in other types of pneumonia or acute respiratory distress syndrome.

High resolution CT scan of the chest may be helpful.

Gallium scan may show increased uptake over the lungs even when the chest X-ray appears relatively normal. Arterial blood gas (ABG) studies detect hypoxia and an increased A-a gradient.

New research is being done to develop a blood test, the ß-glucan assay, that would identify PCP. This test seems promising, but more studies are needed.[2]

Treatment

PCP may respond to drug therapy with co-trimoxazole. Other agents used to treat PCP include pentamidine, trimethoprim-dapsone, clindamycin, primaquine, and atovaquone. Corticosteroids are frequently used as well. However, because of immune system impairment, many patients with PCP who also have HIV tend to experience severe adverse reactions to drug therapy. Giving weekly doses of trimethoprim/sulfamethoxazole may be an effective prophylactic regimen for *P. carinii* pneumonia in pediatric patients with leukemia and lymphoma.[3] Supportive measures, such as oxygen therapy, mechanical ventilation, adequate nutrition, and fluid balance, are important adjunctive therapies. Oral morphine sulfate solution may reduce the respiratory rate and anxiety, thereby enhancing oxygenation.

Special considerations

▶ Implement standard precautions to prevent contagion.
▶ Frequently assess the patient's respiratory status, and monitor ABG levels every 4 hours.
▶ Administer oxygen therapy as ordered. Encourage the patient to ambulate as well

as to perform deep-breathing exercises and incentive spirometry to facilitate effective gas exchange.
▶ Administer antipyretics as ordered to relieve fever.
▶ Monitor the patient's intake, output, and daily weight to evaluate fluid balance. Replace fluids as ordered.
▶ Provide diversionary activities, and coordinate health care team activities to allow adequate rest periods between procedures.
▶ Teach the patient energy-conservation techniques.
▶ Supply nutritional supplements as needed. Encourage the patient to eat a high-calorie, protein-rich diet. Offer small, frequent meals if the patient cannot tolerate large amounts of food.
▶ Reduce anxiety by providing a relaxing environment, eliminating excessive environmental stimuli, and allowing ample time for meals.
▶ Give emotional support, and help patient identify and use meaningful support systems.
▶ Instruct the patient about the medication regimen, especially about the adverse effects.
▶ Emphasize the importance of continuing chemoprophylaxis for those patients at high risk of developing PCP.
▶ If the patient will require oxygen therapy at home, explain that an oxygen concentrator may be most effective.
▶ Because this infection is usually associated with acquired immune deficiency syndrome (AIDS), provide the patient with resources and support organizations for both AIDS and HIV.
▶ Emphasize the importance of regular follow-up care to prevent secondary infection.

REFERENCES

1. Miguez-Burbano, M. J., et al. "Increased Risk of Pneumocystis Carinii and Community-Acquired Pneumonia with Tobacco Use In HIV Disease," *International Journal of Infectious Diseases* 9(4):208–17, July 2005.

2. Medscape. (2007 December 9). "A Quick Blood Test for PCP?" [Online]. Available at *www.medscape.com*.

3. Lindemulder, S., Albano, E. "Successful Intermittent Prophylaxis with Trimethoprim/ Sulfamethoxazole 2 Days Per Week for *Pneumocystis Carinii* (Jiroveci) Pneumonia in Pediatric Oncology Patients," *Pediatrics* 120(1):47–51, July 2007.

PSEUDOMONAS INFECTIONS

Pseudomonas is a small gram-negative bacillus that produces nosocomial infections, superinfections of various parts of the body, and a rare disease called melioidosis. This bacillus is also associated with bacteremia, endocarditis, and osteomyelitis in drug addicts. In local *Pseudomonas* infections, treatment is usually successful and complications rare; however, in patients with any type of lowered immunity—premature neonates; elderly patients; patients with debilitating disease, burns, or wounds; or patients receiving chemotherapy or radiation therapy— septicemic *Pseudomonas* infections are serious and commonly fatal.

Causes and incidence

The most common species of *Pseudomonas* is *P. aeruginosa*. It is noted to be a major virulent pathogen implicated in many syndromes. *P. aeruginosa* infections can have an overall mortality rate of 45% and higher in patients who are immunocompromised.[1] Other species that typically cause disease in humans include *Xanthomonas maltophilia* (formerly known as *P. maltophilia*), *Burkholderia cepacia* (formerly known as *P. cepacia*), *P. fluorescens*, *P. testosteroni*, *P. acidovorans*, *P. alcaligenes*, *P. stutzeri*, *P. putrefaciens*, and *P. putida*. These organisms are commonly found in liquids that have been allowed to stand for a long time, such as benzalkonium chloride, saline solution, penicillin, water in flower vases, and fluids in incubators, humidifiers, and inhalation therapy equipment. *P. aeruginosa* is associated with chronic obstructive pulmonary disease. *B. cepacia* is the organism most closely associated with cystic fibrosis, although *P. aeruginosa* is also associated with it. In elderly patients, *Pseudomonas* infection usually enters through the genitourinary tract; in neonates and infants, through the umbilical cord, skin, and GI tract. Also, hot tub rash infections are often caused by the germ *Pseudomonas aeruginosa*.[2]

Signs and symptoms

The most common infections associated with *Pseudomonas* include skin infections (such as burns and pressure ulcers), urinary tract infections, infant epidemic diarrhea and other diarrheal illnesses, bronchitis, pneumonia, bronchiectasis, meningitis, corneal ulcers, mastoiditis, otitis externa, otitis media, endocarditis, and bacteremia.

Drainage in *Pseudomonas* infections has a distinct, sickly sweet odor and a greenish blue pus that forms a crust on wounds. Other symptoms depend on the site of infection. (See *Melioidosis.*) For example, when it invades the lungs, *Pseudomonas* causes pneumonia with fever, chills, and a productive cough.

Complications

▶ Septic shock
▶ Death
▶ Severe mucopurulent pneumonia
▶ Septicemic-inflammatory response syndrome
▶ Multiple organ dysfunction

Diagnosis

Diagnosis requires isolation of the *Pseudomonas* organism in blood, spinal fluid, urine, exudate, or sputum culture.

Treatment

In the debilitated or otherwise vulnerable patient with clinical evidence of *Pseudomonas*

Melioidosis

Melioidosis results from wound penetration, inhalation, or ingestion of the gram-negative bacteria *Pseudomonas pseudomallei*. Although it was once confined to Southeast Asia, Central America, South America, Madagascar, and Guam, incidence in the United States has risen as a result of the influx of Southeast Asians.

Melioidosis occurs in two forms: chronic melioidosis, which causes osteomyelitis and lung abscesses, and the rare acute melioidosis, which causes pneumonia, bacteremia, and prostration. Acute melioidosis is commonly fatal; however, most melioidosis infections are chronic and asymptomatic, producing clinical symptoms only with accompanying malnutrition, major surgery, or severe burns.

Diagnostic measures consist of isolation of *P. pseudomallei* in a culture of exudate, blood, or sputum; serology tests (complement fixation, passive hemagglutination); and chest X-ray (findings resemble tuberculosis). Treatment includes oral tetracycline and co-trimoxazole, abscess drainage and, in severe cases, chloramphenicol until X-rays show resolution of primary abscesses.

The prognosis is good because most patients have a mild infection and acquire permanent immunity; aggressive use of antibiotics and sulfonamides has improved the prognosis in acute melioidosis.

infection, treatment should begin immediately, without waiting for results of laboratory tests. Antibiotic treatment includes aminoglycosides, such as gentamicin or tobramycin, combined with an antipseudomonal penicillin, such as ticarcillin or piperacillin. An alternative combination is amikacin and a similar penicillin or imipenem and cilastatin. Such combination therapy is necessary because *Pseudomonas* quickly becomes resistant to ticarcillin alone.

Local *Pseudomonas* infections or septicemia secondary to wound infection requires 1% acetic acid irrigations; topical applications of colistimethate, polymyxin B, and silver sulfadiazine cream; and debridement or drainage of the infected wound.

Pseudomonas keratitis infections are of concern especially in patients who use extended-wear lenses. Industry and research groups are investigating antimicrobial contact lenses to reduce bacterial colonization.[3]

Special considerations

▶ Observe and record the character of wound exudate and sputum.

▶ Before administering antibiotics, ask the patient about a history of drug allergies, especially to penicillin. If combinations of piperacillin or ticarcillin and an aminoglycoside are ordered, schedule the doses 1 hour apart (ticarcillin may decrease the antibiotic effect of the aminoglycoside). Don't give both antibiotics through the same administration set.

▶ Monitor the patient's renal function (output, blood urea nitrogen level, specific gravity, urinalysis, and creatinine level) during treatment with aminoglycosides. Obtain drug levels to ensure effectiveness.

▶ Protect immunocompromised patients from exposure to this infection. Proper hand hygiene and sterile techniques prevent further spread.

▶ To prevent *Pseudomonas* infection, maintain proper endotracheal and tracheostomy suctioning technique. Use strict sterile technique when caring for I.V. lines, catheters, and other tubes. Discard suction bottles, irrigating fluid, and open bottles of saline solution every 24 hours. Be sure to change I.V. tubing according to hospital policy and to empty ventilator water reservoirs before refilling them with sterile water. Remember to use suction catheters only once.

REFERENCES

1. Giamarellou, H. "Prescribing Guidelines for Severe Pseudomonas Infections," *Journal of Antimicrobial Chemotherapy* 49(2):229–33, February 2002.
2. Centers for Disease Control and Prevention. (2007 May 2). "Hot Tub Rash Pseudomonas Dermatitis/Folliculitis." [Online]. Available at *www.cdc.gov/healthyswimming/derm.htm*.
3. Willcox, M. D. P. "New Strategies to Prevent Pseudomonas Keratitis," *Eye and Contact Lens* 33(6 Pt 2):401–3, November 2007.

RABIES

Rabies, also known as hydrophobia, is an acute central nervous system (CNS) infection caused by a virus that's transmitted by the saliva of an infected animal (especially wild animals). If symptoms occur, rabies is almost always fatal. Treatment soon after exposure, however, may prevent fatal CNS invasion.

Causes and incidence

The rabies virus is usually transmitted to a human through the bite of an infected animal. The virus begins to replicate in the striated muscle cells at the bite site. Then it spreads up the nerve to the CNS and replicates in the brain. Finally, it moves through the nerves into other tissues, including the salivary glands. Occasionally, airborne droplets and infected-tissue transplants can transmit the virus.

Rabies symptoms appear earlier if the head or face is severely bitten. If the bite is on the face, the risk of developing rabies is about 60%; on the upper extremities, 15% to 40%; and on the lower extremities, about 10%.[1]

While human deaths from rabies are rare in the United States, the disease remains a public and animal health problem that results in 50,000 to 70,000 human deaths worldwide annually. In the United States, dog vaccinations have reduced the incidence of rabies transmission to humans. Approximately 92% of the rabies cases involved wild animals, and 8% were in domestic animals.[2]

During 2006, 49 states and Puerto Rico reported 6,940 cases of rabies in animals and three cases in humans to the Centers for Disease Control and Prevention, representing an 8.2% increase from the 6,417 cases in animals and 1 case in a human reported in 2005.[2]

Signs and symptoms

After an incubation period from 1 to 3 months, rabies typically produces local or radiating pain or burning and a sensation of cold, pruritus, and tingling at the bite site. It also produces prodromal signs and symptoms, such as a slight fever (100° to 102° F [37.8° to 38.9° C]), malaise, headache, anorexia, nausea, sore throat, and persistent loose cough. After this, the patient begins to display nervousness; anxiety; irritability; hyperesthesia; photophobia; sensitivity to loud noises; pupillary dilation; tachycardia; shallow respirations; pain and paresthesia in the bitten area; and excessive salivation, lacrimation, and perspiration.

About 2 to 10 days after the onset of prodromal symptoms, a phase of excitation begins. It's characterized by agitation, marked restlessness, anxiety, and apprehension and cranial nerve dysfunction that causes ocular palsies, strabismus, asymmetrical pupillary dilation or constriction, absence of corneal reflexes, weakness of facial muscles, and hoarseness. Severe systemic symptoms include tachycardia or bradycardia, cyclic respirations, urine retention, and a temperature of about 103° F (39.4° C).

About 50% of affected patients exhibit hydrophobia (literally, "fear of water"). Forceful, painful pharyngeal muscle spasms expel liquids from the mouth and cause dehydration and, possibly, apnea, cyanosis, and death. Difficulty swallowing causes

frothy saliva to drool from the patient's mouth. Eventually, even the sight, mention, or thought of water causes uncontrollable pharyngeal muscle spasms and excessive salivation. Between episodes of excitation and hydrophobia, the patient commonly is cooperative and lucid. After about 3 days, excitation and hydrophobia subside, and the progressively paralytic, terminal phase of this illness begins. The patient experiences progressive, generalized, flaccid paralysis that ultimately leads to peripheral vascular collapse, coma, and death.

Complications
Untreated rabies
► Respiratory failure
► Peripheral vascular collapse
► Central brain failure

Late complications
► Inappropriate secretion of antidiuretic hormone
► Diabetes insipidus
► Cardiac arrhythmias
► Vascular bleeding
► Thrombocytopenia
► Paralytic ileus

Diagnosis
Because rabies is fatal unless treated promptly, always suspect rabies in any person who suffers an unprovoked animal bite until you can prove otherwise.

Virus isolation from the patient's saliva or throat and examination of his blood for fluorescent rabies antibody (FRA) are diagnostic.

Other results typically include elevated white blood cell count, with increased polymorphonuclear and large mononuclear cells; and elevated urinary glucose, acetone, and protein levels.

Confinement of the suspected animal for 10 days of observation by a veterinarian also helps support this diagnosis. If the animal appears rabid, it should be killed and its brain tissue tested for FRA and Negri

bodies (oval or round masses that conclusively confirm rabies).

Treatment
Treatment consists of wound care and immunization as soon as possible after exposure. Thoroughly wash all bite wounds and scratches with soap and water to remove any infected saliva. (See *First aid in animal bites.*) Check the patient's immunization status, and administer tetanus-diphtheria prophylaxis if needed. Take measures to control bacterial infection as ordered. If the wound requires suturing, special treatment and suturing techniques must be used to allow proper drainage.

After rabies exposure, a patient who has not been immunized before must receive passive immunization with rabies immune globulin (RIG) and active immunization with human diploid cell vaccine (HDCV). If the patient has received HDCV before and has an adequate rabies antibody titer, he doesn't need RIG immunization, just an HDCV booster.

Special considerations
► When injecting rabies vaccine, rotate injection sites on the upper arm or thigh. Watch for and symptomatically treat red-

---

First aid in animal bites

Immediately wash the bite vigorously with soap and water for at least 10 minutes to remove the animal's saliva. As soon as possible, flush the wound with a viricidal agent, followed by a clear-water rinse. After cleaning the wound, apply a sterile dressing. If possible, don't suture the wound, and don't immediately stop the bleeding (unless it's massive) because blood flow helps to clean the wound.

Question the patient about the bite. Ask if he provoked the animal (if so, chances are it isn't rabid) and if he can identify it or its owner (because the animal may be confined for observation).

ness, itching, pain, and tenderness at the injection site. Half of the RIG should be infiltrated into and around the bite wound, with the remainder given I.M.

▶ Cooperate with public health authorities to determine the vaccination status of the animal. If the animal is proven rabid, help identify others at risk.

If rabies develops:

▶ Monitor cardiac and pulmonary function continuously.

▶ Isolate the patient. Wear a gown, gloves, and protection for the eyes and mouth when handling saliva and articles contaminated with saliva. Take precautions to avoid being bitten by the patient during the excitation phase.

▶ Keep the room dark and quiet.

▶ Establish communication with the patient and his family. Provide psychological support to help them cope with the patient's symptoms and probable death.

To help prevent rabies:

▶ Stress the need for vaccination of household pets that may be exposed to rabid wild animals.

▶ Warn people not to try to touch wild animals, especially if they appear ill or overly docile (a possible sign of rabies).

▶ Assist in the prophylactic administration of rabies vaccine to high-risk people, such as farm workers, forest rangers, spelunkers (cave explorers), and veterinarians.

REFERENCES

1. U.S. Department of Agriculture. "Controlling Wildlife Vectors of Bovine Tuberculosis and Rabies." [Online]. Available at *www.aphis. usda.gov/ws/researchreports/report15.pdf.*
2. Blanton, J. D., et al. "Rabies Surveillance in the United States during 2006," *Journal of the American Veterinarian Medical Association,* 231(4):540–56, August 2007.

RUBELLA

Rubella, commonly called German measles (although it is not really measles and is caused by a different virus called Rubivirus) is an acute, mildly contagious viral disease that produces a faint, but distinctive 2- to 3-day rash and lymphadenopathy.[1] It usually occurs among children ages 5 to 9, adolescents, and young adults. Rubella flourishes worldwide during the spring (particularly in big cities), and epidemics occur sporadically. Fifty percent of rubella cases are asymptomatic.[1] The disease is self-limiting, with an excellent prognosis.

Causes and incidence

The rubella virus is transmitted through contact with the blood, urine, stools, or nasopharyngeal secretions of infected people and, possibly, by contact with contaminated articles of clothing. Transplacental transmission, especially in the first trimester of pregnancy, can cause serious birth defects, such as microcephaly, mental retardation, patent ductus arteriosus, glaucoma, and bone defects. When infection occurs during pregnancy, especially during the first trimester, the risk of fetal infection may be as high as 90%, often resulting in congenital rubella syndrome.[1] (See *Congenital rubella syndrome.*) Humans are the only known hosts for the rubella virus. The disease is contagious from about 10 days before the rash appears until 5 days after it has appeared.

Signs and symptoms

In children, after an incubation period of 14 to 21 days, an exanthematous, maculopapular rash erupts abruptly. In children, the Rubella rash is usually the first manifestation—a prodrome phase is rare. (See *Incubation and duration of common rash-producing infections,* page 466.) In adolescents and adults, prodromal signs

Congenital rubella syndrome

Congenital rubella is by far the most serious form of the disease. Intrauterine rubella infection, especially during the first trimester, can lead to spontaneous abortion or stillbirth as well as single or multiple birth defects. (As a rule, the earlier the infection occurs during pregnancy, the greater the damage to the fetus.)

The combination of cataracts, deafness, and cardiac disease characterizes congenital rubella syndrome. Low birth weight, microcephaly, and mental retardation are other common manifestations. However, researchers now believe that congenital rubella can cause more disorders, many of which don't appear until later in life. These include dental abnormalities, thrombocytopenic purpura, hemolytic and hypoplastic anemia, encephalitis, giant-cell hepatitis, seborrheic dermatitis, and diabetes mellitus. Indeed, it now appears that congenital rubella may be a lifelong disease. This theory is supported by the fact that the rubella virus has been isolated from urine 15 years after its acquisition in the uterus.

Neonates born with congenital rubella should be isolated immediately because they excrete the virus for several months to a year after birth. Cataracts and cardiac defects may require surgery. The prognosis depends on the particular malformations that occur. The overall mortality for neonates with rubella is 6%, but it's higher for neonates born with thrombocytopenic purpura, congenital cardiac disease, or encephalitis. Parents of affected children need emotional support and guidance in finding help from community resources and organizations.

and symptoms—headache, malaise, anorexia, low-grade fever, coryza, lymphadenopathy and, sometimes, conjunctivitis—are the first to appear. Suboccipital, postauricular, and postcervical lymph node enlargement is a hallmark of this disease and precedes the rash.

Typically, the rubella rash begins on the face and spreads rapidly, in many cases covering the trunk and extremities within hours. Small, red, petechial macules on the soft palate (Forschheimer spots) may precede or accompany the rash but are not diagnostic of rubella. By the end of the second day, the facial rash begins to fade, but the rash on the trunk may become confluent and be mistaken for scarlet fever. The rash continues to fade in the downward order in which it appeared. It generally disappears on the third day, but it may persist for 4 to 5 days—sometimes accompanied by mild coryza and conjunctivitis. The rapid appearance and disappearance of the rubella rash distinguishes it from rubeola. In rare cases, rubella can occur without a rash. Low-grade fever may accompany the rash (99° to 101° F [37.2° to 38.3° C]), but it usually doesn't persist after the first day of the rash; rarely, temperature may reach 104° F (40° C).

Although complications are rare in children with rubella, they can occur just as the rash is fading. The complications usually subside spontaneously within 5 to 30 days. Fever may recur.

Fifty percent of rubella cases are asymptomatic.[1]

Complications
▶ Transient arthritis
▶ Hemorrhagic problems
▶ Encephalitis
▶ Myocarditis
▶ Thrombocytopenia
▶ Hepatitis

Diagnosis
The rubella rash, lymphadenopathy, other characteristic signs, and a history of exposure to infected people usually permit clinical diagnosis without laboratory tests. The rubella rash has been confused with scarlet fever, measles (rubeola), infectious mononucleosis, roseola, erythema infectiosum, and other viral exanthems. Therefore, without exposure history, laboratory confirma-

Incubation and duration of common rash-producing infections

INFECTION	INCUBATION (DAYS)	DURATION (DAYS)
Herpes simplex	2 to 12	7 to 21
Roseola infantum	10 to 15	3 to 6
Rubella	14 to 21	3
Rubeola	8 to 14	5
Varicella	14 to 17	7 to 14

tion is beneficial. Cell cultures of the throat, blood, urine, and cerebrospinal fluid can confirm the virus' presence. Convalescent serum that shows a fourfold rise in antibody titers corroborates the diagnosis.

The Centers for Disease Control and Prevention identifies two categories to look at when confirming rubella diagnosis: clinical case definition and laboratory criteria.

Clinical case definition identifies the following characteristics: acute onset of generalized maculopapular rash, temperature greater than 99°F (37.2°C), arthralgia or arthritis, lymphadenopathy, or conjunctivitis. Laboratory findings are consistent as follows: positive serologic test for rubella immunoglobulin M (IgM) antibody, significant rise between acute and convalescent-phase titers in serum, rubella immunoglobulin G antibody level by any standard serologic assay, isolation of rubella virus and detection of virus by reverse transcription polymerase chain reactions.[1]

Treatment

Because the rubella rash is self-limiting and only mildly pruritic, it doesn't require topical or systemic medication. Treatment con-sists of aspirin for fever and joint pain. Bed rest isn't necessary, but the patient should be isolated until the rash disappears.

Immunization with live virus vaccine RA27/3 is necessary for prevention and appears to be more immunogenic than previous vaccines. The rubella vaccine should be given with measles and mumps vaccines at age 15 months to decrease the cost and number of injections. The rubella vaccine is contraindicated in pregnancy.[2] After the emergence of the Wakefield et al, report in 1998, many parents in the United States refused the measles-mumps-rubella (MMR) vaccine for their infants and children. The report suggested that there may be a correlation between the onset of inflammatory bowel disease and pervasive developmental disorders such as autism with MMR vaccines.[3]

IN THE NEWS *The American Academy of Pediatrics and the Institute of Medicine of the National Academy of Sciences conducted independent reviews of the available information regarding the MMR vaccine and autism and concluded that the available evidence does not support the hypothesis that MMR vaccine causes autism or its associated*

disorders and that there is no causal relationship between the MMR vaccine and autism.[3]

Special considerations

▶ Make the patient with active rubella as comfortable as possible. If the patient is a child, give him children's books or games to keep him occupied.

▶ Explain to the patient why droplet precautions are necessary. Congenital rubella requires contact precautions until age 1. Make sure the patient—or his parents—understand how important it is to avoid exposing women who are pregnant to this disease.

▶ Report confirmed cases of rubella to local public health officials.

Before giving the rubella vaccine:

▶ Obtain a history of allergies, especially to neomycin. If the patient has this allergy or has had a reaction to immunization in the past, check with the physician before giving the vaccine.

▶ Ask women of childbearing age if they are pregnant. If they are or think they may be, don't give the vaccine until after you perform a pregnancy test and confirm that the woman is not pregnant. Warn women who receive rubella vaccine to use an effective means of birth control for at least 3 months after immunization.

▶ Give the vaccine at least 3 months after any administration of immune globulin or blood, which could have antibodies that neutralize the vaccine.

▶ Don't vaccinate patients who are immunocompromised, patients with immunodeficiency diseases, or those receiving immunosuppressive, radiation, or corticosteroid therapy. Instead, administer immune serum globulin as ordered to prevent or reduce infection in susceptible patients.

After giving the rubella vaccine:

▶ Observe the patient for signs of anaphylaxis for at least 30 minutes. Keep epinephrine 1:1000 handy.

▶ Warn the patient about possible mild fever, slight rash, transient arthralgia (in adolescents), and arthritis (in elderly patients). Suggest aspirin or acetaminophen for fever.

▶ If swelling persists after the initial 24 hours, suggest a cold compress to promote vasoconstriction and prevent antigenic cyst formation.

REFERENCES

1. Centers for Disease Control and Prevention. (2008 January 7). "Rubella: Make Sure Your Child Is Fully Immunized." [Online]. Available at *www.cdc.gov/Features/Rubella/*.
2. Centers for Disease Control and Prevention. (2007 July 18). "Guidelines for Vaccinating Pregnant Women." [Online]. Available at *www.cdc.gov/vaccines/pubs/preg-guide.htm*.
3. Katz, S. L. "Has the Measles-Mumps-Rubella Vaccine Been Fully Exonerated?" *Pediatrics* 118(4):1744–45, October 2006.

RUBEOLA

Rubeola, also known as the measles or morbilli, is an acute, highly contagious paramyxovirus infection that may be one of the most common and most serious of all communicable childhood diseases. Use of the vaccine has reduced the occurrence of measles during childhood; as a result, measles is becoming more prevalent in adolescents and adults. (See *Administering measles vaccine,* page 468.) In the United States, the prognosis is usually excellent; however, measles is a major cause of death in children in underdeveloped countries. The largest reported recent outbreak of measles occurred in 2005 in Indiana from a 17-year-old unvaccinated Romanian girl who was incubating measles. This outbreak, in which 34 others contracted the disease, was caused by the importation of measles into a population of children whose parents had refused

Administering measles vaccine

• Ask the patient about known allergies, especially to neomycin (each dose contains a small amount). However, a patient who is allergic to eggs may receive the vaccine because it contains only minimal amounts of albumin and yolk components.

• Avoid giving the vaccine to a pregnant woman (ask for date of last menstrual period). Warn female patients to avoid pregnancy for at least 3 months following vaccination.

• Don't vaccinate children with untreated tuberculosis, immunodeficiencies, leukemia, or lymphoma, or those receiving immunosuppressants. If such children are exposed to the virus, recommend that they receive gamma globulin (gamma globulin won't prevent measles but will lessen its severity). Older unimmunized children who have been exposed to measles for more than 5 days may also require gamma globulin. Be sure to immunize them 3 months later.

• Delay vaccination for 8 to 12 weeks after administration of whole blood, plasma, or gamma globulin because measles antibodies in these components may neutralize the vaccine.

• Watch for signs of anaphylaxis for 30 minutes after vaccination. Keep epinephrine 1:1000 handy.

• Warn the patient or his parents that possible adverse effects are anorexia, malaise, rash, mild thrombocytopenia or leukopenia, and fever. Advise them that mild reactions may occur, usually within 7 to 10 days. If swelling occurs within 24 hours after vaccination, tell the patient to apply cold compresses to the injection site to promote vasoconstriction and to prevent antigenic cyst formation.

• Generally, one bout of measles provides immunity (a second infection is extremely rare and may indicate a misdiagnosis); infants younger than age 4 months may be immune because of circulating maternal antibodies. Under normal conditions, measles vaccine isn't administered to children younger than age 15 months. However, during an epidemic, infants as young as 6 months may receive the vaccine and then be reimmunized at age 15 months. An alternative approach calls for administering gamma globulin to infants between ages 6 and 15 months who are likely to be exposed to measles.

to have them vaccinated because of safety concerns about the vaccine.[1]

Causes and incidence

Measles is spread by direct contact or by contaminated airborne respiratory droplets. The portal of entry is the upper respiratory tract. In temperate zones, incidence is highest in late winter and early spring. Before the availability of measles vaccine, epidemics occurred every 2 to 5 years in large urban areas.

Signs and symptoms

Incubation period of measles from exposure to rash onset is from 7 to 14 days. Patients are usually contagious from 4 days before until 4 days after the onset of the rash.[2]

Initial symptoms begin and greatest communicability occurs during the prodromal phase, about 11 days after exposure to the virus. This phase lasts from 4 to 5 days; signs and symptoms include fever, photophobia, malaise, anorexia, conjunctivitis, coryza, hoarseness, and hacking cough.

At the end of the prodrome, Koplik's spots, the hallmark of the disease, appear. These spots look like tiny, bluish white specks surrounded by a red halo. They appear on the oral mucosa opposite the molars and occasionally bleed. About 5 days after Koplik's spots appear, temperature rises sharply, spots slough off, and a slightly pruritic rash appears. This characteristic rash starts as faint macules behind the ears and on the neck and cheeks. The macules become papular and erythematous, rapidly

spreading over the entire face, neck, eyelids, arms, chest, back, abdomen, and thighs. When the rash reaches the feet (2 to 3 days later), it begins to fade in the same sequence that it appeared, leaving a brownish discoloration that disappears in 7 to 10 days. (See *Incubation and duration of common rash-producing infections,* page 466.)

The disease climax occurs 2 to 3 days after the rash appears and is marked by a fever of 103° to 105° F (39.4° to 40.6° C), severe cough, puffy red eyes, and rhinorrhea. About 5 days after the rash appears, other symptoms disappear and communicability ends. Symptoms are usually mild in patients with partial immunity (conferred by administration of gamma globulin) or infants with transplacental antibodies. More severe symptoms and complications are more likely to develop in young infants, adolescents, adults, and patients who are immunocompromised than in young children.

Atypical measles may appear in patients who received the killed measles vaccine. These patients are acutely ill with a fever and maculopapular rash that's most obvious in the arms and legs or with pulmonary involvement and no skin lesions.

Severe infection may lead to secondary bacterial infection and to autoimmune reaction or organ invasion by the virus, resulting in otitis media, pneumonia, and encephalitis. Subacute sclerosing panencephalitis, a rare and invariably fatal complication, may develop several years after measles, but it is less common in patients who have received the measles vaccine.

Complications
▶ Secondary bacterial infection
▶ Autoimmune reaction
▶ Organ invasion
▶ Otitis media
▶ Cervical adenitis
▶ Laryngitis
▶ Laryngotracheitis
▶ Pneumonia

▶ Encephalitis
▶ Subacute sclerosing panencephalitis (rare and fatal)
▶ Immunosuppressive measles encephalitis
▶ Progressive neurologic deterioration (may be fatal)

Diagnosis
Diagnosis rests on distinctive clinical features, especially the pathognomonic Koplik's spots. Mild measles may resemble rubella, roseola infantum, enterovirus infection, toxoplasmosis, and drug eruptions; laboratory tests are required for a differential diagnosis. If necessary, measles virus may be isolated from the blood, nasopharyngeal secretions, and urine during the febrile period. Serum antibodies appear within 3 days after onset of the rash and reach peak titers 2 to 4 weeks later.

Treatment
There is no specific antiviral therapy for measles, and the basic treatment consists of providing necessary supportive therapy to relieve symptoms such as hydration and antipyretics and treating complications such as pneumonia. Prevention of spreading the disease through droplet isolation throughout the communicable period is necessary. Vaporizers and a warm environment help reduce respiratory irritation, and antipyretics can reduce fever. Don't give aspirin to children because of the risk of Reye's syndrome—a rare but potentially fatal disease.[3] Cough preparations and antibiotics are generally ineffective. Young children with severe infections may benefit from taking vitamin A.[3]

Special considerations
▶ Teach the patient's parents supportive measures, and stress the need for isolation, plenty of rest, and increased fluid intake. Advise them to cope with photophobia by darkening the room or providing sunglasses, and to reduce fever with antipyretics and tepid sponge baths.

▶ Warn the patient's parents to watch for and report the early signs and symptoms of complications, such as encephalitis, otitis media, and pneumonia.

REFERENCES

1. Parker, A. A., et al. "Implications of a 2005 Measles Outbreak in Indiana for Sustained Elimination of Measles in the United States," *New England Journal of Medicine,* 355(5): 447–455, August 2006.
2. Centers for Disease Control and Prevention (January, 8 2008). "Measles (Rubeola)." [Online]. Available at *www.cdc.gov/travel/ yellowBookCh4-Measles.aspx.*
3. Mayo Clinic (April 9, 2008). "Measles." [Online]. Available at *www.mayoclinic.com/ health/measles/DS00331.*

SALMONELLOSIS

A common infection in the United States, salmonellosis is caused by gram-negative bacilli of the genus *Salmonella,* a member of the Enterobacteriaceae family. It occurs as enterocolitis, bacteremia, localized infection, typhoid, or paratyphoid fever. Nontyphoidal forms usually produce mild to moderate illness with low mortality. (See *Types of salmonellosis.*)

Salmonellosis is about 20 times more common in patients with acquired immunodeficiency syndrome than in the general population and is associated with an increased incidence of bacteremia and a tendency for recurrence following treatment.

Typhoid, the most severe form of salmonellosis, usually lasts from 1 to 4 weeks. Mortality is about 3% in patients who are treated. In those who are untreated, 10% of cases result in fatality, usually as a result of intestinal perforation or hemorrhage, cerebral thrombosis, toxemia, pneumonia, or acute circulatory failure. An attack of typhoid confers lifelong immunity, although the patient may become a carrier. Salmonellosis is 20 times more common in patients with acquired

immunodeficiency syndrome. Features are increased incidence of bacteremia, inability to identify the infection source, and tendency of infection to recur after therapy is stopped.

Causes and incidence

Of an estimated 1,700 serotypes of *Salmonella,* 10 cause the diseases most common in the United States; all 10 can survive for weeks in water, ice, sewage, or food. Nontyphoidal salmonellosis generally follows the ingestion of contaminated or inadequately processed foods, especially eggs, chicken, turkey, and duck. Other causes include contact with infected people or animals or ingestion of contaminated dry milk, chocolate bars, or drugs of animal origin. According to a recent study, children infected with *Salmonella* were less likely to have been breast-fed and more likely to have had exposure to reptiles, to have ridden in a shopping cart next to meat or poultry, or to have consumed concentrated liquid infant formula during the 5-day exposure period. Travel outside the United States was associated with illness in infants.

Attending day care with a child with diarrhea was associated with salmonellosis in infants older than 6 months of age.[1] Enterocolitis and bacteremia are common (and more virulent) among infants, elderly persons, and people already weakened by other infections; paratyphoid fever is rare in the United States.

A review of cases in California between 1990 and 1999 found 56,660 reported cases, 11,102 hospitalizations, and 74 deaths attributed to *Salmonella*[2] with an estimated cost of $200 million. Disproportionately affected were the very young and the elderly. Typhoid usually results from drinking water contaminated by the excretions of someone infected with typhoid, or from ingesting contaminated shellfish. (Contamination of shellfish occurs by leakage of sewage from offshore disposal depots.) Most typhoid patients are younger than age 30; most carriers are females older than age 50. Incidence of typhoid in the United States is increasing as a

Types of salmonellosis

TYPE	CAUSE	CLINICAL FEATURES
Bacteremia	Any *Salmonella* species, but most commonly *S. choleraesuis*. Incubation period: variable	Fever, chills, anorexia, weight loss (without GI symptoms), and joint pain
Enterocolitis	Any species of nontyphoidal *Salmonella,* but usually *S. enteritidis.* Incubation period: 6 to 48 hours	Mild to severe abdominal pain, diarrhea, sudden fever of up to 102° F (38.9° C), nausea, and vomiting; usually self-limiting, but may progress to enteric fever (resembling typhoid), local abscesses (usually abdominal), dehydration, and septicemia
Localized infections	Usually follows bacteremia caused by *Salmonella* species	Site of localization determines symptoms; localized abscesses may cause osteomyelitis, endocarditis, bronchopneumonia, pyelonephritis, and arthritis
Paratyphoid	*S. paratyphi* and *S. schottmuelleri* (formerly *S. paratyphi B*). Incubation period: 3 weeks or more	Fever and transient diarrhea; generally resembles typhoid but less severe
Typhoid fever	*S. typhi* enters the GI tract and invades the bloodstream via the lymphatics, setting up intracellular sites. During this phase, infection of the biliary tract leads to intestinal seeding with millions of bacilli. Involved lymphoid tissues (especially Peyer's patches in the ilium) enlarge, ulcerate, and necrose, resulting in hemorrhage. Incubation period: usually 1 to 2 weeks	Symptoms of enterocolitis may develop within hours of ingestion of *S. typhi;* they usually subside before onset of typhoid fever symptoms. *First week:* gradually increasing fever, anorexia, myalgia, malaise, headache, and slow pulse. *Second week:* remittent fever up to 104° F (40° C) usually in the evening, chills, diaphoresis, weakness, delirium, increasing abdominal pain and distention, diarrhea or constipation, cough, moist crackles, tender abdomen with enlarged spleen, and maculopapular rash (especially on abdomen). *Third week:* persistent fever, increasing fatigue and weakness; usually subsides by end of third week, although relapses may occur. *Complications:* intestinal perforation or hemorrhage, abscesses, thrombophlebitis, cerebral thrombosis, pneumonia, osteomyelitis, myocarditis, acute circulatory failure, and chronic carrier state

result of travelers returning from endemic areas.

Signs and symptoms

Clinical manifestations of salmonellosis vary but usually include fever, abdominal pain, and severe diarrhea with enterocolitis. Headache, increasing fever, and constipation are more common in typhoidal infection.

Complications

- Intestinal hemorrhage
- Intestinal perforation
- Cerebral thrombosis
- Pneumonia
- Endocarditis
- Myocarditis
- Meningitis
- Pyelonephritis

- Osteomyelitis
- Cholecystitis
- Hepatitis
- Septicemia
- Acute circulatory failure

Diagnosis

Generally, diagnosis depends on isolation of the organism in a culture, particularly blood (in typhoid, paratyphoid, and bacteremia) or feces (in enterocolitis, paratyphoid, and typhoid). Other appropriate culture specimens include urine, bone marrow, purulent wound or abscess drainage, and vomitus. In endemic areas, clinical symptoms of enterocolitis allow a working diagnosis before the cultures are positive. The presence of *Salmonella typhi* in stool one or more years after treatment indicates that the patient is a carrier, which is true of 3% of patients.

Widal's test, an agglutination reaction against somatic and flagellar antigens, may suggest typhoid with a fourfold rise in titer. However, drug use or hepatic disease can also increase these titers and invalidate test results. Other supportive laboratory values may include transient leukocytosis during the first week of typhoidal salmonellosis, leukopenia during the third week, and leukocytosis in local infection.

Treatment

Antimicrobial therapy for typhoid, paratyphoid, and bacteremia depends on organism sensitivity. Ciprofloxacin or ceftriaxone are antibiotics of choice, with azithromycin as a primary alternative. Increasing resistance has been noted with the use of trimethoprim-sulfamethoxazole and chloramphenicol. Dexamethasone should be administered before antibiotics if shock is present. Localized abscesses typically require surgical drainage. Enterocolitis requires a short course of antibiotics only if bacteremia or prolonged fever is present, or for infants or immunocompromised persons. Supportive treatment includes fluid and electrolyte replacement

and bed rest as needed. Careful administration of small doses of narcotics, kaolin with pectin (Kaopectate), or diphenoxylate with atropine (Lomotil) may be helpful in relieving diarrhea and controlling cramps in patients who must remain active.

Special considerations

- All infections caused by *Salmonella* must be reported to the state health department.
- Follow contact precautions if the patient is incontinent or diapered; otherwise, standard precautions are appropriate. Always wash your hands thoroughly before and after any contact with the patient, and advise other facility personnel to do the same. Teach the patient to use proper hand hygiene, especially after defecating and before eating or handling food. Wear gloves and a gown when disposing of feces or fecally contaminated objects. Continue precautions until three consecutive stool cultures are negative—the first one taken 48 hours after antibiotic treatment ends, followed by two more at 24-hour intervals.
- Observe the patient closely for signs and symptoms of bowel perforation from erosion of intestinal ulcers; sudden pain in the lower right side of the abdomen and abdominal rigidity, possibly after one or more rectal bleeding episodes; sudden fall in temperature or blood pressure; or rising pulse rate (indicating shock).
- During acute infection, plan care and activities to allow the patient as much rest as possible. Protect from falls due to delirium or orthostatic problems by using side rails and other safety measures. Use of a room deodorizer may help minimize odor from diarrhea and provide a more comfortable atmosphere for the patient.
- Provide good skin and mouth care. Turn the patient frequently, and perform mild passive exercises, as indicated. Apply mild heat to the abdomen to relieve cramps.
- Administer antipyretics with caution, and monitor fever closely. These mask fever and lead to possible hypothermia. Instead, to

promote heat loss through the skin without causing shivering (which keeps fever high by vasoconstriction), apply tepid, wet towels (don't use alcohol or ice) to the patient's groin and axillae. To promote heat loss by vasodilation of peripheral blood vessels, use additional wet towels on the arms and legs, wiping with long, vigorous strokes.

▶ After drainage of a joint abscess, provide a clean wound dressing. Applications of heat, elevation, and passive range-of-motion exercises may help decrease swelling and maintain joint mobility.

▶ If the patient has positive stool cultures at the time of discharge, advise thorough hand washing after using the bathroom and avoidance of food handling. Persons employed in food service occupations may not work in that capacity until cultures are negative.

▶ Prevention of food contamination is the most effective deterrent to this group of infections. Foods may become contaminated during processing, handling, storage, or preparation. Salmonella can also be spread through the feces of some pets, especially if diarrhea is present. Reptiles, such as iguanas, are likely to harbor salmonella within their scales and can spread this through direct contact (e.g., handling), or by contamination of surfaces (e.g., carpeting, terrariums). Advise persons at high risk for typhoid (e.g., laboratory workers, travelers) to seek vaccination.

REFERENCES

1. Jones, T. F., et al. "A Case-Control Study of the Epidemiology of Sporadic Salmonella Infection in Infants," *Pediatrics* 118(6): 2380–2387, December 2006.
2. Trevejo, R. T., et al. "Epidemiology of Salmonellosis in California, 1990–1999: Morbidity, Mortality, and Hospitalization Costs," *American Journal of Epidemiology* 157:48–57, January 2003.

SEPTIC SHOCK

Second only to cardiogenic shock as the leading cause of shock-related death, septic shock causes inadequate tissue perfusion, abnormalities of oxygen supply and demand, metabolic changes, and circulatory collapse. It typically occurs among hospitalized patients, usually as a result of bacterial infection. About 25% of patients who develop gram-negative bacteremia go into shock. Unless vigorous treatment begins promptly, preferably before symptoms fully develop, septic shock rapidly progresses to death (in many cases within a few hours) in up to 80% of these patients. Septic shock is the most common cause of death in acute care units in the United States.

Causes and incidence

In two-thirds of patients, septic shock results from infection with the gram-negative bacteria *Escherichia coli, Klebsiella, Enterobacter, Proteus, Pseudomonas,* or *Bacteroides;* in a few, from the gram-positive bacteria *Streptococcus pneumoniae, Streptococcus pyogenes, Staphylococcus aureus,* or *Actinomyces.* Infections with viruses, rickettsiae, chlamydiae, and protozoa may be complicated by shock.

These organisms produce septicemia in people whose resistance is already compromised by an existing condition; infection also results from translocation of bacteria from other areas of the body through surgery, I.V. therapy, and catheters. Septic shock commonly occurs in patients hospitalized for primary infection of the genitourinary, biliary, GI, or gynecologic tract. Other predisposing factors include immunodeficiency, advanced age, trauma, burns, diabetes mellitus, cirrhosis, and disseminated cancer.

Signs and symptoms

Signs and symptoms of septic shock vary according to the stage of shock, the organ-

ism causing it, and the patient's immune response and age:

▶ early stage—oliguria, sudden fever (over 101° F [38.3° C]), and chills; tachypnea; tachycardia; full bounding pulse; hyperglycemia; nausea; vomiting; diarrhea; and prostration

▶ late stage—restlessness, apprehension, irritability, thirst from decreased cerebral tissue perfusion, hypoglycemia, hypothermia, and anuria. Hypotension, altered level of consciousness, and hyperventilation may be the only signs among infants and the elderly.

Complications of septic shock include disseminated intravascular coagulation, renal failure, heart failure, GI ulcers, and hepatic dysfunction.

Complications

▶ Disseminated intravascular coagulation (DIC)
▶ Renal failure
▶ Heart failure
▶ GI ulcers
▶ Abnormal liver function
▶ Oliguria, increased specific gravity
▶ Dyspnea
▶ Edema
▶ Tachycardia
▶ Distended neck veins
▶ Hepatic abnormality

Diagnosis

One or more typical symptoms (fever, confusion, nausea, vomiting, and hyperventilation) in a patient suspected of having an infection suggests septic shock and necessitates immediate treatment.

In early stages, arterial blood gas (ABG) levels indicate respiratory alkalosis (low partial pressure of carbon dioxide [$Paco_2$], low or normal bicarbonate [HCO_3^-], and high pH). As shock progresses, metabolic acidosis develops with hypoxemia, indicated by decreasing $Paco_2$ (may increase as respiratory failure ensues); partial pressure of oxygen; HCO_3^-, and pH.

The following tests support the diagnosis and determine the treatment:

▶ blood cultures to isolate the organism
▶ decreased platelet count and leukocytosis (15,000 to 30,000/µl)
▶ increased blood urea nitrogen and creatinine levels, decreased creatinine clearance
▶ abnormal prothrombin consumption and partial thromboplastin time
▶ simultaneous measurement of urine and plasma osmolalities for renal failure (urine osmolality below 400 mOsm/kg, with a ratio of urine to plasma below 1.5)
▶ decreased central venous pressure (CVP), pulmonary artery pressure, and pulmonary artery wedge pressure (PAWP); decreased cardiac output (in early septic shock, cardiac output increases); low systemic vascular resistance
▶ on electrocardiogram, ST-segment depression, inverted T waves, and arrhythmias resembling myocardial infarction.

Treatment

The first goal of treatment is to monitor for and then reverse shock through volume expansion with I.V. fluids and insertion of a pulmonary artery catheter to check PAWP. Early, aggressive fluid resuscitation in children is critical to improve survival.[1] It is recommended that children in septic shock receive an intravenous isotonic fluid infusion greater than 40 mL/kg within the initial hour of presentation to lower mortality and to improve survival outcomes.[1] Administration of whole blood or plasma can then raise the PAWP to a slightly elevated level of 14 to 18 mm Hg. A ventilator may be necessary to overcome hypoxia. Urinary catheterization allows accurate measurement of hourly urine output.

Treatment also requires immediate administration of I.V. antibiotics to control the infection. Depending on the organism, the antibiotic combination usually includes an aminoglycoside (such as amikacin, gentamicin, or tobramycin) for gram-negative bacteria combined with a penicillin (such as ticarcillin or

piperacillin). Sometimes treatment includes a cephalosporin or vancomycin for suspected staphylococcal infection. Therapy may include chloramphenicol for nonsporulating anaerobes (Bacteroides), which may cause bone marrow depression, and clindamycin, which may produce pseudomembranous enterocolitis. Metronidazole can also be used for anaerobic infection. Appropriate antibiotics for other causes of septic shock depend on the suspected organism. Other measures to combat infection include surgery to drain and excise abscesses, and debridement.

If shock persists after fluid infusion, treatment with vasopressors such as dopamine maintains adequate blood perfusion in the brain, liver, GI tract, kidneys, and skin. In adults with severe sepsis who have a high risk of death, drotrecogin alfa may be used to interrupt the sepsis cascade. Other treatment includes I.V. bicarbonate to correct acidosis and corticosteroids (especially in patients with gram-negative septic shock). In 2001, the Food and Drug Administration approved the first biologic treatment for the most serious, life-threatening forms of sepsis in adults. It is a medication that mimics a naturally occurring human protein, Activated protein C, which hinders a dangerous response to severe infection—blood clot formation that can lead to organ failure and death.[2] Other experimental treatments include opioid antagonists, prostaglandin inhibitors, and calcium channel blockers, which are used to block the rapid inflammatory process.

Special considerations

Determine which of your patients are at high risk for developing septic shock. Know the signs of impending septic shock, but don't rely solely on technical aids to judge the patient's status. Consider any change in mental status and urine output as significant as a change in CVP. Report such changes promptly.

▶ Carefully maintain the pulmonary artery catheter. Check ABG levels for adequate oxygenation or gas exchange, and report any changes immediately.

▶ Record intake, output and daily weight. Maintain adequate urine output (0.5 to 1 ml/kg/hour) and systolic pressure. Avoid fluid overload.

▶ Monitor serum antibiotic levels, and administer drugs as ordered.

▶ Watch closely for known signs of complications: DIC (abnormal bleeding); renal failure (oliguria, increased specific gravity); heart failure (dyspnea, edema, tachycardia, distended neck veins); GI ulcers (hematemesis and melena); and hepatic abnormality (jaundice, hypoprothrombinemia, and hypoalbuminemia).

REFERENCES

1. Kirby, A., and Goldstein, B. "Improved Outcomes Associated with Early Resuscitation in Septic Shock: Do We Need to Resuscitate the Patient or the Physician?," *Pediatrics* 112(4):976–77, October 2003.

2. U.S. Food and Drug Administration. (2001 November 21). "FDA Approves First Biologic Treatment for Sepsis." [Online]. Available at *www.fda.gov/bbs/topics/NEWS/2001/NEW007 80.html.*

SHIGELLOSIS

Shigellosis, also known as bacillary dysentery, is an acute intestinal infection caused by the bacteria Shigella, a short, nonmotile, gram-negative rod. Shigella can be classified into four groups, all of which may cause shigellosis: group A (*S. dysenteriae*), which is most common in Central America and causes particularly severe infection and septicemia; group B (*S. flexneri*), group C (*S. boydii*), and group D (*S. sonnei*). Typically, shigellosis causes a high fever (especially in children), acute self-limiting diarrhea with tenesmus (ineffectual straining at stool) and, possibly, electrolyte imbalance and dehydration. It's most com-

mon in children ages 1 to 4; however, many adults acquire the illness from children.

The prognosis is good. Mild infections usually subside within 10 days; severe infections may persist for 2 to 6 weeks. With prompt treatment, shigellosis is fatal in fewer than 1% of cases, although in severe *S. dysenteriae,* epidemic, mortality may reach 8%.

Causes and incidence

Transmission occurs through the fecal-oral route, by direct contact with contaminated objects, or through ingestion of contaminated food or water. Occasionally, the housefly is a vector.

Shigellosis is endemic in North America, Europe, and the tropics. In the United States, about 18,000 cases appear annually, usually in children or in elderly, debilitated, or malnourished people. Shigellosis commonly occurs among confined populations, such as those in mental institutions or day-care centers.

Signs and symptoms

The main sign of shigella infection is diarrhea, which often is bloody.[1] After an incubation period of 1 to 7 days (3 days is the average), the bacteria remain active during the illness and for a week or two after recovery. It's possible to be asymptomatic while still carrying the shigella germ and pass the illness to others.[1]

Shigella organisms invade the intestinal mucosa and cause inflammation. In children, shigellosis usually produces high fever, diarrhea with tenesmus, nausea, vomiting, irritability, drowsiness, and abdominal pain and distention. Within a few days, the child's stool may contain pus, mucus, and—from the superficial intestinal ulceration typical of this infection—blood. Without treatment, dehydration and weight loss are rapid and overwhelming. In adults, shigellosis produces sporadic, intense abdominal pain, which may be relieved at first by passing formed stools. Eventually, however, it causes rectal irritability, tenesmus and, in severe infection, headache and prostration. Stools may contain pus, mucus, and blood. Fever may be present.

Complications of shigellosis are uncommon, but may be life-threatening in children and patients who are debilitated. About 3% of patients with shigellosis will later develop Reiter's Syndrome, involving intermittent episodes of painful joints, conjunctivitis, and urethritis, which may recur for years. A genetic predisposition to Reiter's Syndrome has been identified.

Complications

- ► Electrolyte imbalance (especially hypokalemia)
- ► Metabolic acidosis
- ► Shock
- ► Conjunctivitis
- ► Iritis
- ► Arthritis
- ► Rectal prolapse
- ► Secondary bacterial infections
- ► Acute blood loss from mucosal ulcers
- ► Toxic neuritis

Diagnosis

Positive shigella bacteria in the stool is the confirming diagnosis.

Fever (in children) and diarrhea with stools containing blood, pus, and mucus point to this diagnosis; microscopic bacteriologic studies and culture help confirm it.

Microscopic examination of a fresh stool may reveal mucus, red blood cells, and polymorphonuclear leukocytes; direct immunofluorescence with specific antisera will demonstrate Shigella. Severe infection increases hemagglutinating antibodies. Sigmoidoscopy or proctoscopy may reveal typical superficial ulcerations.

Diagnosis must rule out other causes of diarrhea, such as enteropathogenic *Escherichia coli* infection, malabsorption diseases, and amebic or viral diseases.

Treatment

Treatment of shigellosis includes oral or intravenous fluid and electrolyte replacement, a low-residue diet, and use of enteric precautions. Antibiotics are sometimes used and include ampicillin and trimethoprim-sulfamethoxazole. Antibiotic resistance is developing, and in mild infections, therefore, antibiotics are often avoided. A person usually recovers quickly. Antidiarrheal agents, such as loperamide (Imodium) and diphenoxylate with atropine (Lomotil), may worsen symptoms and should be avoided.

A preventive vaccine containing attenuated strains of Shigella is under investigation for general applications and is in use in laboratories. The U.S. Department of Agriculture is testing the effectiveness in using ionizing irradiation as an intervention to reduce the microbial population of the shigella organism on fresh vegetables.[2]

Special considerations

Supportive care can minimize complications and increase patient comfort.

▶ To prevent dehydration, administer I.V. fluids as ordered. Measure intake and output (including stools) carefully.

▶ Correct identification of Shigella requires examination and culture of fresh stool specimens. Therefore, hand carry specimens directly to the laboratory. Because shigellosis is suspected, include this information on the laboratory slip.

▶ Topical heat such as with a heating pad may relieve abdominal discomfort, and schedule care to conserve patient strength.

▶ To help prevent spread of this disease, maintain enteric precautions until microscopic bacteriologic studies confirm that the stool specimen is negative. If a risk of exposure to the patient's stools exists, put on a gown and gloves before entering the room. Keep the patient's (and your own) nails short to avoid harboring organisms. Change soiled linen promptly, and store in an isolation container.

▶ During shigellosis outbreaks, obtain stool specimens from all potentially infected staff, and instruct those infected to remain away from work until two stool specimens are negative.

▶ Report cases to the local health department.

REFERENCES

1. Mayo Clinic (2008 April 12). "Shigella Infection" [Online]. Available at *www.mayoclinic.com/health/shigella/DS00719*.
2. U.S. Department of Agriculture. (2008 March 31). "Non-Thermal and Advanced Thermal Food Processing Intervention Technologies" [Online]. Available at *www.ars.usda.gov/research/projects/projects.htm?ACCN_NO=410263*.

STREPTOCOCCAL INFECTIONS

Streptococci are small gram-positive bacteria, spherical to ovoid in shape and linked together in pairs or chains. Several species occur as part of normal human flora in the respiratory, GI, and genitourinary tracts. Although researchers have identified 21 species of streptococci, three classes—groups A, B, and D—cause most of the infections.[1] (See *Comparing streptococcal infections,* pages 478 to 485.) Organisms belonging to groups A and B beta-hemolytic streptococci are associated with a characteristic pattern of human infections. Most disorders due to group D streptococcus are caused by *Enterococcus faecalis,* formerly called *Streptococcus faecalis,* or *S. bovis.* Group C and group G streptococci have been identified as the etiologic agent in such infections as bacteremia, meningitis, pharyngitis, osteomyelitis, and neonatal sepsis.[3]

Clinically, there are three states of streptococcal infection: carrier, acute, and delayed nonsuppurative complications. In the carrier state, the patient is infected with a disease-causing species of streptococci with-

(Text continues on page 484.)

Comparing streptococcal infections

CAUSES AND INCIDENCE	SIGNS AND SYMPTOMS

Streptococcus pyogenes (group A streptococcus)

Streptococcal pharyngitis (strep throat)

- Accounts for 95% of all cases of bacterial pharyngitis[1]
- Equal number of females and males affected
- Most common in children ages 5 to 10, from October to April[2]
- Spread by direct person-to-person contact via droplets of saliva or nasal secretions
- Organism usually colonizes in the throats of those with no symptoms
- Up to 20% of school children may be carriers.
- Pets also may be carriers.

- After a 1- to 5-day incubation period: temperature of 100° to 104° F (38.3° to 40° C), sore throat with severe pain on swallowing, beefy red pharynx, tonsillar hypertrophy exudate, and uvula, swollen glands along the jaw line, generalized malaise and weakness, anorexia, occasional abdominal discomfort[2]
- Up to 40% of small children have symptoms too mild for diagnosis.
- Fever abates in 3 to 5 days; nearly all symptoms subside within a week.

Scarlet fever (scarlatina)

- Usually follows streptococcal pharyngitis; may follow wound infections or puerperal sepsis
- Caused by streptococcal strain that releases an erythrogenic toxin
- Most common in children ages 2 to 10
- Spread by large respiratory droplets or direct contact with items soiled with respiratory secretions

- Streptococcal sore throat, fever, strawberry tongue, fine erythematous rash that blanches on pressure and resembles sunburn with goose bumps; usually appears on the second clinical day of illness[1]
- Rash usually appears first on upper chest, then spreads to neck, axillae, abdomen, groin, legs, and arms, elbows, and knees (deep red lines called Pastia's lines) sparing soles and palms; flushed cheeks, pallor around mouth.

Erysipelas (St. Anthony's Fire)

- Occurs primarily in infants and adults older than age 30
- Usually follows streptococcal pharyngitis
- Exact mode of spread to skin unknown
- Risk factors include impaired lymphatic or venous drainage (mastectomy, saphenous vein harvesting), and immunocompromised patients

- Sudden onset with reddened, swollen, raised lesions (skin looks like an orange peel), usually on face and scalp, bordered by areas that often contain easily ruptured blebs filled with yellow-tinged fluid; lesions sting and itch; lesions on the trunk, arms, or legs usually affect incision or wound sites. Desquamation of affected area may occur 7 to 10 days afterward.[1]
- Other symptoms include vomiting, fever, headache, cervical lymphadenopathy, and sore throat.

DIAGNOSIS	COMPLICATIONS	TREATMENT AND SPECIAL CONSIDERATIONS
• Clinically indistinguishable from viral pharyngitis • Rapid antigen detection tests detect the presence of group A antigen directly from throat swabs; results in minutes. These are more than 95% specific, and throat culture is then not necessary.[1] • Throat culture showing group A beta hemolytic streptococci (carriers have positive throat culture) • Elevated white blood cell (WBC) count • Serology showing a fourfold rise in streptozyme titers during convalescence	• Acute otitis media or acute sinusitis occurs most frequently • Rarely, bacteremic spread may cause arthritis, endocarditis, meningitis, osteomyelitis, or liver abscess • Poststreptococcal sequelae; acute rheumatic fever or acute glomerulonephritis • Reye's syndrome	• Penicillin or erythromycin, analgesics, and antipyretics may be ordered. • Saltwater gargles and fluids may help. • Stress the need for bed rest and isolation from other children for 24 hours after antibiotic therapy begins; the patient should finish his prescription, even if symptoms subside; abscess, glomerulonephritis, and rheumatic fever can occur. • Tell the patient not to skip doses and to properly dispose of soiled tissues. • Recurrent infection may be caused by reinfection from others in the home. • Group A streptococcus vaccines are presently in various stages of development.[1]
• Characteristic rash and strawberry tongue • Culture and gram stain showing *S. pyogenes* from nasopharynx[1] • Granulocytosis	• Although rare, complications may include high fever, arthritis, jaundice, pneumonia, pericarditis, and peritonsillar abscess.	• Penicillin or erythromycin may be ordered. • Keep the patient in isolation for the first 24 hours. • Carefully dispose of purulent discharge. • Stress the need for prompt and complete antibiotic treatment.
• Typical reddened lesions • Complete blood count with elevated WBC, positive blood cultures in 5% of patients • Culture taken from edge of lesions showing group A beta hemolytic streptococci • Throat culture almost always positive for group A beta hemolytic streptococci	• Abscesses, gangrene, thrombophlebitis, metastatic infection • Untreated lesions on trunk, arms, or legs may involve large body areas and lead to death.	• Penicillin or erythromycin I.V. or by mouth may be ordered; oral dicloxacillin, I.V. nafcillin or oxacillin may be used for facial erysipelas. • Cold packs, analgesics, topical anesthetics, and elevation of affected limbs may be methods to increase comfort. • Prevention includes prompt treatment of streptococcal infections and drainage and secretion precautions. • Infection recurrence is common.

(continued)

Comparing streptococcal infections *(continued)*

CAUSES AND INCIDENCE	SIGNS AND SYMPTOMS

Impetigo (streptococcal pyoderma)

- Common in children ages 2 to 5; in hot, humid weather; high rate of familial spread
- Predisposing factors; close contact in schools, overcrowded living quarters, poor skin hygiene, minor skin trauma
- May spread by direct contact environmental contamination, or arthropod vector
- Bullous is most common form in infants and children; nonbullous form is most common in children ages 2 to 5 years and in warm climates with poor hygiene.

- Small macules rapidly develop into vesicles, then become pustular and encrusted, causing pain, surrounding erythema, regional adenitis, cellulitis, and itching; scratching spreads infection.
- Lesions commonly affect the face, heal slowly, and leave depigmented areas.
- Regional lymphadenopathy with nonbullous form is common.

Streptococcus agalactiae (Group B streptococcus)

Neonatal streptococcal infections

- Incidence of early onset infection (age 6 days or younger): 2/1,000 live births
- Incidence of late onset infection (age 7 days to 3 months: 1/1,000 live births
- Spread by vaginal delivery or hands of nursery staff[4]
- Predisposing factors: maternal genital tract colonization, membrane rupture over 24 hours before delivery, crowded nursery[4]
- The Centers for Disease Control and Prevention recommends universal prenatal screening for vaginal group B streptococcus at 35 to 27 weeks' gestation.[4]

- Early onset: bacteremia, pneumonia, and meningitis; mortality from 14% for infants weighing more than 1,500 g at birth to 61% for infants weighing less than 1,500 g at birth
- Late onset: bacteremia with meningitis, fever, and bone and joint involvement; mortality 15% to 20%
- Other signs and symptoms, such as skin lesions, depend on the site affected.

Adult group B streptococcal infection

- Most adult infections occur in postpartum females, usually in the form of endometritis or wound infection following cesarean section.
- Other risk factors include being older than age 60, cardiac disease, alcoholism, renal failure, previous stroke, neurogenic bladder, pressure ulcers, corticosteroid therapy, or nursing home residency.
- Incidence of group B streptococcal endometritis is 1.3/1,000 live births.[4]

- Fever, malaise, and uterine tenderness
- Change in lochia
- Bacteremia and pneumonia patients can exhibit neurologic symptoms such as a change in mental status.

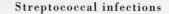

DIAGNOSIS	COMPLICATIONS	TREATMENT AND SPECIAL CONSIDERATIONS
• Characteristic lesions with honey-colored crust • Culture and Gram stain of swabbed lesions showing *S. pyogenes*	• Septicemia (rare) • Ecthyma, a form of impetigo with deep ulcers	• Penicillin I.V. or oral erythromycin, dicloxacillin, cephalexin, azithromycin • Perform frequent washing of lesion to remove crusts with antiseptics, such as povidone-iodine or antibacterial soap, followed by thorough drying. • Keep fingernails cut short. • Isolate a patient with draining wounds. • Instruct patient not to share towels, washcloths, or bath soap. • Prevention includes good hygiene and proper wound care. • Children in day care should wait 48 to 72 hours after antibiotic initiation before returning.
• Isolation of group B streptococcus from blood, cerebrospinal fluid, or skin • Chest X-ray showing massive infiltrate similar to that of respiratory distress syndrome or pneumonia	• Overwhelming pneumonia, sepsis, meningitis, and death	• Penicillin or ampicillin and an aminoglycoside IV may be ordered. • Patient isolation is unnecessary unless an open draining lesion is present, but proper hand hygiene is essential; for a draining lesion, take drainage and secretion precautions. • Group B streptococcus prophylaxis may be ordered for females who are pregnant if vaginal or rectal cultures are positive at 35 to 37 weeks gestation or if the patient meets other criteria, such as delivery earlier or later than 3 weeks of term, amniotic fluid rupture for 18 hours or more, or an intrapartum temperature greater than or equal to 100.4° F (38° C).
• Isolation of group B streptococcus from blood or infection site	• Bacteremia followed by meningitis or endocarditis	• Ampicillin, penicillin, vancomycin, teicoplanin I.V. may be ordered. • Perform careful observation for symptoms of infection following delivery. • Follow drainage and secretion precautions.

(continued)

Comparing streptococcal infections *(continued)*

CAUSES AND INCIDENCE	SIGNS AND SYMPTOMS
• Group B streptococcal bacteremia and pneumonia occur in elderly patients and commonly in patients with diabetes. • Invasive group B streptococcal infection occurs in patients with human immunodeficiency virus.	

Streptococcus pneumoniae

Pneumococcal pneumonia
• Accounts for 7% of all cases of bacterial pneumonias
• Leading cause of community-acquired pneumonia, 80% of infections in children age 6 years or younger, and 5% in people of other ages
• More common in males, elderly people, Blacks, and Native Americans in winter and early spring
• Spread by droplets and contact with infective secretions
• Transmission occurs during coughing and sneezing within 6 feet of the carrier.[4]
• Predisposing factors: trauma, viral infection, underlying pulmonary disease, overcrowded living quarters, chronic diseases, asplenia, and immunodeficiency
• Among the 10 leading causes of death in the United States

• Sudden onset with severe shaking, chills, temperature of 102° F (38.9° C), bacteremia, cough, (with thick, scant, blood tinged sputum) accompanied by pleuritic pain
• Malaise, weakness, and prostration common
• Tachypnea, anorexia, nausea, and vomiting less common
• Severity of pneumonia usually due to host's cellular defenses, not bacterial virulence

Otitis media
• High incidence with about 76% to 95% of all children having otitis media at least once (*S. pneumoniae* causes half of these cases.)

• Ear pain, ear drainage, hearing loss, fever, lethargy, and irritability
• Other possible symptoms: vertigo, nystagmus, tinnitus

Meningitis
• Can follow bacteremic pneumonia, mastoiditis, sinusitis, skull fracture, or endocarditis
• Mortality (30% to 60%) highest in infants and elderly people

• Fever, headache, nuchal rigidity, vomiting, photophobia, lethargy, coma, wide pulse pressure, and bradycardia

DIAGNOSIS	COMPLICATIONS	TREATMENT AND SPECIAL CONSIDERATIONS
• Gram-stain of sputum showing gram-positive diplococci; culture showing *S. pneumoniae* • Chest X-ray showing lobular consolidation in adults; bronchopneumonia in children and elderly patients • Elevated WBC count • Blood cultures usually positive for *S. pneumoniae*	• Pleural effusion (occurs in 25% of patients) • Pericarditis (rare) • Lung abscess (rare) • Bacteremia • Empyema (most common complication) • Disseminated intravascular coagulation • Death possible if bacteremia is present	• Penicillin or erythromycin I.V. or I.M. may be ordered. • Monitor and support respirations, as needed. • Record sputum color and amount. • Prevent dehydration. • Avoid sedatives and opioids to preserve cough reflex. • Carefully dispose of all purulent drainage (standard precautions); advise high-risk patients to receive a vaccine and to avoid infected people. • Effective hand-washing technique is required. • Educate family/caregiver in prevention of cross-contamination. • Prevention is through receiving pneumococcal vaccines: pneumococcal conjugate vaccine is recommended for all children less than 24 months and for children between ages 24 and 59 months who are at high risk; pneumococcal polysaccharide vaccine is recommended for children and older adults at risk.[5]
• Fluid in middle ear • Isolation of *S. pneumoniae* from aspirated fluid if necessary	• Recurrent attacks (may cause hearing loss)	• Amoxicillin or ampicillin and analgesics may be ordered. • Tell the patient to report a lack of response to therapy after 72 hours.
• Isolation of *S. pneumoniae* from cerebrospinal fluid (CSF) blood culture • Increased CSF cell count and protein level; decreased CSF glucose level • Computed tomography scan of head • EEG	• Persistent hearing deficits, seizures, hemiparesis, or other nerve deficits • Encephalitis	• Penicillin I.V. or chloramphenicol may be ordered. • Monitor the patient closely for neurologic changes. • Watch for symptoms of septic shock, such as acidosis and tissue hypoxia.

(continued)

Comparing streptococcal infections *(continued)*

CAUSES AND INCIDENCE	SIGNS AND SYMPTOMS
Group D streptococcus	
Endocarditis • Group D streptococcus (enterococcus) causes 10% to 20% of all bacterial endocarditis. • Most common in elderly people and in those who abuse I.V. substances • Typically follows bacteremia from an obvious source, such as a wound infection, urinary tract infection, or I.V. insertion site infection • Most cases are subacute • Also causes urinary tract infection	• Weakness, fatigue, irritability, weight loss, fever, night sweats, anorexia, arthralgia, splenomegaly, and new systolic murmur

out evidence of infection. In the acute form, streptococci invade the tissues and cause physical symptoms. In the delayed nonsuppurative complications state, specific signs and symptoms associated with streptococcal infection occur. These include those associated with the inflammatory state of acute rheumatic fever, chorea, and glomerulonephritis. If further complications occur, they usually appear about 2 weeks after the acute illness, but they may be evident after a nonsymptomatic illness.[3]

REFERENCES

1. Ferri, F. *Ferri's Clinical Advisor 2007: Instant Diagnosis and Treatment,* 9th ed. St. Louis, Mo: Mosby, 2007.
2. National Institute of Allergy and Infectious Disease. (2007 September 19). "Group A Streptococcal Infections." [Online]. Available at *www.3niaid.nih.gov.*
3. Mandell, B., and Dolin, R. "Principles and Practices of Infectious Diseases, 6th Ed., chapter 80," *JAMA,* 293(18), May 11, 2005.
4. Centers for Disease Control and Prevention. (2002 August 16). "Prevention of Perinatal GBS Disease." [Online]. Available at *www.cdc.gov.*
5. Centers for Disease Control and Prevention (2008 February 12). "Pneumococcal Vaccination" [Online]. Available at: *http://www.cdc.gov/vaccines/vpd-vac/pneumo/default.htm.*

TETANUS

Tetanus, also known as lockjaw, is an acute exotoxin-mediated infection caused by the anaerobic, spore-forming, gram-positive bacillus *Clostridium tetani*. It causes seizures and severe muscle spasms that are strong enough to cause bone fractures in the spine.[1] This infection is usually systemic; less commonly, localized. Tetanus is fatal in up to 60% of unimmunized people, usually within 10 days of onset. When symptoms develop within 3 days after exposure, the prognosis is poor.

Causes and incidence

Normally, transmission occurs through a puncture wound that is contaminated by soil, dust, or animal excreta containing *C. tetani,* or through burns and minor

DIAGNOSIS	COMPLICATIONS	TREATMENT AND SPECIAL CONSIDERATIONS
• Anemia, increased erythrocyte sedimentation rate and serum immunoglobulin level, and positive blood culture for group D streptococcus • Echocardiogram showing vegetation on valves	• Embolization • Pulmonary infarction • Osteomyelitis	• Penicillin for *Streptococcus bovis* (nonenterococcal group D Streptococcus) may be ordered. • Penicillin or ampicillin and an aminoglycoside for enterococcal group D streptococcus may be ordered.

wounds. After *C. tetani* enters the body, it causes local infection and tissue necrosis. It also produces toxins that then enter the bloodstream and lymphatics and eventually spread to central nervous system tissue.

Tetanus occurs worldwide, but is more prevalent in agricultural regions and developing countries that lack mass immunization programs. It's one of the most common causes of neonatal deaths in developing countries, where infants of unimmunized mothers are delivered under unsterile conditions. In such infants, the unhealed umbilical cord is the portal of entry.

Diphtheria and tetanus antibodies are known to appear within 3 to 6 months after end of treatment as a sign of immune recovery and the reinstatement of immunological memory.

In the United States, about 75% of all cases occur between April and September.

Signs and symptoms
The incubation period varies from 3 to 4 weeks in mild tetanus to less than 2 days in severe tetanus. When symptoms occur

within 3 days after injury, death is more likely. If tetanus remains localized, signs of onset are spasm and increased muscle tone near the wound.

If tetanus is generalized (systemic), indications include marked muscle hypertonicity, hyperactive deep tendon reflexes, tachycardia, profuse sweating, low-grade fever, and painful, involuntary muscle contractions:
▶ neck and facial muscles, especially cheek muscles—locked jaw (trismus); painful spasms of masticatory muscles; difficulty opening the mouth; and risus sardonicus, a grotesque, grinning expression produced by a spasm of facial muscles
▶ somatic muscles—arched-back rigidity (opisthotonos), boardlike abdominal rigidity
▶ intermittent tonic seizures lasting several minutes, which may result in cyanosis and sudden death by asphyxiation.

Despite such pronounced neuromuscular symptoms, cerebral and sensory functions remain normal. Complications can include atelectasis, pneumonia, pulmonary emboli,

acute gastric ulcers, flexion contractures, and cardiac arrhythmias.

Neonatal tetanus is always generalized. The first clinical sign is difficulty in sucking, which usually appears 3 to 10 days after birth. It progresses to total inability to suck with excessive crying, irritability, and nuchal rigidity.

Complications
▶ Atelectasis
▶ Pneumonia
▶ Pulmonary emboli
▶ Airway obstruction
▶ Acute gastric ulcers
▶ Seizures
▶ Flexion contractures
▶ Cardiac arrhythmias

Diagnosis
In many cases, diagnosis must rest on clinical features, a history of trauma, and no previous tetanus immunization. Blood cultures and tetanus antibody tests are often negative; only a third of patients have a positive wound culture. Cerebrospinal fluid pressure may rise above normal. Diagnosis must also rule out meningitis, rabies, phenothiazine or strychnine toxicity, and other conditions that mimic tetanus.

Treatment
Within 72 hours after a puncture wound, a patient with no previous history of tetanus immunization first requires tetanus immune globulin (TIG) or tetanus antitoxin to neutralize the toxins and to confer temporary protection. Next, he needs active immunization with tetanus toxoid. If he hasn't received tetanus immunization within 10 years, a booster injection of tetanus toxoid is necessary. Tetanus toxoid (Td) and diphtheria (DT) immunizations are sometimes given in combination doses depending on age. From birth to 6 weeks, neither Td nor DT is recommended. From 6 weeks through 7 years

old, only DT is recommended. For children 7 years and older and in geriatric patients, only Td is recommended.[1] If tetanus develops despite immediate postinjury treatment, the patient will require airway maintenance and a muscle relaxant, such as diazepam, to decrease muscle rigidity and spasm. If muscle contractions aren't relieved by muscle relaxants, a neuromuscular blocker, such as metocurine iodide, may be prescribed. The patient with tetanus needs high-dose antibiotics (penicillin administered I.V. if he isn't allergic to it or such alternatives as clindamycin, erythromycin, and metronidazole.) If a patient presents with an infected wound, the possibility of a retained foreign body should be considered.[2] The source of the toxin needs to be removed and destroyed through surgical exploration and wound debridement. A time limit should be set to explore the wound. Wounds should be treated with plain water irrigation and complete removal of retained fragments.[2]

Special considerations
▶ Thoroughly debride and clean the injury site with 3% hydrogen peroxide, and check the patient's immunization history. Record the cause of injury. If it's an animal bite, report the case to local public health authorities.
▶ Before giving penicillin and TIG, antitoxin, or toxoid, obtain an accurate history of allergies to immunizations or penicillin. If the patient has a history of allergies, keep epinephrine 1:1000 and resuscitation equipment available.
▶ Stress the importance of maintaining active immunization with a booster dose of tetanus toxoid every 10 years.

After tetanus develops:
▶ Maintain an adequate airway and ventilation to prevent pneumonia and atelectasis. Suction often, and watch for signs of respiratory distress. Keep emergency airway equipment on hand because the pa-

tient may require artificial ventilation or oxygen administration.

► Maintain an I.V. line for medications and emergency care, if necessary.

► Monitor the electrocardiogram frequently for arrhythmias. Record intake and output accurately, and check vital signs often.

► Turn the patient frequently to prevent pressure ulcers and pulmonary stasis.

► Because even minimal external stimulation provokes muscle spasms, keep the patient's room quiet and only dimly lighted. Warn visitors not to upset or overly stimulate the patient.

► If urine retention develops, insert an indwelling urinary catheter.

► Give muscle relaxants and sedatives as ordered, and schedule patient care—such as passive range-of-motion exercises—to coincide with periods of heaviest sedation.

► Insert an artificial airway, if necessary, to prevent tongue injury and maintain airway during spasms.

► Provide adequate nutrition to meet the patient's increased metabolic needs. The patient may need nasogastric feedings or total parenteral nutrition.

REFERENCES

1. Mayo Clinic. (2007 April 1). "Diphtheria and Tetanus Toxoid (Parenteral Route)." [Online]. Available at *www.mayoclinic.com/health/drug-information/DR602279.*
2. Halaas, G. W. "Management of Foreign Bodies in the Skin," *American Family Physician* 76(5):683–8, September 2007.

VANCOMYCIN-RESISTANT *ENTEROCOCCUS* INFECTION

Vancomycin-resistant *Enterococcus* (VRE) is a mutation of a common bacterium normally found in the GI tract that's spread easily by direct person-to-person contact. Facilities in more than 40 states have reported VRE infection, with 30% of enterococcus infections in intensive care units (ICUs) and 25% of enterococcus infections in non–ICU areas reporting as vancomycin-resistant.

Patients most at risk for VRE infection include:

► immunosuppressed patients or those with severe underlying disease

► patients with a history of taking vancomycin, third-generation cephalosporins, antibiotics targeted at anaerobic bacteria (such as *Clostridium difficile*), or multiple courses of antibiotics

► patients with indwelling urinary or central venous catheters

► elderly patients, especially those with prolonged or repeated hospital admissions

► patients with cancer or chronic renal failure

► patients undergoing cardiothoracic or intra-abdominal surgery or organ transplant

► patients with wounds opening into the pelvic or intra-abdominal area, including surgical wounds, burns, and pressure ulcers

► patients with enterococcal bacteremia, typically associated with endocarditis

► patients exposed to contaminated equipment or to another VRE–positive patient.

Causes and incidence

VRE enters health care facilities through an infected or colonized patient or a colonized health care worker. It can also develop following treatment with vancomycin. VRE spreads through direct contact between the patient and caregiver or between patients. It can also spread through patient contact with contaminated surfaces such as an overbed table, where it's capable of living for weeks. VRE has also been detected on patient gowns, bed linens, and handrails.

Signs and symptoms

There are no specific signs and symptoms related to VRE infection. The causative agent may be found incidentally with culture results.

Complications
▶ Sepsis
▶ Multisystem dysfunction
▶ Death (immunocompromised patients)

Diagnosis
Persons with no signs or symptoms of infection are considered colonized if VRE can be isolated from stool or a rectal swab.

Once colonized, a patient is more than 10 times as likely to become infected with VRE, for example through a breach in the immune system.

Treatment
New antimicrobials, such as linezolid, quinupristin, and dalfopristin, are available for treatment of VRE infection. However, in a recent study done in a tertiary care medical center, linezolid-resistant VRE was isolated along with some of the associated risk factors, such as peripheral vascular disease and/or the receipt of a solid organ transplant, total parenteral nutrition, piperacillin-tazobactam, and/or cefepime. From this, the institution decided to improve its infection-control practices and to reassess its antibiotic choices.[1]

Patients who are already colonized with VRE usually aren't treated with antimicrobials. Instead, the physician may stop all antibiotics and simply wait for normal bacteria to repopulate and replace the VRE strain. Combinations of various drugs also may be used, depending on the source of the infection. To prevent the spread of VRE, some facilities perform weekly surveillance cultures on at-risk patients in the intensive care or oncology units and on patients who have been transferred from a long-term care facility. Any colonized patient is then placed in contact isolation until culture-negative or until discharged. Colonization can last indefinitely; no protocol has been established for the length of time a patient should remain in isolation. The Centers for Disease Control and Prevention has set limits and guidelines for the use of vancomycin and other glycopeptides. The use of vancomycin prophylactically as a preoperative antibiotic for surgical site infections is not recommended.[2]

Special considerations
▶ Hand hygiene before and after care of the patient is crucial. Good hand hygiene is the most effective way to prevent VRE from spreading.
▶ Use an antiseptic soap such as chlorhexidine. Bacteria have been cultured from workers' hands after they've washed with milder soap. Alcohol-based hand sanitizers are effective as well.
▶ Use contact precautions when in contact with the patient or his support equipment. Provide the patient with a private room and dedicated equipment. Disinfect the environment and the equipment frequently.
▶ Change gloves when contaminated or when moving from a "dirty" area of the body to a clean one.
▶ Don't touch potentially contaminated surfaces such as an overbed table after removing your gown and gloves.
▶ Be particularly prudent in caring for a patient with an ileostomy, colostomy, or draining wound that isn't contained by a dressing.
▶ Instruct the patient's family and friends to wear protective garb when they visit him, and teach them how to dispose of it. Instruct them on proper hand hygiene.
▶ Provide teaching and emotional support to the patient and his family members.
▶ Consider grouping ("cohorting") infected or colonized patients together and assigning the same nursing staff to them.
▶ Don't lay equipment used on the patient on the bed or on the overbed table. Wipe the equipment with the appropriate disinfectant before leaving the room.
▶ Ensure judicious and careful use of antibiotics. Encourage physicians to limit their use.

▶ Instruct patients to take antibiotics for the full period prescribed, even if they begin to feel better.

REFERENCES

1. Pogue, J. M., et al. "Determination of Risk Factors Associated with Isolation of Linezolid-Resistant Strains of Vancomycin-Resistant Enterococcus," *Infection Control and Hospital Epidemiology* 28(12):1382–8, December 2007.
2. Centers for Disease Control and Prevention. (2001 December 8). "Clinical Consequences and Cost of Limiting Use of Vancomycin for Perioperative Prophylaxis: Example of Coronary Artery Bypass Surgery." [Online]. Available at *www.cdc.gov/ncidod/eid/ vol7no5/zanetti1G2.htm*.

VARICELLA

Varicella, commonly known as chickenpox, is a common, acute, and highly contagious infection caused by the herpesvirus varicella-zoster, the same virus that, in its latent stage, causes herpes zoster (shingles).

Causes and incidence

Chickenpox can occur at any age, but it's most common in children ages 2 to 8. Congenital varicella may affect infants whose mothers had acute infections in their first or early second trimester. Neonatal infection is rare, probably because of transient maternal immunity. However, neonates born to mothers who develop varicella 5 days before delivery or up to 2 days after delivery are at risk for developing severe generalized varicella. Second attacks are also rare. This infection is transmitted by direct contact (primarily with respiratory secretions; less commonly, with skin lesions) and indirect contact (airborne). The incubation period usually lasts 14 to 17 days but can be as short as 10 days and as long as 20 days. (See *Incubation and duration of common rash-producing infections,* page 466.) Chickenpox is probably communicable from 1 day before lesions erupt to 6 days after vesicles form (it's most contagious in the early stages of eruption of skin lesions).

Chickenpox occurs worldwide and is endemic in large cities. Outbreaks occur sporadically, usually in areas with large groups of susceptible children. It affects all races and both sexes equally. Seasonal distribution varies; in temperate areas, incidence is higher during late autumn, winter, and spring.

Most children recover completely. Potentially fatal complications may affect children on corticosteroids, antimetabolites, or other immunosuppressants, and those with leukemia, other neoplasms, or immunodeficiency disorders. Congenital and adult varicella may also have severe effects.

Signs and symptoms

Chickenpox produces distinctive signs and symptoms, notably a pruritic rash. During the prodromal phase, the patient has slight fever, malaise, and anorexia. Within 24 hours, the rash typically begins as crops of small, erythematous macules on the trunk or scalp. It progresses to papules and then clear vesicles on an erythematous base (the so-called dewdrop on a rose petal). These become cloudy and break easily; then scabs form.

The rash spreads to the face and over the trunk of the body, then to the limbs, buccal mucosa, axillae, upper respiratory tract, conjunctivae and, occasionally, the genitalia. New vesicles continue to appear for 3 or 4 days, so the rash contains a combination of red papules, vesicles, and scabs in various stages.

Complications

▶ Severe pruritus
▶ Skin infection with excessive scratching
▶ Scarring
▶ Impetigo
▶ Furuncles
▶ Cellulitis

▶ Reye's syndrome (rare)
▶ Pneumonia
▶ Myocarditis
▶ Bleeding disorders
▶ Arthritis
▶ Nephritis
▶ Hepatitis
▶ Acute myositis

Congenital varicella causes:

▶ Hypoplastic deformity
▶ Limb scarring
▶ Retarded growth
▶ Central nervous system problems
▶ Eye problems.

Diagnosis

Diagnosis rests on the characteristic clinical signs and usually doesn't require laboratory tests. However, the virus can be isolated from vesicular fluid within the first 3 to 4 days of the rash; Giemsa stain distinguishes varicella-zoster from vaccinia and variola viruses. Serum contains antibodies 7 days after onset. Varicella zoster can be isolated in the saliva of patients with herpes zoster and without a rash. This information could be helpful in the diagnosis of neurological disease produced by varicella zoster virus without rash.[1]

Treatment

Chickenpox calls for droplet and contact isolation until all vesicles and most of the scabs are dry (no new lesions; usually 1 week after the onset of the rash). Children with only a few remaining scabs are no longer contagious and can return to school. Congenital chickenpox requires no isolation.

In most cases, treatment consists of local or systemic antipruritics: lukewarm oatmeal baths, calamine lotion, or diphenhydramine (or another antihistamine). Antibiotics are unnecessary unless bacterial infection develops. Salicylates are contraindicated because of their link with Reye's syndrome. Susceptible patients may need special treatment. When

given up to 72 hours after exposure to varicella, varicella-zoster immunoglobulin may provide passive immunity. Acyclovir, valacyclovir, and famciclovir, antiviral agents, may slow vesicle formation, speed skin healing, and control the systemic spread of infection. However, according to the Centers for Disease Control and Prevention, only acyclovir is currently licensed for use in treating varicella.[2]

In a research study done at a well-known children's hospital, varicella zoster virus immunization was effective in preventing both primary varicella zoster virus and herpes zoster in HIV-infected children.[3]

Special considerations

Care is supportive and emphasizes patient and family teaching and preventive measures.

▶ Teach the child and his family how to apply topical antipruritic medications correctly. Stress the importance of good hygiene.
▶ Tell the patient not to scratch the lesions. However, because the need to scratch may be overwhelming, parents should trim the child's fingernails or tie mittens on his hands.
▶ Warn parents to watch for and immediately report signs of complications. Severe skin pain and burning may indicate a serious secondary infection and require prompt medical attention.
▶ Varicella vaccine, part of the recommended childhood immunization schedule, effectively prevents infection. It is also effective if given up to 5 days post-exposure.
▶ To help prevent chickenpox, don't admit a child exposed to chickenpox to a unit that contains children who receive immunosuppressants or who have leukemia or immunodeficiency disorders. A vulnerable child who has been exposed to chickenpox should be evaluated for administration of varicella-zoster immunoglobulin to lessen the severity of the disease.

REFERENCES

1. Mehta, S. K., et al. "Varicella-Zoster Virus in the Saliva of Patients with Herpes Zoster," *Journal of Infectious Diseases,* Feb 8, 2008.
2. Centers for Disease Control and Prevention. (2007 May 11). "Varicella Treatment Questions & Answers." [Online]. Available at *www.cdc.gov/vaccines/vpd-vac/varicella/dis-faqs-gen-treatment.htm.*
3. Wood, S. M., et al. "Primary Varicella and Herpes Zoster among HIV-Infected Children from 1989 to 2006," *Pediatrics* 121(1):e150–6, January 2008.

WEST NILE ENCEPHALITIS

West Nile encephalitis is categorized as an infectious disease that primarily causes an inflammation or "encephalitis" of the brain.

West Nile virus (WNV) is a flavivirus causing illness in humans (as well as birds and other animals, especially horses), which may range from very mild to severe or even fatal. It is spread by infected mosquitoes, with birds serving as a reservoir. Most WNV infections (greater than 80%) produce no or very mild symptoms, so that a person may not even recognize illness. In rare cases (less than 1%), WNV infection may result in inflammation of the brain (encephalitis), spinal cord (myelitis), or the tissue surrounding these structures (meningitis), causing severe illness, which may be fatal in anywhere from 3% to 15% of cases.

The virus had not been previously documented in the Western hemisphere until 1999, when it was definitively identified in numerous dead birds in New York, New Jersey, and Connecticut. Scientists in the United States discovered the strain initially in and around the Bronx Zoo and believe that infected birds may have carried the disease and that it spread as mosquitoes fed on them.

Causes and incidence

WNV is transmitted to humans (and animals) by the bite of a mosquito (primarily the Culex species) infected with the virus. Mosquitoes become infected via feeding on contaminated birds. Anyone exposed to and bitten by mosquitoes is at risk for contracting the illness. In temperate areas of the world, WNV cases peak in summer and early fall, during months of greatest mosquito activity. In southern climates, where temperatures are milder, WNV infections may occur year round. Persons over 50 and those with compromised immune systems are at greatest risk for developing severe illness (e.g. encephalitis) or complications. As of July 18, 2006, a total of 10 states had reported 15 cases of human WNV illness to the Centers for Disease Control and Prevention (CDC). Nine cases (60%) for which such data were available occurred in males; median age of patients was 50 years. The date of illness onset ranged from January to July; no deaths were reported.[1]

The CDC reported that there is no current evidence that a person can contract the virus from handling live or dead infected birds. They advise persons to contact local public health department officials to report all findings of dead birds (without obvious traumatic cause). Local health departments may have specific guidelines on disposal of carcasses; if not, it is prudent to avoid direct contact when handling dead animals, including birds; wear gloves, and dispose of carcasses in double plastic bags.

There is no evidence of WNV transmission from person to person through casual contact.

In 2002, it was documented that WNV could be spread to humans through four novel routes: blood transfusion, organ transplantation, transplacental transfer, and breast-feeding.

Rarely, however, WNV has been shown to spread through blood transfusions and organ transplants. Since the WNV entered

North America in 1999 and in 2002, blood-donor screening was started in 2003 before the mosquito season. It is estimated that blood donor screening in North America has prevented close to 2,200 recipient infections and potential clinical disease.[2]

It is uncertain and under evaluation as to whether WNV may spread through breast milk, or in pregnancy from mother to fetus. As one study indicates, transmission of WNV through breast-feeding seems to be rare, but more studies need to be conducted.[3]

Signs and symptoms

The incubation period for WNV infection is about 3 to 14 days postexposure. Mild infection occurs in about 20 percent of persons and produces symptoms such as fever; headache; body aches; nausea; vomiting; swollen lymph nodes; or a skin rash on the chest, abdomen, and back. Illness may last from a few days to several weeks. About 80% of infected persons do not develop any symptoms. It is estimated that about 1 in 150 persons infected with WNV will develop severe infection, such as encephalitis, meningitis, or myelitis, manifested by high fever, headache, neck stiffness, stupor, disorientation, coma, tremors, seizures, weakness, stupor, numbness, paralysis, and other neurologic deficits. Patients who have had WNV complain of long-term problems such as multiple somatic effects, tremors, and motor skill abnormalities.[1]

Complications

▶ Progression to coma
▶ Tremors
▶ Occasional convulsions
▶ Paralysis
▶ Death (rare)

Diagnosis

In symptomatic persons, testing for WNV may include an immunoglobulin M (IgM) antibody test, done on blood or cerebrospinal fluid from a lumbar puncture. This test is unreliable early in the illness, but most infected persons will have a positive result within 8 days of the onset of symptoms. Confirmatory testing may be done on the same or a different specimen. An additional confirmatory test, the plaque reduction neutralization test (PRNT) may be done through state laboratory agencies or the CDC. The PRNT requires viral growth and may take a week or more to conduct. In mild cases, no testing may be pursued, but the diagnosis then is also not confirmed. Other viral or bacterial infections may also cause encephalitis, meningitis, or myelitis (including St. Louis encephalitis, a similar virus that may cause a false-positive WNV test), and in suspected cases with severe symptoms, testing must be pursued.

Treatment

There is no specific therapy to treat WNV and no known cure. Treatment is therefore supportive, with intravenous fluids, control of fever, protection from secondary infections (e.g., pneumonia or urinary tract infections), and ventilator or respiratory support when needed. Mild cases may need little supportive care, and most persons recover fully within a few days to several weeks. Severe cases require intensive hospitalized treatments.

Special considerations

▶ Obtain an extensive history of the patient's whereabouts within the past 2 to 3 weeks (especially around bodies of water, such as lakes and ponds), the presence of dead birds, and recent mosquito bites acquired.
▶ Perform a comprehensive physical assessment, and report signs of fever, headache, lymphadenopathy, and a maculopapular rash.
▶ Perform a complete neurological examination, and report any signs of confusion, lethargy, weakness, or slurred speech.
▶ Maintain adequate hydration with I.V. fluids.
▶ Monitor strict intake and output.

▶ Use fever control methods, such as cooling blankets and acetaminophen as ordered.

▶ Provide respiratory support measures when applicable.

▶ West Nile encephalitis isn't transmitted from person to person, but use standard precautions when handling body fluids and blood.

▶ Report any suspected cases of West Nile encephalitis to the applicable state health department.

▶ Prevention of mosquito breeding grounds and mosquito bites are the most effective deterrents to WNV. Recommend that standing water, which acts as a breeding pool for mosquito larvae, be eliminated (such as old tires, tire swings, unused wading pools, and planters). This may be as simple as drilling drainage holes or involve removal of the material.

▶ Teach the patient ways to reduce his risk of becoming infected with West Nile encephalitis:

– Stay indoors at dawn, dusk, and in the early evening.

– Wear long-sleeved shirts and long pants outdoors.

– Apply insect repellent sparingly to exposed skin. Check the label. An effective repellent will contain 20% to 30% N,N-diethyl-meta-toluamide (DEET). DEET in high concentrations (greater than 30%) may cause adverse effects, particularly in children; avoid products containing more than 30% DEET.

– Repellents may irritate the eyes and mouth, so avoid applying repellent to the hands of children. It is contraindicated to apply insect repellents to children younger than age 3 years. Spray clothing with repellents containing DEET, because mosquitoes may bite through thin clothing.

– Whenever you use an insecticide or insect repellent, be sure to read and follow the manufacturer's directions for use as printed on the product.

REFERENCES

1. Centers for Disease Control and Prevention, Morbidity and Mortality Weekly Report. "West Nile Virus Activity—United States, 2006." [Online]. Available at *www.cdc.gov/mmwr/preview/mmwrhtml/mm5622a3.htm.*

2. Stramer, S. L. "Reacting to an Emerging Safety Threat: West Nile Virus in North America," *Development in Biologicals* 127:43–58, 2007.

3. Hinckley, A. F., et al. "Transmission of West Nile Virus through Human Breast Milk Seems to be Rare," *Pediatrics* 119(3):e666–71, March 2007.

4. Carson, P. J., et al. "Long-Term Clinical and Neuropsychological Outcomes of West Nile Virus Infection," *Clinical Infectious Diseases* 43(6):723–30, September 2006.

Appendices and index

EVIDENCE-BASED NURSING PRACTICE

Evidence-based nursing practice is built on information obtained from research. The basic steps in evidence-based nursing practice include:

► carefully formulating the clinical question
► searching for peer-reviewed evidence-based articles that address the clinical question
► analyzing and comparing data, critically evaluating and comparing the articles
► applying the information from the studies.

Step 1: Formulating the clinical question

Follow these steps to formulate the clinical question:

► Start with a specific and concrete question.
► Formulate the question in terms of a relationship between:
   – a patient or patient population
   – an intervention (typically a treatment, diagnostic test, or nursing procedure)
   – the result of the intervention
   – what else could be done instead.

Step 2: Searching for evidence

Your goal during the database search is to find published reports of the results of research projects. Be sure to use only articles that are published in peer-reviewed journals, which require outside experts to review articles submitted for publication. If the title of the article leaves you uncertain whether the article is a report of a research project, read the abstract carefully. You can find reports of research by using:

► libraries
► Web sites
► electronic databases with Web-based tools such as CINAHL, MEDLINE and PubMed. (See *Evidence-based resources*, page 498.)

The standard format for research reports includes:

► abstract
► introduction or review of the literature (a brief summary of past related research)
► methods
► results
► discussion section.

Step 3: Analyzing and comparing data

Evaluating the quality of a research report can be difficult if you haven't had some training in research methodology. Even seasoned researchers debate the quality of studies and how to interpret and apply the results. However, if you follow a few basic rules, you can make sure that the study you read has met a baseline standard of quality.

► *Validity*—does the research project actually measure what it claims to measure?
► *Reliability*—will the results of the study be repeatable? Ideally, you shouldn't accept the results of any study as true without finding at least one other study that attempted to repeat it and got the same results.

▶ *Randomizing* is a hallmark of high-quality research. Ideally, researchers assign people randomly to either a study or control group.

▶ *Group size* is important. Research on large numbers of subjects produces more reliable results than smaller studies.

However, not all types of research can use randomization, double-blinding, control groups, and large populations. Understanding the acceptable alternatives requires training and experience.

Comparing the studies you have gathered is the next step, and this can be challenging. You must weigh variables, such as patient population characteristics and quality of the study design. Final decisions usually require discussion and compromise.

Levels of evidence

Weighing and leveling the degree of evidence that a study has can be a daunting task. A systematic approach to leveling the evidence can be found below.

Leveling the evidence is based on the following questions:

▶ Was the study randomized?
▶ What was the study population?
▶ What criteria had to be met by participants?
▶ Was the intervention described properly?
▶ Was the study blinded?
▶ How was the data collected?
▶ How was the data analyzed?
▶ What were the end results?
▶ What conclusions were achieved?
▶ Did the study have any limits?

Step 4: Applying the data

After the evidence has been evaluated, the next step is to determine whether the evidence supports rejecting—or implementing—the intervention. If the evidence supports a change, procedures or policies can be changed or created to incorporate the new evidence.

Leveling the evidence

LEVEL AND QUALITY OF EVIDENCE	TYPE OF EVIDENCE
Level 1	Evidence from a systematic review or meta-analysis of all relevant randomized clinical trials (RCTs), or evidence-based clinical practice guidelines based on systematic reviews of RCTs or three or more RCTs of good quality that have similar results.
Level 2	Evidence obtained from at least one well-designed RCT
Level 3	Evidence obtained from well-designed controlled trials without randomization
Level 4	Evidence from well-designed case-control or cohort studies
Level 5	Evidence from systematic reviews of descriptive and qualitative studies
Level 6	Evidence from a single descriptive or qualitative study
Level 7	Evidence from the opinion of authorities and/or reports of expert committees

Adapted from Melnyk, B.M., and Fineout-Overholt, E. *Evidence-Based Practice in Nursing & Healthcare: A Guide to Best Practice.* Philadelphia: Lippincott Williams & Wilkins, 2005.

EVIDENCE-BASED RESOURCES

Academic Center for Evidence-Based
Nursing:
www.acestar.uthscsa.edu/About.htm

American Academy of Pediatrics:
www.aap.org/policy/paramtoc.html

American Association of Clinical
Endocrinologists:
www.aace.com/clin/guidelines

American Association of Critical Care
Nurses:
*www.aacn.org/AACN/practiceAlert.nsf/
vwdoc/pa2?opendocument*

American Association of Respiratory Care:
www.rcjournal.com/cpgs/#evidence

American Cancer Society:
*www.cancer.org/docroot/ped/content/
ped_2_3x_acs_cancer_detection_
guidelines_36.asp?sitearea=ped*

American College of Cardiology:
*www.acc.org/qualityandscience/clinical/
statements.htm*

American College of Physicians:
*www.acponline.org/clinical_information/
guidelines/*

American Medical Directors Association:
www.amda.com/tools/guidelines.cfm

American Psychiatric Association:
*www.psych.org/MainMenu/Psychiatric
Practice/PracticeGuidelines_1.aspx*

Association of Women's Health, Obstetric
and Neonatal Nurses:
http://awhonn.org

Clinical Trials:
www.clinicaltrials.gov

CMA InfoBase:
http://mdm.ca/cpgsnew/cpgs/index.asp

Cochrane Library:
www.cochrane.org

Education Resources Information Center:
www.eric.ed.gov

Guidelines Advisory Committee:
www.gacguidelines.ca

Guidelines International Network:
www.G-I-N.net

Health Services/Technology Assessment
Text:
http://hstat.nlm.nih.gov

Healthlinks at University of Washington:
http://healthlinks.washington.edu

Infusion Nursing Society:
www.ins1.org

Institute for Clinical Systems Improvement:
www.icsi.org/guidelines_and_more/

Joanna Briggs Institute:
*http://www.joannabriggs.edu.au/about/
home.php*

Ministry of Health Services, British
Columbia, Canada:
*www.healthservices.gov.bc.ca/msp/
protoguides*

National Association of Neonatal Nurses:
www.nann.org

National Cancer Institute:
www.cancer.gov/search/cancer_literature/

National Guideline Clearinghouse (NGC):
www.guideline.gov

National Institute for Clinical Excellence
(NICE):
www.nice.org.uk/catcg2.asp?c=20034

National Kidney Foundation:
*www.kidney.org/professionals/doqi/
guidelineindex/cfm*

New York Academy of Medicine:
www.ebmny.org/cpg.html

NLM Gateway:
http://gateway.nlm.nih.gov/gw/Cmd

Oncology Nursing Society:
www.ons.org

Ovid MEDLINE:
*www.ovid.com/site/products/ovidguide/
nursing.htm*

Primary Care Clinical Practice Guidelines:
*http://medicine.ucsf.edu/resources/
guidelines/*

PubMed:
www.pubmed.gov

Registered Nurses Association of Ontario:
www.rnao.org/bestpractices

Resources for Evidence-Based Nursing at
McMaster University:
*http://hsl.lib.mcmaster.ca/education/
nursing/ebn/index.htm*

Scottish Intercollegiate Guideline Network:
www.sign.ac.uk/guidelines/index.html

Teaching/Learning Resources for Evidence-
Based Practice:
*www.mdx.ac.uk/www/rctsh/ebp/
main.htm*

Thomson Scientific:
http://scientific.thomson.com/isi/

University of Iowa Gerontological Nursing
Interventions Research Center:
*http://www.nursing.uiowa.edu/excellence/
nursing_interventions/*

Veterans Administration:
www.oqp.med.va.gov/cpg/cpg.htm

Virginia Henderson International Nursing
Library:
www.nursinglibrary.org/portal/main.aspx

Wound, Ostomy, and Continence Nurses
Society:
*www.wocn.org/WOCN_Library/
Position_Statements*

INDEX

i refers to an illustration; t refers to a table.

i refers to an illustration; t refers to a table.

i refers to an illustration; t refers to a table.

i refers to an illustration; t refers to a table.

i refers to an illustration; t refers to a table.

i refers to an illustration; t refers to a table.